Handbook of
HUMAN
IMMUNOLOGY

Handbook of HUMAN IMMUNOLOGY

Edited by

Mary S. Leffell, Ph.D.
Johns Hopkins University
School of Medicine
Baltimore, MD

Albert D. Donnenberg, Ph.D.
University of Pittsburgh
Cancer Institute
Pittsburgh, PA

Noel R. Rose, M.D., Ph.D.
Johns Hopkins University
Schools of Medicine and of Public Health
Baltimore, MD

CRC Press
Boca Raton   New York

Cover Art — Artist Kate Bazis received her Bachelor of Fine Arts degree from Carnegie Mellon University. She lives and works in Pittsburgh, PA.

Publisher:	Robert B. Stern
Project Editor:	Renee Taub
Marketing Manager:	Susie Carlisle
Direct Marketing Manager:	Becky McEldowney
Cover design:	Denise Craig
PrePress:	Kevin Luong
Manufacturing:	Sheri Schwartz

Library of Congress Cataloging-in-Publication Data

Handbook of human immunology / edited by Mary S. Leffell, Albert
    D. Donnenberg, Noel R. Rose.
        p. cm.
    Includes bibliographical references and index.
    ISBN 0-8493-0134-3 (alk. paper)
    1. Immune system.   2. Immunology.   I. Leffell, Mary S.
    II. Donnenberg, Albert David.   III. Rose, Noel R.
    [DNLM: 1. Immunity, Cellular.   2. Immune System.   3. Immunologic
Techniques.   QW 568 C911 1997]
    QR181.C77   1997
    616.07'9--DC21
    DNLM/DLC
    for Library of Congress   96-45395
                                                                        CIP

PREFACE

The importance of immunological processes in clinical medicine has been well appreciated for over 20 years, but within the past few years the application of molecular genetic techniques has not only increased our understanding of immunopathogenesis, but has also revolutionized laboratory tests applicable to the diagnosis and monitoring of diseases involving the immune system. The primary goal of the *Handbook of Human Immunology* has been to provide an accessible, "user-friendly" reference to molecular and cellular immunology for practicing clinicians.

Introductory chapters present an overview of the molecular basis of immune responses and immunological disorders, focusing on the role of cell receptors, accessory molecules, and cytokines in these processes. Emphasis has been placed on immunological parameters which are useful clinically. The basic principles underlying assays of the immune system in autoimmune disorders and in immunodeficiencies are discussed, but the emphasis is on the application and interpretation of immune tests. The *Handbook* provides normal ranges for immunoglobulins and their age-dependent concentrations, as well as to the complement system. Cellular immunology is discussed from the perspectives of lymphocyte functional parameters, as well as through immunophenotyping of lymphocytes and other leukocytes. Both the serological and molecular diagnosis of infectious diseases and autoimmune disorders are reviewed. The *Handbook* also contains up-to-date information on the exciting developments in immunogenetics, covering the application of T-cell receptor genes and the HLA alleles in disease associations and transplantation. Finally, comprehensive coverage is given to humoral allosensitization to HLA antigens which may result from pregnancy, transfusion, and transplantation and to how such sensitization can be analyzed and overcome in transplantation.

While new developments are taking place at such a rapid pace that no book can realistically claim to be absolutely current, the editors believe that the approach to this *Handbook*, based on underlying principles, will provide a timely and useful guide to the application of molecular immunology in clinical practice.

THE EDITORS

Mary S. Leffell, Ph.D., is Co-Director of the Immunogenetics Laboratory and is an Associate Professor of Medicine of the Johns Hopkins University School of Medicine, Baltimore, Maryland. She holds a joint appointment as an Associate Professor in the Department of Molecular Microbiology and Immunology, School of Public Health and Hygiene, the Johns Hopkins University.

Dr. Leffell graduated in 1968 from the University of Tennessee, Knoxville, Tennessee with a B.S. degree in Microbiology (Summa Cum Laude). Dr. Leffell was named a Woodrow Wilson fellow in 1968 and obtained her Ph.D. degree in Immunology in 1973 from the University of North Carolina, Chapel Hill.

Dr. Leffell is a member of the American Society for Histocompatibility and Immunogenetics, American Association of Immunologists, American Society of Transplant Physicians, American College of Allergy and Immunology, and the International Transplantation Society. She was President of the American Society for Histocompatibility and Immunogenetics from 1994–1995 and has served two terms on the Board of Directors and on the Executive Committee of the national organ procurement and transplantation network, the United Network for Organ Sharing. She has been a member of the American Board of Histocompatibility and Immunogenetics and is currently a member of the American Board of Medical Laboratory Immunology. Dr. Leffell has been an invited faculty member and on the program committee for a graduate-level course in histocompatibility and immunogenetics sponsored by the Southeastern Organ Procurement Foundation since the beginning of that course in 1983.

Dr. Leffell has presented nine invited lectures at national meetings and has organized three regional and national scientific meetings. Her research interests are in transplantation immunology and immunogenetics, as well as in clinical immunology. She has published numerous research papers and several book chapters in these areas.

Albert D. Donnenberg, Ph.D., is an Associate Professor of Medicine and Director of Laboratory Research at the University of Pittsburgh School of Medicine, Division of Hematology/Bone Marrow Transplantation (BMT). He is also Co-Director of the University of Pittsburgh Cancer Institute (UPCI) Hematopoiesis and Hematologic Malignancies Program.

Dr. Donnenberg graduated from the University of Colorado in 1973, with a B.A. in Philosophy. In 1980, he earned a Ph.D. from the Johns Hopkins University School of Hygiene and Public Health in Infectious Disease Epidemiology. He completed a Research Fellowship at the JHU School of Medicine, Department of Oncology. From 1982 through 1991, he was an instructor in Oncology, and Immunology and Infectious Diseases, becoming an Assistant Professor in 1983 and an Associate Professor in 1989.

Among the many societies to which Dr. Donnenberg belongs are the International Society for Experimental Hematology, the American Association of Immunologists, the American Society of Hematology, and the Clinical Immunology Society. His honors include Delta Omega Honorary Public Health Society and Carter-Wallace Fellowship for AIDS Research. He was a University of Pittsburgh Faculty Honoree in 1993.

Dr. Donnenberg's publishing credits include 60 refereed articles and 18 book chapters. He has presented over 50 invited lectures at national and international meetings, universities and institutes. He has been the recipient of grants from the National Institutes of Health, Department of Defense, and private organizations. His research interests in human immunology/experimental hematology include the development of new approaches to bone marrow transplantation and analysis of multiparameter flow cytometry data. His basic science research centers on the mechanisms of lymphocyte replacement in both healthy and immunodeficiency states.

Noel R. Rose, M.D., Ph.D., is Professor of Pathology and Director of the Division of Immunology at The Johns Hopkins University School of Medicine and Professor of Molecular Microbiology and Immunology and Director of the World Health Organization Collaborating Center for Autoimmune Diseases at The Johns Hopkins University School of Hygiene and Public Health. He also holds joint appointments in the Departments of Medicine and Environmental Health Sciences.

Dr. Rose received his M.D. degree from The State University of New York at Buffalo and his Ph.D. from The University of Pennsylvania. He also holds an honorary M.D. from The University of Cagliari and an honorary Sc.D from The University of Sasseri. He was elected to Alpha Omega Alpha, the honorary medical society; Sigma Xi, the honorary scientific society, and Delta Omega, the honorary public health society. He is a member of The Academy of Scholars of Wayne State University and has received the Distinguished Award and the Board of Governors Faculty Recognition Award from Wayne State, as well as the Distinguished Medical Alumnus Award from The State University of New York at Buffalo. He is a Fellow of The College of American Pathologists, The American Society of Clinical Pathologists, The American Academy of Microbiology, The American Academy of Allergy, Asthma and Immunology, and The American Public Health Association. He has received the Abbott Award of The American Society for Microbiology and the Research Medal of The University of Pisa. He has served as President of The Clinical Immunology Society, a member of the Board of Governors of The American Academy of Microbiology and The Society for Experimental Biology and Medicine, and chaired the Immunology Committees of The International Union of Immunological Societies and The Food and Drug Administration. He has also been a member of the Board of Scientific Visitors of The National Toxicology Program and The National Eye Institute.

In the past, Dr. Rose was Professor of Microbiology and Director of The Center for Immunology at The State University of Buffalo and Director of The Erie County Laboratories. Later, he was Professor and Chairman of the Department of Microbiology and Immunology at Wayne State University School of Medicine and Professor and Chairman of the Department of Immunology and Infectious Diseases at The Johns Hopkins University School of Hygiene and Public Health.

Dr. Rose has been Editor-in-Chief of all five editions of *The Manual of Clinical Laboratory Immunology* and serves as Editor-in-Chief of *Clinical Immunology and Immunopathology*, Section Editor of *Clinical and Diagnostic Laboratory Immunology* and is on the Editorial Board of seventeen additional publications. He has edited or co-edited 19 books.

Dr. Rose's research interests are primarily in the area of self/nonself discrimination and autoimmune diseases. He has published approximately 540 articles in this field.

CONTRIBUTORS

Pradip N. Akolkar
Division of Molecular Medicine
North Shore University Hospital
Manhasset, New York

Barbara Detrick
Department of Pathology
George Washington University
Medical Center
Washington, D.C.

Albert D. Donnenberg
University of Pittsburgh Cancer Institute
Pittsburgh, Pennsylvania

Steven D. Douglas
Immunology Section
Division of Allergy, Immunology,
and Infectious Diseases
Children's Hospital of Philadelphia
Philadelphia, Pennsylvania

James D. Folds
Clinical Immunology Laboratory
University of North Carolina Hospitals
Chapel Hill, North Carolina

Beena Gulwani-Akolkar
Division of Molecular Medicine
North Shore University Hospital
Manhasset, New York

Robert G. Hamilton
Clinical Immunology
Johns Hopkins University
School of Medicine
Baltimore, Maryland

John M. Hart
Immunogenetics Laboratory
Department of Medicine
Johns Hopkins University
School of Medicine
Baltimore, Maryland

John J. Hooks
Immunology and Virology Section
National Eye Institute
National Institutes of Health
Bethesda, Maryland

Carolyn Katovich Hurley
Department of Microbiology and
Immunology
Georgetown University
School of Medicine
Washington, D.C.

Naynesh R. Kamani
Division of
Hematology/Oncology/Immunology
Department of Pediatrics
University of Texas HSC at San Antonio
San Antonio, Texas

Kimberly L. Kane
Northside Medical Laboratory
Western Reserve Care System
Youngstown, Ohio

Mary S. Leffell
Immunogenetics Laboratory
Johns Hopkins University
School of Medicine
Baltimore, Maryland

Robert H. McLean
Department of Pediatrics
University of Maryland
    School of Medicine
Baltimore, Maryland

Preeti Pancholi
Department of Virology and Parasitology
New York Blood Center
New York, New York

David Persing
Division of Clinical Microbiology
    and Experimental Pathology
Mayo Clinic
Rochester, Minnesota

Noel R. Rose
Johns Hopkins University
    Schools of Medicine and
    of Public Health
Baltimore, Maryland

Jack Silver
Division of Molecular Medicine
North Shore University Hospital
Manhasset, New York

Thomas R. Welch
Division of Pediatric Nephrology
Children's Hospital Medical Center
Cincinnati, Ohio

Theresa Whiteside
University of Pittsburgh Cancer
    Institute
Pittsburgh, Pennsylvania

Alan Winkelstein (deceased)
University of Pittsburgh
    School of Medicine
University of Pittsburgh
    Cancer Institute
Pittsburgh, Pennsylvania

Andrea A. Zachary
Immunogenetics Laboratory
Department of Medicine
Johns Hopkins University
    School of Medicine
Baltimore, Maryland

TABLE OF CONTENTS

Chapter 1

AN OVERVIEW OF THE IMMUNE SYSTEM: THE MOLECULAR BASIS FOR IMMUNE RESPONSES

Mary S. Leffell

CONTENTS

0-8493-0134-3/97/$0.00+$.50

I. INTRODUCTION

The immune system, as fully evolved in higher vertebrates, is truly a remarkable defense against pathogenic microorganisms. It is capable of responding with exquisite specificity and adaptability; moreover, upon secondary challenge, the response is accelerated, heightened, and has specific memory for the original insult. A crucial characteristic of the immune system is the ability to discriminate "self" from "nonself" — an ability which is essential not only for defense against pathogens, but also for immune surveillance against malignant cells. In the 1970s and 1980s, much was learned about the phenomena of immune responses. Clinically, it was appreciated that immune mechanisms were involved in a wide range of conditions besides host defense. Immune processes were defined in allergic or atopic disorders; in autoimmune and other immunopathologic diseases; in specific immunodeficiency syndromes, both congenital and acquired; and in rejection of transplanted tissues and organs. An appreciation of immunology has pervaded every specialty area in medicine. Today, thanks to the spectacular advances in genetic technology, our understanding of immune reactions is at the molecular level. Immune processes can be dissected as the interactions of cellular ligands and/or soluble mediators with specific receptors on target cells.

The purpose of this handbook is to provide a quick reference to the elements of the human immune system, their normal values in health, and their aberrations in disease. Because technologies have advanced so rapidly, the principles of assays utilized in clinical immunology laboratories are also presented, along with guidelines for their appropriate applications. This immediate chapter provides a brief overview of the immune system from our current, molecular perspective.

II. CELLS OF THE IMMUNE SYSTEM AND HOST DEFENSE[1-3]

The cells involved in host defense and specific immune response can be broadly categorized into three types: nonspecific accessory cells; antigen processing and presenting cells; and mediators of specific, adaptable immunity. Phagocytic cells, particularly the polymorphonuclear leukocytes, including neutrophils, eosinophils, and basophils, are examples of nonspecific accessory cells. Blood monocytes and tissue macrophages are also important phagocytic cells, but, as will be discussed below, they have additional and vital functions as antigen processing cells. The so-called K (killer) and NK (natural killer) cells, which do not display a unique antigen specificity, but which are broadly specific for a range of target cell antigens, may also be placed in the group of accessory cells. This group may be thought of as the first line of host defense: the phagocytes providing an immediate response against invading microorganisms and the NK cells functioning in immune surveillance against intracellular pathogens and malignancies. Monocytes, macrophages, K, and NK cells may also function as specific effector cells, attacking and destroying target cells when activated and "armed" with antibodies against appropriate target cell antigens.

Specific immune responses begin with antigen processing and presentation.[4] It is now appreciated that foreign antigens must be presented in an appropriate conformation to evoke a humoral or antibody response. Stimulation of a cellular response requires "processing " of antigens into small peptides, followed by an appropriate presentation of these peptides to immunologically competent cells. Antigen-presenting/processing cells (APC), of which monocytes and macrophages are the prototypes, comprise the second category of cells in immunity. They literally prepare antigens by proteolytic degradation into small peptides, then display or present them on their cell surface to stimulate the third category of cells, the lymphocytes.

Lymphocytes are the principal mediators of immune processes. There are two major classes of lymphocytes: B lymphocytes and T lymphocytes, which are responsible for humoral and cellular immunity, respectively. T lymphocytes are further classified into two major subclasses which are defined by the presence of either of two cell surface molecules, CD4 or CD8. Although not absolute, in general, CD4+ T cells provide "helper" function in the induction of immune responses, while CD8+ cells are mediators of cellular immunity through the cytotoxic destruction of other cells. The lymphocyte response, which is triggered by binding of a ligand to a membrane receptor, is restricted to a limited set of structurally similar antigens. Lymphocytes respond only to small portions of foreign antigens. These portions, which are usually small peptides no more than 6 to 30 residues in length, are the antigenic determinants or epitopes. In general, B lymphocytes recognize epitopes with a specific conformation, and this specificity is reflected in the antibodies produced against those epitopes. In contrast, T lymphocytes respond to "processed" peptides, from 8 to 30 residues in length. T lymphocyte responses are also "restricted" in that the peptides can be recognized by the T cells only when they are bound to another molecule, specifically one of the host's own histocompatibility or HLA molecules. Histocompatibility molecules are encoded in a gene complex termed the major histocompatibility complex (MHC), and the human molecules are referred to as the human leukocyte antigens or HLA system. The requirement for antigen presentation of peptides by histocompatibility molecules is called MHC restriction.

A. Hematopoietic Leukocytes

All of the leukocytes involved in host defense and immunity are derived during hematopoiesis from stem cells in the bone marrow. It is generally accepted that the lymphoid, monocyte/myeloid, and megakaryocytic lines of leukocytes diverge and differentiate from a common, pluripotential stem cell.[5] The cells in these major lineages, along with their general types of cell receptors and functions are summarized in Table 1.

B. Nonhematopoietic Accessory Cells

Other nonhematopoietic cells may function in immune responses, particularly in antigen presentation.[6] Their function generally depends upon the expression of MHC molecules and in some cases may be

TABLE 1

Hematopoietic Cells of the Immune System and Host Defense

Cell Lineage	Specificity	Membrane Receptors	Functions
Lymphoid			
T lymphocyte	Antigen specific	TCR/CD3 complex CD4, CD8 Coreceptors Various adhesion molecules	Cytokine production; recruitment and activation of other cells; "help" for B cells; MHC-restricted cytotoxic activity; regulation and suppression
B lymphocyte	Antigen specific	Surface immunoglobulin (SIg) Various adhesion molecules	Humoral Immunity — production of specific antibodies; antigen presentation to T cells
NK, K cells ("3rd population" of lymphocytes)	Broad specificity for a range of cell antigens	NK target cell receptor Fc receptors (Fc$_\gamma$RIII) Various adhesion molecules	Non-MHC-restricted, natural killer(NK) cytotoxic defense; antibody dependent cytotoxicity (ADCC) by "killer" (K) cells; lymphokine-activated killer (LAK) cells; cytokine production
Monocytic/myeloid:			
Monocytes, tissue macrophages	Ususally nonspecific; may display specificity through antibodies bound by Fc receptors	Various accessory and adhesion molecules Fc receptors Complement receptors	Phagocytic defense; antigen processing and presentation; cytokine production; regulation through cytokines, prostaglandins, and leucotrienes
Neutrophils	Nonspecific	Fc receptors Complement receptors Various adhesion molecules	1st line phagocytic defense *vs.* extracellular pathogens
Eosinophils	Nonspecific	Fc receptors (Fc$_\epsilon$RI, Fc$_\gamma$R)	Acessory cell in allergic/atopic reactions; production/release of inflammatory, allergic mediators; parasitic defense
Basophils, mast cells	Nonspecific	Fc receptors (Fc$_\epsilon$RI, Fc$_\gamma$R)	Acessory cell in allergic/atopic reactions; production/release of inflammatory, allergic mediators

dependent upon induced or enhanced expression of MHC molecules subsequent to inflammation. Dendritic cells are important, nonhematopoietic cells that function with B cells and macrophages as the primary, "professional" APC in the lymph nodes.[7] Various other cells, such as astrocytes and endothelial cells, can serve as APC under the right circumstances. These cells are sometimes called "nonprofessional" APC, since their role in immune response can be considered a secondary function.

C. General Principles of Cell Interactions and Induction of Responses[1-3]

The cells of host defense and the immune system interact through a complex system of cell receptors and soluble mediators, generically termed cytokines. The primary stimulus or trigger for a cellular response usually is binding of an appropriate ligand which may be a soluble factor or another receptor on another cell. Cytokines generally provide secondary signals to amplify the response by binding to their respective cell membrane receptors. Nonspecific responses, such as phagocytosis, may be triggered by the mere physical contact of bacteria or foreign particles with the phagocyte membrane. Phagocytosis, however, is greatly enhanced when particles are coated or "opsonized" with antibody or complement components. Antibodies or complement components then facilitate phagocytosis by binding to receptors for the Fc portion of immunoglobulins or for key complement components, such as C3b. Lymphocytes respond through antigen-specific receptors: surface immunoglobulin (SIg) for B cells and the T-cell receptor (TCR) for T cells. Clones of lymphocytes, derived from single precursor cells, are limited in response to a small set of closely related antigenic determinants or epitopes which can be bound to their specific antigen receptors. Following the primary and secondary cell receptor binding events, biochemical signals (discussed below) are transduced from the receptors to the cell nucleus, activating the cell for effector functions which may involve further differentiation, acquisition of enhanced functions, synthesis of new proteins, release of granule-contained mediators, and cell division.

III. CELL MEMBRANE RECEPTORS AND ADHESION MOLECULES

As with the cells involved in immunity, the cellular receptors can be classified into general categories based on their functions. These functions include: binding of specific antigens; promotion of cellular

interaction by facilitating membrane-to-membrane contact of interacting cells; binding of soluble mediators; and transduction of activation
signals. Broadly categorized, the principal types of receptors are the
lymphocyte antigen receptors and coreceptors, adhesion molecules,
and cytokine and complement receptors. The nomenclature of cell
receptors is often confusing to nonimmunologists, for various names
and acronyms are used interchangeably. This has resulted because earlier names coined by investigators often described the functions that
were attributed to these molecules. For example, ICAM stands for
"intracellular adhesion molecule" and LFA for "leukocyte function
antigen." Many cell surface molecules have been identified by monoclonal antibodies (Mabs), which are specific for antigens found on cells
of different hematopoietic lineages and at different stages of differentiation. An international committee, sponsored by the World Health
Organization (WHO) meets periodically and determines if there is
sufficient consensus among investigators to give a molecule, defined
by one or more Mabs, an official designation. These names are CD
designations or "clusters of differentiation," based on their order of
designation and their patterns of antibody reactivity.[8] As much as possible in this chapter, the CD nomenclature will be used, except when
an acronym for the molecule is more commonly known or more obvious as to function.

A. The Immunoglobulin Superfamily Receptors

The immunoglobulin (Ig) superfamily is comprised of a number
of molecules which are all believed to have evolved from an ancestral
gene encoding a basic unit of structure, the immunoglobulin domain.[9]
The basic domain is a peptide about 90 residues in length. There are
three types of immunoglobulin domains, based on their folding patterns: the C or constant domain; the V or variable domain; and the
"β-pleated sheet and α-helix" domain. The various members of the
superfamily differ structurally in their combinations of types of
domains. For example, immunoglobulin chains are composed of varying numbers of C domains with a single V domain at the N–terminal
end. Similar combinations of C and V domains are utilized in the chains
of the TCR, and adhesion molecules, including CD4, CD8, CD2, and
ICAM-1(CD54). MHC chains have C-type domains and the sheet and
helix type of domains.

Most of the immunoglobulin family members which serve as cell
receptors are heterodimers of subunit chains, as illustrated in Figure 1.
The predominant form of the TCR is compsed of α and β chains.[10] A
small percentage of T cells express another TCR comprised of γ and δ
chains.[11] The TCR is tightly associated in the cell membrane with the

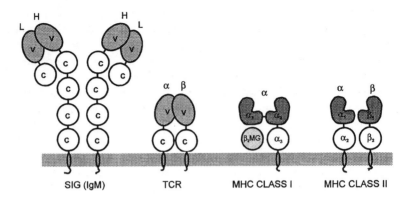

Figure 1
Domain structure of the immunoglobulin family receptors. The Immunoglobulin (Ig) family of receptors includes the antigen receptors for B and T lymphocytes, surface immunoglobulin (SIg), and the T-cell receptor (TCR), respectively. SIg is a heterodimer of two Ig heavy (H) and two Ig light (L) chains. The H chains are comprised of multiple constant (C) domains and one variable (V) domain. The Ig light chain consists of one V and one C domain. The interaction of the NH-terminal V domains from the H and L chains forms the antigen binding site. The TCR consists of an α and β chain, each of which is comprised of one C and one V domain. Similarly to Ig, the interaction of the V domains forms the antigen binding site of theTCR. The MHC molecules, which provide MHC restriction for T lymphocytes, share the constant domain structure with other members of the Ig family, but have a different structure for their NH-terminal domains. These domains are formed by the folding of portions of the molecule into β pleated sheets and α helices. The α_1 and α_2 domains of the class I heavy chain form the peptide binding site or groove for class I antigen presentation to T cells. The peptide binding groove for class II MHC molecules is produced by the interaction of the α_1 and β_1 domains of the class II α and β chains.

CD3 complex, composed of from 3 to 5 different chains (γ, δ, ϵ, ζ, η). MHC molecules are also heterodimers. Class I MHC molecules are composed of an chain with three domains (one C type and two sheet and helix types) and a small chain of one C type domain, called β_2 microglobulin (β_2M).[12] Class II MHC molecules are composed of two chains, nearly equal in weight and which both have one constant and one sheet and helix-type domains.[13] SIg, the antigen receptor for B lymphocytes, is composed of two Ig heavy chains which determine the Ig isotype or class, and two light chains. The N–terminal domains of both heavy and light Ig chains are the variable or V type.[14]

In addition to their extracellular domains, all members of the superfamily which serve as cell receptors have transmembrane and cytoplasmic segments that serve to anchor the receptor in the membrane and to facilitate internal signaling. As mentioned above, the TCR and SIg serve as the antigen specific receptors for T and B lymphocytes, respectively. Class I and class II MHC molecules function in antigen presentation or MHC restriction of T cells. CD4 and CD8 are critical coreceptors for T lymphocytes, acting as adhesion molecules, accessory molecules in signaling, and in MHC restriction of the two major T-cell subclasses.[15] Other members of the Ig family, such as ICAM-1(CD54), ICAM2, and LFA-3(CD58), serve primarily as adhesion molecules. CD2(LFA-2) serves both in adhesion and in internal signaling, while the CD3 complex of chains serves to transduce an activation signal from the TCR. The major members of the Ig superfamily important in immune reactions are summarized in Table 2.

B. Adhesion Molecules of the Selectin, Addressin, Integrin, and Ig Families[16,17]

Many of the steps in host defense and in the induction of immune responses, from phagocytosis to lymphocyte activation, require cell-to-cell contact. Moreover, leukocytes continually circulate throughout the body from the blood stream into the tissues and regional lymph nodes, into the lymphatics, and from the lymphatic vessels back into the blood stream via the thoracic duct. As lymphocytes mature and leave the primary lymphoid organs, the bone marrow and thymus, they populate the secondary lymphoid tissues, i.e., the lymph nodes and spleen. Lymphocytes then circulate throughout the body as do other leukocytes, but they retain the ability to return selectively to their respective lymphoid organs. Cell adhesion, emigration from the circulation through the endothelium, and homing to lymphoid tissues all are mediated through various adhesion molecules. Adhesion molecules also participate in cell activation and in some effector functions. The tissue distribution, ligands, and functions of some of the major adhesion molecules are listed in Table 3.

1. Selectins and Addressins[18]

The selectins constitute a family of adhesion molecules characterized by extracellular lectin-like domains which bind to specific sugar groups expressed on cell-surface carbohydrates. Selectins are responsible for leukocyte homing to different tissues and are expressed on both leukocytes and vascular endothelium. Specific tissue homing is mediated by recognition of vascular addressins. For example, the ligands for L-selectin are mucin-like molecules, including CD34, GlyCAM-1, and MadCAM-1. CD34 and GlyCAM-1 are expressed in specialized venules in lymph nodes, the high endothelial venules (HEV). Circulating lymphocytes enter the lymph nodes through the HEV and the addressins literally direct these cells into the peripheral lymph nodes. MadCAM-1 plays a similar role in directing lymphocytes into the mucosal lymphoid tissue.

TABLE 2

Receptors and Adhesion Molecules of the Immunoglobulin Superfamily

Receptor	Distribution	Ligand	Functions
CD2 (LFA-2)	T cells, some NK cells	CD58(LFA-3)	Adhesion; alternate signaling pathway
CD58(LFA-3)	T,B cells; EC[a], RBC[b], PMN[c]	CD2(LFA-2)	Adhesion
CD54(ICAM-1)	EC, macrophages, activated B cells, dendritic cells	LFA-1, CD2 (LFA-2), Mac-1 (CD11b/CD18)	Adhesion
B7	B cells, EC, APC[d]	CD28	Adhesion and secondary signaling
CD28	Naive T cells, activated B cells	B7.1(CD70), B7.2(CD80)	Adhesion and secondary signaling
CTLA-4	Activated T cells	B7.1(CD70), B7.2(CD80)	Alternate receptor for B7; binds with higher affinity than CD28
SIg	B cells	Conformational antigen epitopes	Antigen binding; primary activation signal
$TCR_{\alpha\beta}$	Majority of human T cells	Complex of MHC and peptide	Antigen binding; primary activation signal
$TCR_{\gamma\delta}$	Small % of T cells, primarily in skin and mucosal tissues	Unknown	Presumably antigen binding and activation; may be involved in thymic selection, T-cell differentiation; host defense in skin and gut
CD3	T cells	None; associated with TCR	Signal transduction, cell activation
CD4	60–70% of T cells	MHC class II	Coreceptor with $TCR_{\alpha\beta}$; adhesion and signaling
CD8	20–30% of T cells	MHC class I	Coreceptor with $TCR_{\alpha\beta}$; adhesion and signaling
MHC class I	All mature, nucleated cells	$TCR_{\alpha\beta}$	Antigen presentation; MHC restriction of CD8[+] T cells
MHC class II	Constitutive expression on B cells, monocytes and macrophages; inducible on activated T cells, EC, other APC	$TCR_{\alpha\beta}$	Antigen presentation; MHC restriction of CD4[+] T cells

[a] EC = endothelial cells.
[b] RBC = erythrocytes.
[c] PMN = polymorphonuclear leucocytes.
[d] APC = antigen presenting cells.

TABLE 3

Adhesion Molecules of the Selectin, Integrin and Addressin Families

Molecule	Tissue Distribution	Ligand	Functions
Selectins			
L-Selectin	Leukocytes	CD34, GlyCAM-1, MadCAM-1	Leukocyte homing; leukocyte binding and interaction with endothelium
P-Selectin (CD62)	Platelets, activated endothelium	Sialyl lewis x[a]	Leukocyte binding and interaction with endothelium; coagulation
E-Selectin	Activated endothelium	Sialyl lewis x[a]	Leukocyte binding and interaction with endothelium
Addressins			
CD34	Endothelium	L-Selectin	Leukocyte binding and interaction with endothelium
GlyCAM-1	High endothelium venules (HEV)	L-Selectin	Leukocyte binding and interaction with endothelium
MadCAM-1	Endothelium of venules in mucosal lymphoid tissue	L-Selectin, VLA-4	Promotes lymphocyte entry into mucosal lymphoid tissue
Integrins			
LFA-1 (CD11a/CD18)	Lymphocytes and other leukocytes	ICAMs	Strong adhesion to apposing cells and extracellular matrix
Mac-1 (CD11b/CD18)	Macrophages and other leukocytes	ICAMs, iC3b[b]	Strong adhesion to apposing cells and extracellular matrix; binding of complement opsonized particles
CR4 (CD11c/CD18)	Phagocytic cells	iC3b	Promotes phagocytosis through binding of opsonized particles
VLA-4 (CD49d/CD29)	Lymphocytes, monocytes	VCAM-1	Strong adhesion and anchoring to extracellar matrix
VLA-5	T lymphocytes and other leukocytes	Fibronectin	Strong adhesion and anchoring to extracellar matrix

[a] Carbohydrate moiety on cell surface glycoproteins of leukocytes.
[b] iC3b = inactivated form of the split complement component C3b.

2. Integrins and Ig Superfamily Adhesion Molecules[8,19]

While the selectins and addressins direct leukocyte homing, additional adhesion molecules are required to enable cells to cross the endothelial barrier and enter the tissue spaces. Members of the integrin and Ig superfamily are critical for these steps. Integrin and Ig adhesion molecules also are vital to the induction of immune responses by promoting the interaction of lymphocytes with APC and, in the effector stages of an immune response, with their target cells.

The integrins constitute a large family of molecules that are heterodimers of a large α chain and a smaller β chain. The integrins are grouped into families on the basis of common, shared β chains and distinct α chains. For example, LFA-1(CD11a/CD18) and Mac-1(CD11b/CD18) are two important integrins expressed on lymphocytes, macrophages, and other leukocytes. They are both members of the β_2 family, sharing a common β chain (CD18) with distinct α chains (CD11a and CD11b). Integrins function in inflammation and immune responses mediating adhesion of one cell to another or adhesion to the extracellular matrix. Because integrins are important adhesion molecules for neutrophils and macrophages, host defense against extracellular pathogens is severely impaired in a condition known as leukocyte adhesion deficiency, which results from an heritable defect in the β_2 chain.[20] Integrins also function in lymphocyte activation and in interaction with target cells. LFA-1, which is expressed on all T cells, is thought to be especially important in this regard. When lymphocytes are activated, additional members of the integrin family are expressed. Then molecules, such as the VLA (very late antigen) integrins, provide strong and prolonged adhesion of cells to the extracellular matrix or to target cells.

There are several members of the Ig superfamily that serve as adhesion molecules. These include LFA and ICAM molecules. CD2 (LFA-2), which is expressed on all T cells and some NK cells, facilitates the initial interaction between these cells and APC and target cells. The ICAM molecules are found on APC as well as vascular endothelium and, thus, contribute to both cell trafficking and interaction with APC. The specific antigen receptors, SIg and the TCR, as well as the T cell coreceptors and MHC molecules, also can be classified as adhesion molecules. However, as will be discussed below, successful interaction of immune cells with APC and target cells depends upon the sequential and concerted interaction of both the nonspecific and antigen-specific molecules.

C. Cytokines and Their Receptors[21-22]

The soluble protein mediators of immunity which act similarly to hormones are generically called "cytokines." Cytokines exert their effects on target cells via specific membrane receptors. Cytokines are generally rather small polypeptides (around 17 to 20 kDa), with short half-lives. Most cytokines are not stored in secretory granules, but are synthesized as needed. Cytokines exert many influences over the immune system, from controlling the development and differentiation of leukocytes to promoting cell activation and proliferation, and to regulation and suppression of immune responses. Cytokines can be grouped according to their general functions into five categories. The hematopoietins stimulate the development and maturation of leukocytes from progenitor stem cells. The interleukins, as their name implies, provide signals or stimulation among leukocytes, often promoting the expansion and development of particular responses, such as delayed type hypersensitivity or immunoglobulin class switching. In addition to their antiviral effects in host defense, the interferons play a significant role in immune responses by increasing MHC expression and activating certain cells. The chemokines promote the specific migration or chemotaxis of leukocytes into the tissues at the sites of inflammation or infection. A final group contains miscellaneous cytokines as yet unclassified with a general function, but which are believed to be important in immune responses.

The cytokine receptors are transmembrane proteins, usually with an internal signaling domain.[23] Most often the receptors are heterodimers, with both chains singly capable of binding the cytokine, but exhibiting much higher binding affinity when paired. Some cytokine receptors express a third subunit chain which may be shared by different members of a family of receptors.[24] The cytokine receptors can be grouped into five classes based on common structural or functional properties. These include: the hematopoietic, the IFN receptors; the Ig superfamily, the TNF-like, and the G-protein coupled receptors. Cytokines and their receptors will be discussed in detail in Chapter 7, but a brief summary of some of the cytokines important in immunity are summarized here in Table 4.

D. The Complement System and Complement Receptors

The complement system is comprised of a number of soluble plasma proteins, some of which are proteolytic enzymes and others are regulatory and inflammatory proteins.[25,26] The complement system also includes cell receptors which bind activated or proteolytically cleaved complement fragments. The complement system serves several functions in host defense: it acts as a first line of defense against microbial invasion, providing nonspecific defense against many pathogens by cytolysis; it augments humoral immunity, enhancing the clearance of immune complexes and the phagocytosis of antibody-coated microorganisms; and its

TABLE 4

Cytokines and Their Receptors

Family	Cytokine	Producer Cells	Receptor(s)	Functions
Hematopoietins	Erythropoietin (Epo)	Kidney	EpoR	Stimulates erythropoiesis
	IL-2 (T cell growth factor)	T cells	CD25(α), CD122(β), γc[a]	T-cell proliferation
	IL-3 (multicolony CSF)	T cells, thymic epithelial cells	CD123, βc[b]	Stimulates hematopoiesis
	IL-4 (B-cell growth factor)	T cells, mast cells	CD124, γc[a]	B-cell activation; IgE switch
	IL-5	T cells, mast cells	CD125, βc[b]	Eosinophil growth, differentiation
	IL-6 (B cell differentiation factor)	T cells, macrophages	CD126, Cdw130[c]	T, B-cell growth/differentiation; acute phase reaction
	IL-7	Bone marrow	CDw127, γc[a]	Pre-B,T-cell growth
	IL-9	T cells	IL-9R, γc[a]	Mast cell activation
	IL-11	Stromal fibroblasts	IL-11R, CDw130	Synergy with IL-3,IL-4 in hematopoiesis
	IL-13	T cells	IL-13R, γc[a]	B-cell growth/differentiation; inhibits macrophage cytokine production
	IL-15	T cells	Il-15R, γc[a]	T-cell growth factor; IL-2 like
	GM-CSF	Macrophages, T cells	CDw116, βc[b]	Stimulates growth/differentiation of myelomonocytic cells

Family	Cytokine	Source cells	Receptor	Function
Interferons	IFN-α	Leukocytes	CD118	Antiviral; increased class I MHC expression
	IFN-β	Fibroblasts	CD118	Antiviral; increased class I MHC expression
	IFN-γ	T, NK cells	CD119	Macrophage activation; increased MHC expression
TNF family	TNF-α (cachectin)	NK cells, macrophages	p55, p75 CD120	Inflammation, endothelial cell activation
	TNF-β (lymphotoxin)	T, B cells	p55, p75 CD120	Cytotoxicity, endothelial cell activation
	CD40-L (ligand for CD40)	T cells, mast cells	CD40	B-cell activation (co-stimulatory signal); Ig class switch
Chemokines:	Fas ligand	T cells, thymic stroma?	CD95 (Fas)	Apoptosis; Ca^{2+} — independent cytotoxicity
	IL-8	Macrophages	CDw128	Chemotaxis of T cells, neutrophils
	MCP-1, MIP, RANTES	Macrophages, T cells, other cells	Receptors unidentified	Chemotaxis of monocytes, T cells, eosinophils
Miscellaneous (no family assigned)	TGF-β	Monocytes, T cells, chondrocytes	Unidentified	Anti-inflammatory; inhibits cell growth
	IL-1α, IL-1β	Macrophages, epithelial cells	CDw121	T cell and macrophage activation; pyrogenic
	IL-10 (cytokine synthesis inhibitor)	T cells, macrophages	Unidentified	Inhibits cytokine production by macrophages and proliferation of Th1 clones
	IL-12	B cells, macrophages	Unidentified	Activates NK cells; Induces differentiation of Th0 → Th1
	MIF	T cells	Unidentified	Inhibits macrophage migration

a γC = common γ chain shared by multiple cytokine receptors.
b βC = common β chain shared by multiple cytokine receptors.
c "w" indicates designation is provisional from WHO nomenclature workshop.

TABLE 5

Complement Components and Receptors

Native Component	Active Forms	Receptors	Functions
C1	C1q C1r C1s	C1q receptor	Binds immune complexes to phagocytic cells; C1r, C1s cleave next components in pathway
C4	C4b C4a	CR1	Promotes phagocytosis Weak inflammatory mediator
C2	C2b		C3/C5 convertase — cleaves C3 and C5
Factor B Factor D			Activating enzymes in alternate pathway
C3	C3b	CR1	Important opsonin — promotes phagocytosis; binds C5; initiates amplification by alternate pathway
	iC3b C3a	CR2, CR3, CR4	Promotes phagocytosis Inflammatory mediator
C5	C5b C5a		Initiates membrane attack complex Potent inflammatory mediator and chemotactant
C6–C9	Polymerized complex		Membrane attack complex; osmotic lysis of pathogens and cells

components exert powerful inflammatory effects in infected or injured tissues.[27] For its lytic effect on target cells, the complement system can be activated by two pathways, the classical and alternate pathways. In both pathways, the complement components, C1 to C9, factor B (properdin), and factor D, interact in a cascade fashion with one component activating the next, often by cleavage of native factors into active subunits. When complement is activated on a cell surface, the complete cascade generates a "membrane attack complex" on target cell surfaces, which results in osmotic lysis of the cells.[28] Key complement fragments, notably C3a and C5a, generated during the cascade, augment inflammation and promote emigration of leukocytes through chemotaxis.[27] Additionally, leukocytes have specific receptors for certain complement components and binding of leukocytes to cells or particles coated or opsonized with complement fragments promotes phagocytosis.[29] The complement system will be discussed thoroughly in Chapter 8, but a brief summary of key complement proteins and complement receptors is given in Table 5.

E. Receptor-Mediated Signaling[30-32]

Aside from binding its specific ligand, the second critical function common to lymphocyte antigen receptors, cytokine receptors, and many of the adhesion molecules is signal transduction. Engagement of its ligand by a receptor molecule triggers a sequence of events in biochemical signaling pathways which is similar to the signal transduction pathways for other types of cell receptors, such as hormones or neurotransmitters. The signal is passed along the receptor to other cell surface-associated molecules and/or coupling proteins, activating key enzymes and nuclear factors which ultimately turn on quiescent genes in the cell. Optimal signaling generally requires aggregation of multiple receptors. For example, optimal T-cell activation requires coaggregation of the TCR with its coreceptors CD4 and CD8. For B lymphocytes, coaggregation of CD19 with the SIg enhances B-cell signaling. Receptors which transduce activation signals generally have an inherent tyrosine kinase (TK) in their cytoplasmic domains, or they are associated with cytosolic molecules with kinase activity. Phosphorylation of associated molecules by the kinase activity of receptors activates adjacent molecules and thus amplifies the signal transduction. The lymphocyte antigen receptors are closely associated with important coreceptors in a complex on the cell surface. Key T lymphocyte receptors which have TK activity (inherently or by association) include: the CD3 complex, CD4 and CD8. The B lymphocyte coreceptor complex includes: Ig_α and Ig_β associated with SIg; CD19; a membrane-spanning protein called TAPA-1; and the complement receptor CR2. Members of the *src* proto-oncogene family, such as p56[lck] (lck) and p59[fyn] (fyn), serve as important cytosolic kinases for T-cell activation and are associated with CD4 and CD8 (lck) and CD3 (fyn). Another cytosolic protein kinase, called zeta-associated protein 70 (ZAP-70), binds to and activates the ζ chains of the CD3 complex. ZAP-70 is thought to be related to *syk*, which appears to play a similar role in B-cell signaling. Various other tyrosine kinases, including *blk*, *lck*, *fyn*, and *lyn*, are associated with the B-cell coreceptor complex. While up-regulation of many of these kinases may require phosphorylation, some molecules have regulatory sites which require dephosphorylation. Thus, cell activation may be modulated by yet another cell surface molecule, CD45 (also known as the leukocyte common antigen), whose cytoplasmic domain has intrinsic tyrosine phosphatase activity.[33] Coaggregation of CD45 is thought to be involved in activation of coreceptors, such as CD4 and CD8.

Aggregation of cell surface receptors with the resultant activation of their inherent or associated tyrosine kinases can activate many components of signaling pathways, including the second messenger "G" proteins, members of the *ras* family of proto-oncogenes, phospholipase C, phosphatidyl inositol-3-kinase, and other protein kinases, such as protein kinase C (PKC). While the exact steps and interactions have not been clearly established, the following appear to be key steps in lymphocyte activation.[32] Cross-linking or clustering of receptors initiates kinase activity. Association of secondary kinases, such as ZAP-70, fyn (T cells), and syk (B cells) activates phospholipase C, which cleaves phosphatidyl inositol to diacylglycerol (DAG) and inositol triphosphate (IP_3). From DAG and IP_3, two signaling pathways diverge. DAG can activate PKC. The PKC pathway is thought to stimulate the transcription of factors, such as *myc, fos,* and *jun,* which, in turn, serve as transcription factors for other genes. IP_3 binds to the endoplasmic reticulum and induces release of calcium into the cytoplasm. The rise in intracellular Ca^{2+} activates other proteins, notably the calcium-dependent enzyme, calcineurin. Calcineurin is believed to activate and cause the transcription factor $NF-AT_p$ (nuclear factor of activated T cells) to translocate to the nucleus. There $NF-AT_p$ assembles with other nuclear factors in the promoter regions of genes, such as IL-2 and other cytokines. The resultant activation of multiple DNA-binding proteins by the PKC pathway and the increased Ca^{2+} flux induce the transcription of many genes which leads to cell activation, differentiation, and proliferation. A general flow chart of these events is illustrated in Figure 2.

It is important to note that for lymphocyte activation, engagement of the antigen-specific receptor is usually insufficient for optimal signaling and activation. Coaggregation of multiple receptors is required, stressing the importance of accessory, adhesion molecules and/or the cytokine receptors.[35,36] The concomitant action of their kinase activities provides what is termed the "second signal." Since the PKC pathway may be activated by other events, aside from DAG produced in the phospholipase pathway, second signals may enhance PKC activity as well as initiating other signal pathways. Adhesion molecules and their ligands which may provide the second or co-stimulatory signal for T cells include: CD28 and B7; ICAM-1 and LFA-1; CD2 and LFA-3.[34] CD40 and its ligand CD40-L provide co-stimulation for B cells.[37] Cytokines produced by APC, such as IL-1 and IL-6, may also deliver secondary signals when bound to their receptors.[35] Since most immune responses involve at some point direct cell-to-cell interaction, it is now thought that intercellular signaling occurs, and that this reciprocal "conversation," involving multiple interactions of receptors between APC and lymphocytes, is required for the proliferation of antigen-specific clones. In the absence of the appropriate second signals, lymphocyte tolerance or nonresponsiveness may result. Signaling through lymphocyte antigen receptors and accessory molecules stimulates lymphocyte activation, development, and differentiation throughout their lifespan. Signaling events also function in down-regulation of immune responses, as it has been recently shown that signaling of B lymphocytes through Fc receptors provides negative regulation. Such signaling presumably occurs during a humoral response when sufficient antibody has been produced to form circulating immune complexes. Binding of immune complexes cross-links Fc receptors, providing a down-regulatory signal that shuts down antibody production.[38]

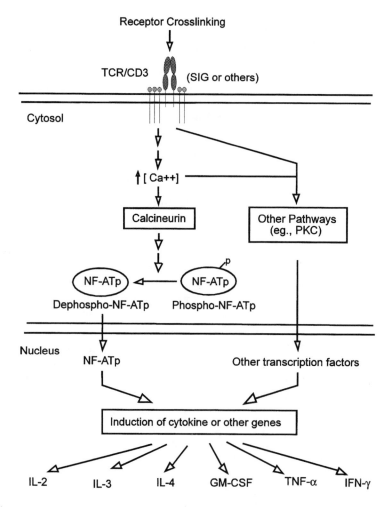

Figure 2

Lymphocyte signal transduction pathways. A series of biochemical events, often involving interrelated pathways, is initiated by the cross-linking of cell surface receptors on
lymphocytes. Clustering of the cytoplasmic domains of the lymphocyte antigen receptor
molecules activates various enzymes which regulate protein phosphorylation. While the
exact steps in the signaling pathways have not been clearly defined, two major effects
appear to be common to different cells: there is an increase in intracellular calcium, and
protein kinase C (PKC) is activated. The rise in intracellular calcium activates the enzyme
calcineurin, which, in turn, activates the transcription factor, $NF-AT_p$ (nuclear factor of
activated T cells). Similarly, activation of PKC or other pathways promotes the activation
of other transcription factors. $NF-AT_p$ and the other transcription factors then translocate
into the nucleus where, after binding to their respective promoter regions, they induce
cytokine and other genes involved in lymphocyte activation, expansion and differentiation.
(Modified from Rao, A., *Immunol. Today*, 15, 274, 1994.)

IV. DEVELOPMENT OF B AND T LYMPHOCYTES

Development and maturation of B and T lymphocytes involves differentiation from the lymphoid stem cells, generation of a repertoire of antigen receptors, and shaping of this repertoire by a process generally called selection. The basic steps of B and T lymphocyte development are diagrammed in Figures 3 and 4.

A. Generation of B and T Lymphocyte Antigen Receptor Repertoires[39-42]

The specificity or commitment of B and T lymphocytes to antigenic epitopes is reflected in their antigen receptors. Individual lymphocytes have 10^6 or more surface receptors, all sharing the same combining site which can bind to a set of antigenic determinants that are closely related in structure. Clones of lymphocytes, which are derived from a single precursor cell, will all share the same surface antigen receptor. As illustrated in Figure 1, the antigen binding sites of SIg and TCR are formed by the interactions of the variable domains of the Ig heavy and light chains for SIg and by the variable domains of the TCR α and β chains. An incredible feature of the immune system is the vast diversity that is found in the range of specific antigen receptors expressed on mature lymphocytes — estimated in excess of 10^9 for both T and B cells. The details of how this diversity is generated in the Ig and TCR genes are beyond the scope of this overview, and only a brief summary will be given here. Generation of diversity in lymphocyte antigen receptors involves gene rearrangement which occurs during the development and maturation of B lymphocytes in the bone marrow and T lymphocytes in the thymus.

The basic steps of gene rearrangement are the same for both types of lymphocytes. The genes for Ig and TCR chains are composed of multiple segments or exons that encode different portions of the proteins. These segments are referred to as V (variable), D (diversity), J (joining), and C (constant). As these molecules are cell membrane receptors, there are also other exons encoding transmembrane and cytoplasmic segments. In germline DNA, the chromosomes containing the Ig and TCR genes have multiple V, D, J, and C genes. In particular for the V genes, depending on the TCR or Ig chain involved, there may be up to 100 different possible V segments. The V segments are usually grouped in families with different D and/or J and C genes downstream and separated by large stretches of intervening DNA. At certain points in lymphocyte development, gene rearrangement commences (Figures 3 and 4). For both T and B cells, gene rearrangement is controlled by the *recombinase* enzymes, RAG-1 and RAG- 2, which bind to highly conserved target sequences in the germline DNA of the Ig and

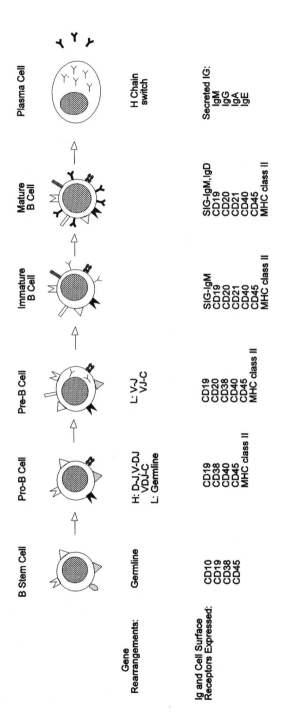

Figure 3

Major stages of B lymphocyte development. The differentiation and development of B lymphocytes can be traced through multiple stages by the expression of various cell surface receptors or differentiation antigens (CD markers). The B lymphocyte antigen receptor or surface immunoglobulin (SIg) repertoire is generated during development in the bone marrow by progressive immunoglobulin (Ig) gene rearrangements. The rearrangement of Ig heavy (H) chain genes occurs first at the pre-B cell stage of development. The D-J gene segments rearrange first, followed by V-DJ joining, and last, by VDJ joining to a constant (C) gene segment. Similar rearrangement occurs for the Ig light (L) chains at the pre-B cell stage. Throughout B lymphocyte development there is a progressive increase in the number of cell receptors or CD markers expressed, culminating with mature, immunocompetent B lymphocytes. After antigen stimulation, selected B lymphocyte clones enter terminal differentiation into plasma cells, which secrete antigen-specific immunoglobulins. The plasma cell is essentially a protein factory, producing specific antibodies, and is virtually devoid of the usual CD markers expressed on mature B cells. Further Ig gene rearrangements can occur at the plasma cell stage, producing the phenomenon of Ig class or isotype switch.

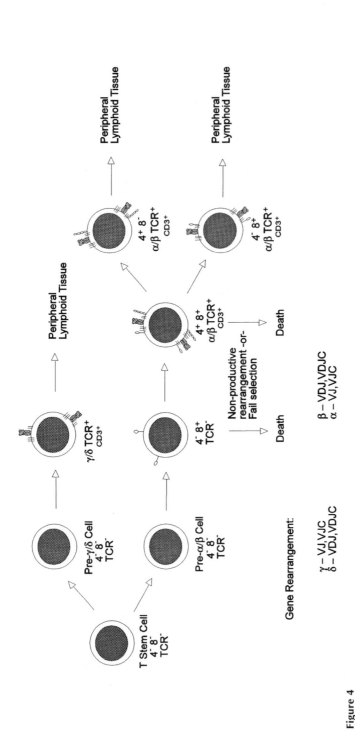

Figure 4

T cell development. Two pathways for T cell development diverge from uncommitted T cell precursors in the thymus. For γ/δ T cells, the γ genes are rearranged, followed by the δ genes. Productive rearrangements lead to expression of γ/δ TCR/CD3. The γ/δ T cells do not express the other T cell markers, CD4 or CD8, and have different functional properties and localizations in the body than do the more numerous α/β T cells. The first T cell-specific marker detectable on α/β T cells is CD8 (8⁺). At this stage, the rearrangement of β chain genes commences. Maturation of α/β T cells continues through a "double-positive" stage when thymocytes express both CD4 and CD8 (4⁺8⁺). The CD3 complex is also detectable at this stage in low concentration and the α TCR genes rearrange. The majority of thymocytes at this stage ultimately die, either from abberant or nonproductive gene rearrangement or from failure of thymic selection (either positive or negative selection). The minority of cells that are successfully selected diverge into single positive cells, i.e., CD4⁺ or CD8⁺. These cells then migrate from the thymus and enter the peripheral circulation and populate the secondary lymphoid organs.

TCR genes.[42] During gene rearrangement, different V genes are randomly joined with D or D/J and C genes to yield a functional gene which can be transcribed and translated into a Ig or TCR chain. As rearrangement progresses, there are additional factors that enhance the diversity of potential receptors, aside from that produced by the random joining of different gene segments. The point of D or D/J joining to the V gene influences the final specificity of an Ig or TCR chain. In many cases, the joining of these segments is imprecise and the original nucleotide sequence is altered. Additionally, DNA repair enzymes sometimes add or delete nucleotides at the joining sites. Finally, as the Ig and TCR receptors are heterodimers of subunit chains, additional diversity is generated by the random pairing of different Ig heavy and light chains and TCR α and β (or TCR γ and δ) chains to form the functional molecules.

B. B- and T-Lymphocyte Selection[43-45]

With the vast repertoire of antigen receptors that can be generated by the random processes of gene rearrangement, it is essential that there is some selection of the developing lymphocytes to prevent the maturation of cells that could be potentially self-reactive. Thus, both B and T lymphocytes undergo a selection during their development which results in the elimination of self-reactive clones. For B lymphocytes, this process occurs in the bone marrow. Immature B cells with receptors for self cell-surface antigens appear to undergo a type of cell suicide or programmed cell death. Morphologically, this process is known as apoptosis, in which the cell nucleus essentially condenses and ultimately disintegrates. Other developing B cells that can bind soluble self antigens are somehow tolerized or rendered anergic (unresponsive) to these antigens. Because this process occurs early in B-cell development and within the marrow where exposure is limited to potential self antigens, only self-reactive cells are eliminated or anergized. Immature cells that do not encounter antigens continue to develop and eventually leave the marrow to populate peripheral lymphoid tissues. It is important to note that, while selection of self-reactive B cells occurs during early development, further diversification of the B-cell SIg repertoire occurs in the periphery. It has been clearly shown that somatic hypermutation (by DNA point mutations) occurs in B lymphocytes following antigenic stimulation. Somatic hypermutation can expand the Ig V gene repertoire and is generally thought to explain the phenomenon of increase in antibody binding affinity during a humoral immune response, but may also provide a source of self-reactive antibodies. Presumably, in normal situations, potentially self-reactive B cells are regulated or suppressed by T-lymphocyte control of the humoral response.[46]

Selective forces also shape the potential T-cell repertoire.[47-49] The T-lymphocyte repertoire, however, is subject to two constraints: the need to eliminate self-reactive cells (negative selection) and the requirement to generate cells with self-MHC restricted receptors (positive selection). Developing T lymphocytes leave the bone marrow early in their development and migrate to the thymus. Within the compartments of the thymus, immature T cells undergo rearrangement of their TCR genes and acquire their coreceptors CD4 and CD8. During the early stages of thymic development, T cells express both CD4 and CD8. Developing T cells are thought to first interact with thymic epithelium, where only cells with receptors which can bind to self-MHC are selected and permitted to mature. Positive selection also occurs for the MHC restriction of the CD4 and CD8 coreceptors and after this step, maturing T cells split into two lineages, CD4+ or CD8+. Positive selection insures that the mature T-cell repertoire will contain "useful T cells," i.e., T cells that can meet the requirements of MHC restriction both to recognize self-MHC antigens and to interact with their respective T-cell populations, i.e., CD4+ cells with MHC class II and CD8+ cells with MHC class I. Negative selection also occurs in the thymus when developing T cells interact with bone marrow-derived APC. T-cell precursors with receptors for self MHC and/or self peptides are eliminated at this stage. Thus, in the two stages, potential T cells are selected which are self-MHC restricted, but not self-reactive. As for B cells, the major mechanism for elimination of self-reactive T cells is a programmed cell death by apoptosis.[50]

V. THE MAJOR HISTOCOMPATIBILITY COMPLEX[51-54]

The major histocompatibility complex (MHC) is a group of closely linked genes which was first appreciated because it contains the structural genes for the histocompatibility or transplantation antigens. The MHC is now recognized to include many other genes for important components that are vital to the induction and regulation of immune responses. A simplified map of the human MHC or HLA system is given in Figure 5. The MHC can be divided into three regions, of which the class I and II regions contain the loci for the human histocompatibility or HLA antigens. The class I region genes encode the α or heavy chain of the major class I human histocompatibility antigens, HLA-A, B, and C. There are several other genes in the class I region, most of which are pseudo genes and not functional. HLA-E and F are known to be transcribed, but no significant tissue expression has yet been documented. HLA-G is expressed transiently on trophoblastic tissue and may be involved in tolerance at the maternal–fetal interface.[55] The organization of genes in the MHC class II region is more complex than

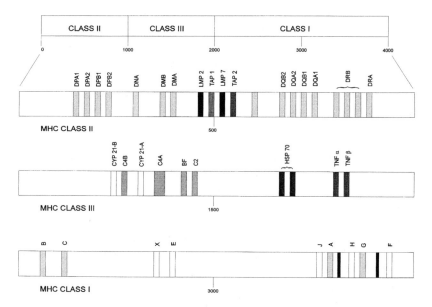

Figure 5

A map of the human major histocompatibility complex (MHC). The major genes of the three subregions of the human MHC or HLA system are shown in the enlarged sections of the MHC map. The HLA gene complex is contained in a 3500-kb segment of DNA and is located on the short arm of chromosome 6. The class II region contains the structural genes for the α and β chains of the major class II HLA molecules, including: DPA and DPB, DQA and DQB, DRA and DRB. While other class II genes, such as DNA and DOB, are transcribed, their actual tissue expression, if any, is limited. The class II region also contains the LMP (low molecular weight proteases) and the TAP (transporters associated with antigen processing) genes, which are believed to be involved in processing of antigenic peptides. The class II region contains the genes for the complement components, C2, C4, and factor B (Bf); the enzyme 21-hydroxylase (CYP-21); members of the heat shock protein 70 family (HSP 70); and tumor necrosis factor α (TNF-α) and tumor necrosis factor β or lymphotoxin (TNF-β). The structural genes for the α or heavy chain of the major HLA class I molecules, HLA-A, B, and C are found in the class I region. A number of additional class I genes are also present in the class I region, but most are pseudogenes, truncated genes, or gene fragments and are, therefore, not expressed. An exception is HLA-G, which is expressed on the trophoblast.

that of class I, as it contains the structural genes for both the α and β chains of the class II molecules. The genes for the class II chains are designated A and B for the respective α and β chains, and the class II region includes the following: 4 DP genes (B2, A2, B1, A1); 1 DN gene (A); 1 DO gene (B); 5 DQ genes (B2,A2,B3,B1,A1); and a varying number of DR genes (B1-B9, A) depending upon the haplotype. The class II region also contains two recently identified types of genes which are thought to be involved in antigen processing. These include two LMP (low molecular weight proteins) genes and two TAP (transporters associated with antigen processing) genes. The LMP genes are thought to include two subunits of a cytoplasmic, multicatalytic complex of proteases or "proteasome." The TAP genes encode proteins that are involved in transporting peptides into the endoplasmic reticulum. The genes in the class III region are a heterogenous group and include a variety of soluble factors important in immune responses. These include: the complement factors C2, C4, and Factor B; members of the heat shock protein (HSP) 70 family; and the tumor necrosis factors, TNFα and TNFβ.

As previously discussed, structurally the class I and II MHC molecules are members of the Ig family (Figure I).[12,13] The class I MHC antigens, HLA-A,B, and C, are constitutively expressed to some extent on all nucleated cells. The density of surface expression does vary with different cells and tissues, but class I molecules are found in high concentrations on leukocytes, particularly on APC and lymphocytes. In man, the class II molecules, HLA-DR, DQ, and DP, are constitutively expressed only on B lymphocytes, monocytes, and macrophages. These molecules are inducible on various cells, particularly by cytokines such as the interferons produced during inflammation. In man, HLA-DR expression is also induced on T lymphocytes following the activation of these cells. The tissue distribution of MHC molecules on APC and lymphocytes parallels their function in antigen presentation and MHC restriction and will be discussed further below.

A.   MHC Restriction[10,56]

The biologic function of MHC antigens is to present antigenic peptides to T lymphocytes. In fact, it is an absolute requirement for T-lymphocyte activation for T cells to "see" the antigenic peptide bound to an MHC molecule. This requirement, known as MHC restriction, distinguishes T cells from B cells. The SIg receptor of B lymphocytes and their stimulated products, i.e., specific antibodies, bind to antigenic epitopes on soluble molecules or on the surfaces of particles — an ability which is well suited to their role in humoral immunity. In contrast, T lymphocytes mediate cellular immunity through direct cell-to-cell contact. MHC restriction provides the mechanism for this intercellular activity.

The molecular basis for MHC restriction was established with the elucidation of the crystalline structures of class I and II MHC molecules.[12,13] As noted above, the N-terminal domains of MHC molecules are formed by the folding of portions of their component chains in β-pleated sheets and α helices. This structure is unique to MHC molecules among the members of the Ig family. The sheet portions form a floor and the helices form the sides of a peptide-binding groove. During antigen processing (see below), peptide fragments of antigens are bound in the grooves of MHC molecules and displayed on the surfaces of APC. The TCR recognizes and binds to the complex of MHC and peptide (Figure 6).[10] The TCR has three points of contact with the MHC:peptide complex, designated as CDR1, CDR2, and CDR3. The CDR3 region reflects complementarity with the bound peptide, while the CDR1 and CDR2 regions depend upon recognition of self-MHC sequences. Comparison of the crystalline structures of class I and class II molecules has revealed overall structural similarity, but with a few significant differences. Class I molecules have a groove with deep anchor pockets at each end.[57] These pockets restrict the binding of peptides to those of 8 to 9 residues in length. The peptide-binding groove of class II molecules is more flexible and is relatively open at one end, which permits binding of larger peptides from 13 to 25 residues in length.[58] For the different MHC alleles of both classes, there is a complementary sequence motif or pattern which determines a set of related peptides that can be bound.[59,60] MHC restriction also determines which of the two subsets of T lymphocytes that can interact. CD8[+] T lymphocytes interact with class I MHC molecules through a specific binding site located on the α_3 domain. Conversely, CD4[+] T lymphocytes interact only with class II molecules through two binding sites, which are thought to be located on the first two domains of the CD4 molecule.[61] The coreceptor binding of CD4 and CD8 to class II and class I MHC molecules is also illustrated in Figures 6A and 6B.

B. Antigen Processing and Presentation[62-67]

T lymphocytes comprise the majority of circulating peripheral blood lymphocytes, and they play a major role in the induction of all immune responses. Their activation depends upon recognition of MHC:peptide complexes on the surfaces of APC, and it is within the APC that the peptide ligands are generated. There are two major pathways of antigen processing and these are adapted to sample proteins derived from intracellular and extracellular sources. The "loading" or binding of peptides to MHC molecules is tied to their biosynthesis, such that when new MHC molecules are transported and expressed on the surfaces of APC, they carry with them peptides for presentation to T cells. In general, class I MHC molecules bind peptides that are synthesized within or derived from cytosolic sources, such as viral proteins or aberrant cellular proteins. This presentation is well suited for the function of the cytotoxic CD8[+] T cells, which are restricted to MHC class I bearing APC and which recognize and destroy virally infected cells or other cells different from normal self cells. In contrast,

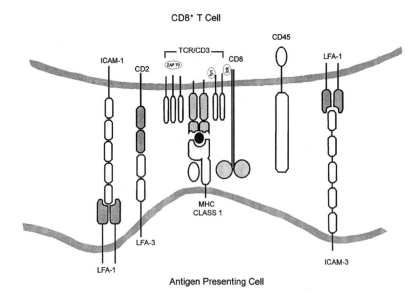

Figure 6(A)

Receptors and adhesion molecules involved in the interaction of CD8+ T cells with MHC class I antigen-presenting cells (APC). The initial binding of T cells to APC is facilitated by adhesion molecules and their ligands, including CD2/LFA-3 (lymphocyte function antigen-3 or CD58) and LFA-1/ICAM-1 (intercellular adhesion molecule-1). These molecules are expressed and function as preliminary adhesion molecules on both the CD8 and CD4 subsets of T lymphocytes. On CD8+ T cells, the CD8 molecule acts both as an adhesion molecule and as a coreceptor with the TCR. If the TCR has sufficient affinity for the MHC class I:peptide complex, stable binding is achieved. Clustering of the CD3 complex and CD8 coreceptors initiates signaling for cell activation. Enzymes involved in signal transduction include the phosphatase inherent in the cytoplasmic domain of CD45 and the cytoplasmic tyrosine kinases ZAP-70, *fyn,* and *lck.*

MHC class II molecules are primarily loaded with peptides derived from extracellular sources. Since CD4+ T cells provide "help" for B cells in antibody production and for the activation of macrophages in the destruction of phagocytized pathogens, presentation of extracellularly derived peptides to class II restricted CD4+ cells promotes defense against extracellular invasion. The major steps in antigen processing can be summarized as follows:

Class I Antigen Processing

1. Cytosolic proteins are degraded by proteasome complexes into small peptides. The LMP genes found in the class II MHC region are thought to encode two subunits of a proteasome complex devoted to antigen processing.

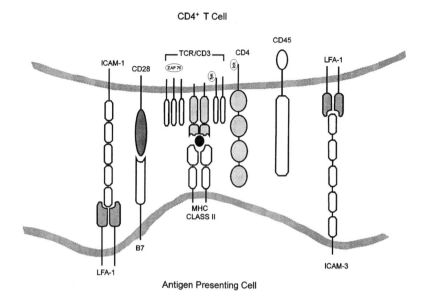

Figure 6(B)
Receptors and adhesion molecules involved in the interaction of CD4+ T cells with MHC class II antigen-presenting cells. The LFA and ICAM adhesion molecules also contribute to the initial interaction of CD4+ T cells with APC. Providing class II MHC restriction, the CD4 molecule functions similarly to CD8 for class I MHC APC, acting both as an adhesion molecule and a coreceptor for the TCR. The molecule CD28 and its ligand, B7, are important in the activation of naive T cells and, as such, may function both for naive (i.e., cells that have not previously encountered antigens) CD4+ and CD8+ T cells. The interaction of B7 and CD28 provides the so-called "second" or costimulatory signal necessary for T-cell activation and clonal expansion. As for the CD8 T cell, signal transduction is initiated by the cross-linking or clustering of multiple receptors with their associated tyrosine kinases.

2. The peptides are transported into the lumen of the endoplasmic reticulum (ER) by the TAP transporter. The TAP 1 and TAP 2 genes, located in the MHC class II region, encode proteins of the ATP-binding cassette family (ABC) of protein transporters. Assembled as a heterodimer, the TAP transporter has cytosolic ATP-binding domains and hydrophobic transmembrane domains which can transport the proteasome degraded peptides into the lumen of the ER.

3. Peptides introduced into the ER interact with newly synthesized class I MHC molecules. Those with complementary sequence motifs to appropriate MHC molecules are bound within the MHC peptide groove.

4. Peptide binding stabilizes the conformation of the new MHC molecules and facilitates their proper folding. Class I molecules with bound peptides are then transported to the cell surface.

Class II Antigen Processing

1. Antigens are endocytosed or taken up by phagocytosis (particulate antigens) into intracellular vesicles (endosomes or phagosomes).

2. Internalized antigens are degraded within the endosome–lysosome compartments by proteases. Some cell surface receptors, such as Fc receptors and complement receptors, may be internalized into the endosomes, where ligands bound to these receptors dissociate and are degraded.

3. Newly synthesized class II molecules in the ER appear to be stabilized by a chaperon-like protein, the invariant chain (Ii). The Ii protects the peptide groove and also is believed to direct the class II molecules to the endosome compartment.

4. Transport vesicles containing the class II molecules fuse with the endosome–lysosome vesicles. Under acidic conditions within the endosome compartment, the Ii dissociates and is itself degraded, permitting the class II molecules to bind appropriate peptides.

5. Class II molecules, stabilized with bound peptides, are transported to the cell surface.

C. MHC Polymorphism[53,68,69]

Because T lymphocytes are MHC restricted, an individual's array of MHC molecules indirectly controls antigen recognition through the peptides which can be bound. MHC molecules differ from one another by different amino acid residues located predominantly in the peptide binding groove. These different substitutions are the result of different alleles or alternate forms of the MHC genes. The importance of MHC control of immune responsiveness was first appreciated in inbred animals, where it was shown that strains lacking certain MHC alleles could not respond to immunization with synthetic peptides. In fact, the genetic control of this responsiveness led to the designation of immune response (IR) genes long before MHC restriction was understood.[70]

Three factors ensure that appropriate antigen presentation and subsequent immune responses can occur at both the individual and population levels. First, each individual MHC molecule can bind a range of peptides. The anchor residues of the peptide binding grooves of both class I and class II molecules largely influence the sequences of peptides that can be bound, but allow some variability. Peptides with exact sequence complementarity bind with high affinity, but other closely related peptides can also bind. The range of peptides bound is great enough that MHC peptide binding has been described as being "promiscuous." Second, because of the multiple loci (HLA-A,B,C and HLA-DR,DQ DP) expressed on cells, the potential for peptide binding is further expanded. Finally, MHC polymorphism provides a vast number of different MHC alleles in the population. Large numbers of different alleles exist for the different MHC loci. For example, sequencing studies of HLA-DRB1 have identified over 100 distinct alleles, and preliminary analysis indicates that this level of polymorphism will be as high for other loci, such as HLA-B.

It is thought that various genetic mechanisms have produced this vast MHC polymorphism throughout evolution, and it is logical that diversification of MHC molecules safeguards the survival of populations by ensuring that some individuals will have the appropriate MHC to present antigens from microbial pathogens.[71,72] This level of allele polymorphism in the population also means that most individuals are heterozygous at the MHC loci, i.e., they have different alleles at each locus. Because expression of MHC alleles is co-dominant, the number of MHC molecules available for antigen presentation is effectively doubled. Moreover, for class II MHC gene products, pairing of α and β chains from different chromosomes can occur, expanding the number of different MHC molecules even further.

While MHC polymorphism assures effective antigen presentation of most microbial pathogens, clinically MHC polymorphism complicates attempts to find histocompatible donors for bone marrow and solid organ transplantation. Recent analyses of registries maintained by the National Marrow Donor Program and the United Network for Organ Sharing have established the extent of heterogeneity in HLA phenotypes, showing that the great majority of individuals have unique phenotypes. Finding "perfect" matches for transplantation, therefore, can require extremely large donor pools of at least several hundred thousand individuals.[73,74]

VI. INDUCTION OF IMMUNE RESPONSES

Induction of immune responses can follow any introduction into the body of foreign material, but may also result from abnormal immune regulation or breakdown in normal self-tolerance. For purposes of this discussion, the sequence of events leading to immunity to infections agents will be used. The sequence begins whenever an infectious agent breaches the external mucosal or epithelial barriers.

A. Initial, Nonspecfic Defenses and Acute Inflammation[1-3,75,76]

Penetration of the epithelium evokes localized inflammation due to damage or activation of tissue mast cells. Degranulation of the mast cell vasoactive amines, histamine and serotonin, cases a localized increase in blood flow and vascular permeability. The resulting fluid accumulation in the tissues brings in the complement plasma proteins. Since the alternate complement pathway can be activated by the cell walls of many microbes, complement activation produces additional inflammatory mediators with the release of C3a and C5a. Polymorphonuclear leukocytes respond to chemotactic stimuli, including C5a, and migrate into the tissues. Pathogens opsonized by C3b may then be quickly phagocytosed and destroyed. Although the neutrophil leukocytes are generally the first cells to enter an inflamed tissue area, they are followed within a few hours by monocytes, NK cells, and eventually lymphocytes. As will be discussed below, the principal sites for lymphocyte stimulation are the peripheral lymph nodes and spleen, but it should be noted that $TCR_{\gamma\delta}$ T cells may play an important part in defense at the mucosal and epithelial barriers.

The importance of the inflammatory mediators initiating host defense should not be minimized. These agents cause an immediate accumulation of phagocytes and plasma proteins, which can contain many infectious agents. These agents can be evoked within minutes to a few hours, compared to the days it takes to evoke a primary, specific immune response. If infection is not contained by the initial wave of polymorphonuclear leukocytes, infiltrating macrophages become activated and release additional inflammatory cytokines, including IL-1, IL-6, IL-8, IL-12, and TNF-α. IL-8 is a chemotactic factor and recruits additional cells, while IL-1 and TNF-α activate vascular endothelium and further increase vascular permeability. Ongoing inflammation and infection in the tissues results in fluid drainage to the regional lymph nodes, which is a usual starting point for the induction of specific, lymphocyte-mediated immunity. Similarly, pathogens originating in the mucosa are concentrated or trapped in the Peyer's patches and tonsils, while blood-borne pathogens accumulate in the spleen.

B. The Role of Adhesion Molecules in Lymphocyte Emigration and Antigen Recognition[77,78]

Lymphocytes continuously circulate between the bloodstream and the lymphoid organs. Because the lymph nodes and spleen entrap microorganisms from the draining lymphatics and blood and because they are also densely populated with "professional" APC, they are ideal sites for the induction of immune responses. The professional APC which are found in lymph nodes include dendritic cells, which are found in the cortex; B lymphocytes, which are located primarily in the follicles; and macrophages, which are found throughout the node. The different types of APC and their distribution in the lymph nodes allow entrapment and antigen processing of many different pathogens and their products.

The migration of lymphocytes from the bloodstream occurs across the walls of the specialized high endothelial venules (HEV). Adhesion molecules, including members of the selectin, integrin, and Ig superfamily contribute to this process (Tables 2 and 3). Mediators of acute inflammation induce the synthesis of new adhesion molecules and activate others such that their binding affinity is increased. Lymphocyte homing to specific lymphoid tissues is influenced particularly by the selectins which recognize the mucin-like adressins on vascular endothelium. L-Selectin expression promotes attachment of leukocytes to vascular enodthelium, but by itself, only transiently. Additional adhesion molecules must be engaged for lymphocytes to cross the endothelial barrier into the lymphoid organs. The integrins LFA-1 and VLA-4 are important for T-cell adhesion to the endothelium, while Mac-1 functions for macrophages. Once inside the lymphoid tissue, lymphocytes must interact with APC via their antigen-specific receptors and additional adhesion molecules. Certain Ig family members, including CD2, LFA-3 (CD58), ICAM-1, and ICAM-3, facilitate this interaction.

As lymphocytes, particularly T cells, pass through the secondary lymphoid organs, adhesion molecules promote a transient binding of these cells to APC. This adhesion is crucial for T cells whose antigen receptors must encounter and recognize small peptides bound to MHC molecules. Given that the frequency of T cell with a TCR for a given peptide antigen is usually 1 in 10^5, the sampling process must allow sufficient adhesion to allow the TCR to contact and bind appropriate MHC:peptide complexes. When the TCR is engaged, signal transduction from the TCR activates a conformational change in the integrin LFA-1 which causes it to bind its ligands, ICAM 1-3, with greater affinity.[79] This increased adhesion prolongs the association of the T cell and APC until the T cell can be fully activated. The T-cell coreceptors, CD4 and CD8, also contribute to adhesion, as well as providing MHC class I or II restriction and costimulation. Some of the important coreceptors and adhesion molecules in T cell and APC interactions are illustrated in Figures 6A and 6B. Similar adhesion interactions promote the interaction of B lymphocytes with T cells and APC.

C. Lymphocyte Activation and Clonal Expansion[1-3]

In addition to facilitating the initial binding of lymphocyte TCR and SIg receptors with antigen, many of the adhesion molecules are required to provide costimulation or secondary signaling (Table 2 and

Figure 2) before lymphocytes can be fully activated. As signal trans-duction was previously discussed, it will suffice to reiterate that appro-priate lymphocyte activation induces the transcription of several new genes which are necessary to promote further lymphocyte differentia-tion and cell division. The proliferation of clones of lymphocytes from individual precursors stimulated by specific antigens is a key feature of adaptive immune responses. This feature allows the selective expan-sion of selected lymphocyte clones from the entire lymphocyte reper-toire with the appropriate antigenic specificity for the inciting antigens. Some of the critical genes which are turned on during the activation process include key cytokines, IL-2, IL-4, and IL-6, among others. Under the influence of these cytokines (Table 4), activated precursor lymphocytes differentiate and proliferate, producing clones of lympho-cytes with the same antigenic specificity. Importantly, two types of progeny cells emerge: effector cells, which mediate immediate immune reactivity, and memory cells, which revert to a resting state and are long-lived, staying in the circulation until subsequent reexposure to the inciting antigens evokes their reactivation. Because the initial clonal expansion increases the frequency of memory cells with specific antigen receptors, compared to the initial lymphocyte repertoire, subsequent antigen exposure evokes a quicker response since there are more pre-cursor cells capable of responding. Thus, memory cells explain the phenomenon of the quickened, secondary (anamnestic) response or "immunologic memory".

Aside from memory cells, the effector cells for T lymphocyte, or cell-mediated immune responses, are generated in the two major T-cell populations. CD4+ effector T cells are largely cytokine-producing cells, providing "help" for the B lymphocytes in antibody production and supplying the cytokines of delayed hypersensitivity reactions, activat-ing and recruiting other lymphocytes, macrophages, and NK cells. The CD8+ population of effector T cells is comprised mainly of cytotoxic cells (CTL). The CD8+ CTL are responsible for the destruction of virally infected cells, allogenic cells in organ transplantation, and potentially malignant cells in immune surveillance. For B lymphocytes, activation results in differentiation to plasma cells which actively synthesize and secrete antibodies of various Ig classes specific for the inciting anti-gen(s). T-lymphocyte "help," via the cytokines produced by CD4+ lym-phocytes, is critical for a humoral immune response. During the course of a complete humoral immune response, the B lymphocyte progeny plasma cells not only produce initial antibodies of the IgM isotype, but subsequently "switch" by a further gene rearrangement and begin producing antibodies of the IgG, IgA, or IgE classes. It is now known that the regulation for the Ig class switch is largely under the influence of certain T-cell-derived cytokines, including IL-4 and IL-10.

D. The Central Role of CD4⁺ T Lymphocytes: Th1 and Th2 Cytokines[80]

CD4⁺ T lymphocytes play a primary role in all adaptive immune responses, controlling and driving the differentiation of other lymphocytes into the three major effector types: the B lymphocyte humoral response, the CD4⁺ delayed type hypersensitivity response, and the CD8⁺ CTL response. Although many leukocytes secrete cytokines, CD4⁺ T cells are the principal producers. It is now appreciated that the types of cytokines produced by CD4⁺ T cells can change during an immune response. Early on in a primary response, CD4⁺ cells (Th0) produce a variety of cytokines, but with prolonged antigenic stimulation, the cytokines secreted become more restricted and assume what is called a Th1 or Th2 pattern. The principal cytokines produced by the Th0 cells are IL-2, IL-4, and IFN-γ. The Th1 cytokines include IFN-γ, TNF-β, GM-CSF, IL-3, and IL-2, while the Th2 cytokines consist of IL-4, IL-5, IL-6, and IL-10. CD4 cells which produce predominantly Th1 cytokines are said to be inflammatory T cells and potentiate cell-mediated immunity. The Th1 cytokines activate macrophages and NK cells, and through IL-2, help expand and activate CD8 T cells. The Th1 T cells are thought to express a membrane bound form of TNF, which when bound to a receptor on macrophages, promotes their activation. On the other hand, CD4 cells which produce Th2 cytokines are the helper T cells, which are essential for development of humoral immunity. Th2 T cells also express the CD40 ligand on their cell surface. Binding of this ligand to CD40 on B cells induces proliferation of Th2 T cells. The Th1 and Th2 cytokines appear to be mutually inhibitory and cross-regulatory. For example, IL-10 suppresses cytokine production by Th1 clones and IFN-γ inhibits proliferation of Th2 clones.[81]

VII. IMMUNE EFFECTOR MECHANISMS

As noted above, lymphocyte-mediated, specific immune responses can be grouped into three categories: humoral or antibody-mediated; T-cell-mediated cytotoxicity; and T-cell-driven, delayed hypersensitivity. These divisions are also useful classifications of host defense against microbial pathogens and malignant cells. A summary of the mechanisms and effector molecules important in these three types of immune defense is given in Table 6.

A. T and NK Cell-Mediated Cytotoxicity[82,83]

Cytotoxic T cells (CTL) are vital in host defense against viruses, certain types of intracellular or cytoplasmic bacteria, some protozoa, and malignant cells. Both the stimulation and effector phases of the CTL response are MHC restricted and require interaction with class I MHC molecules on target cell surfaces. Once activated, CTL destroy target cells by inducing them to undergo apoptosis. In this process, CTL bind to the target cells through the interaction of the TCR with class I MHC and through other adhesion molecules. The CTL then release the contents of their secretory granules, including perforin, TNF-β (LT), and granzymes (serine proteases). Perforin molecules polymerize in the membrane of the target cell, forming a pore which is thought to act as a conduit for the other granule contents, while granzymes induce apoptosis when they contact the target cell surface.[83,84] CTL are also thought to express a membrane form of TNF, the *fas* ligand, which can interact with the *fas* on target cell membranes.[85] Activation of *fas* on target cells serves as a second mechanism for inducing apoptosis. Activated CTL are extremely effective and selective "killer" cells. Their specific interaction with infected cells is mediated by the TCR and MHC restriction. This specific binding to target cells ensures that the membrane interactions and the release of CTL granule components affect only the target cells, sparing uninfected neighboring cells.

NK cells may also exert cytotoxic activity by similar mechanisms to CTL. However, NK cells are not MHC restricted and do not possess a specific receptor like the TCR.[86] NK cells do appear to have receptors which allow recognition of some features of virally infected cells and tumor cells. Additionally, NK cells possess an Fc receptor for IgG (FcγRIII), which enables them to participate in antibody-dependent, cell-mediated cytotoxicity (ADCC). NK cells can be activated by cytokines, in particular IL-12 and TNF-α, and, once activated, can themselves produce significant amounts of IFN-γ. Through their cytotoxic activity and IFN-γ production, NK cells mediate potent cytotoxicity against virally infected cells and some tumor cells and, thus, serve as important accessory cells to T-cell-mediated cytotoxicity. NK defense is especially important in early stages of host defense, functioning in the period before specific CTL can be recruited and activated.

B. T-Cell-Mediated Delayed Hypersensitivity[75,87]

The delayed hypersensitivity response evoked by the inflammatory CD4 cells is a vital defense against intracellular pathogens, such as the mycobacteria, which can survive in the vesicles of macrophages. Activated CD4 inflammatory cells produce the Th1 pattern of cytokines, which both recruit and activate macrophages, causing them to become highly effective in killing intracellular organisms. The principal Th1 cytokines involved in macrophage recruitment are IL-3, GM-CSF, macrophage chemotactic factor (MCF), and migration inhibition factor (MIF). IFN-γ and the membrane form of TNF-α are the cytokines involved in macrophage activation. Upon activation, macrophages undergo a series of changes which enhance their antimicrobial activity. Notably, the production of nitric oxide and oxygen radicals, which are critical to the intracellular killing of microorganisms, is significantly enhanced. In addition to recruiting and activating macrophages, CD4 T cells can themselves exert limited cytotoxicity and may function to kill effete, infected macrophages or other target cells. The CD4 inflammatory cells also participate in the sequelae of delayed hypersensitivity reactions, e.g., the granuloma formation seen in chronic infections, e.g., tuberculosis.

C. B-Lymphocyte-Mediated Humoral Immunity[88]

Upon activation by antigens, B lymphocytes differentiate into plasma cells which secrete specific antibodies. While B lymphocytes and their plasma cell progeny are, therefore, the principal mediators of humoral immunity, their response is highly dependent upon and tightly regulated by the CD4 T cells, in particular, the Th2 cytokines.

There are four major mechanisms through which antibodies serve in host defense: neutralization of microbial toxins or microbial receptors; opsonization of microbes for phagocytosis; activation of complement; and arming of accessory cells through Fc receptors. Neutralization of bacterial toxins can occur by steric hindrance and/or through clearance by phagocytes and cells of the reticuloendothelial system. Specific antibodies against bacterial and viral receptors can effectively prevent adherence or entry of pathogens into target cells. Opsonization or antibody coating of microorganisms facilitates phagocytosis by cells with Fc receptors for IgG (FcγRI,II). Complement activation by antibody-coated microbes also promotes phagocytosis through complement receptors and can further result in bacterial lysis through the complement cascade. Finally, various accessory cells can be armed with specific antibodies through Fc receptors. Thus, NK cells participate in ADCC by way of their FcγRIII receptors and the FcγR and FcϵR on eosinophils may be important in defense against parasites. Tissue mast cells and circulating basophils possess high affinity receptors for IgE (FcϵRI). Arming of these cells with IgE antibodies is the first step in the release of their potent inflammatory mediators in protective local inflammation and, pathologically, in acute allergic reactions. A thorough discussion of the different immunoglobulin isotypes, their functions, measurement, and normal ranges is given in Chapter 3.

TABLE 6

Effector Mechanisms in Immune Responses

Cytotoxicity: Defense against Viruses and Tumor Cells

Lymphocytes	Effector Molecules	Functions
CD8+ CTL	Perforin	Pore formation in target cell membranes
	TNF-β (LT)	Induces apoptosis
	Granzymes	Serine proteases which participate in killing
	Fas ligand	Induces apoptosis
Accessory Cells		
NK cells	Similar to CTL	Similar to CTL

Delayed Hypersensitivity: Defense against Intracellular Pathogens

Lymphocytes	Effector Molecules	Functions
CD4+ Th1	GM-CSF, IL-3	Macrophage recruitment
	IFN-γ	Macrophage activation
	Membrane TNF	Macrophage activation
Accessory Cells	**Effector Molecules**	**Functions**
Macrophages	Nitric oxide, oxygen radicals	Intracellular killing of pathogens
	Antibacterial peptides	Bactericidal activity
	Lysosomal enzymes	Antibacterial activity, degradation

Humoral Immunity: Defense against Extracellular Pathogens

Lymphocytes	Effector Molecules	Functions
B cells → plasma cells	IgG	Opsonization; complement activation; neutralization; ADCC; transplacental transfer; diffusion into extravascular sites
	IgM	Complement activation; neutralization; agglutination
	IgA	Major Ig in mucosal secretions; neutralization; opsonization; complement activation
	IgE	Sensitization of mast cells; diffusion into extravascular sites

Accessory Cells	Effector Molecules	Functions
Macrophages	FcγRI-III	Phagocytosis; ADCC
Neutrophils	FcγRI-III	Phagocytosis
Eosinophils	FcγRI-III, Fcε RII	Anti-parasitic immunity; phagocytosis
Mast cells	Fcε RI	Sensitization for release of inflammatory mediators

VIII. REGULATION OF IMMUNE RESPONSES[81,89-92]

As with many other biologic systems, there are inherent regulatory mechanisms which prevent uncontrolled activation of the immune system. The importance of these self-regulatory mechanisms is evident when there is absence or dysfunction of control, as is believed to occur in some autoimmune syndromes. The following list briefly describes the major mechanisms of normal immunoregulation:

1. **Antigen concentration.** The continuing presence or decline of antigen is itself a major regulatory factor. Immune responses are evoked by the introduction of antigens and generally increase with continued antigenic exposure. Following the clearance of antigens, the immune response usually is down-regulated by various self-regulatory mechanisms.

2. **Idiotypic networks.** First proposed by Niels Jerne for control of antibody production, it is now thought that idiotypic networks regulate both humoral and cell-mediated immunity. The term "idiotype" refers to the unique portions of the antigen binding sites of antibodies or of lymphocyte receptors. In the network theory, the variable regions of antibodies or receptors can induce the formation of a second set of antibodies or cell receptors with specificity against the first set. The second set of receptors or antibodies are called anti-idiotypes, and they can suppress production of the original set. Subsequent anti-idiotypes can then be formed against the second set and, as the process continues with formation of additional anti-idiotypes, these interactions produce a regulatory network. Anti-idiotypic responses for antibodies have been demonstrated both experimentally and in certain immune disorders, while evidence for anti-receptor idiotypic responses have been shown only experimentally.

3. **T suppressor cells.** The function of antigen-specific T suppressor cells is controversial despite abundant experimental evidence that T cells, primarily from the CD8+ population, can suppress other B- and T-lymphocyte responses. To date, no clear mechanism for T cell suppressor activity has been established. Two basic mechanisms are currently considered possible. The first is that CD8 cells can suppress CD4 cells via cytokines that down-regulate the CD4 response. This mechanism would be similar to that for the cross-regulation of CD4 Th1 and Th2 cells and would likely involve similar cytokines. The second proposal is that CD4 cells could be directly eliminated by CD8 cytotoxic cells. Experimental evidence for both hypotheses has been obtained with animal models.

4. **Th1–Th2 regulation.** As has already been mentioned, an important regulation in the induction of immune responses is the selective activation of the helper or inflammatory CD4 T cells. Because certain of the cytokines produced by these CD4 subsets are mutually inhibitory, as the immune response progresses, one type of response generally predominates.

While many of the details and exact steps of immune regulation need better definition, it is likely with current molecular technology that full understanding of these mechanisms will be forthcoming. This knowledge may well initiate a new era in clinical immunology by providing the basis for improved immunotherapy, immunomodulation, and immunosuppression in allergic disorders, autoimmunity, and graft rejection.

REFERENCES

1. Paul, W.E., The immune system: An introduction, in *Fundamental Immunology*, 3rd ed., Paul, W.E., Ed., Raven Press, New York, 1993, 1.
2. Unanue, E.R., Overview of the immune system, in *Samter's Immunologic Diseases*, 5th ed., Vol. 1, Frank, M.M., Austen, K.F., Claman, H.N., and Unanue, E.R., Eds., Little, Brown, Boston, 1995, 3.
3. Janeway, C.A., Jr. and Travers, P., *Immunobiology: The Immune System in Health and Disease*, Current Biology/Garland Publishing, New York, 1994, chap.1.
4. Unanue, E.R., Macrophages, antigen-presenting cells, and the phenomena of antigen handling and presentation, in *Fundamental Immunology*, 3rd ed., Paul, W.E., Ed., Raven Press, New York, 1993, 111.
5. Ikuta, K., Uchida, N., Freidman, J., and Weissman, I.L., Lymphocyte development from stem cells, *Annu. Rev. Immunol.*, 10, 759, 1992.
6. Knight, S.C. and Stagg, A.J., Antigen presenting cell types, *Curr. Opin. Immunol.*, 5, 374, 1993.
7. Steinman, R.M. The dendritic cell and its role in immunogenicity, *Annu. Rev. Immunol.*, 9, 271, 1993.
8. Schlossman, S.F., Boumsell, L., Gilks, W., Harlan, J.M., Kishimoto, T., Morimoto, C., Ritz, J., Shaw, S., Siverstein, R.L., Springer, T.A. et al., CD antigens 1993, *Immunol. Today*, 15, 98, 1993.
9. Williams, A. F. and Barclay, A.N., The immunoglobulin superfamily — domains for cell surface recognition, *Annu. Rev. Immunol.*, 6, 381, 1988.
10. Davis, M.M. and Bjorkman, P.J., T-cell antigen receptor genes and T-cell recognition, *Nature*, 334, 395, 1988.
11. Haas, W., Pereira, P., and Tonegawa, S., Gamma/delta cells, *Annu. Rev. Immunol.*, 11, 637, 1993.
12. Bjorkman, P.J., Saper, M.A., Samraoui, B., Bennet, W.S., Strominger, J.L., and Wiley, D.C. Structure of the human class I histocompatibility antigen HLA-A2, *Nature*, 329, 506, 1987.
13. Brown, J.H., Jardetzy, T.S., Gorja, J.C., Stern, L.J., Urban, R.G., Strominger, J.L., and Wiley, D.C., The three-dimensional structure of the human class II histocompatibility antigen HLA-DR1, *Nature*, 364, 33, 1993.
14. Reth, M., Antigen receptors on B lymphocytes, *Annu. Rev. Immunol.*, 10, 97, 1992.
15. Janeway, C.A., Jr., The T-cell receptor as a multicomponent signaling machine: CD4/CD8 coreceptors and CD45 in T-cell activation, *Annu. Rev. Immunol.*, 10, 645, 1992.
16. Dustin, M.L. and Springer, T.A., The role of lymphocyte adhesion receptors in transient interactions and cell locomotion, *Annu. Rev. Immunol.*, 9, 27, 1993.
17. Hogg, N. and Landis, R.C., Adhesion molecules in cell interactions, *Curr. Opin. Immunol.*, 5, 383, 1993.

18. Bevilacqua, M., Butcher, E., Furie, B. et al., Selectins: a family of adhesion receptors, *Cell*, 67, 233, 1991.

19. Shimizu, Y., van Seventer, G., Horgan, K.J., and Shaw, S., Roles of adhesion molecules in T cell recognition: fundamental similarities between four integrins on resting human T cells (LFA-1, VLA-4, VLA-5, VLA-6) in expression, binding and costimulation, *Immunol. Rev.*, 114, 109, 1990.

20. Etzioni, A., Harlan, J.M., Pollack, S., Phillips, L.M., Gershoni-Baruch, R., and Paulson, J.C., Leukocyte adhesion deficiency (LAD) II: a new adhesion defect due to absence of sialyl Lewis X, the ligand for selectins, *Immunodeficiency*, 4, 307, 1993.

21. Arai, K., Lee, F., Miyajima, A., Miyatake, S., Arai, N., Yokota, T., Cytokines: coordinators of immune and inflammatory responses, *Annu. Rev. Biochem.*, 59, 783, 1990.

22. Oppenheim, J.J., Zachariae, C.O.C., Mukaida, N., and Matsushima, K., Properties of the novel proinflammatory supergene intercrine cytokine family, *Annu. Rev. Immunol.*, 9, 817, 1993.

23. Gerard, C. and Gerard, N.P., The pro-inflammatory seven transmembrane spanning receptors of the leukocyte, *Curr. Opin. Immunobiol.*, 6, 140, 1994.

24. Leonard, W.J., Noguchi, M., Russel, S.M., and McBride, O.W., The molecular basis of X-linked severe combined immunodeficiency: the role of the interleukin-2 receptor gamma chain as a common gamma chain, gamma c, *Immunol. Rev.*, 138, 61, 1994.

25. Tomlinson, S., Complement defense mechanisms, *Curr. Opin. Immunol.*, 5, 83, 1993.

26. Cooper, N.R., The classical complement pathway. Activation and regulation of the first complement component, *Adv. Immunol.*, 37, 151, 1985.

27. Frank, M.M. and Fries, L.F., The role of complement in inflammation and phagocytosis, *Immunol. Today*, 12, 322, 1991.

28. Esser, A.F., Big MAC attack: complement proteins cause leaky patches, *Immunol. Today*, 12, 316, 1991.

29. Ahearn, J.M. and Fearon, D.T., Structure and function of the complement receptors of CR1 (CD35) and CR2 (CD21), *Adv. Immunol.*, 46, 183, 1989.

30. Chan, A.C., Desai, D.M., and Weiss, A., The role of protein tyrosine kinases and protein tyrosine phosphatases in T cell antigen receptor signal transduction, *Annu. Rev. Immunol.*, 12, 555, 1994.

31. Pleiman, C.M., D'Ambrosio, D., and Cambier, J.C., The B-cell antigen receptor complex: structure and signal transduction., *Immunol. Today*, 15, 393, 1994.

32. Rao, A., NF-ATp: a transcription factor required for the coordinate induction of several cytokine genes, *Immunol. Today*, 15, 274, 1994.

33. Trowbridge, I.S. and Thomas, M.L., CD45: An emerging role as a protein tyrosine phosphatase required for lymphocyte activation and development, *Annu. Rev. Immunol.*, 12, 85, 1994.

34. Fraser, J.D., Irving, B.A., Crabtree, G.R., and Weiss, A., Regulation of interleukin-2 gene enhancer activity by the T cell accessory molecule CD28, *Science*, 251, 313, 1991.

35. Taniguchi, T., Cytokine signaling through nonreceptor protein tyrosine kinases, *Science*, 268, 251, 1995.

36. Clark, E.A. and Brugge, J.S., Integrins and signal transduction pathways: the road taken, *Science*, 268, 233, 1995.

37. Banchereau, J., Bazan, F., Blanchard, D., Brière, Galizzi, J.P., van Kooten, C., Liu, Y.J., Rousset, F., and Saeland, S., The CD40 antigen and its ligand, *Annu. Rev. Immunol.*, 12, 881, 1994.

38. D'Ambrosio, D., Hippen, K.L., Minskoff, S.A., Mellman, I., Pani, G., Siminovitch, K.A., and Cambier, J.C., Recruitment and activation of PTP1C in negative regulation of antigen receptor signaling by FcRIIB1, *Science*, 268, 293, 1995.

39. Blackwell, T.K. and Alt, F.W., Mechanism and developmental program of immunoglobulin gene rearrangement in mammals, *Annu. Rev. Genet.*, 23, 605, 1989.

40. Shatz, D.G., Oettinger, M.A., and Schlissel, M.S., V(D)J recombination: molecular biology and regulation, *Annu. Rev. Immunol.*, 10, 359, 1993.

41. Winoto, A. and Baltimore, D., Separate lineages of T cells expressing the αβ and γδ receptors, *Nature*, 338, 430, 1989.

42. Oettinger, M.A., Schatz, D.G., Gorka, C., and Baltimore, D., RAG-1 and RAG-2, adjacent genes that synergistically activate V(D)J recombination, *Science*, 248, 1517, 1990.

43. von Boehmer, H., Kisielow, P., Lishi, H., Scott, B., Borgulya, P., and Teh, H.S., The expression of CD4 and CD8 accessory molecules on mature T cells is not random but correlates with the specificity of the αβ receptor for antigen, *Immunol. Rev.*, 109, 143, 1989.

44. Goodnow, C.C., Crosbie, J., Adelstein, S., Lavoie, T.B., Smith-Gill, S.J., Brink, R.A., Pritchard-Briscoe, H., Wotherspoon, J.S., Loblay, R.H., Raphael, K., Trent, R.J., and Basten, A., A transgenic mouse model of immunological tolerance: absence of secretion and altered surface expression of immunoglobulin in self-reactive B lymphocytes, *Nature*, 334, 676, 1988.

45. von Boehmer, H., The developmental biology of T lymphocytes, *Annu. Rev. Immunol.*, 6, 309, 1993.

46. Becker, R.S. and Knight, K.L., Somatic diversification of immunoglobulin heavy-chain VDJ genes: evidence for somatic gene conversion in rabbits, *Cell*, 63, 987, 1990.

47. Sprent, J., Lo, D., Gao, E.K., and Ron, Y., T cell selection in the thymus, *Immunol. Rev.*, 10, 57, 1989.

48. Kappler, J.W., Roehm, N., and Marrack, P., T cell tolerance by clonal elimination in the thymus, *Cell*, 49, 273, 1987.

49. Ashton-Rickardt, P.G., Van Kaer, L., Schumacher, T.N.M., Ploegh, H.L., and Tonegawa, S., Peptide contributes to the specificity of positive selection of CD8[+] T cells in the thymus, *Cell*, 73, 1041, 1993.

50. Núñez, G., Merino, R., Grillot, D., and González-García, M., Bcl-2 and Bcl-x: regulatory switches for lymphoid death and survival, *Immunol. Today*, 15, 582, 1994.

51. Bjorkman, P.J. and Parham, P., Structure, function and diversity of class I major histocompatibility complex molecules, *Annu. Rev. Biochem.*, 59, 253, 1990.

52. Klein, J., Satta, Y., and O'hUigin, C., The molecular descent of the major histocompatibility complex, *Annu. Rev. Immunol.*, 11, 269, 1993.

53. Bodmer, J.G., Marsh, S.G.E., Albert, E.D., Bodmer, W.F., Dupont, B., Erlich, H.A., Mach, B. et al. Nomenclature for factors of the HLA system, 1994, *Tissue Antigens*, 44, 1, 1994.

54. Campbell, R.D. and Trowsdale, J., Map of the human MHC, *Immunol. Today*, 14, 349, 1993.

55. Schmidt, C.M. and Orr, H.T., Maternal/fetal interactions: the role of the MHC class I molecule HLA-G, *Crit. Rev. Immunol.*, 13, 207, 1993.

56. Zinkernagel, R.M. and Doherty, P., MHC-restricted cytotoxic T cells: studies on the biological role of polymorphic major transplantation antigens determining T cell restriction–specificity, function, and responsiveness, *Adv. Immunol.*, 27,51, 1979.

57. Fremont, D.H., Matsumura, M., Stura, E.A., Peterson, P.A., and Wilson, I., Crystal structures of two viral peptides in complex with murine MHC class I H-2k[b], *Science*, 257, 919, 1992.

58. Stern, L.J., Brown, J.H., Jardetsky, T.S., Gorga, J.C., Urban, R.G., Strominger, J.L., and Wiley, D.C., Crystal structure of the human class II MHC protein HLA-DR1 complexed with and influenza virus peptide, *Nature*, 368, 215, 1994.

59. Falk, K., Rotzsche, O., Stevanovic, S., Jung, G., and Rammensee, H.-G., Allele-specific motifs revealed by sequencing of self peptides eluted from MHC molecules, *Nature*, 351, 290, 1991.

60. Hunt, D.F., Henderson, R.A., Shabanowitz, J, Sakaguchi, K., Michel, H., Sevilir, N., Cox, A.L., Appella, E., and Engelhard, V.H., Characterization of peptides bound to the class I MHC molecule HLA-A2.1 by mass spectrometry, *Science*, 255, 1261, 1992.

61. Janeway, C.A., Jr., The T-cell receptor as a multicomponent signaling machine: CD4/CD8 coreceptors and CD45 in T-cell activation, *Annu. Rev. Immunol.*, 10, 645, 1992.

62. Brodsky, F.M. and Guagliardi, L.E., The cell biology of antigen processing and presentation, *Annu. Rev. Immunol.*, 9, 70, 1991.

63. Goldberg, A.L. and Rock, K.L., Proteolysis, proteasomes and antigen presentation, *Nature*, 348, 375, 1992.

64. Monaco, J.J., Genes in the MHC that may affect antigen processing, *Curr. Opinion Immunol.*, 4, 70, 1992.

65. Germain, R.N. and Margoulies, D.H.A., *Annu. Rev. Immunol.*, 11, 403, 1993.

66. Amigorena, S., Drake, J.R., Webster, P., and Mellman, I., Transient accumulation of new class II MHC molecules in a novel endocytic compartment in B lymphocytes, *Nature*, 12, 113, 1994.

67. Tulp, A., Verwoerd, D., Dobberstein, B., Ploegh, H.L., and Pieters, J., Isolation and characterization of the intracellular MHC class II compartment, *Nature*, 12, 120, 1994.

68. Parham, P., Chen, B.P., Clayberger, C., Ennis, P.D., Krensky, A.M., Lawlor, D.A., Littman, D.R., et al., Diversity of class I HLA molecules: functional and evolutionary interactions with T cells, *Cold Spring Harbor Symp. Quant. Biol.*, 54, 529, 1989.

69. Howard, J., Fast forward in the MHC, *Nature*, 357, 284, 1992.

70. Schwartz, R.H., Immune response (Ir) genes of the murine major histocompatibility complex, *Adv. Immunol.*, 38, 31, 1958.

71. Erlich, H.A. and Gyllensten, U.B., Shared epitopes among HLA class II alleles: gene conversion, common ancestry and balancing selection, *Immunol. Today*, 12, 411, 1991.

72. Hill, A.V., Elvin, J., Willis, A.C., Aidoo, M., Allsopp, C.E.M., Gotch, F.M., Gao, X.M. et al., Molecular analysis of the association of B53 and resistance to severe malaria, *Nature*, 360, 434, 1992.

73. Leffell, M.S., Steinberg, A.G., Bias, W.B., Machan, C.H., and Zachary, A.A., The distribution of HLA antigens and phenotypes among donors and patients in the UNOS Registry, *Transplantation*, 58, 1119, 1994.

74. Beatty, P. G., Mori, M., and Milford, E., Impact of racial genetic polymorphism upon the probability of finding an HLA-matched donor, *Transplantation*, 60, 778, 1995.

75. Dinarello, C.A., Role of interleukin-1 and tumor necrosis factor in systemic responses to infection and inflammation, in *Inflammation — Basic Principles and Clinical Correlates*, Gallin, J.I., Goldstein, I.M., and Synderman, R., Eds., Raven Press, New York, 1992, 211.

76. Miller, M.D. and Krangel, M.S., Biology and biochemistry of the chemokines: a family of chemotactic and inflammatory cytokines, *Crit. Rev. Immunol.*, 12, 30, 1992.

77. Bevilacqua, M.P., Endothelial leukocyte adhesion molecules, *Annu. Rev. Immunol.*, 11, 767, 1993.

78. Springer, T.A., Traffic signals for lymphocyte recirculation and leukocyte emigration: the multi-step paradigm, *Cell*, 76, 301, 1994.

79. Dustin, M.L. and Springer, T.A., T-cell receptor cross-linking transiently stimulates adhesiveness through LFA-1, *Nature*, 341, 619, 1989.

80. Mosmann, T.R. and Coffman, R.L., Th1 and Th2 cells: different patterns of lymphokine secretion lead to different functional properties, *Annu. Rev. Immunol.*, 11, 145, 1993.

81. Sher, A., Gazzinelli, R.T., Oswald, I.P., Clerici, M., Kullberg, M., Pearce, E.J., Berzofsky, J.A. et al., Role of T cell cytokines in the downregulation of immune responses in parasitic and retroviral infection, *Immunol. Rev.*, 127, 183, 1992.

82. Apasov, S., Redegeld, F., and Sitkovsky, M., Cell-mediated cytotoxicity: contact and secreted factors, *Curr. Opin. Immunol.*, 5, 404, 1993.

83. Podack, E.R., Hengartner, H., and Lichtenheld, M.G., A central role of perforin in cytolysis?, *Annu. Rev. Immunol.*, 9, 129, 1993.

84. Smyth, M.A. and Trapani, J.A., Granzymes: exogenous proteinases that induce target cell apoptosis, *Immunol. Today*, 16, 202, 1995.

85. Nagat, S. and Suda, T., Fas and Fas ligand: *lpr* and *gld* mutations, *Immunol. Today*, 16, 39, 1995.

86. Yokoyama, W.M. and Seaman, W.E., The Ly-49 and NKR-P1 gene families encoding lectin- like receptors on natural killer cells: the NK gene complex, *Annu. Rev. Immunol.*, 11, 613, 1993.

87. Paulnock, D.M., Macrophage activation by T cells, *Curr. Opin. Immunol.*, 4, 344, 1992.

88. MacLennan, I.C., Liu, Y.J., and Johnson, G.D., Maturation and dispersal of B cell clones during T cell-dependent antibody responses, *Immunol. Rev.*, 126, 143, 1992.

89. Dorf, M.E. and Benacerraf, B., Suppressor cells and immunoregulation, *Annu. Rev. Immunol.*, 2, 127, 1984.

90. Fridman, W.H., Regulation of B cell activation and antigen presentation by Fc receptors, *Curr. Opin. Immunol.*, 5, 355, 1993.

91. Perelson, A. S., Immune network theory, *Immunol. Rev.*, 110, 5, 1989.

92. Powrie, F. And Coffman, R.L., Cytokine regulation of T cell function: potential for therapeutic intervention, *Immunol. Today*, 14, 270, 1993.

Chapter 2

AN OVERVIEW OF THE IMMUNE SYSTEM: IMMUNOLOGICAL MECHANISMS IN IMMUNE DEFICIENCY AND AUTOIMMUNITY

Albert D. Donnenberg

CONTENTS

0-8493-0134-3/97/$0.00+$.50

I. INTRODUCTION

As described in Chapter 1, host defense and immunopathologic
disease can be viewed as two sides of the same coin. We live in a hostile
environment filled with microbial and parasitic agents programmed to
thrive without regard to our health. The same effector mechanisms that
allow us to successfully defend ourselves can also function to our
detriment when the boundaries between self and nonself become
blurred, inflammatory processes proceed without appropriate regulation, or key components of the immune system are eliminated or dis-
rupted. This introductory chapter will briefly treat these dual aspects
of the immune system and hopefully provide a context for the practical
information which is to follow in this text.

II. IMMUNODEFICIENCIES

Perhaps the most seemingly straightforward of the immunopathologic processes are states of immune deficiency. In these disorders, one
or more of the components of the immune system are absent or rendered ineffective as the result of heredity or disease. However, primary
immune deficiencies are relatively rare. Decades before the present
epidemic of acquired immune deficiency syndrome, it was noted that
"despite the fascinating theoretic implications of the primary immunologic deficiency diseases…, the secondary immunologic deficiency syndromes are encountered much more frequently in clinical practice."[1]
This is true even more so today. Nevertheless, the primary immunodeficiencies, as "experiments of nature," have helped define the role of
individual components of the immune system by revealing unique

---

* The author is indebted to Dr. Timothy Wright, Chief of Rheumatology, Department of
Medicine, University of Pittsburgh School of Medicine, for the material in the section on
scleroderma.

pathologic consequences associated with the absence or dysfunction of particular components of the immune system. Practical aspects concerning the diagnosis of several such disorders will be treated in subsequent chapters, including deficiencies in complement components, adhesion molecules, and immunoglobulin synthesis. Recently, the ability to experimentally *knock out* particular genes encoding immunologically important products has made it possible to create murine models of specific immune deficiencies.[2] Many of these controlled experiments have revealed a remarkable robustness of the immune system. Through redundancy and compensatory mechanisms, the host is often able to offset, at least in part, the deletion of demonstrably important gene products in response to challenge with experimental pathogens.[3] Thus, in man, clinically significant immune deficiencies can be viewed as critical lesions of the immune system: alterations of genes, or depletion of cells, which have far-reaching consequences often affecting multiple arms of the immune system. Several excellent reviews have recently been published which discuss the causes and consequences of primary immunodeficiency diseases.[4-6] Some of the major disorders, which have recently been elucidated at the molecular level, are examined here.

A. X-Linked or Bruton Type Agammaglobulinemia

X-Linked or Bruton type agammaglobulinemia (XLA) is a hereditary pure B-cell deficiency disease affecting male children. The defect has been localized to mutations of a single gene, *btk* (Bruton thymidine kinase), localized on the long arm of the X chromosome, which appears to be essential for maturation of early B, but not T lymphocytes.[7] Pre-B cells are present in the bone marrow, albeit in reduced number and with reduced mitotic indices. Mature B cells are virtually absent from the bone marrow, lymphoid tissue, and peripheral blood, indicating a failure of B lymphopoiesis. In the phenotypically normal maternal carrier, X-chromosome inactivation, which is random in non-B cells, excludes B cells with the defective allele. Thus, pre-B cells with defective *btk* are not viable in the maternal carrier either. The disease manifests itself in the first year of life, after maternal immunoglobulin has waned. Since T-cell immunity and granulocyte and monocyte function are unaffected by the *btk* mutation, the disease manifestations virtually define the roles of B cells in protective immunity. Affected children are susceptible to recurrent pyogenic infections, persistent enterovirus infection, giardia enteritis, and mycoplasma arthritis. Cases of live-vaccine associated poliomyelitis have also been reported. Prophylactic treatment with intravenous immunoglobulin ameliorates the pan-immunoglobulin deficiency resulting from this disorder and has become standard therapy.

B. Hyper-IGM Syndrome

Hyper-IgM syndrome, like XLA, also maps to a defect on the X-chromosome in the majority of cases, although autosomal and acquired disorders with similar clinical manifestations have also been reported. As the name implies, it is characterized by elevated (or sometimes high normal) IgM levels with little or no IgG, IgA, or IgE. IgD levels are also elevated. Lymphocyte numbers (B cell and T cell) are usually within normal limits, although germinal centers are strikingly absent in lymphoid tissue. As discussed in Chapter 5, immunoglobulin class switching occurs sequentially in the course of a normal B-cell response. B cells bearing the early immunoglobulins IgM and IgD can "switch" heavy chains without changing the antigen specificity of their receptors. The switch to IgG isotypes, IgA or IgE, changes the biological properties of the secreted antibodies. Early studies showed that patient B cells could be induced to undergo class switch *in vivo*, when cocultured with constitutively activated Sézary syndrome T cells.[8] The conclusion of these investigators that the defect may lie in T rather than B lymphocytes proved to be well founded when, several years later, the defect was found to reside in the gene encoding CD40 ligand (CD40L).[9] CD40L is a T-cell activation marker which is transiently expressed during the early phases of T-cell activation. The interaction of CD40 and CD40L, expressed on B cells and activated T cells, respectively, has been shown to be one of the major contact-dependent interactions between these two lymphocyte populations, and one of the major mediators of T-cell-dependent B-cell activation.[10] The finding that deletions or mutations of the CD40L gene were responsible for the hyper-IgM syndrome confirmed the pivotal role of the gene product in B-cell maturation and germinal center development. The spectrum of diseases associated with this disorder emphasizes the role of B cells (and their ability to class switch) in combating pyogenic infections. The prevalence of antibody-mediated autoimmune disorders (hemolytic anemia, thrombocytopenia, recurrent neutropenia), as well as increased susceptibility to opportunistic agents that are usually associated with T cell deficiencies (*Pneumocystis carinii*), points to other important consequences of CD40L deficiency.

C. Wiskott-Aldrich Syndrome

Wiskott-Aldrich syndrome (WAS) is also inherited as an X-linked recessive trait. Although the defective gene has been identified,[11] the function of the protein encoded by this gene, termed Wiskott-Aldrich protein (WASP) has not yet been determined. In addition to an immunodeficiency characterized by progressively increasing B-cell numbers, decreasing T cells, compromised T-cell function, immunoglobulin abnormalities, and poor antibody responses, affected children have a pathognomonic, profound platelet deficiency with atypically small platelets. Interestingly, a severe X-linked platelet deficiency with small platelets but without immunodeficiency has recently been traced to different mutations in the same gene.[12] In keeping with the notion that WASP exerts an important effect on multiple hematopoietic lineages, only T cells, B cells, monocytes, and granulocytes expressing the normal X chromosome survive in heterozygous maternal carriers. WAS patients respond to aggressive management which includes splenectomy, antibiotics, and immunoglobulin therapy, but usually die in the second or third decade of life from infections, bleeding, or cancer. HLA-matched sibling bone marrow transplantation, when feasible, is considered the treatment of choice and can be curative.[13]

D. Common Variable Immunodeficiency

"Common variable immunodeficiency" (CVID) is used to describe the most common but variably expressed of the immunoglobulin deficiency disorders. Since the diagnosis is made by ruling out other known causes of hypogammaglobulinemia, it probably encompasses a variety of etiologically distinct entities. Despite its status as the most common primary immune deficiency, it is still a relatively rare disease with an estimated incidence between 1:50,000 to 1:200,000.[6] CVID usually presents in the second or third decade of life, affecting males and females equally. The extent of the immunoglobulin defect is variable, with IgG and IgA deficits common. Blunted cell mediated immunity may also accompany this syndrome, as evidenced by depressed delayed-type hypersensitivity (as measured by skin test) or *in vitro* responsiveness to recall antigens or mitogens. Since there has been no convincing demonstration of an inherent B cell defect, the "common thread" of this disorder may well be a signaling defect (or a family of defects) affecting helper T cells. Although CD4+ T cells from affected individuals are often hyporesponsive to antigens and mitogens, they proliferate and produce cytokines in response to phorbol esters plus ionomycin (stimuli which bypass receptor mediated signal transduction by directly activating protein kinase c and increasing intracellular calcium levels). Peripheral T-cell and B-cell counts, as determined by flow cytometry, are likewise variable in CVID and may range from hypo- to hypercellular.

In the case shown in Figure 1, the patient presented with high numbers of phenotypically normal B cells, and an increase in CD4+ and CD8+ T cells, but a virtual absence of resting naive CD4+/CD45RA+

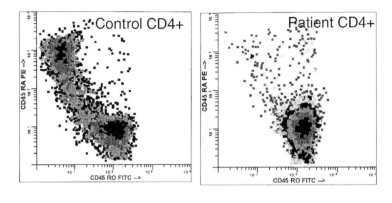

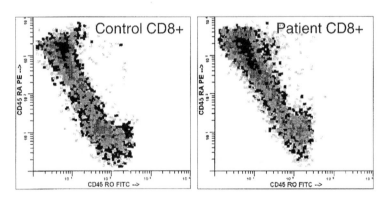

Figure 1

Expression of CD45 isoforms on T cells from a healthy control subject and a patient with common variable hypogammaglobulinemia. Three-color flow cytometry (described in detail in Chapter 11 on flow cytometry) was used to examine CD45 expression on CD4+ T cells and CD8+ T cells. In the control subject, T cells (CD4+ and CD8+) can be divided into two major populations (CD45RO+/CD45RA- and CD45RO-/CD45+). The diagonal between these two clusters probably represents cells undergoing switching between these isoforms. Note that the patient has normal representation of both CD45 isoforms among CD8+ T cells, but lacks a CD45RO-/CD45RA+ population among his CD4+ T cells. The absence of this population, which represents mature naive helper T cells, may play a significant role in the manifestations of his immune deficiency.

T cells. The vast majority of CD4+ cells were CD45RO+ (usually associated with memory T cells) and CD38+ (usually associated with activated T cells), but were completely negative for CD25 (IL-2 receptor), a marker constitutively expressed at low levels on resting memory cells and up-regulated during antigen-driven activation. These CD4+ T cells also uniformly expressed high levels of CD95 (fas or APO-1). In short-term, unstimulated culture (24 h), more than 80% of these cells underwent

apoptosis. Peripheral blood mononuclear cells from this patient prolif-
erated in response to the super-antigen staphylococcus enterotoxin B
(SEB) and to the phorbol ester TPA (in combination with the calcium
ionophore ionomycin), but not to the recall antigen tetanus toxoid, as
measured by a thymidine uptake assay. It has been suggested that the
constellation of activation and "memory" markers seen in this patient
(which also predominates in bone marrow transplant recipients early
after transplant and in HIV-1–infected subjects late in disease) may
represent a stage of T-cell maturation preceding that of the stable naive
T cell. Such pre-naive T cells may become prominent in the peripheral
circulation in conditions where T-cell half-life is short and lymphopoiesis and apoptosis are prominent.[14] Such cells have not been selected by
antigen and are therefore not competent to provide antigen specific
B-cell help. If this interpretation is correct, it may in part, explain why
B cells fail to undergo class switch in the presence of an abundance of
"activated" CD4[+] T cells.

E. Severe Combined Immunodeficiency

Severe combined immunodeficiency (SCID) is an X-linked disorder
in the majority of cases (60%). Lymphocyte counts are characteristically
low (<1000 cells/μl) with a complete absence of T lymphocytes. NK
cells can be normal or elevated; B cells, when present, are not functional. Unlike the conditions discussed above, SCID is rapidly fatal and
requires early intervention in the form of bone marrow transplantation,
which, when successful, is corrective.[15] Without therapy, affected
infants quickly succumb to opportunistic fungal or viral infection. The
discovery that the gamma chain of the IL-2 receptor (IL-2Rγ) mapped
to Xq13 made it an attractive candidate for the XSCID gene, a hypothesis that was subsequently confirmed.[16] That the mutation of a single
chain of a cytokine receptor gene could result in such far-reaching and
catastrophic consequences was explained when IL-2Rγ was found to
be a common subunit of receptors for IL-4, IL-7, IL-9, IL-13, and IL-15.
The heterodimerization of this protein with the IL-2β chain is required
for IL-2–mediated signal transduction. This relationship may also hold
for the other cytokine receptors. The presence of the XSCID mutation
is lethal to T cells; in the maternal carrier, only T cells with the normal
X chromosome survive. The other major cause of the SCID syndrome
is transmitted as an autosomal recessive trait and results from an
entirely different mechanism: mutations in the genes encoding adenos-
ine deaminase or purine nucleoside phosphorylase. In both T and
B lymphocytes, these enzymes are essential for clearance of otherwise
toxic purine metabolites.

F. MHC Expression Defects

MHC expression defects constitute a class of primary immune deficiencies also known as the "bare lymphocyte syndrome." MHC class I molecules are expressed by somatic cells and provide an avenue for presentation of intrinsic antigens (e.g., intracellular viral proteins expressed in infected cells). Intracellular proteins are degraded into peptides, captured by MHC class I and "displayed" on the cell surface, where antigenic peptides can be recognized by CD8+ T cells. MHC class II is predominantly expressed on specialized antigen presenting cells (APC) which can process extrinsic and intrinsic antigens and display peptide fragments for the benefit of CD4+ T cells. Deficiencies have been documented in both MHC classes. Both lead to immune deficiency states that are inherited as autosomal recessive traits. MHC class II deficiency is not due to a defect in the genes encoding the MHC class II molecules. Rather, it has been traced to an MHC class II-specific transcription activator which is postulated to serve as an "on-off" switch for other downstream interactors which limit the transcription of these genes.[17] Affected individuals suffer a severe combined immunodeficiency and have greatly reduced numbers of circulating CD4+ T cells. Like MHC class II deficiency, MHC class I deficiency does not result from a defect in the genes encoding the MHC class I proteins (α chain and β_2-microglobulin), but from a mutation in the gene encoding one of two transporter proteins associated with antigen processing (TAP) and MHC class I assembly.[18] A mutation in TAP2, which normally forms a heterodimer with TAP1, prevents transport of cytoplasmic peptide fragments across the Golgi where they are required for the assembly of the MHC class I heterodimer. In the absence of peptide fragment bound in the cleft of the α chain (see Chapter 1), MHC class I molecules are unstable and are only weakly expressed on the cell surface. Individuals affected by MHC class I deficiency have reduced numbers of CD8+ T cells and suffer from recurrent infections.

G. T-Cell Activation Deficiencies

T-Cell activation deficiencies represent a new class of immune deficiencies. Cases have recently been described in which immune impairments have been explained by defects in early or later events in T-cell activation. Examples of the former include apparent defects in ZAP-70 tyrosine kinase activity or calcium influx.[19] Deficiencies in cytokine gene transcription[20] represent the latter.

III. AUTOIMMUNITY

A. Autoimmunity and Tolerance

The term **autoimmunity** emphasizes the notion that the same mechanisms which protect us from potential pathogens can also cause disease when turned against *self*. Almost a century ago, Ehrlich coined the term **horror autotoxicus** to describe the immune system's natural aversion to such responses.[21] In the intervening decades, we have learned that the immune system is programmed to discriminate between **self** and **nonself** by selective expansion, deletion, or inactivation of T cells bearing receptors that are literally generated at random by recombination of the genes encoding the antigen receptor (see Chapter 1). Yet, even in healthy individuals, the barrier against anti-self response is not absolute. Autoantibodies can be demonstrated in the absence of disease, and normal T cells can respond against potential autoantigens such as topoisomerase I (discussed below).

These problems and others are pointed out by Fuchs in Matzinger's article which emphasizes the role of **danger** signals (tissue destruction, disruption of normal architecture, and activation of innate antigen nonspecific immune mechanisms) as the first line instigators of adaptive immunity.[22] The thesis that "tolerance or activation to a peripheral antigen is not determined by the self or nonself origin of the antigen but rather by the conditions under which it is introduced"[23] has precedent in the ideas of Bretscher, Schwartz, and others who recognized that antigen dose[24] and mode of presentation[25] could make the difference between an immunogenic and tolerogenic encounter. Matzinger expands on this notion, emphasizing the importance of the **second signal** provided by professional APC (the first signal being engagement of the antigen receptor on the T or B cell) in the initiation of primary immune responses. She argues that the most important determining factors may relate more to the conditions under which T and B lymphocytes receive or fail to receive permission to respond to antigen than to their idiotypic specificities. The vast majority of self tissues with which lymphocytes regularly come into contact are intrinsically invisible to newly generated CD4+ T cells because they (normally) lack MHC class II expression. They are tolerogenic to CD8+ T cells because, despite the presence of MHC class I on their surface, they display potentially antigenic peptides in the absence of **second signal**. APC themselves normally go unrecognized, since their own MHC-antigen profile (MAP) drives clonal deletion of autoreactive T cells in the thymus. Here, the APC's MAP consists of both intrinsic peptides and extrinsic peptides scavenged from the environment. According to this hypothesis,

TABLE 1

Alteration of the MHC/Antigen Profile of APCs by Display of *Cryptic Self*

Stimulus	Response: Consequences
Cellular stress	Differences in intracellular peptides including heat shock proteins (hsp): facilitated binding of self peptides to MHC by hsp.
Activation of APC	Increased MHC class II: increased concentration of normally subimmunogenic self peptides. Increased expression of adhesion molecules (ICAM, LFA-1): reduced threshold for T cell response. Change in protease profile: altered peptide spectrum.
Viral infection of APC	Expression of viral and viral induced cellular proteins; down-regulation of other host proteins: shift in peptides competing for MHC binding; activation of APC.

Adapted from Lehman, P.V. et al., *Immunol. Today,* 14(5), 203, 1993.

the only way in which a primary response can be initiated is when a newly generated mature T cell (a *virgin* T cell) encounters an APC-displaying cognate peptide that is not normally part of its MAP. How then is autoimmunity initiated and maintained in such a well-ordered system? Matzinger and Fuchs postulate that "autoimmunity may not be a defect in the immune response, but in the expression of antigen, either in its concentration, location or the way in which it is presented."[22]

Lehmann et al. have emphasized the importance of presentation of previously cryptic self-antigens as the initial event inciting autoimmune response.[26] According to their interpretation, autoimmunity does not represent the loss of self tolerance, but rather the initiation of responses to self antigens to which the host was never tolerant (immunologic ignorance, discussed below). They hypothesize that a nascent autoimmune response to **cryptic self**, although initially very restricted in the repertoire of responding T cells, could propagate to cells that recognize other epitopes on the nominal autoantigen, or to other self molecules, by a chain of events which they have called **determinant spreading**. They picture clinically apparent autoimmune disease as a vicious cycle of cytokine-driven up-regulation of previously cryptic autoantigen presentation, leading to ongoing T-cell stimulation, further T-cell recruitment, determinant spreading, and greater cytokine production. This process of diversification may obscure the identity of the original inciting antigen, which may have been cryptic self, cross-reactive nonself (molecular mimicry), or perhaps an entirely foreign determinant. Table 1 illustrates a variety of ways in which external factors may alter presentation of previously cryptic self determinants such that they are presented in an immunogenic manner.

B. Immune Response to Topoisomerase I in Systemic Sclerosis

Systemic sclerosis (SSc) or scleroderma is a systemic autoimmune disease in which important target antigens have been identified and T- and B-cell responses to a potential autoantigen, topoisomerase I (topo I) have been well studied in both healthy and affected individuals. For the purposes of this introductory chapter, SSc serves as an illustration of the principles discussed above. SSc is an idiopathic disorder of connective tissue characterized by increased production and deposition of collagen in the skin and internal organs such as the lungs, gastrointestinal tract and kidneys. The prevalence of SSc in the U.S. is estimated to be 0.5/1000,[27] which is similar to the estimates for many other autoimmune diseases including multiple sclerosis, type I diabetes mellitus, and systemic lupus erythematosus. It is a disease that affects women approximately three times more frequently than men (the female to male ratio is as high as 15:1 in childbearing years), and its incidence increases with age.[27]

1. Tissue Inflammation in SSc

At the level of gene expression in the affected tissue, SSc pathogenesis is characterized by increased production and deposition of collagen which results, at least in part, from increased transcription rates of procollagen type I, III, and VI genes and increased accumulation of the collagen mRNAs by dermal fibroblasts.[28] The regulation of other genes is also altered in SSc. For example, SSc dermal fibroblasts overexpress interleukin-6 (IL-6), a cytokine with known pro-inflammatory properties.[29] In addition, IL-1 receptor (IL-1R) numbers are increased on the surface of SSc fibroblasts and IL-1R mRNA levels are also elevated.[30] Mononuclear cells have been shown to infiltrate scleroderma skin[31,32] and to elaborate a variety of cytokines to which fibroblasts are responsive. Thus the pathogenesis of SSc is believed to be driven by an active immune process involving the activation of resident and infiltrating cells including macrophages, T lymphocytes, and mast cells. The importance of the interaction between the mononuclear cells, fibroblasts, and other cells found in the lesions is further supported by the findings that ICAM-1 expression is elevated on a subpopulation of fibroblasts in SSc lesions,[33,34] while β1 and β2 integrin expression is increased on the surface of the infiltrating mononuclear leukocytes.[35] Intralesional activated endothelial cells display increased surface expression of ELAM-1 and ICAM-1,[35] which may facilitate trafficking of leukocytes across the endothelium. Although the factors responsible for initiating this process have not been identified, epidemiologic studies point to the effects of a variety of environmental insults and certain drugs in individuals rendered susceptible, at least in part, by the ability of their MHC determinants to present autoantigen.

2. T and B Cell Responses to Topo I

Although the target antigen(s) of the T cells in the dermis of SSc skin is as yet unknown, there is considerable evidence that the immune response is directed at a systemic level toward specific autoantigens. This evidence is provided by analysis of patient sera for the presence of antinuclear antibodies (ANAs), a major immunopathological feature of SSc found in the sera of more than 90% of SSc patients.[36] The antigens to which these autoantibodies bind include DNA topoisomerase I; centromere/kinetochore; RNA polymerases I, II, and III; U3 ribonucleoprotein; and Th ribonucleoprotein.[37-39] Particular ANA specificities are highly associated with clinical subsets of SSc. Anti-topo I is associated with diffuse cutaneous involvement and high frequencies of pulmonary interstitial fibrosis and peripheral vascular disease,[38,39] anticentromere antibody with limited cutaneous involvement,[38] and anti-RNA polymerase antibodies with diffuse cutaneous, as well as heart and kidney involvement.[37,39] These clinical associations provide evidence that the production of SSc-specific ANAs may be causally linked to the pathogenesis of this disease. The association of anti-topo I with diffuse skin involvement is likely to represent an integral part of the disease process, since this autoantibody is found only in SSc sera and not in the sera of patients with other autoimmune diseases. While there is controversy over the pathogenicity of antibodies directed towards intracellular antigens, the T cells driving autoantibody production have the potential for direct involvement in the inflammatory process leading to tissue fibrosis. As such, autoantibodies serve as markers for the autoantigen-specific T cells that are activated in this disease. Wright et al. have reported that production of anti-topo I antibody is dependent on antigen-dependent activation of T cells and reciprocal T–B interactions similar to those involved in response to foreign antigen.[40] Their data also indicate that T cells from both SSc patients and normal individuals with certain MHC class II alleles (see below) are capable of responding to the topo I *in vitro*. However, T cells from SSc patients proliferate with accelerated kinetics consistent with recent or ongoing antigen exposure *in vivo*.[41]

3. Immunogenetic Associations of Anti-Topo I Responses

There are several reports describing immunogenetic associations with autoantibody production in SSc patients. Reveille et al.[42] showed that the broad specificity HLA-DQ3 (DQB1*0301, *0302, and *0303) was most strongly associated with the anti-topo I response in Caucasian and American Black SSc patients, and the remaining DQ3-negative patients had DQB1*0601, *0602, *0604, or *0402. They concluded that a tyrosine at position 30 and the amino acid sequence Thr, Arg, Ala, Glu, Leu, Asp, and Thr comprising positions 71 to 77 in the DQB1 β1 domain were associated with the anti-topo I response. Morel et al.[43] reported that 87% of SSc patients with anti-topo I had DR11-related alleles. In particular, DRB1*1104 was most strongly associated with the presence of anti-topo I antibody. Recently, Kuwana et al.[44] found that the DRB1*1502-DRB5*0102-DQB1*0601 haplotype was detected in 75% of Japanese SSc patients with anti-topo I and that this frequency was significantly increased compared to SSc patients without anti-topo I and race-matched healthy controls. It was also noted that all anti-topo I-positive SSc patients had either the DQB1*0601 or *0301 allele, which share a tyrosine residue at position 26 in the second hypervariable region in the β1 domain of the DQ molecule, as opposed to a glycine or a leucine in the other known DQB1 alleles. From these results, it is likely that both HLA-DR and DQ genes, not a single HLA-DR or DQ allele, regulate the autoimmune response to topo I by controlling the binding of the MHC class II molecule with the processed topo I peptide(s).

4. Tolerance and Anti-Topo I Responses

Since the antigens recognized by SSc T cells and autoantibodies are endogenous, the development of an immune response must involve either a breach of self-tolerance or, alternatively, the immunogenic presentation of peptides that previously escaped detection of the immune system as a tolerogen. As discussed above, there are several possible mechanisms for such responses. First, an immunogenic foreign protein resembling the autoantigen may result in a breach of self-tolerance by molecular mimicry. This protein may be a component of a microbial pathogen and could be present only at the onset of the autoimmune response. In support of this mechanism, Mamula et al.[45] recently demonstrated that immunization of mice with a mixture of human and murine small nuclear ribonucleoproteins (snRNP, an autoantigen implicated in systemic lupus erythematosis) resulted in the development of autoreactive T cells and autoantibodies specific for murine snRNP. Murine snRNPs alone were not immunogenic. A second potential mechanism predisposing to the development of autoantibody responses may result from the limited tissue distribution or rapid degradation of the potential antigen, precluding inclusion in the APC's MAP (described above) and resulting in a lack of negative selection. Thus, the host is **immunologically ignorant** of the antigen, rather than immunologically tolerant. In this regard, Wright and others have found that topo I, a major autoantigen in SSc, is highly susceptible to proteolytic degradation[41,46,47] and thus may not normally be available to act as a tolerogen. A third related pathway is the altered expression or processing of the target proteins, which may occur by several mechanisms. In systemic lupus erythematosis (SLE) there is increased expression and release of SLE-associated autoantigens from cells undergoing apoptosis. In an experimental model of viral infection and autoimmune disease, autoantigens and viral antigens were shown to co-localize in apoptotic blebs which are released from dying cells. This may present viral and host determinants in a new and potentially immunogenic context.[48] Alteration of posttranslational modifications such as phosphorylation, oxidation, hapten modification, or complex formation could affect the immunogenicity of self proteins by altering their resistance to proteolysis. For example, autoreactive T cells and autoantibodies specific for the tumor suppressor protein p53 were found in mice immunized with purified murine p53 complexed with the SV40 large T antigen.[49] In addition, the exposure and immune recognition of previously cryptic antigenic determinants could occur as a consequence of inflammation, such as has been proposed for the interphotoreceptor retinoid binding protein, an autoantigen implicated in certain types of ocular autoimmune disease.[50]

C. Animal Models of Autoimmunity

Like the immunodeficiency diseases discussed above, animal models of autoimmunity and genetic tools such as the creation of transgenic strains, have permitted dissection of murine counterparts to human diseases such as SLE and insulin-dependent diabetes mellitus (IDS) at the molecular level. Unlike the immunodeficiency disorders, molecular explanations of these apparently polygenic human diseases are proving more difficult. For a more complete overview of the immunological and genetic components of autoimmune disease the reader is referred to several excellent review articles.[51-55]

REFERENCES

1. Shuster, J., in *Clinical Immunology*, Freeman, S.O., Ed., Harper and Row, New York, 1971, 342.
2. Sharpe, A.H., Analysis of lymphocyte costimulation *in vivo* using transgenic and 'knockout' mice [review], *Curr. Opin. Immunol.*, 7(3), 389, 1995.
3. Kaufmann, S.H. and Ladel, C.H., Application of knockout mice to the experimental analysis of infections with bacteria and protozoa [review], *Trends Microbiol.*, 2(7), 235, 1994.

4. Rosen, F.S., Cooper, M.D., and Wedgwood, R.J., The primary immunodeficiencies [review], *N. Engl. J. Med.*, 333(7), 431, 1995.

5. Belmont, J.W., Insights into lymphocyte development from X-linked immune deficiencies [review], *Trends Genetics*, 11(3), 112, 1995.

6. Rosen, F.C., chairman, World Health Organization scientific group, Primary immunodeficiency diseases. Report of a WHO Scientific Group [review], *Clin. Exp. Immunol.*, 99(Suppl. 1), 1, 1995.

7. Smith, C.I., Baskin, B., Humire-Greiff, P., Zhou, J.N., Olsson, P.G., Maniar, H.S., Kjellen, P., Lambris, J.D., Christensson, B., Hammarstrom, L. et al., Expression of Bruton's agammaglobulinemia tyrosine kinase gene, BTK, is selectively down-regulated in T lymphocytes and plasma cells, *J. Immunol.*, 152(2), 557, 1994.

8. Mayer, L., Kwan, S.P., Thompson, C., Ko, H.S., Chiorazzi, N., Waldmann, T., and Rosen, F., Evidence for a defect in "switch" T cells in patients immunodeficiency and hyperimmunoglobulinemia M, *N. Engl. J. Med.*, 314(7), 409, 1986.

9. Ramesh, N., Morio, T., Fuleihan, R., Worm, M., Horner, A., Tsitsikov, E., Castigli, E., and Geha, R.S., CD40-CD40 ligand (CD40L) interactions and X-linked hyper IgM syndrome [review], *Clin. Immunol. Immunopathol.*, 76(3 Pt 2), S208, 1995.

10. Aversa, G., Punnonen, J., Carballido, J.M., Cocks, B.G., and de Vries, J.E., CD40 ligand-CD40 interaction in Ig isotype switching in mature and immature human B cells [review], *Semin. Immunol.*, 6(5), 295, 1994.

11. Derry, J.M., Ochs, H.D., and Francke, U., Isolation of a novel gene mutated in Wiskott-Aldrich syndrome, *Cell*, 78(4), 635, 1994.

12. Villa, A., Notarangelo, L., Macchi, P., Mantuano, E., Cavagni, G., Brugnoni, D., Strina, D., Patrosso, M.C., Ramenghi, U., Sacco, M.G. et al. X-linked thrombocytopenia and Wiskott-Aldrich syndrome are allelic diseases with mutations in the WASP gene, *Nature Genetics*, 9(4), 414, 1995.

13. Mullen, C.A., Anderson, K.D., and Blaese, R.M., Splenectomy and/or bone marrow transplantation in the management of the Wiskott-Aldrich syndrome: long-term follow-up of 62 cases *Blood*, 82(10), 29616, 1993.

14. Donnenberg, A.D., Margolick, J.B., and Donnenberg, V.S., Lymphopoiesis, apoptosis and immune amnesia, *Ann. N.Y. Acad. Sci.*, 770, 213, 1996.

15. O'Reilly, R.J., Keever, C.A., Small, T.N., and Brochstein, J., The use of HLA-non-identical T-cell-depleted marrow transplants for correction of severe combined immunodeficiency disease [review], *Immunodef. Rev.*, 1(4), 273, 1989.

16. Noguchi, M., Yi, H., Rosenblatt, H.M., Filipovich, A.H., Adelstein, S., Modi, W.S., McBride, O.W., and Leonard, W.J., Interleukin-2 receptor gamma chain mutation results in X-linked severe combined immunodeficiency in humans, *Cell*, 73(1), 147, 1993.

17. Zhou, H. and Glimcher, L.H., Human MHC class II gene transcription directed by the carboxyl terminus of CIITA, one of the defective genes in type II MHC combined immune deficiency, *Immunity*, 2(5), 545, 1995.

18. de la Salle, H., Hanau, D., Fricker, D., Urlacher, A., Kelly, A., Salamero, J., Powis, S.H., Donato, L., Bausinger, H., Laforet, M. et al., Homozygous human TAP peptide transporter mutation in HLA class I, *Science*, 265(5169), 237, 1994.

19. Le Deist, F., Hivroz, C., Partiseti, M., Rieux-Laucat, F., Debatin, K.M., Choquet, D., De Villartay, J.P., and Fischer, A., T-cell activation deficiencies [review], *Clin. Immunol. Immunopathol.*, 76(3), S163, 1995.

20. Castigli, E., Pahwa, R., Good, R.A., Geha, R.S., and Chatila, T.A. Molecular basis of a multiple lymphokine deficiency in a patient with severe combined immunodeficiency, *Proc. Nat. Acad. Sci. U.S.A.*, 90(10), 4728, 1993.

21. Ehrlich, P. and Morgenroth, J., On hemolysins, fifth communication, *Berl. Klin. Wochenschr.*, 1901, reprinted in *The Collected papers of Paul Ehrlich*, Pergamon Press, London, 1957, 246.

22. Matzinger, P., Tolerance, danger and the extended family, *Annu. Rev. Immunol.*, 12, 991, 1994.
23. Ridge, J.P., Fuchs, E.J., and Matzinger, P., Neonatal tolerance revisited: turning on newborn T cells with dendritic cells, *Science*, 271, 1723, 1996.
24. Bretscher, P. and Cohn, M., A theory of self-nonself discrimination, *Science*, 169(950), 1042, 1970.
25. Jenkins, M.K. and Schwartz, R.H., Antigen presentation by chemically modified splenocytes induces antigen-specific T cell unresponsiveness *in vitro* and *in vivo*, *J. Exp. Med.*, 165(2), 302, 1987.
26. Lehman, P.V., Sercarz, E.E., Forsthuber, T., Dayan, C.M., and Gammon, G., Determinant spreading and the dynamics of the autoimmune T cell repertoire, *Immunol. Today*, 14(5), 203, 1993.
27. Medsger, T.A., Jr., Epidemiology of systemic sclerosis, *Clin. Dermatolog.*, 12, 207, 1994.
28. Unemori, E.N. and Amento, E.P. Connective tissue metabolism including cytokines in scleroderma, *Curr. Opin. Rheumatol.*, 3, 953, 1991.
29. Feghali, C.A., Bost, K.L., Boulware, D.W., and Levy, L.S. Mechanisms of pathogenesis in scleroderma. I. Overproduction of interleukin 6 by fibroblasts cultured from affected skin sites of patients with scleroderma, *J. Rheumatol.*, 19, 1207, 1992.
30. Kawaguchi, Y., Harigai, M., Hara, M., Suzuki, K., Kawakami, M., Ishizuka, T., Hidaka, T., Kitani, A., Kawagoe, M., and Nakamura, H., Increased interleukin 1 receptor, type I, at messenger RNA and protein level in skin fibroblasts from patients with systemic sclerosis, *Biochem. Biophys. Res. Commun.*, 184, 1504, 1992.
31. Fleischmajer, R., Perlish, H.S., and Reeves, J.R.T., Cellular infiltrates in schleroderma skin, *Arthritis Rheum.*, 20, 975, 1977.
32. Ishikawa, O. and Ishikawa, H., Macrophage infiltration in the skin of patients with systemic sclerosis, *J. Rheumatol.*, 19, 1202, 1992.
33. Needleman, B., Increased expression of intercellular adhesion molecule 1 on the fibroblasts of scleroderma patients, *Arthritis Rheum.*, 33, 1847, 1990.
34. Abraham, D., Lupoli, S., McWhirter, A., Plater-Zyberk, C., Piela, T.H., Korn, J.H., Olsen, I. and Black, C., Expression and function of surface antigens on scleroderma fibroblasts, *Arthritis Rheum.*, 34, 1164, 1991.
35. Sollberg, S., Peltonen, J., Uitto, J., and Jimenez, S.A., Elevated expression of b1 and b2 integrins, intercellular adhesion molecule 1, and endothelial leukocyte adhesion molecule, in the skin of patients with systemic scloerosis of recent onset, *Arthritis Rheum.*, 35, 290, 1992.
36. Silman, A.J., Epidemiology of scleroderma, *Ann. Rheum. Dis.*, 50, 846, 1991.
37. Okano, Y., Steen, V.D., and Medsger, T.A., Jr., Autoantibody reactive with RNA polymerase III in systemic sclerosis, *Ann. Int. Med.*, 119, 1005, 1993.
38. Steen, V.D., Powell, D.L., and Medsger, T.A., Jr., Clinical correlations and prognosis based on serum autoantibodies in patients with systemic sclerosis, *Arthritis Rheum.*, 31, 196, 1988.
39. Kuwana, M., Okano, Y., Kaburaki, J., Tojo,T., and Homma, M., Clinical and prognostic associations based on serum antinuclear antibodies in Japanese patients with systemic sclerosis, *Arthritis Rheum.*, 37, 75, 1994.
40. Kuwana, M., Medsger, T.A., and Wright, T.M., T-B cell collaboration is essential for the autoantibody response to DNA topoisomerase I in systemic sclerosis, *J. Immunol.*, 155, 2703, 1995.
41. Kuwana, M., Medsger, T.A., and Wright, T.M., T cell proliferative response induced by DNA topoisomerase I in patients with systemic sclerosis and healthy donors, *J. Clin. Invest.*, 96, 586, 1995.

42. Reveille, J.D., Durban, E., MacLeod-St. Clair, M.J., Goldstein, R., Moreda, R., Altman, R.D., and Arnett, F.C., Association of amino acid sequences in the HLA-DQB 1 first domain with antitopoisomerase I autoantibody response in scleroderma (progressive systemic sclerosis), *J. Clin. Invest.*, 90, 973, 1992.

43. Morel, P.A., Chang, H., Tweardy, D.J., and Medsger, T.A., Jr., Systemic sclerosis with diffuse scleroderma is associated with DRB1*1104, *Arthritis Rheum.*, 34, S137, 1991.

44. Kuwana, M., Kaburaki, J., Okano, Y., Inoko, H., and Tsuji, K., The HLA-DR and DQ genes control the autoimmune response to DNA topoisomerase I in systemic sclerosis (scleroderma), *J. Clin. Invest.*, 92, 1296, 1993.

45. Mamula, M.J., Fatenejad, S., and Craft, J., B cells process and present lupus autoantigens that initiate autoimmune T cell responses, *J. Immunol.*, 152(3), 1453, 1994.

46. Kuwana, M., Medsger, T.A., and Wright, T.M., Detection of anti-DNA topoisomerase I antibody by an enzyme-linked immunosorbent assay using overlapping recombinant polypeptides, *Clin. Immunol. Immunopath.*, 76, 266, 1995.

47. Samuels, D.S. and Shimizu, N., The predominant form of mammalian DNA topoisomerase I *in vivo* has a molecular mass of 100 kDa, *Mol. Biol. Rep.*, 19, 99, 1994.

48. Rosen, A., Casciola-Rosen, L., and Ahearn, J., Novel packages of viral and self-antigens are generated during apoptosis, *J. Exp. Med.*, 181(4), 1557, 1995.

49. Dong, X., Hamilton, H.J., Satoh, M., Wang, J. and Reeves, W.H., Initiation of autoimmunity to the p53 tumor suppressor protein by complexes of p53 and SV40 large T antigen, *J. Exp. Med.*, 179, 1243, 1994.

50. Lipham, W.J., Redmond, T.M., Takahashi, H., Berzofsky, J.A., Wiggert, B., Chader, G.J. and Gery, I., Recognition of peptides that are immunopathogenic but cryptic. Mechanisms that allow lymphocytes sensitized against cryptic peptides to initiate pathogenic autoimmune processes, *J. Immunol.*, 146, 3757, 1991.

51. Theofilopoulos, A.N., The basis of autoimmunity. I. Mechanisms of aberrant self-recognition [review], *Immunol. Today*, 16(2), 90, 1995.

52. Theofilopoulos, A.N., The basis of autoimmunity. II. Genetic predisposition [review], *Immunol. Today*, 16(3), 150, 1995.

53. Tan, E.M. and Chan, E.K., Molecular biology of autoantigens and new insights into autoimmunity [review], *Clin. Invest.*, 71(4), 327, 1993.

54. Esch, T., Clark, L., Zhang, X.M., Goldman, S., and Heber-Katz, E., Observations, legends, and conjectures concerning restricted T-cell receptor usage and autoimmune disease [review], *Crit. Rev. Immunol.*, 11(5), 249, 1992.

55. Burek, C.L. and Rose, N.R., Autoimmune thyroid disease and the major histocompatibility complex, *Clin. Immunol. Newsl.*, 16(1-2), 21, 1996.

Chapter 3

HUMAN IMMUNOGLOBULINS

Robert G. Hamilton

CONTENTS

0-8493-0134-3/97/$0.00+$.50

I. INTRODUCTION

The human immunoglobulins are a family of proteins that confer humoral immunity and perform vital roles in promoting cellular immunity. Five distinct classes or **isotypes** of immunoglobulins (IgG, IgA, IgM, IgD, and IgE) have been identified in human serum on the basis of their structural, biological and antigenic differences.[1-4] IgG and IgA have been further subdivided into IgG1, IgG2, IgG3, and IgG4 or IgA1 and IgA2 on the basis of unique antigenic determinants.[5,6] Multiple **allotypic** determinants in the constant region domains of human IgG and IgA molecules as well as kappa light chains indicate inherited genetic markers. Finally, there are several immunoglobulin-associated polypeptides such as secretory component and J chain that have no structural homology with the immunoglobulins, but serve important functions in immunoglobulin polymerization and transport across membranes into a variety of secretions (e.g., saliva, sweat, nasal secretions, breast milk, and colostrum). This diversity of the immunoglobulin components of the humoral immune system provides a complex network of protective and surveillance functions.

From a clinical perspective, quantitative levels of these analytes in serum can aid in the diagnosis and management of immunodeficiency, abnormal protein metabolism, and malignant states (e.g., multiple myeloma). As such, they provide a differential diagnosis as to possible causes of recurrent infections and can indicate a strategy for subsequent therapeutic intervention. However, the reported target ranges of each immunoglobulin vary widely as a result of differences in the quantitation methods and reagents employed and populations studied. To date, no compendium of information is available that summarizes the levels of immunoglobulins in healthy pediatric and adult populations, in an attempt to provide a consensus for reference intervals upon which action levels can be based.

The goals of this chapter are threefold. First, primary structural and biological properties of human immunoglobulins will be overviewed to highlight their antigenic diversity, which is the basis upon which they are quantified. Second, the design and performance of the clinical laboratory methods that are used in the quantification of immunoglobulins will be discussed within the context of available commercial and research reagents and their performance in interlaboratory proficiency surveys. Finally, a reference compendium has been prepared which summarizes the ranges of the immunoglobulins in the serum, urine, and cerebral spinal fluid (CSF) of healthy populations, where possible as a function of age and sex and other demographic variables.

II. PROPERTIES OF HUMAN IMMUNOGLOBULINS

A. General Immunoglobulin Structural Properties

Immunoglobulins may be functionally defined as glycoproteins that possess the ability to bind to substances (antigens) which have elicited their formation. Tables 1 and 2 summarize many of the known physical and biological properties of the human immunoglobulin heavy and light chains, secretory component, J chain, and the five classes of intact immunoglobulins. As a group, the immunoglobulins are composed of 82 to 96% polypeptides and 4 to 18% carbohydrate, and they account for approximately 20% of all proteins in plasma.[3-5] When placed in porous agarose gels together with other serum proteins under current and selected ionic conditions, most immunoglobulins

TABLE 1

Human Immunoglobulin Chain Characteristics

Property Designation	Light Chains		Heavy Chains					Secretory Component SC	J Chain J
	Kappa	Lambda	Alpha	Delta	Epsilon	Gamma	Mu		
Associated isotypes	All	All	IgA	IgD	IgE	IgG	IgM	IgA	IgA-IgM
Subclasses or subtypes	—	1,2,3,4	1-2	—	—	1,2,3,4	1-2	—	—
Allotypes	Km(1)-(3)	—	A2m(1)-(2)	—	—	Gm(1)-(25)	—	—	—
Molecular weight (Da)[a]	23,000	23,000	55,000	62,000	70,000	50,000 60,000 = g3	70,000	70,000	15,000
V region subgroups	V_κI-IV	V_λI-VI	V_HI-IV	V_HI-IV	V_HI-IV	V_HI-IV	V_HI-IV	—	—
Carbohydrate ave %	0	0	8-10	18	18	3-4	12-15	16	8
No. of oligosaccharides	0	0	2-3	NA	5	1	5	NA	1

Note: NA = not available.

[a] Approximate molecular weights.

TABLE 2

Structural and Biological Properties of Human Immunoglobulins

	IgA1	IgA2	IgD	IgE	IgG1	IgG2	IgG3	IgG4	IgM
Heavy chain class	Alpha 1	Alpha 2	Delta	Epsilon	Gamma 1	Gamma 2	Gamma 3	Gamma 4	Mu
Light chain type	K and λ	K and λ	K and λ	K and λ	K and λ	K and λ	K and λ	K and λ	K and λ
Averaged Ig light chain K/λ ratio[12]	1.4	1.6			2.4	1.1	1.4	8.0	3.2
Molecular weight (Da) of secreted form[a]	160,000 m 300,000 d	160,000 m 350,000 d	180,000 m	190,000 m	150,000 m	150,000 m	160,000 m	150,000 m	950,000 p
H chain domain #	4	4	4	5	4	4	4	4	5
Hinge (amino acids)	18	5	Yes	None	15	12	62	12	None
Interchain disulfide bonds per monomer					2	4	11	2	
pI range mean (SD)					8.6 (0.4)	7.4 (0.6)	8.3 (0.7)	7.2 (0.8)	
Tail piece	Yes	Yes	Yes	No	No	No	No	No	Yes
Allotypes	None	A2m(1) A2m(2)	None	Em1	G1m: a(1), x(2), f(3), z(17)	G2m: n(23)	G3m: b1(5), c3(6), b5(10),b0(11) b3(13),b4(14) s(15), t(16), g1(21), c5(24), u(26),v(27), g5(28)	G4m Gm4a(i) Gm4b(i)	None
Distribution: % intravascular[12]	55 ± 4	57 ± 2	75	50	45	45	45	45	80
Biological half-life (days)[3,12]	5.9 ± 0.5	4.5 ± 0.3	2–8	1–5	21–24	21–24	7–8	21–24	5–10
Fractional catabolic rate (% intravascular pool catabolized/day)	24 ± 2	32 ± 4	37	71	7	7	17	7	8.8
Synthetic rate (mg/kg/day)[3,12]	24 ± 5	4.3 ± 1	0.4	0.002	33	33	33	33	3.3

TABLE 2 (continued)

Structural and Biological Properties of Human Immunoglobulins

	IgA1	IgA2	IgD	IgE	IgG1	IgG2	IgG3	IgG4	IgM
Approximate % total Ig in adult serum	11–14%	1–4%	0.2%	0.004%	45–53%	11–15%	0.03–0.06%	0.015–0.045%	10%
Adult range: age 16–60 in serum g/l[b]	1.81	0.22	—	—	5–12	2–6	0.5–1	0.2–1	0.25–3.1
Functional valency	2, 4	2, 4	2	2	2	2	2	1–2	5–10
Transplacental transfer	0	0	0	0	++	+	++	++	0
Binding to phagocytic cells	—	—	—	—	++	+	++	±	0
Complement activation classical path	0	0	0	0	++	+	+++	0	+++

[a] Approximate molecular weight (m = monomer, d = dimer, t = trimer of IgA are produced, p = pentamer).

[b] Ranges of immunoglobulins in serum are examined in detail in the text. These ranges are provided as a general indication of target levels. Immunoglobulin rates of metabolism were extracted from: Waldmann, T.A., Strober, W., and Blaese, R.M., Metabolism of immunoglobulins, in *Progress in Immunology,* Amos, B., Ed., Academic Press, New York, 1971, 891.

migrate together with C-reactive protein toward the cathode, forming a broad band that has been labeled the classical gamma globulin region. Heterogeneity in their composition and net charge causes some immunoglobulins to also migrate more toward the anode, overlapping with hemopexin, transferrin, and a variety of other proteins in the beta globulin region.[4]

As a family, the human immunoglobulins share a basic structural unit that is comprised of four polypeptide chains that are held together by both noncovalent forces and covalent disulfide bonds between their heavy chains, and with the exception of IgA2, also between their heavy and light chains.[1,3-5] Each four-chain unit is bilaterally symmetrical, containing two structurally identical **heavy** (H) chains and two identical **light** (L) chains (e.g., H_2L_2). Each polypeptide chain is composed of a number of domains comprised of 100 to 110 amino acids residues, each forming a loop as a result of intrachain disulfide bonds. The N-terminal domain of each chain contains the area designated as the variable or V region. The V region contains several highly variable or hypervariable regions, which together form the antigen-binding pocket that confers the property of antigen specificity on the immunoglobulin molecule. The COOH-terminal domains (CH1, hinge, CH2, CH3, CH4) have been collectively defined as the constant region, because the polypeptide backbone is generally invariant (with exception of allotypic differences) within a particular class of immunoglobulin. From a clinical laboratory point of view, the constant region structure is vital to the design of immunoglobulin quantification methods. Assays are constructed using poly- and monoclonal antibody (Mab) reagents that bind to nonallotypic, invariant, isotype-unique determinants in the immunoglobulin constant region domains.

1. Human Light Chains

Human light chains are approximately 23,000-Da proteins that contain no oligosaccharides.[4] They have been classified into two types: kappa (K) and lambda (λ), based on their unique antigenic determinants that result from structural differences in their constant region domains. Lambda light chains have been further subdivided into four subtypes based on structural and antigenic differences. The combination of a light chain with a heavy chain is a random process, and thus a complete repertoire of light chains can be found bound to every immunoglobulin isotype heavy chain. It is the heavy chain, therefore, that determines the isotype of the immunoglobulin. The kappa to lambda ratio (K/λ) in the serum of healthy humans is approximately 2 to 1; however, it can reportedly vary from 1.1 to 8.0, depending on the human immunoglobulin isotype (Table 2).

2. Human Heavy Chains

The principal structural characteristics of the five major classes of heavy chains are summarized in Table 1. Heavy chains vary in their molecular weight (50,000 to 70,000 Da), the percentage of carbohydrates (4 to 18%), and number of oligosaccharides (1 to 5), number of respective subclasses (IgG1-4, IgA1,2) and allotypes (Gm1-25, A2m1-2), number of constant region domains, and number of interchain disulfide bonds. Further details about the structural aspects of the human heavy chains are beyond the scope of this chapter and are presented elsewhere.[3-5] Most importantly to this discussion, the unique determinants on the heavy chain define the isotype of an immunoglobulin and thus form the basis upon which the different classes of immunoglobulins are antigenically differentiated and quantified in the immunoassays discussed subsequently.

3. Secretory Component

Human secretory component (SC) is a 90,000-MW glycoprotein that is expressed as an integral protein on the basolateral membrane of mucosal epithelial cells.[3,6-7] SC is either released into mucosal secretions as a 70,000-MW soluble fragment or bound to polymers of IgA through strong noncovalent interactions. Structurally, it shares no homology with human heavy or light polypeptide chains or the human J chain. It contains a high carbohydrate content and serves as a receptor to transport IgA across mucosal tissues into various human secretions. Secreted human IgA is composed of two IgA monomers, a J chain linker, and a molecule of secretory component. Mucosal secretions contain a mixture of secretory IgA and free SC.[8] Highly specific murine monoclonal antibodies are available (Table 3) which bind to selected determinants on the secretory component and allow its quantification in serum and mucosal secretions.[9]

4. J Chain

The J chain is an elongated glycoprotein of approximately 15,000 Da that can be distinguished by its unusually high quantity of glutamic acid and aspartic acid residues.[3,10] It reportedly serves as a facilitator of polymeric immunoglobulin (e.g., IgM, IgA) polymerization. A single J chain has been identified in each pentameric IgM or polymeric IgA molecule, covalently bound to the penultimate cysteine residue of mu or alpha heavy chains. From a clinical point of view, the J chain is rarely quantified unless a structural or functional abnormality of this protein is suspected or it is required as a marker to distinguish multiple myeloma from benign gammopathy (see Reference 10).

TABLE 3

Human Immunoglobulin Specific Murine Monoclonal Antibodies

Clone	Mouse Isotype	Human Ig Specificity	Epitope Specificity[b]
HP6000[a]	IgG2b	IgG-PAN	Fc-CH2
HP6017	IgG2a	IgG-PAN	Fc-CH2
HP6043	IgG2b	IgG-PAN	Fc-CH2
HP6045	IgG1	IgG-PAN	Fd-CH1
HP6046[a]	IgG1	IgG-PAN	Fd-CH1
HP6069[a]	IgG1	IgG1	Fc-CH2
HP6070	IgG1	IgG1	Fc-CH2
HP6091	IgG1	IgG1	Fc-CH2
HP6002[a]	IgG2b	IgG2	Fc-CH2
HP6014[a]	IgG1	IgG2	Fd-CH1
HP6047[a]	IgG1	IgG3	Fd-Hinge
HP6050	IgG1	IgG3	Fd-Hinge
HP6023	IgG3	IgG4	Fc-CH3
HP6025[a]	IgG1	IgG4	Fc-CH3
HP6019[a]	IgG1	IgG1,3,4	Fc-CH2
HP6030[a]	IgG1	IgG2,3,4	Fc-CH2
HP6058[a]	IgG1	IgG1,2,3	Fc-CH2
HP6029	IgG1	IgE	Fc
HP6061	IgM	IgE	Fc
HP6081	IgG1	IgM	Fc
HP6083	IgG1	IgM	Fc
HP6084	IgG1	IgM	Fc
HP6086	IgG1	IgM	Fc
HP6111	IgG1	IgA-PAN	Fc
HP6123	IgG1	IgA-PAN	Fd
HP6054	IgG2a	Lambda light chain	—
HP6062	IgG3	Kappa light chain	—
HP6130	IgG1	Secretory component	—
HP6141	IgG1	Secretory component	—

[a] Mabs specific for human IgG that were selected as components for the poly-monoclonal antihuman IgG reagent.[34]

[b] Designation of the domain to which the IgG-specific Mabs bind have been obtained from References 25–30. The Fd refers to the heavy chain of the $F(ab')_2$.

B. Isotype-Unique Structural and Biological Properties

Immunoglobulins are bifunctional molecules that bind antigen through their V region. This binding process can elicit a variety of secondary effector functions (e.g., complement activation leading to bacteriolysis and augmentation of phagocyte chemotaxis and opsonization and histamine release from mast cells), which are independent of the immunoglobulin's antigen specificity and depend on C-region determinants (Table 2). While all five major isotypes of human immunoglobulins share the common structural features of the 4-chain monomer subunits discussed above, they vary among themselves in terms of minor structural aspects that confer some special biological properties.

1. Human IgA

Polymeric secretory IgA is composed of two 4-chain basic units and one molecule each of secretory component and J chain (approximately 400,000 MW).[3-4] It is the predominant immunoglobulin in colostrum, saliva, tears, bronchial secretions, nasal mucosa, prostatic fluid, vaginal secretions, and mucous secretions of the small intestine.[6-7] In contrast, 10% of the circulating serum IgA is polymeric, while 90% is monomeric (160,000 MW). Together, they constitute approximately 15% of the total serum immunoglobulins. Two subclasses of IgA have been identified (IgA1 and IgA2).[11] Apart from the 13-amino acid deletion in the IgA2 hinge region, IgA1 and IgA2 constant region domains vary only by 20 amino acid substitutions. IgA2 is present in two allotypic forms: IgA2m(1) and IgA2m(2). The two human IgA PAN* specific murine Mabs listed in Table 3 react to either the Fc** or Fab of both subclasses of IgA and both allotypic forms of IgA2. IgA2 lacks proteolytically sensitive epitopes, which makes it particularly resistant to cleavage by enzymes produced by a variety of bacteria (*Clostridium* spp., *S. pneumoniae*, *S. sanguis*, *H. influenzae*, *N. gonorrhoeae*, *N. meningitidis*) that otherwise readily cleave IgA1 into Fab and Fc fragments. The polymeric nature and presence of SC on IgA in secretions adds to its resistance to bacterial proteolysis. The light chains of IgA2m(2) are linked together by disulfide bonds, rather than to their respective alpha heavy chain; however, no special biological function has been associated with this unique structural difference.[11-12]

In terms of complement activation, IgA poorly activates the classical pathway.[6] This process has been hypothesized as a host mechanism for attenuating inflammatory responses induced by IgG antibodies at the mucosal surface. In contrast, IgA reportedly activates the alternative pathway of complement to provide some direct protective functions. IgA, once bound to a bacterial or parasitic surface antigen, may bind receptors on inflammatory cells, leading to their destruction by means of antibody-dependent cell-mediated cytotoxicity (ADCC). Moreover, its binding to viral or microbial surface antigens may restrict the mobility of microorganisms and prevent their binding onto mucosal epithelium. Finally, secretory IgA can play an important first line of defense in antigen clearance by binding to antigens that leak across an epithelium and transporting them back across to prevent their entry.[7] To

---

* PAN = an antibody that binds to **all** allotypic forms and subclasses of a particular isotype of human immunoglobulin (e.g., IgG PAN reactive Mab = antibody that binds to all allotypic forms of human IgG1, IgG2, IgG3, and IgG4 molecules).

** Fc = immunoglobulin fragment that binds complement.

summarize, the unique structure of IgA resists proteolysis and it functions to block uptake of antigen, bacterial, or viral attachment, limit inflammation induced by classical pathway complement activation, and promote microbial destruction through ADCC by binding to leukocyte receptors.

2. Human IgD

IgD is a 4-chain monomer of approximately 180,000 MW. While IgD is normally present in serum in trace amounts (0.2% of total serum immunoglobulin), it is predominantly found with IgM on the surface of human B lymphocytes.[3] Despite suggestions that IgD may be involved in B-cell differentiation, its principal function is as yet unknown. As such, IgD is rarely quantitated in a general workup of an individual suspected of a humoral immune deficiency or a B-cell dyscrasia.

3. Human IgE

IgE (190,000 MW) exists in serum in a 4-chain monomeric form. While IgE constitutes only 0.004% of the total serum immunoglobulins, it possesses a clinically significant biological function by binding through its Fc region to high affinity receptors on mast cells and basophils.[13] Upon subsequent exposure to relevant protein allergens from trees, grasses, weeds, pet dander, molds, foods, or insect venoms, IgE antibodies on mast cells become cross-linked. This process triggers the production and release of vasoactive mediators (e.g., histamine, prostaglandins, leukotrienes) that can induce mild to severe immediate type I hypersensitivity reactions in sensitized atopic individuals. Clinical diagnostic allergy laboratories focus on the quantitation of total serum IgE and allergen-specific IgE to identify an individual's propensity to develop a spectrum of type I reactions upon exposure to a defined panel of 400 to 500 known allergenic substances.[14] Total serum IgE is commonly expressed in international units per milliliter (IU/ml) or converted to mass units, using 1 IU = 2.4 ng of protein. More recently, System Internationale Units have been used in which 1 SI = 1 µg/liter.

4. Human IgG

In healthy adults, the four-polypeptide chain IgG monomer (150,000 MW) constitutes approximately 75% of the total serum immunoglobulins.[3-4] IgG is approximately equally distributed between intravascular and extravascular serum pools. One important biological function of IgG is its unique ability to cross the placenta, which affords protection for the fetus and newborn. Human IgG has been divided into four subclasses on the basis of unique antigenic determinants. Table 2 summarizes major structural and biological differences among the IgG subclasses. Relative subclass percentages of the total IgG in serum are: IgG1, 60 to 70%; IgG2, 14 to 20%; IgG3, 4 to 8%; and IgG4, 2 to 6%.[3,5,15] While IgG1, IgG2, and IgG4 possess a molecular weight of approximately 150,000, IgG3 is heavier (160,000 MW) as a result of an extended 62-amino acid hinge region which contains 11 interchain disulfide bonds. The highly rigid hinge region of IgG3 promotes accessibility of proteolytic enzymes to sensitive Fc cleavage sites, which results in an increased fractional catabolic rate and a shorter biological half-life (7 to 8 days) than has been observed for IgG1, IgG2, and IgG4 (21 to 24 days). In terms of complement activation, IgG1 and IgG3 are most effective, while IgG4, due to its apparent compact structure, does not appear to activate the classical pathway of complement. IgG4 antibodies are unique in that they appear to be functionally monovalent due to their compact nature. This knowledge has led researchers in the field of allergy to speculate that IgG4 antibodies serve to scavange antigen, prevent mast cell bound IgE antibody from being cross-linked by antigen, and thus block IgE-mediated hypersensitivity reactions in atopic individuals who have undergone immunotherapy. Other important structural and biological differences among the human IgG sub-classes that relate to Fc receptor binding and binding sites on the constant region domains for rheumatoid factors, complement components, and bacterial proteins (protein A, protein G) are beyond the scope of this overview. The reader is directed to several reviews that discuss these differences in detail.[5,15-16]

5. Human IgM

IgM is a pentameric immunoglobulin of about 900,000 MW that constitutes about 10% of serum immunoglobulins in healthy individuals. IgM antibodies are clinically significant because they predominate in early immune responses to most antigens. Along with IgD, IgM is a major immunoglobulin that is expressed on the surface of B cells. With a theoretical functional valency of 10, IgM antibodies are highly efficient in activating the classical pathway of the complement cascade.[3,17]

III. CLINICAL APPLICATIONS

An immunological workup of an individual that presents with the complaint of chronic or recurrent infections, sometimes with unusual infecting agents, commonly involves examination for one or more defects in the patient's antibody-mediated (B cell), cell-mediated

(T cell), phagocytic, or complement segments of the immune system. The level of serum immunoglobulins are commonly measured to identify an underlying defect in the humoral immune system.[18-19]

There are a variety of primary immunodeficiency disorders that can produce immunoglobulin patterns ranging from a complete absence of all isotypes of immunoglobulin (e.g., hypogammaglobulinemia) to a selective decrease in a single isotype (selective IgA deficiency). Sometimes, a deficiency in one or several isotypes (e.g., IgG and IgA) can be associated with an elevated level of a third isotype (e.g., IgM). The immunoglobulin profiles of the major primary immunodeficiency diseases are presented in Table 4. In the case of hyper-IgE syndrome, levels of IgE in excess of 12,000 ng/ml can be accompanied by diminished antibody responses following immunization. A spectrum of secondary causes of decreased serum immunoglobulin levels may include malignant neoplastic diseases (e.g., myeloma), protein losing states (e.g., nephrotic syndrome and protein losing enteropathy), and immunosuppressive treatment (e.g., transient decrease from corticosteroids). A detailed description of the common symptoms, laboratory findings, and other immune markers used in the differential diagnosis of these and other immunodeficiency disorders are presented in detail elsewhere.[19]

On the other extreme from immunodeficiency states are hematological diseases such as plasma cell dyscrasias that can lead to gross elevations in one or several immunoglobulin isotypes as a result of malignant proliferation of one or several clones of B cells.[20] As a group, these conditions are also referred to as paraproteinemias or monoclonal gammopathies, and they can be distinguished by the presence of a monoclonal immunoglobulin in the patient's serum or urine. The laboratory investigation of paraproteinemias involves a variety of hematologic (e.g., complete blood count with differential), routine clinical chemistry (e.g., total protein, albumin, globulin, calcium, phosphate, electrolytes, uric acid), hemostatic (e.g, clotting time, platelet count), serum viscosity, radiological examination, and renal function tests. Immunological tests are then performed, beginning with a total serum immunoglobulin and ending with a serum protein electrophoresis with immunofixation if a paraprotein is suspected.[20-21] A quantitative measurement of serum kappa to lambda light chains has been proposed as a simpler alternative method to electrophoresis-immunofixation for identifying monoclonal proteins. In theory, a serum K/λ light chain ratio that is above or below a reference range for healthy adults may indicate the presence of a paraprotein.[22] However, because serum levels of immunoglobulins other than the myeloma isotype are highly variable and commonly significantly lower than the adult reference ranges in most patients, the observed serum K/λ ratio may be decreased, normal, or increased in individuals with known paraprotein. Thus, a

TABLE 4

Serum Immunoglobulin Levels in Primary Immunodeficiency Disorders

Disease	Total Ig	IgA	IgD	IgE	IgG	IgM
X-linked infantile hypogammaglobulinemia (Bruton's agammaglobulinemia)	<2.5 g/l	<	<	<N	<2.0 g/l	<
Transient hypogammaglobuminemia of infancy[a]	<3.0 g/l	<	<	<	<2.5g/l	<
Common, variable immunodeficiency (acquired hypogammaglobulinemia: 15–35 years of age)	<3.0 g/l	<N	<	<	<2.5 g/l	<N
Immunodeficiency with hyper-IgM	<	<	<	<N	<	>
Selective IgA deficiency[b]	N>	<0.05 g/l	N>	N>	N>	N>
Selective IgM deficiency (rare)	N	N	N	N	N	<
Severe combined B/T cell immunodeficiency[c]	<	<	<	<	<M	<
Cellular immunodeficiency with abnormal immunoglobulin synthesis (Nezelof's Syndrome)[d]	<N>	<N>	<N>	<N>	<N>	<N>
Immunodeficiency with thrombocytopenia, eczema, and recurrent infection (Wiskott-Aldrich syndrome)	?	>	?	>	N	<

Note: < = below age-adjusted reference range or nondetectable; N = normal level for age group; > = above age-adjusted reference range; M = maternal IgG transferred through the placenta; ? = unknown.

a   Most infants go through a period of hypogammaglobulinemia at approximately 5 to 6 months of age as infant shifts from exogenous IgG (maternal through placenta) to endogenously produced immunoglobulin. During this period the infant can experience recurrent respiratory tract infections.

b   Selective IgA deficiency has been also associated with an IgG2 deficiency in some individuals; some patients have normal levels of serum IgA levels < 0.05 g/l and either normal or low secretory IgA. Rarely, normal serum IgA levels can be accompanied by low secretory IgA, possibly as a result of an absence of secretory component.

c   Onset of symptoms by 6 months of age with recurrent viral, bacterial, fungal, and protozoal infection. The presence of placentally delivered material IgG can make diagnosis difficult.

d   Various degrees of B cell immunodeficiency produce decreased, normal, or increased (<N>) immunoglobulin levels.

normal serum K/λ light chain ratio does not guarantee the absence of a paraprotein. Abnormal serum K/λ ratios are generally followed by protein electrophoresis with immunofixation to confirm the presence and the type of the paraprotein(s).[23] Bence-Jones protein (light chains) can be detected in the urine of about half of all patients with multiple myeloma. About 20% of these myeloma patients have only Bence-Jones proteinuria as the sole distinguishing feature. Waldenstrom's macroglobulinemia is a special disease state in which the patients experience hyperviscosity of the blood as a result of excess monoclonal IgM production. While the monoclonal IgM is often a pentamer, monomeric IgM has also been observed in this abnormal immunological state.

IgE is a special immunoglobulin isotype in terms of its clinical utility. A moderately elevated total serum IgE positively reinforces the differential diagnosis of atopic disorders such as allergic rhinitis, allergic asthma, and atopic dermatitis. Very high serum IgE levels are necessary for the diagnosis of hyper-IgE syndrome in patients with an increased susceptibilty to infections and dermatitis. Many parasitic infections can produce extremely elevated total serum IgE levels, and thus a high IgE in the absence of other explanations strongly suggests the possibility of parasitism. A normal IgE level makes the diagnosis of parasitism less likely as a cause of eosinophilia, which otherwise is a common feature of nonallergic asthma. Normal total serum IgE levels can identify nonallergic or intrinsic asthma and exclude bronchopulmonary aspergillosis.

This chapter deals with immunoglobulin levels in health and disease. Several notes of caution are warranted when measuring immunoglobulins in clinical specimens from individuals with disease. First, clinical immunoglobulin assays are designed to measure immunoglobulins at levels that are commonly observed in healthy children and adults. However, some clinical assays may not have the analytical sensitivity required to detect low levels of immunoglobulins in pediatric sera. Second, paraproteins are often structurally atypical immunoglobulins that may produce inaccurate results in some clinical immunoglobulin assays. This can be a problem, for instance, in polyclonal antibody-based immunodiffusion assays where the size of the immunoglobulin (e.g., IgM-pentamer or monomer) will affect its rate of migration and thus the resultant diameter of the immunoprecipitation ring. It may also be a problem in poly- and monoclonal antibody-based immunoassays which use antisera that fail to recognize altered structural determinants on some atypical paraproteins. Finally, an individual may have an immunoglobulin level which fluxuates about its norm for that individual. When it varies significantly from the individual's norm, it may still be within the population reference intervals and thus be considered "normal," when it is actually abnormal for that individual. This has contributed to a hightened interest in identifying an

antibody deficiency as opposed to simply an **immunoglobulin deficiency** in the identification of causes of recurrent infectious disease. In other words, an individual with a serum immunoglobulin within the reference range for an age-adjusted healthy population may be unable to mount a specific antibody response against a panel of protein or carbohydrate antigens. Other sections in this volume will discuss the issue of antibody detection, functional antibody deficiencies, and reference ranges for antibody responses.

IV. METHODS OF QUANTITATION

A. Specimen Types

Human immunoglobulins have been detected in a variety of human body fluids. The most extensively studied and reproducible clinical specimen between individuals of different sexes and races is serum (plasma).[18] Urine is evaluated for heavy and/or light chains and occasionally intact immunoglobulins if kidney dysfunction and plasma cell dyscrasias are suspected. The level of IgG and presence of oligoclonal bands in cerebral spinal fluid (CSF) is evaluated in the workup of an individual suspected of multiple sclerosis. Finally, immunoglobulins (e.g., secretory IgA) are occasionally investigated on a research basis in other human body fluids such as tears, sweat and peritoneal fluid, colostrum, saliva, bronchial secretions, nasal mucosa, prostatic fluid, vaginal secretions, and mucous secretions of the small intestine. The reference ranges presented in this chapter will focus on immunoglobulin levels that have been reported in serum, urine, and CSF.

B. Reagents

A variety of immunological reagents are used in clinical assays to quantitate human immunoglobulins. The majority of these are polyclonal antibodies, which lend themselves to assays involving immunoprecipitation. More recently, well-documented murine monoclonal antibodies have become available that are highly specific for the human immunoglobulins and especially useful in the quantitation of the human IgG and IgA subclasses where maximal specificity is a requirement.

1. Polyclonal Antibodies

Assays involving the formation of an immune complex which is subsequently detected visually or by light-scatter techniques (e.g., immunodiffusion, nephelometry, turbimetry) almost always require the use of highly avid polyclonal antibody reagents to achieve sufficient analytical sensitivity. A majority of clinical laboratories measuring human immunoglobulins purchase an "approved" assay that has been through a lengthy documentation process conducted by the Food and Drug Administration (e.g., 510K). In these cases, the specificity of antibody reagents used in the assay have been documented by cross-reactivity analyses. Cross-reactivity for heterologous immunoglobulin isotypes of at least <0.01% should be demonstrated. For researchers interested in establishing their own assays, potential vendors of polyclonal antibody reagents are listed in compendia such as *Linscott's Directory of Immunological and Biological Reagents.*[24]

2. Monoclonal Antibodies

There are selected clinical assays, such as those that measure IgG and IgA subclass levels in serum, where the specificity possible only with Mabs has become a requirement. International collaborative studies have documented available murine Mabs for their specificity and utility in the detection of the human IgG subclasses.[25-26] A IUIS collaborative study[92] has also documented the specificity of murine Mabs specific for the human IgA subclasses and human secretory component. A variety of highly specific and inexpensive murine Mabs specific for human IgG PAN, IgG subclasses 1 to 4,[25-28] IgA PAN, IgA1-2,[29] IgM, IgE,[30] secretory piece and kappa and lambda light chains[25] have become available from multiple vendors.[24] The mouse isotype, human immunoglobulin specificity, and clone number of a selected panel of such Mabs are presented in Table 3 for illustration. HP6014, for example, describes a mouse IgG1 antihuman IgG2 Fab that is the hybridoma product of clone 6014. The term "PAN" has been used in the documentation studies to reflect the fact that a particular MAb does bind to all subclasses and allotypic forms of a particular human immunoglobulin isotype. Thus, HP6017 is a IgG Fc PAN-reactive MAb that has been shown to react to the Fc region of all four subclasses and allotypic forms of human IgG. Many of these Mabs have been purified from ascites by immunochemical techniques such as sequential anion exchange resin and hydroxylapatite chromatography. Occasionally, they are labeled with biotin or an enzyme and then quality controlled by electrophoretic-blotting methods such as isoelectric focusing (IEF) immunoblot analysis.[31] Their degree of immunoreactivity and cross-reactivity is studied with human paraproteins to confirm their consistency and restricted specificity.[25,26] Of the antibodies listed in Table 3, Mabs produced from clones HP6043 (antihuman IgG Fc PAN), HP6083 (antihuman IgM Fc) and HP6123 (antihuman IgA Fd* PAN) have been identified by

---

* Fd = immunoglobulin heavy chain of the F(ab')$_2$ fragment.

investigators in the U.S. as reference antibodies for the detection of human IgG, IgA, and IgM antibodies in infectious disease serological immunoassays.

3. International and National Reference Proteins and Serum Standards

A. Reference Proteins for Specificity Analysis

International collaborative studies of human immunoglobulin-specific monoclonal antibodies have been the most recent application of human reference immunoglobulins which are supplied by investigators to agencies such as the World Health Organization. Their use has been invaluable in documenting the restricted isotype specificity and lack of allotype selectivity of human immunoglobulin-specific immunochemical reagents. The majority of these so-called reference immunoglobulins are myeloma paraproteins that have been isolated from human serum and characterized in terms of their light chain type and heavy chain isotype. As such, they may be considered atypical immunoglobulins. The use of multiple paraproteins of the same heavy and light chain type and allotype can minimize biases that may result from possible structural differences caused during transcription or translation of the paraprotein from the myeloma cell line.

Modern molecular engineering techniques have been used to produce two panels of useful human–mouse chimeric antibodies that possess human immunoglobulin constant region domains and a defined V-region specificity for the haptens nitrophenyl (NP) or dansyl.[32-33] While these are not currently internationally recognized reference proteins, they have been successfully applied to the documentation of the isotype-restricted specificity of the panel of human immunoglobulin-specific murine Mabs in Table 3.[34] In some cases, their ability to bind to a defined insolubilized antigen and present their C-region determinants in an orientation that would mimic human antibodies binding to their insolubilized antigen has made them candidates as calibration proteins for future human antibody standards.[35]

B. Human Serum Pools

Over the years, a number of internationally recognized human serum pools have been calibrated by value transfer or consensus procedures for use as reference sera to calibrate clinical human serum immunoglobulin assays. Primary reference sera for calibrating human IgG, IgA, and IgM assays include the World Health Organization International Reference Preparation (WHO 67/86; WHO 67/97), the United States–National Reference Preparation (USNRP-IS1644), Netherlands Red Cross Reference Preparation (NRCRP-H0002), International Federation of

Clinical Chemistry Immunoglobulin Standard (IFCC) 71/4, and College of American Pathologists (CAP) Reference Preparation for Serum Proteins (CAP-RPSP-4).[36-38] The WHO International Reference Preparation for human IgD (WHO 67/37) and IgE (WHO 75/502) have been used to calibrate total serum IgD and IgE assays, respectively.[39-40] A new international serum protein standard has been jointly finalized by the International Federation of Clinical Chemistry (IFCC) and the CAP and was released in 1993 as the CAP/BCR*/IFCC Reference Preparation for proteins in Human Serum (RPPHS).

C. Assay Designs

Of the immunoglobulins discussed above, human IgG, IgA, IgM, and IgE and the light chains are those that are routinely measured in the clinical immunology laboratory. Abnormal serum IgD concentrations have not been clearly associated with any particular disease state, and thus IgD is rarely measured, except when an IgD paraprotein is suspected. Secretory component and J chain are considered research analytes. Three basic types of assays are currently used by clinical immunology laboratories to quantitate human IgG, IgA, IgM, IgE, and the kappa and lambda light chains. These are immunodiffusion assays, nephelometric–turbimetric assays, and immunoassays.[41]

1. Immunodiffusion

The radial immunodiffusion assay as originally described in 1965 by Mancini et al.[42] employs polyclonal antisera or, in rare cases, a carefully constructed mixture of monoclonal antibodies, in a porous agarose gel into which a small quantity of serum (5 to 10 μl) is pipetted. As the serum proteins migrate through the gel, immune-complexed proteins form a visible white precipitin ring with a diameter that is proportional to the concentration of the particular analyte specific for the antiserum in the gel. The ring diameter is measured either at a defined time such as 18 to 20 h (Fahey-McKelvey technique[43]) or at maximal endpoint equivalence (Mancini technique) and interpolated from a dose-response curve constructed with multiple dilutions of a reference serum. Immunodiffusion assays are used in smaller clinical laboratories that have fewer specimens and can accept a 2 to 3 day turnaround time. In the 1992 Diagnostic Immunology Series 1 Proficiency Survey conducted by the CAP, approximately 7% of the 994 participating clinical laboratories that measured human IgG, IgA, and IgM used immunodiffusion assays.[44] Performance of these laboratories in the CAP survey in terms of accuracy and variance was equivalent

---

* BCR = Bureau Communitaire de Réference.

(e.g., interlaboratory variation <8% CV) to laboratories using other assay methods. Gel-based immunodiffusion methods are limited in their analytical sensitivity (1 µg/ml[41]) and thus they are not clinically useful in the measurement of immunoglobulins that are normally in low concentrations in serum (e.g., IgE). Variance in the immunodiffusion assay is primarily dependent on the accuracy with which the test and reference sera are pipetted and the precipitin ring diameters are measured.

2. Nephelometric–Turbidimetric Assays

Both nephelometric and turbidimetric assays function on a similar principle in which serum (containing variable amounts of the analyte) is added to a reaction chamber containing a constant amount of optically clear immunoglobulin G-, A-, or M-specific antiserum. The extent of immune complex formation varies as a function of the quantity of the particular immunoglobulin being measured. The rate or extent of immunoglobulin–anti-immunoglobulin complex formation is then measured by the extent of light incident on the reaction chamber (a) that is scattered or reflected toward a detector that is not in the direct path of the transmitted light (nephelometry); or (b) that is attenuated (decreased) in intensity as measured by a detector in the direct path of the transmitted light as a result of scattering, reflectance, and absorption (turbidimetry).[45] Light scatter or turbidity increases immediately following the mixture of antigen and antibody to a maximum value (equivalence) and then decreases. The extent of scatter or absorption obtained with dilutions of a reference serum containing known quantities of IgG, IgA, or IgM allow construction of a reference serum from which response results obtained with test sera are interpolated. Early nephelometric assays generally exhibited a lower analytical sensitivity than turbidimetric assays, due to difficulty in accurately and precisely measuring small changes in light absorbance in the forward direction.[46] However, newer stable, high resolution photometric systems have made the two methods competitive. Both assays suffer from inaccuracies caused when the immunoglobulin (antigen) is in a molar excess relative to the anti-immunoglobulin (antiserum); however, computer algorithms are designed to flag antigen excess automatically. Finally, any particles or solvents, as well as serum macromolecules, can scatter light artifactually. The advantages of these two methods reside in their speed and relative simplicity. High levels of lipoproteins in lipemic serum, hemoglobulin concentrations >5.0 g/l in hemolyzed blood and bilirubin levels >0.15 g/l in icteric serum may cause interference in both nephelometric and turbidimetric assays.[47] Of the 994 participating clinical laboratories in the 1992 CAP Diagnostic Immunology Series 1 Proficiency Survey, 13% used one of the two commercially available turbidometic assays, while 80% used one of four commercially available nephelometric assays for the measurement of human IgG, IgA, and IgM in serum.[44]

3. Immunoassay

The human immunoglobulins in low concentrations in serum, urine, and other body fluids are most commonly measured by immunoassays which can achieve analytical sensitivities of 1 ng/ml.[41] More specifically, human IgG1, IgG2, IgG3, and IgG4,[48-49] human IgA1 and IgA2, secretory component,[9,11] J chain[10] and IgE[50] can be effectively measured by monoclonal antibody-based two-site immunometric assays. In general, these assays use an insolubilized capture antibody to bind the immunoglobulin isotype of interest from serum, urine, or other body fluids and a biotin-, enzyme-, fluorophor-, or radio-labeled polyclonal, poly-monoclonal,[51] or monoclonal antibody specific for different immunoglobulin epitopes to detect bound immunoglobulin. Analysis of multiple dilutions of a reference serum permits the construction of a reference curve from which response values obtained with test specimens can be interpolated in mass/volume units of immunoglobulin. Due to the available sensitivity, serum specimens are normally diluted 1:10 (IgE) to over 1:10,000 (IgG1 to 4) and thus hemolysis, bilirubin, and lipemia rarely cause interference. Immunoassays are technically more complex than immunodiffusion and immunoprecipitation (nephelometric and turbimetric) assays, and they generally require more replicates and dilutions of the unknown specimen to obtain accurate results. Immunoassays are, however, an important clinical method for immunoglobulin measurement, as evidenced by the fact that all 234 laboratories participating in the 1992 SE Diagnostic Allergy CAP survey measured total serum IgE by a commercially available immunoassay.[52]

V. REFERENCE VALUES

In an ideal world, laboratory personnel would select an immunoglobulin quantitation method and then establish reference ranges for a population whose demographics closely resemble the expected patient population that will be tested. This, however, can be difficult to accomplish for clinical immunology laboratories which perform interstate commerce and thus receive specimens from large geographical areas that contain a spectrum of individuals with varying ages and ethnic backgrounds. The alternative strategy has been to adopt published reference intervals that are suggested by the manufacturer. A compendium of reported human immunoglobulin mean and 95-percentile reference intervals is thus presented below to aid the laboratorian in the interpretation of immunoglobulin measurements. One common denominator among these published studies has been the use of specimens from **healthy individuals** to establish the reference range. A healthy individual may be defined as one with "a state of complete physical, mental and social well being and not merely the absence of disease or infirmity." Individuals satisfying this definition can be difficult to find. Thus, with all their potential flaws, the published reference intervals which are summarized in Tables 5 to 9 may be the best information available for those laboratories that have not determined their own reference ranges upon which to assign action levels for immunoglobulin concentrations in serum, urine, and CSF.

A. Factors Influencing Immunoglobulin Levels

There are multiple factors that influence immunoglobulin levels in humans. Age is possibly the most important personal attribute that determines serum immunoglobulin levels. Other suggested factors include the subject's sex, ethnic backgorund, history of allergies and recurrent infections, and whether the individual lives in a geographic region where parasites are endemic. For purposes of this report, the reference ranges extracted from the literature have been partitioned based on the study population's age, sex, and/or specimen type. In one early study of immunoglobulin levels in approximately 300 healthy individuals (1/3 black, 2/3 Caucausian/Hispanic) using immunodiffusion methods, no racial differences were suggested by the data, and thus results were grouped according to age and sex only.[53] In a similar manner, subsequently reported reference immunoglobulin ranges have also been grouped according to the study population's age and occasionally its sex. The impact of genetic factors (race or ethnic origin, blood groups, histocompatibility antigens), physiological factors (stage in menstrual cycle or pregnancy, physical condition), or socioeconomic, environmental, or chronobiological factors on the level of immunoglobulins in healthy study populations has not been definitively determined.

B. Immunoglobulin Reference Intervals

1. Serum IgG, IgA, IgM, and IgD

B cells are reportedly produced starting at the 8th week of gestation. At full term (38 weeks), the healthy newborn has a complete complement of B cells containing surface immunoglobulin of all isotypes.[51] In 1965, Stiehm and Fudenberg reported the first quantitative

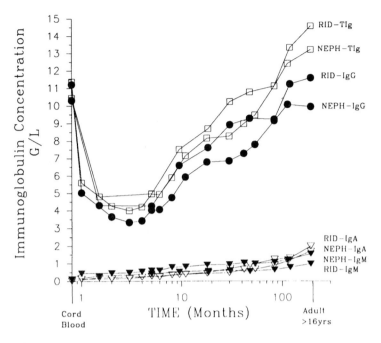

Figure 1

Mean total serum IgG (closed circles), IgA (open inverted triangles), IgM (closed inverted triangles), and immunoglobulin (open boxes) concentrations, as measured by immunodiffusion[53] or nephelometry[58] from birth (cord blood) to adult levels (>192 months). IgE and IgD are not presented as they comprise <1% of the total immunoglobulin in serum. Levels of almost exclusively maternal IgG in cord serum decrease to a minimum by 3 to 5 months and then progressively increase to adult levels by age 16 for IgG and IgM or early adulthood for IgA. Table 5 presents the associated 95-percentile intervals associated with these mean estimates. Data extracted from References 53 and 58.

study of serum IgG, IgA, and IgM levels in humans as a function of age that were measured in mass per volume units (g/l) rather than in previously used arbitrary units or titers.[53] These quantitative immunoglobulin measurements were measured by immunodiffusion, using polyclonal antiserum produced in their own facility and serum collected from 296 children and 30 adults that were clinically healthy at the time of their study. A second study reported by Jolliff et al. in 1982[58] used nephelometric methods to measure IgG, IgA, and IgM in the serum of 25 boys and 25 girls who were bled at defined intervals from birth to 10 years of age. The mean serum IgG, IgA, and IgM concentrations for both of these studies are depicted in Figure 1 and presented together with their 95-percentile reference intervals in Table 5. Both studies demonstrated that the mean umbilical cord serum IgG level was 10.3 to 11.2 g/l, which constituted approximately 90% of the total immunoglobulins measurable in the cord blood. Moreover, cord serum

TABLE 5

Total Human IgG, IgA and IgM Levels in Serum as a Function of Age[a]

Age	N	IgG mean (g/l)	IgG 95 Perc. Range		IgA mean (g/l)	IgA 95 Perc. Range		IgM mean (g/l)	IgM 95 Perc. Range		TIg mean (g/l)	Total Ig 95 Perc. Range		Ref No.	Assay Method
Cord blood	22	10.31	6.31	14.31	0.02	0.000	0.080	0.11	0.01	0.21	10.44	6.42	14.46	53	RID
1–3 months	29	4.30	1.92	6.68	0.21	0.000	0.47	0.30	0.08	0.52	4.81	2.27	7.35	53	RID
4–6 months	33	4.27	0.55	7.99	0.28	0.000	0.64	0.43	0.09	0.77	4.98	0.90	9.06	53	RID
7–12 months	56	6.61	2.23	10.99	0.37	0.010	0.73	0.54	0.08	1.00	7.52	2.68	12.36	53	RID
13–24 months	59	7.62	3.44	11.80	0.50	0.020	0.98	0.58	0.12	1.04	8.70	3.54	13.86	53	RID
25–36 months	33	8.92	5.26	12.58	0.71	0.000	1.45	0.61	0.23	0.99	10.24	6.14	14.34	53	RID
3–5 years	28	9.29	4.73	13.85	0.93	0.390	1.47	0.56	0.20	0.92	10.78	5.88	15.68	53	RID
6–8 years	18	9.23	4.11	14.35	1.24	0.340	2.14	0.65	0.15	1.15	11.12	5.23	16.98	53	RID
9–11 years	9	11.24	6.54	15.94	1.31	0.110	2.51	0.79	0.13	1.45	13.34	8.26	18.42	53	RID
12–16 years	9	9.46	6.98	11.94	1.48	0.220	2.74	0.59	0.19	0.99	11.53	8.15	14.91	53	RID
Adults	30	11.58	5.48	17.68	2.00	0.780	3.22	0.99	0.45	1.53	14.57	7.51	21.63	53	RID

	n														n	
Cord blood	50	11.21	6.36	16.06	0.023	0.014	0.036	0.13	0.06	0.25	11.36	6.44	16.35	58	Neph
1 month	50	5.03	2.51	9.06	0.13	0.013	0.53	0.45	0.20	0.87	5.61	2.72	10.46	58	Neph
2 months	50	3.65	2.06	6.01	0.15	0.028	0.47	0.46	0.17	1.05	4.26	2.26	7.53	58	Neph
3 months	50	3.34	1.76	5.81	0.17	0.046	0.46	0.49	0.24	0.89	4.00	2.05	7.16	58	Neph
4 months	50	3.43	1.96	5.58	0.23	0.044	0.73	0.55	0.27	1.01	4.21	2.27	7.32	58	Neph
5 months	50	4.03	1.72	8.14	0.31	0.081	0.84	0.62	0.33	1.08	4.96	2.13	10.06	58	Neph
6 months	50	4.07	2.15	7.04	0.25	0.081	0.68	0.62	0.35	1.02	4.94	2.58	8.74	58	Neph
7–9 months	50	4.75	2.17	9.04	0.36	0.11	0.90	0.80	0.34	1.26	5.91	2.62	11.20	58	Neph
10–12 months	50	5.94	2.94	10.69	0.40	0.16	0.84	0.82	0.41	1.49	7.16	3.51	13.02	58	Neph
1 year	50	6.79	3.45	12.13	0.44	0.14	1.06	0.93	0.43	1.73	8.16	4.02	14.92	58	Neph
2 years	50	6.85	4.24	10.51	0.47	0.14	1.23	0.95	0.48	1.68	8.27	4.86	13.42	58	Neph
3 years	50	7.28	4.41	11.35	0.66	0.22	1.59	1.04	0.47	2.00	8.98	5.10	14.94	58	Neph
4–5 years	50	7.80	4.63	12.36	0.68	0.25	1.54	0.99	0.43	1.96	9.47	5.31	15.86	58	Neph
6–8 years	50	9.15	6.33	12.80	0.90	0.33	2.02	1.07	0.48	2.07	11.12	7.14	16.89	58	Neph
9–10 years	50	10.07	6.08	15.72	1.13	0.45	2.36	1.21	0.52	2.42	12.41	7.05	20.50	58	Neph
Adult	120	9.94	6.39	13.49	1.71	0.70	3.12	1.56	0.56	3.52	13.21	7.65	20.13	58	Neph

a Results are presented as the mean serum immunoglobulin level in g/l and the 95th percentile range (2.5–97.5 percentile: mean ±2 SD)
Data extracted with permission from References 53 and 58 that used immunodiffusion (RID) or nephelometry (Neph) assays, respectively.

contained a trace quantities of IgM (0.11 to 0.13 g/l) and IgA (0.02 g/l) which could be elevated by *in utero* infections. The transplacentally transferred IgG in the serum of healthy newborns decreased to a minimum by 3 to 5 months as neonatal IgM production began to increase (Figure 1). No differences in immunoglobulin levels were detected in their study between male and female infants during the first year of life in the Stiehm study, and thus they combined these values for clinical use. Adult IgG and IgM levels are generally achieved by age 16 while levels of IgA can increase into early adulthood.[53] Table 6 summarizes the mean and 95-percentile reference intervals for IgG, IgA, and IgM that have been reported for healthy adults in these and five additional population studies. The demographics of the study populations (number, sex, age range, race, clinical testing, environment), assay, and statistical methods employed are summarized where available. The two adult ranges determined by immunodiffusion are broader than those obtained by the nephelometric and turbidometric assays (Figures 2 to 4). These reports cover most of the commercial assays that are employed clinically for human IgG, IgA, and IgM measurements as assessed by review of the CAP Diagnostic Immunology Survey.[44] While several immunoassays for total human serum IgG are available, none are used by clinical laboratories participating in the CAP surveys, possibly because they are more technically complex and labor intensive than immunodiffusion and nephelometric and turbidometric assays.

2. Serum IgG Subclasses

Of the five immunoglobulin isotypes, IgG has achieved special importance because it is the sole immunoglobulin that is transported across the placenta and thus can confer humoral immunity on the neonate. Concentrations of the individual IgG subclasses in human serum have therefore been extensively studied as a function of age, using a variety of immunodiffusion and immunoassays. Figure 5 presents a composite of the age-dependent profiles of human mean IgG1, IgG2, IgG3, and IgG4 levels in the serum of children and adults as measured by eight groups, using a variety of polyclonal and monoclonal antibody reagents. Trends in the mean levels of IgG1, IgG2, IgG3, and IgG4 are in general agreement, with a characteristic valley in all four subclasses occurring at 3 to 6 months as maternally derived IgG is replaced by immunoglobulin synthesized by the infant. IgG1 and IgG3 synthesis occurs earlier and is more rapid in early childhood than is synthesis of IgG2 and IgG4. IgG1 concentrations increase to adult levels at 5 to 7 years, in contrast to IgG3 at 7 to 9 years, IgG2 at 8 to 10 years and IgG4 at 9 to 11 years.[71-72] Differential exposure to environmental antigens is thought to combine with natural biological variation in the rate of achieving immunological maturity and inherited genetic

TABLE 6

Adult Human Serum IgG, IgA and IgM Levels in Serum Reference Intervals[a]

Author/Ref	N Adults	Age Range	IgG mean (g/l)	IgG 95 Percentile Interval (g/l)	IgA mean (g/l)	IgA 95 Percentile Interval (g/l)	IgM mean (g/l)	IgM 95 Percentile Interval (g/l)	IgD mean (g/l)	Total IgD 95 Percentile Interval (g/l)	Company Name	Assay Name	Assay Method
Weeke[54]	200	15–93	10.40	6.80 16.00	1.37	0.54 3.50	0.55	0.21 1.44	NA	NA NA	Dansk	Laurell	IEP
Stiehm[53]	30	>16	11.60	5.60 17.60	2.00	0.78 3.22	0.99	0.47 1.50	NA	NA NA	NA	None	RID
Bulletin[57]	300	>16	10.47	5.64 17.65	1.77	0.85 3.85	1.26	0.45 2.50	0.04	0.00 0.14	Sanofi	Quanticlone	RID
Jolliff[58]	120	16–62	9.94	6.39 13.49	1.71	0.70 3.12	1.56	0.56 3.52	NA	NA NA	Beckman	ICS	NEPH
Dati[56]	773 M	>16	12.00	8.00 17.00	2.30	1.00 4.90	1.40	0.50 3.20	NA	NA NA	Behring	BN-100	NEPH
Dati[56]	680 F	>16 M/F Combined	NA		2.10	0.85 4.50	1.55	0.60 3.70	NA	NA NA	Behring	BN-100	NEPH
Bulletin[59]	349	>16	NA	6.78 17.14	NA	0.73 4.22	NA	0.54 2.96	NA	NA NA	Abbott	TDx	NEPH
Hutson[55b]	213	17–65	NA	5.68 14.83	NA	0.57 4.14	NA	0.20 2.74	NA	NA NA	DuPont	ACA	TURB
Intermethod mean[a]	=		11.00		1.95		1.30		0.04				
Intermethod 1SD	=		0.96		0.27		0.24		NA				
Intermethod CV	=		8.7%		13.8%		18.6%		NA				
Maximum of range	=			17.65		4.90		3.70		0.14			
Minimum of range	=			5.60		0.57		0.20		0.00			
N	=		4		4		4		1				

a IEP results not included in inter-method analyses.

b Population consisted of 149 M and 64 F with a race distribution of 91% Caucasian, 6% black, and 3% Hispanic in study by Huston et al.[55]

NA = data not reported; M = male; F = female; IEP = immunoelectrophoresis; TURB = turbidometric assay; NEPH = nephelometric assay; RID = radial immunodiff. Results are presented as the mean serum immunoglobulin level in g/l and the 95th percentile range (2.5–97.5 percentile: mean ± 2 SD).

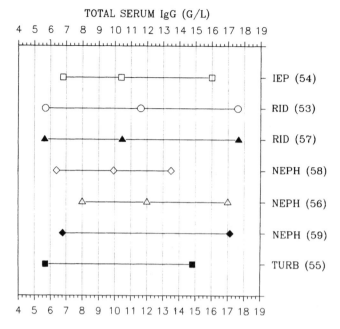

Figure 2

Mean and 95-percentile reference intervals (mean ± 2 SD) for total serum IgG in adults as reported by seven groups using the available commercial assays. See Table 6 for actual data. Despite the use of three different assay procedures and seven unique sets of immunochemical reagents, the group mean total serum IgG levels determined in adult sera were 11.0 g/l, with an acceptable variance of 8.7% CV. The group total serum IgG maximum was 17.65 g/l and the minimum was 5.60 g/l.

factors to produce the variation observed in adult IgG subclass concentrations in serum. The 95-percentile reference intervals for human IgG as defined using a monoclonal antibody-based immunoassay are presented in Table 7 as an illustration of representative target ranges.

3.   Urinary IgG, IgA, and IgM

The glomeruli of the kidney function as ultrafilters for plasma proteins and normally exclude high MW proteins such as IgM from reaching the glomerular filtrate, except in trace amounts. The passage of high MW proteins into the urine (proteinuria) can occur as a result of (a) increased glomerular permeability, (b) defective tubular reabsorption, (c) overload of a particular serum protein (e.g., Bence-Jones light chains), or (d) postrenal protein secretion.[61] Urine can be clinically evaluated by electrophoresis-immunofixation for light chains when a plasma cell dyscrasia is suspected as a result of condition "c." Both immunoglobulins (IgG, IgA) and/or light chains may also be quantitatively measured as evidence of kidney damage. IgG and IgA are

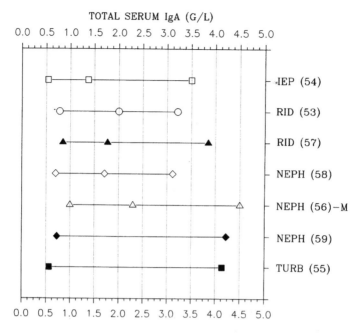

TOTAL SERUM IgA (G/L)

Figure 3

Mean and 95-percentile reference intervals (mean ± 2 SD) for total serum IgA in adults as reported by seven groups using the available commercial assays. See Table 6 for actual data. Despite the use of three different assay procedures and seven unique sets of immunochemical reagents, the group mean total serum IgA levels determined in adult sera were 1.95 g/l with an acceptable variance of 13.8% CV. The group total serum IgA maximum was 4.90 g/l and the minimum was 0.57 g/l.

normally present in urine at total levels from 1.2 to 6.5 mg (IgG) and 1.3 to 5.0 mg (IgA) in a 24-h urine specimen (Table 8).[61,82] Levels above this range are considered evidence of kidney disfunction.

4. Cerebrospinal Fluid (CSF) IgG, IgA, and IgM

CSF is secreted by the choroid plexuses, around the cerebral vessels and along the walls of the ventricles of the brain. It fills the ventricles and bathes the spinal cord. Eventually CSF is reabsorbed into the blood through the arachnoid villi. Because CSF is principally an ultrafiltrate of plasma, its protein (typically 0.15 to 0.45 g/l in lumbar fluid) is comprised primarily of low molecular weight prealbumin, albumin, and transferrin. CSF from healthy adults also normally contains low IgG concentrations that range from undetectable to 0.086 g/l, depending on the report, method of measurement, and study group's age (Table 7). In one study, a gradual age-dependent increase was observed by Tibbling et al. up to 40 years of age.[63] IgA concentrations in the CSF of healthy adults ranged from undetectable to 0.006 g/l. IgG and IgA

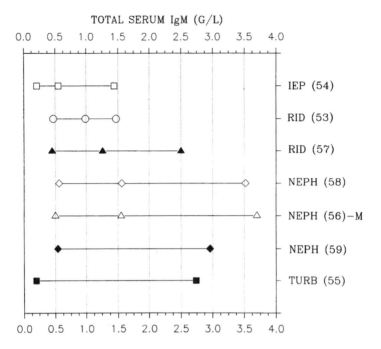

Figure 4
Mean and 95-percentile reference intervals (mean ± 2 SD) for total serum IgM in adults
as reported by seven groups using the available commercial assays. See Table 6 for actual
data. Despite the use of three different assay procedures and seven unique sets of
immunochemical reagents, the group mean total serum IgM levels determined in adult
sera were 1.30 g/l with a variance of 18.6% CV. The group total serum IgM maximum
was 3.70 g/l and the minimum was 0.20 g/l.

can be detected in the CSF presumably as a result of immunoglobulin
synthesis by B cells that infiltrate demyelinated lesions within the central nervous system. An elevation in CSF IgG concentrations and the
presence of oligoclonal bands by electrophoresis-immunofixation are
clinically used markers of increased permeability of the blood/brain
barrier (capillary endothelium of vessels of the central nervous system)
that may occur in patients with active multiple sclerosis, subacute
sclerosing panencephalitis, and acute aseptic meningitis. The CSF
IgG/albumin ratio or immunoglobulin index is used to determine
whether there is an increased permeability or increased local IgG production, or both. Decreased CSF IgG levels have been seen in individuals with active systemic lupus erythematosus with central nervous
system involvement. In the few studies where IgM was measured in
CSF from healthy adults, it was undetectable (<0.002 g/l). Thus, IgM
is not routinely measured in CSF.

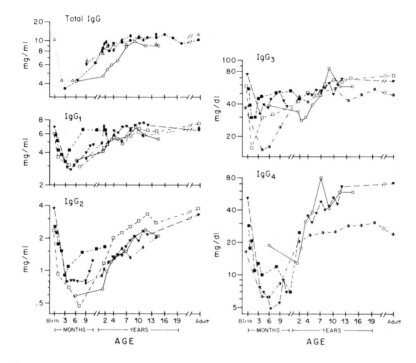

Figure 5

Mean total IgG, IgG1, IgG2, IgG3, and IgG4 concentrations as measured by immuno-diffusion or immunoassay in serum collected from children at birth (cord blood) through adult (>16) ages. Table 7 presents the associated 95-percentile intervals associated with one of these mean estimates from Reference 64. Data for figure extracted from references 64 (Schur et al.; open circles; 65 (Allansmith et al., closed circles, 53 (Stiehm and Fudenberg; open triangles, total IgG only); 66-67 (Zegers et al. and Van der Giessen et al.; closed inverted triangles; 68 (Shakelford et al., closed diamonds; 69 (Oxelius and Svenningsen, open boxes; 70 (Morell et al., closed boxes; and 71 (Lee et al., closed circles. All studies demonstrate a decrease in all four subclasses of IgG during the first 3–5 months of observation. (From Lee, S.I., Heiner, D.C., and Wara, D., *Monogr. Allergy*, 19, 108, 1986. S. Karger AG, Basel. With permission.)

5. *Serum IgE*

As with the other immunoglobulin isotypes, the concentration of IgE in the serum is highly age dependent. The concentration of IgE in cord serum is low, usually <2 kU/l (<4.8 µg/l), because it does not cross the placental barrier in significant amounts.[73-76] Mean serum IgE levels progressively increase in healthy children up to 10 to 15 years of age. The rise in serum IgE toward adult levels is slower than that of IgG, but comparable to that of IgA. Atopic infants have an earlier and steeper rise in serum IgE levels during their early years of life as compared with non-atopic controls.[76] An age-dependent decline in total serum IgE may occur from the second through eighth decades of life.

TABLE 7

Human IgG Subclass Levels as a Function of Age

Age Group	Human IgG1 (g/l)	Human IgG2 (g/l)	Human IgG3 (g/l)	Human IgG4 (g/l)
Cord blood	4.35–10.84	1.43–4.53	0.27–1.46	<0.01–0.47
0–2 months	2.18–4.96	0.40–1.67	0.04–0.23	<0.01–0.33
3–5 months	1.43–3.94	0.23–1.47	0.04–1.00	<0.01–0.14
6–8 months	1.90–3.88	0.37–0.60	0.12–0.62	<0.01
9–24 months	2.86–6.80	0.30–3.27	0.13–0.82	<0.01–0.65
3–4 years	3.81–8.84	0.70–4.43	0.17–0.90	<0.01–1.16
5–6 years	2.92–8.16	0.83–5.13	0.08–1.11	<0.01–1.21
7–8 years	4.22–8.02	1.13–4.80	0.15–1.33	<0.01–0.84
9–10 years	4.56–9.38	1.63–5.13	0.26–1.13	<0.01–1.21
11–12 years	4.56–9.52	1.47–4.93	0.12–1.79	<0.01–1.68
13–14 years	3.47–9.93	1.17–4.40	0.23–1.17	<0.01–0.83
Adult	3.10–9.10	0.72–4.10	0.17–0.72	0.02–0.65

Data extracted with permission from Reference 64.

In contrast to IgG, IgA, IgM, and IgD levels that are routinely compared against 95 percentile reference intervals obtained with serum from healthy individuals, serum IgE levels must be judged against intervals established with serum from an age-adjusted healthy and **non-atopic** individuals.

Representative serum IgE concentrations as measured in the serum of non-atopic children and adults are presented in Table 9. After 14 years of age, serum IgE levels >333 kU/l (800 µg/l) are considered abnormally elevated and strongly associated with atopic disorders such as allergic rhinitis, extrinsic asthma, and atopic dermatitis. The overlap between IgE levels in atopic and non-atopic populations, however, is considerable.[73-77] One study of adults with allergic asthma demonstrated a mean serum IgE level of 1589 µg/l (range 55 to 12,750 µg/l), with only about one half of them having IgE concentrations above the 800 µg/l upper limit for non-atopic individuals. In a different study, very high levels of serum IgE (mean: 978 kU/l; range 1.3 to 65,208 kU/l) were observed in approximately 90% of patients with atopic dermatitis.

6. Immunoglobulins in Other Fluids

Of the gut-associated lymphoid tissue, bronchus-associated lymphoid tissue, and human small intestinal lamina propria-associated B cells, approximately 85% contain surface IgA, while only 5% and 10%, respectively, contain surface IgG and IgM. Since the surface immunoglobulin reflects the isotype of plasma cells derived from B cell precursors, secretory IgA is the predominant immunoglobulin produced in these tissues and associated secretions. Moreover, secretory IgA is

TABLE 8

Human Urine and CSF Immunoglobulin G/A/M Reference Intervals

Assay Neme	Total Urinary Human IgG (mg/24 h volume)	Total Urinary Human IgA (mg/24 h volume)	Total Urinary Human IgM (mg/24 h volume)	Author/Ref.
LC-Partigen RID Behring	1.2–6.5	1.3–5.0	Undetectable	Ritzmann[61] Manuel[82]

Assay Neme	Total CSF Human IgG (g/l)	Total CSF Human IgG (g/l)	Total CSF Human IgM (g/l)	Author/Ref.
LC-Partigen RID-Behring	UD to 0.055	0.0015 to 0.006	<0.001	Ritzmann[61]
RIA	0.035 to 0.058 (15-60 year)	<0.002	<0.002	Tietz[62]
RID	0.017 ± 0.004[a] (17–30 year)	ND	ND	Tibbling[63]
N = 93	0.021 ± 0.007 (31–40 year)			
(17–60)	0.024 ± 0.008 (41–50 year)			
	0.027 ± 0.009 (51–60 year)			
	0.026 ± 0.009 (61–77 year)			
Quanticlone RID Sanofi Pasteur	UD to 0.086	ND	ND	Sanofi Tech Bull.[57]

Note: UD = undetectable, ND = not done.

a Mean ± 1 SD

TABLE 9

Human Serum IgE Non-Atopic Reference Ranges[a]

Total N	Sex M/F	Age Range	Total Human IgE (Geometric Mean kU/l)	Total Human IgE (Upper 95% Confidence limit kU/l)	Author/Ref.
26	M (15), F (11)	Cord	0.22	1.28	Kjellman,[75]
21	M (7), F (14)	6 week	0.69	6.12	Scandinavian children [b]
20	M (14), F (6)	3 month	0.82	3.76	
20	M (10), F (10)	6 month	2.68	16.3	
20	M (14), F (6)	9 month	2.36	7.3	
18	M (14), F (4)	1 year	3.49	15.2	
20	M (13), F (7)	2 year	3.03	29.5	
11	M (6), F (5)	3 year	1.80	16.9	
9	M (6), F (3)	4 year	8.58	68.9	
19	M (10), F (9)	7 year	12.9	161	
20	M (11), F (9)	10 year	23.7	570	
22	M (15), F (7)	14 year	20.1	195	
175	Not specified	17–85 year	13.2	114	Zetterstrom,[82] Swedish adults
72	M	6–14 year	42.7	527	Barbee,[76]
73	F	6–14 year	43.3	344	white adults in U.S.
109	M	15–24 year	33.6	447	
121	F	15–24 year	18.6[c]	262	
108	M	25–34 year	16.8	275	
89	F	25–34 year	16.6	216	
62	M	35–44 year	21.7	242	
67	F	35–44 year	19.3	206	
88	M	45–54 year	19.2	254	
97	F	45–54 year	13.3	177	
105	M	55–64 year	21.3	354	
172	F	55–64 year	11.7[c]	148	
145	M	65–74 year	21.2	248	
199	F	65–74 year	11.5[c]	122	
69	M	75+ year	18.4	219	
87	F	75+ year	9.2[c]	124	
758	M	6–75 year	22.9	317	
905	F	6–75 year	14.7[c]	189	

[a] M = male, F = female. All total serum IgE levels reported in this table were measured with a noncompetitive paper disk radioimmunosorbent test marketed by Kabi-Pharmacia Diagnostics.
[b] Study performed with sera from children with no history of atopic disease or first-degree atopic relatives.
[c] Mean serum IgE for females is significantly lower than for males.

the predominant immunoglobulin in secretions emanating from mucosal tissues in middle ear, urogenital tract, mammary gland, conjunctiva, and salivary glands. IgA in saliva, for instance, appears to reach adult levels (approximately 0.11 g/l) by about 6 weeks of development.[62] Reports of immunoglobulins other than IgA in body fluids such as tears, sweat and peritoneal fluid, colostrum, saliva, bronchial secretions, nasal mucosa, prostatic fluid, vaginal secretions, and mucous secretions of the small intestine are rare.

Most recently, IgE levels in tears may become a routine measurement in the opthamology clinic. A monoclonal antibody-based solid phase immunoassay has become available that has been designed to analyze the level of IgE in tears that have been collected from the inferior marginal tear duct using a 2-µl capillary tube. Tear IgE levels are reportedly increased in individuals with giant papillary conjunctivitis, secondary to wearing contact lenses.[78] The mean total IgE levels in the tears of allergic symptomatic patients have been also shown to be statistically elevated as compared to tears of nonallergic symptomatic and asymptomatic subjects.[79]

C. Human Light Chain Reference Intervals

As indicated above, an alteration in the kappa to lambda light chain ratio in serum has been proposed as a marker of monoclonal or M-component-related immunoglobulin abnormalities. Kappa chains containing immunoglobulins normally predominate in healthy individuals, with an average reported K/λ light chain ratio of 1.8 to 1.9.[23,56,80-83] Table 10 presents the patient demographics, methods, and published kappa, lambda levels in serum for selected studies that compute the serum K/λ ratio. The mean immunoglobulin kappa/lambda ratios among these studies of healthy subjects varied from 1.8 to 1.9: 1.84,[22] 1.83 ± 0.3,[23] 1.86,[56] 1.87 ± 0.23,[80] 1.9 ± 0.3,[82] 1.83.[83] Possibly the most interesting study involved the examination of 10 sequential sera from 12 healthy subjects to study intra-individual biological variation as distinct from methodologic analytical variation.[80] These authors concluded that high inter-individual variability in the light chain ratios makes their measurement more well-suited for monitoring changes rather than as a replacement for serum protein electrophoresis in the early detection of monoclonal gammopathies.

D. Total Serum IgG Levels during Gammaglobulin Therapy

As indicated above, a total IgG <2.5 g/l with nondetectable IgA and IgM in serum can aid in the identification of patients with primary hypo- or agammaglobulinemia (Table 4). Once identified, the patient, especially a child, may be put on exogenous immune globulin replacement therapy. The total serum IgG can be useful to determine the optimal dose required for administration and to document the biological half-life and total achieved level of IgG in the particular patient.

TABLE 10
Human Serum Light Chain Reference Intervals

N	Sex M/F	Age Range	Statistics	Instrument and Reagents	Assay	Kappa Light Chain Range (g/l)	Lambda Light Chain Range (g/l)	Kappa/Lambda Ratio Ref. Interval	Author/Ref.
30	F	19–57	Normal[a]	Behring Diagnostics	NEPH	1.86–4.92	0.86–2.80	1.40–2.45	Seppo,[22] Finland
70	M	20–65	Logarithmic			Mean = 3.12	Mean = 1.68	Mean = 1.84 Median = 1.82	
50	ND	Adults	ND	Behring Diagnostics	NEPH	Mean = 2.72	Mean = 1.47	1.35–2.65[b] 1.83 ± 0.3[b]	Lievens,[23] Belgium
1453	773 M 680 F	Adults	2.5–97.5 Percentile	Behring Diagnostics	NEPH	2.0–4.40 Mean = 3.00	1.10–2.40 Mean = 1.60	Mean = 1.86	Dati et al.[56]
12	6M 6F	23–48	Mean ± 2 SD	Cobas Fara Hoffman LaRoche	TURB	Mean = 7.9	Mean = 4.23	(Mean ± SD) 1.87 ± 0.23	Ford[78]

[a] Serum K/λ ratios kept closely to a logarithmic normal distribution with a positive skewness.
[b] Mean ± SD.

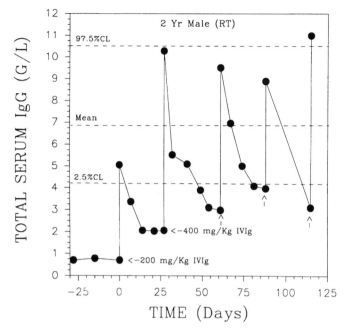

Figure 6

Changes in total serum IgG levels measured by immunoassay in sequential sera collected from a single 2-year-old male (RT) with primary immunodeficiency (Bruton's agamma-globulinemia). Specimens were collected prior to and during a period when monthly injections of IV-immunoglobulin (IVIg) were administered. Low IgG levels (<1 g/l) were detected prior to administration of 200 mg/kg of IV gammaglobulin. IgG levels increased to 5 g/l and then diminished, with a biological half-life of 10 to 11 days. Higher doses of IV Ig (400 mg/kg) were then administered in the second through fourth doses depicted to achieve an average IgG level around the mean for 2-year-old infants. The biological half-life appeared to decrease to 5–6 days on these subsequent doses.

Figure 6 illustrates one such evaluation in which total IgG was mea-sured in sequential sera collected from a 2-year-old male with Bruton's disease who had a total IgG of 0.7 g/l and nondetectable IgA and IgM prior to therapy. Following administration of 200 mg/kg of IV-immune globulin (IV-Ig), the total IgG increased to 5 g/l, but rapidly declined with a biological half-life of 10 to 11 days. The decision was made based on these results to increase the dose to 400 mg/kg, which in four subsequent administrations was able to maintain the total serum IgG level between the 2.5 and 97.5 percentile interval for a 2-year-old child. The biological half-life decreased to 5 to 6 days with the increased level of administered IgG. This study serves to illustrate the utility of repet-itive total serum IgG measurements for monitoring IV-Ig therapy and for making adjustments in dose to optimize circulating levels of IgG into the range appropriate for the age of the patient.

TABLE 11

External Proficiency Surveys for Immunoglobulins and Light Chains[a]

Variable	IgG	IgG1-4	IgA	IgM	IgE	IgD	K/μl Ratio
Survey code	SM, S	S	SM	SM	SM, SE	S	S
Provider agency	CAP	CAP, UKNEQAS	CAP	CAP	CAP	CAP	CAP
No of cycles per year	3, 3	3, 6	3	3	3, 3	3	3
No. of sera per cycle	5, 1	1, 2	5	5	5, 5	1	1
No. of assay methods	12, 9	2, 5	11	12	7, 10	2	3
Laboratories participating	1,072; 545	66, 45	1,072	1,074	367; 214	63	157

[a] The number of participating laboratories, methods, and other parameters presented in this table were extracted from reports of the College of American Pathologists (CAP) SM, S, and SE surveys for cycle 1 of 1993.

VI. EXTERNAL PROFICIENCY SURVEYS

In the U.S., the most widely subscribed external proficiency survey for human immunoglobulins and light chains is conducted by the College of American Pathologists. The design (e.g., number of participating laboratories, cycles per year, sera per cycle, and reporting specimen) for the three surveys of relevance to the diagnostic immunology laboratory are summarized in Table 11. The Diagnostic Immunology Series 1 (SM; code S1) and Series 2 (S; code S2) Surveys provide 15 specimens per year for the evaluation of laboratory methods that are used to measure serum IgG, IgG subclasses 1 to 4, IgA, IgM, IgE, IgD, and human kappa/lambda light chain ratios. There is no available survey for human IgA subclasses. In addition to the immunoglobulins, these surveys also provide external proficiency testing for assays that measure other immunological analytes, such as complement components 3 and 4, rheumatoid factor, C-reactive protein, serum hCG, alpha-1 antitrypsin, ceruloplasmin, haptoglobin, prealbumin, and a panel of antibodies against bacterial, viral, and autoantigens. Discussion of these nonimmunoglobulin analytes is beyond the scope of this chapter. The diagnostic allergy CAP survey called "SE" provides 15 sera per year to laboratories performing total serum IgE and allergen-specific IgE antibody assays. The diagnostic allergy (SE) survey has been favorably contrasted to the proficiency program coordinated in Europe by British scientists.[85] For those analytes, such as the human IgG subclasses, where only few specimens are submitted by the CAP surveys,[86] American laboratorians can elect to supplement their proficiency testing program by participating in other programs, such as those conducted by the U.K. External Quality Assessment Scheme for Autoimmune

Serology (UKEQAS). The CAP surveys are generally designed to include three cycles per year and five specimens per cycle, which fulfills the requirements for regulated analytes that are measured by highly complex tests as specified by U.S. Public Law 100-578, the Clinical Laboratory Improvement Amendments of 1988 (CLIA '88). For the CAP surveys, a 1 to 2 week turnaround time from receipt of the specimens to submission of results is expected for all participants. Once compiled, a summary of the mean, standard deviation, coefficient of variation, median, low value, and high values for each assay method and a pass/fail designation for regulated analytes is returned to the participating laboratory and state licensing agencies. The general performance of the assays for the immunoglobulins has been difficult to summarize in a clear manner, due to the vast quantity of information. Those laboratories producing measurements outside the 95 percentile (mean ± 2 SDs) of the group data can be considered out of control, providing the number of laboratories is sufficiently large to make statistical inferences. Due to the availability of excellent, stable primary reference sera, the interlaboratory agreement for total serum IgG, IgA IgM, and IgE measurements between laboratories, using the same assay method and reagents is generally within acceptable levels (<10% coefficient of variation). Differences in immunoglobulin assignments that occur between laboratories that use different methods can generally be traced to the use of an inappropriate calibration serum by the manufacturer or laboratory.

VII. INTERFERENCES

Despite the excellent interlaboratory and interassay agreement of immunoglobulin levels performed in clinical laboratories using FDA-approved commercial products, there are occasionally outlier results that can not be traced to hemolysis, lipemia, or high levels of bilirubin. An overview of published work linking human rheumatoid factors to spuriously high or low immunoglobulin levels as a result of immunological method interference is presented elsewhere.[87] This problem can only become more common place as murine and engineered chimeric (human-mouse) antibodies are increasingly used to diagnose and treat human diseases.[88-89] In addition to exogenously administered heterologous, chimeric or humanized antibodies that may elicit human rheumatoid factors, the presence of naturally occurring anti-immunoglobulin autoantibodies is also well known.[90] These autoantibodies are thought to play a role in regulating the level of total serum immunoglobulins. They can also be considered potential interferring factors in immunological assays (see Section V.C) that are employed by clinical laboratories to quantitate human immunoglobulins. Difficulty in documenting the role of these autoantibodies in assay interference in part stems from the fact that human immunoglobulin-specific autoantibodies are heterogeneous, and they are difficult to quantitate when circulating in a complexed form, bound to their respective immunoglobulin. The use of purified human immunoglobulins and engineered chimeric autoantibodies (e.g., human IgG1 antihuman IgE Fc) are being used as research tools to construct families of dose-response curves by varying either the autoantibody (IgG anti-IgE) or ligand (IgE) concentration in a serum protein matrix.[91] By doing so, reference calibration curves may be established from which the concentration of human immunoglobulin-specific autoantibodies can be estimated. The use of these calibration curves should allow more definitive identification of their presence and role in altering the accuracy of immunological assays that measure total immunoglobulin concentrations in human serum.

VIII. SUMMARY

The immunoglobulins are among the most important human serum proteins as they confer humoral immunity, promote cellular immunity, and facilitate complement activation. By these actions, immunoglobulins pay a key role in the immunological defense of the human against infectious agents. This chapter has examined structural details of immunoglobulins that serve as determinants for immunological reagents that are used in clinical assays for their measurement in human body fluids. Future trends in this specialized area of clinical immunology will no doubt involve the use of more uniform assay methods, increasingly stable and better-characterized reference sera as calibrators, and ultraspecific (monoclonal) reagents. These gradual changes should ultimately translate to more accurate analytical measurement of immunoglobulin levels in serum, urine, CSF, and other body fluids that are performed in hospitals, reference laboratories, and research environments throughout the world.

ACKNOWLEDGMENTS

The author extends his appreciation to Dr. Deborah Fawcett and Dr. Stephen Buescher of the University of Texas School of Medicine in Houston, Texas, who obtained the sequential sera from the 2-year-old immunodeficiency patient that were subsequently used to examine the utility of total serum IgG measurements in monitoring IV-gammaglobulin therapy for dose optimization.

REFERENCES

1. Putnam, F.W., *The Plasma Proteins*, Academic Press, New York, 1977, 1.
2. Kabat, E.A., The structural basis of antibody complementarity, *Adv. Protein Chem.*, 32, 1, 1978.
3. Goodman J.W., Immunoglobulins I. Structure and Function, in *Basic and Clinical Immunology*, Stites, D.P., Stobo, J.D., and Wells, J.V., Eds., Appleton & Lange, Norwalk, CT, 1987, chap. 4.
4. Kabat, E.A., Heterogeneity and structure of immunoglobulins and antibodies, in *Structural Concepts in Immunology and Immunochemistry*, Kabat, E.A., Ed., Holt, Rinehart and Winston, New York, 1976, chap. 9.
5. Jefferis, R., Structure-function relationships of IgG subclasses, in *The human IgG subclasses: molecular analysis of structure, function and regulation*, Shakib, F., Ed., Pergamon Press, New York, 1990, 93.
6. Heremans, J.F., Biochemical features and biological significance of immunoglobulin A, in *Immunoglobulins, Biological Aspects and Clinical Uses*, Merler, E., Ed., National Academy of Sciences, Washington, D.C., 1970, 52.
7. Tomasi, T.B., Jr., The gamma A globulins: first line of defense, in *Immunology, Current Knowledge of Basic Concepts in Immunology and Their Clinical Application*, Good, R.A. and Fisher, D.W., Eds., Sinauer Associates, Stanford, CT, 1971, 76.
8. Brandtzaeg, P., Human secretory immunoglobulins. 4. Quantitation of free secretory piece, *Acta Path. Microbiol. Scand.*, 79, 189, 1971.
9. Jones, C., Mermelstein, N., Kincaid-Smith, P., Powell, H., and Roberton, D., Quantification of human serum polymeric IgA, IgA1 and IgA2 immunoglobulin by enzyme immunoassay, *Clin. Exp. Immunol.*, 72, 344, 1988.
10. Mestecky J, Moldoveanu, Z., Julian, B.A., and Prichal, J.T., J chain disease: a novel form of plasma cell dyscrasia, *Am. J. Med.*, 88, 411, 1990.
11. Mesteky, J. and Russell, M.W., IgA Subclasses, *Monogr. Allergy*, 19, 277, 1986.
12. Morell, A., Skvaril, F., Noseda, G., and Bbarandun, S., Metabolic properties of human IgA subclasses, *Clin. Exp. Immunol.*, 13, 521, 1973.
13. Ishizaka, K., Ishizaka, T., and Lee, E.H., Biologic functions of the Fc fragment of E myeloma protein, *Immunochemistry*, 7, 687, 1970.
14. Hamilton, R.G. and Adkinson, N.F., Jr., Serological methods in the diagnosis and management of human allergic disease, *Crit. Rev. Clin. Lab. Sci.*, 21, 1, 1984.
15. Spiegelberg, H.L., Biological activities of immunoglobulins of difference classes and subclasses, *Adv. Immunol.*, 19, 259, 1974.
16. Burton, D.R., Gregory, L., and Jefferis, R., Aspects of molecular structure of IgG subclasses. *Monogr. Allergy*, 19, 7, 1986.
17. Turner, M.W., Structure and function of immunoglobulins, in *Immunochermistry: an Advanced Textbook*, Glynn, L. E. and Steward, M. W., Eds., John Wiley, Chichester, 1977.
18. Whicher, J.T., The role of immunoglobulin assays in clinical medicine, *Ann. Clin. Biochem.*, 21, 461, 1984.
19. Ammann, A.J., Immunodeficiency diseases, in *Basic and Clinical Immunology*, Stites, D.P., Stobo, J.D., and Wells, J.V., Eds., Appleton & Lange, Norwalk, CT, 1987, chap. 20.
20. Wells, J.V., Isbister, J.P., and Ries, C.A., Hematologic diseases, in *Basic and Clinical Immunology*, Stites, D.P., Stobo, J.D., and Wells, J.V., Eds., Appleton & Lange, Norwalk, CT, 1987, chap. 22.
21. Fifield, R. and Keller, I., An immunochemical evaluation for the identification and typing of monoclonal proteins, *Ann. Clin. Biochem.*, 27, 327, 1990.
22. Seppo, T.L., Soppi, E.T., and Morsky, P.J., Critical evaluation of the serum kappa/lambda light chain ratio in the detection of M proteins, *Clin. Chim. Acta*, 207, 143, 1992.

23. Lievens, M.M., Medical and technical usefulness of measurement of kappa and lambda immunoglobulin light chains in serum with an M-component, *J. Clin. Chem. Clin. Biochem.*, 27, 519, 1989.

24. Linscott, W.D., Directory of immunological and biological reagents, 1993, 1(415-383-2666).

25. Jefferis, R., Reimer, C.B., Skvaril, F., De Lange, G., Ling, N.R., Lowe, J., Walker, M.R., Phillips, D.J., Aloiso, C.H., Wells, T.W., Vaerman, J.P., Magnusson, C.G., Kubagawa, H., Cooper, M., Vartdal, F., Vandvik, B., Haaijnan, J.J., Makela, O., Sarnesto, A., Lando, Z., Gergely, J., Rajnavolgyi, E., Laszlo, G., Radl, J., and Molinaro, G., Evaluation of monoclonal antibodies having specificity for human IgG subclasses: result of an IUIS/WHO collaborative study, *Immunol. Lett.*, 10, 223, 1985.

26. Hamilton, R.G., Production and epitope location of monoclonal antibodies to the human IgG subclasses, in *The Human IgG Subclasses: Molecular Analysis of Structure, Function and Regulation*, Shakib, F., Ed., Pergamon Press, New York, 1990, 79.

27. Reimer, C.B., Phillips, D.J., Aloisio, C.H., Moore, D.D., Galland, G.G., Wells, T.W., Black, C.M., and McDougal, J.S., Evaluation of thirty-one mouse monoclonal antibodies to human IgG epitopes, *Hybridoma*, 3, 263, 1984.

28. Phillips, D.J., Wells, T.W., and Reimer, C.B., Estimation of association constants of monoclonal antibodies to human IgG epitopes using fluorescent sequential saturation assays. *Immunol. Lett.*, 17, 159, 1987.

29. Reimer, C.B., Phillips, D.J., Aloisio, C.H., Black, C.M., and Wells, T.M., Specificity and association constants of 33 monoclonal antibodies to human IgA epitopes, *Immunol. Lett.*, 21, 209, 1989.

30. Reimer C.B., Five hydridomas secreting monoclonal antibodies against human IgE, *Monoclonal Antibody News*, 4, 2, 1986.

31. Hamilton R.G., Roebber M., Reimer C.B., and Rodkey S.L., Isoelectric focusing patterns of mouse monoclonal antibodies to the four human IgG subclasses, *Electrophoresis*, 9, 127, 1987.

32. Neuberger, M.S., Williams, G.T., Mitchell, E.B., Joubal, S.S., Flanagan, J.G., and Rabbitts, T.H., A hapten-specific chimeric IgE antibody with human physiological effector function, *Nature*, 314, 268, 1985.

33. Morrison, S.L., Johnson, J.J., Herzenberg, L.A., and Oi, V.T., Chimeric human antibody molecules: mouse antigen-binding domains with human constant region domains, *Proc. Natl. Acad. Sci. U.S.A.*, 81, 6851, 1984.

34. Hamilton R.G. and Morrison S.L., Epitope mapping of human immunoglobulin specific murine monoclonal antibodies with domain switched, deleted, and point-mutated chimeric antibodies, *J. Immunol. Methods*, 158, 107, 1993.

35. Hamilton, R.G., Application of engineered chimeric antibodies to the calibration of human antibody standards, *Ann. Biol. Clin.*, 49, 242, 1991.

36. Rowe, D.S., Grab, B., and Anderson, S.G., An international reference preparation for human serum immunoglobulins G, A and M: content of immunoglobulins by weight, *Bull WHO*, 46, 67, 1972.

37. Reimer, C.B., Smith S.J., Wells, T.W., Nakamura, R.M., Keitges P.W., Ritchie, R.F., Williams, G.W., Hanson, D.J., and Dorsey, D.B., Collaborative calibration of the U.S. National and the College of American Pathologists reference preparations for specific serum proteins, *Am. J. Clin. Pathol.*, 77, 12, 1982.

38. Whicher, J.T., Hunt, J., and Perry, D.E. Method specific variations in the calibration of a new immunoglobulin standard suitable for use in nephelometric techniques, *Clin. Chem.*, 24, 531, 1978.

39. Rowe, D.S., Anderson, S.G., and Tackett, L., A research standard for human serum immunoglobulin D., *Bull. W. H. O.*, 43, 607, 1970.

40. *WHO ECBS Tech. Rep.*, Series No. 658, 23, 21, 1981.

41. Whicher, J.T., Warren, C., and Chambers, R.E., Immunochemical assays for immunoglobulins, *Ann. Clin. Biochem.*, 21, 78, 1984.
42. Mancini, G., Carbonara A.O., and Heremans J.F., Immunochemical quantitation of antigens by single radial immunodiffusion, *Immunochemistry*, 2, 235, 1965.
43. McKelvey, E.M. and Fahey, J.F., Immunoglobulin changes in disease: quantitation on the basis of heavy polypeptide chains, IgG, IgA, and IgM and of light polypeptide chains, *J. Clin. Invest.*, 44, 1778, 1965.
44. College of American Pathologists, Diagnostic Immunology Series 1 Survey, Northfield, IL, 1992.
45. Sternberg, J., A rate nephelometer for measuring specific proteins by immunoprecipitin reactions, *Clin. Chem.*, 23, 1456, 1977.
46. Hills, L.P. and Tiffany, T.O., Comparison of turbimetric and light scattering measurements of immunoglobulins by use of a centrifugal analyzer with absorbance and fluorescence/light scattering optics, *Clin. Chem.*, 26, 1459, 1980.
47. Normansell, D.E., Quantitation of serum immunoglobulins, *Crit. Rev. Clin. Lab. Sci.*, 17, 103, 1982.
48. Hamilton, R.G., Wilson, R., Spillman, T., and Roebber, M., Monoclonal antibody based immunoenzymetric assays for quantification of human IgG and its four subclasses, *J. Immunoassay*, 9, 275, 1988.
49. Papadea, C., Check, I.J., and Reimer, C.B., Monoclonal antibody based solid phase immunoenzymetric assays for quantifying human immunoglobulin G and its subclasses in serum, *Clin. Chem.*, 31, 1940, 1985.
50. Hamilton, R.G. and Adkinson, N.F., Jr., Measurement of total serum immunoglobulin E and allergen-specific immunoglobulin E antibody, in *Manual of Clinical Immunology*, Rose, H.R., de Macario, E.C., Fahey, J.L., Friedman, H., and Penn, G.M., Eds., American Society for Microbiology, Washington, D.C., 1992, 689.
51. Stites, D.P. and Channing Rodgers, R.P., Clinical laboratory methods for detection of antigens and antibodies, in *Basic and Clinical Immunology*, Stites, D.P., Stobo, J.D., and Wells, J.V., Eds., Appleton & Lange, Norwalk, CT, 1987, chap. 17.
52. College of American Pathologists, Diagnostic Allergy Survey (SE), Northfield, IL, 1992.
53. Stiehm, E.R. and Fudenberg, H.H., Serum levels of immune globulins in health and disease, *Pediatrics*, 37, 717, 1966.
54. Weeke, B. and Krasilnikoff, P.A., The concentrations of 21 serum proteins in normal children and adults, *Acta Med. Scand.*, 192, 149, 1972.
55. Hutson, D.K., The performance characteristics of the immunoglobulin method for the Du Pont ACA discrete clinical analyzer, technical bulletin, E-61050, Du Pont Company, Wilmington, DE, 1983.
56. Dati, F., Lammers, M., Adam, A., Sontag, D., and Stienen, L., Reference values for 18 plasma proteins on the Behring Nephelometer System, *Sonderdruck Lab. Med.*, 13, 87, 1989.
57. Technical bulletin, Sanofi Diagnostics Pasteur, 0630891, Chaska, MN.
58. Jolliff, C.R., Cost, K.M., Stivrins, P.C., Grossman, P.P., Nolte, C.R., Franco, S.M., Fijan, K.J., Fletcher, L.L., and Shriner, H.C., Reference intervals for serum IgG, IgA, IgM, C3 and C4 as determined by rate nephelometry, *Clin. Chem.*, 28, 126, 1982.
59. TDxFLxTM Assay Manual for Immunoglobulin G, Immunoglobulin A and Immunoglobulin M, Abbott Laboratories, Abbott Park, IL, R-107, 1991.
60. Herbeth, B., Henny, J., and Siest, G., Biological variations and reference values of transferrin, immunoglobulin A and orosmucoid, *Ann. Biol. Clin.*, 41, 23, 1983.
61. Ritzmann, S.E., Immunoglobulin abnormalities, in *Serum Proteins Abnormalities, Diagnostic and Clinical Aspects*, Ritzmann, S.E. and Daniels, J.C., Eds., Alan R. Liss, New York, 1982, 351.

108 HANDBOOK OF HUMAN IMMUNOLOGY

62. Tietz, N.W., Ed., *Clinical Guide to Laboratory Tests,* Saunders, Philadelphia, 1983.
63. Tibbling, G., Link H., and Ohman, S., Principles of albumin and IgG analysis in neurological disorders. I. Establishment of reference values, *Scand. J. Clin. Lab. Invest.,* 37, 385, 1977.
64. Schur, P.H., Rosen, F., and Norman, M.E., Immunoglobulin G subclasses in normal children, *Pediatr. Res.,* 13, 181, 1979.
65. Allansmith, M., McClellan, B.H., Butterworth, M., and Maloney, J.R., The development of immunoglobulin levels in man, *J. Pediatr.,* 72, 276, 1968.
66. Zegers, B.J., van der Giessen, M., Reerink-Brongers, E.E., and Stoop, J.W., The serum IgG subclass levels in healthy infants of 13–62 weeks of age, *Clin. Chim. Acta,* 101, 265, 1980.
67. van der Giessen, M., Roussow, E., Algra-van Veen, T., Van Loghem, E., Zegers, B.J.M., and Sander, P.C., Quantitation of IgG subclasses in sea of normal adults and healthy children between 4 and 12 years of age, *Clin. Exp. Immunol.,* 21, 501, 1975.
68. Shakelford, P.G., Granoff, D.M., and Hahm, M.G., Relation of age, race and allotype to immunoglobulin subclass concentrations, *Pediatr. Res.,* 19, 846, 1985.
69. Oxelius, V.A. and Svenningsen, N.W., IgG subclass concentrations in preterm neonates, *Acta Pediatr. Scand.,* 73, 626, 1984.
70. Morell, A., Skvaril, F., Hitzig, W.G., and Barandun, S., IgG subclasses: development of the serum concentrations in normal infants and children, *J. Pediatr.,* 80, 960, 1972.
71. Lee, S.I, Heiner, D.C., and Wara, D., Development of serum IgG subclasses levels in children, *Monogr. Allergy,* 19, 108, 1986.
72. Black, C.M., Plikaytis, B.D., Wells, T.W., Ramirez, R.M., Carlone, G.M., Chilmoncyk, B.A., and Reimer, C.B., Two site immunoenzymetric assays for serum IgG subclass infant/maternal ratios at full term, *J. Immunol. Methods,* 106, 71, 1988.
73. Dati, F. and Ringel, K.P., Reference values for serum IgE in healthy non-atopic children and adults, *Clin. Chem.,* 28, 1556, 1982.
74. Ringel, K. P. Dati, F., and Buchhqiz, E., IgE-Normalwerte bei Kindem, *Laboratorumblatter,* 32, 25, 1982.
75. Saarinen, U.M., Juntunen, K., Kajosarri, J., and Bjorksten F., Serum immunoglobulin E in atopic and non-atopic children aged 6 months to 5 years, *Acta Paediatr. Scand.,* 71, 489, 1982.
76. Barbee, R.A., Halomen, M., Lebowitz, M., and Burrows, B., Distribution of IgE in a community population sample: correlations with age, sex and allergen skin test reactivity, *J. Allergy Clin. Immunol.,* 68, 106, 1981.
77. Wittig, H.J., Belloit, J., DeFillippi, I., and Royal, G. Age-related serum IgE levels in healthy subjects and in patients with allergic disease, *J. Allergy Clin. Immunol.,* 66, 305, 1980.
78. Insler, M.S., Lim, J.M., Queng, J.T., Wanissorn, C., and McGovern, J.P., Tear and serum IgE concentrations by tandem R immunoradiometric assay in allergic patients, *Opthalmology,* 94, 945, 1987.
79. McClellan, B.H., Whitney, C.R., Newman, L.P., and Allansmith, M.R., Immunoglobulins in tears, *Am. J. Opthalmol.,* 76, 89, 1973.
80. Ford, R.P., Mitchell, P.E.G., and Fraser, C.G., Desirable performance characteristics and clinical utility of immunglobulin and light chain assays derived from data on biological variation, *Clin. Chem.,* 34, 1733, 1988.
81. Lammers M. and Gressner, A.M., Immunoglobulin light chain determination in serum and urine by use of a fully mechanized immunonephelometric method, *J. Clin. Chem. Clin. Biochem.,* 24, 786, 1986.
82. Skvaril, F., Barandum, S., Morell, A., Kuffer, F., and Probst, M., Imbalances of kappa/lambda immunoglobulin light chain ratios in normal individuals and in immunodeficient patients, in *Protides of Biological Fluids,* Peeters, H., Ed., 23, Pergamon Press, New York, 415, 1975.

83. Sun, T., de Szalay, H., Lien, Y.Y., and Chang, V., Quantitation of kappa and lambda light chains for the detection of monoclonal gammopathy, *J. Clin. Lab. Anal.*, 2, 84, 1988.

84. Manuel, Y., Revillard, J.P., and Betuel, H., *Proteins in Normal and Pathological Urine*, S. Karger, Basel, 1970, 11.

85. Fifield, R. and Hamilton, R.G., Inter-laboratory "external" quality assessment programs for the diagnostic allergy laboratory, *J. Clin. Immunoassay*, 16, 144, 1993.

86. Hamilton, R.G., Inter-laboratory quality control program for IgG subclass protein immunoassays in North America, in *Protides of the Biological Fluids*, Peeters, H., Ed, Vol. 36, Pergamon Press, New York, 127–131, 1989.

87. Hamilton, R.G., Autoantibodies to immunoglobulins: rheumatoid factor interference in immunological assays, *Monogr. Allergy*, 26, 27, 1989.

88. Hamilton, R.G., Monoclonal antibodies in the diagnosis and therapy of human diseases, *Ann. Biol. Clin.*, 47, 575, 1989.

89. Chang, T.W., Davis, F.M., Sun, N.C., Sun, C.R.y., MacGlashan, D.W., and Hamilton, R.G., Monoclonal antibodies specific for human IgE producing B-cells: a potential therapeutic for IgE mediated allergic diseases, *Biotechnology*, 9, 122, 1990.

90. Lichenstein, L.M., Kagey-Sobotka, A., White J.M., and Hamilton, R.G., Anti-human IgG causes basophil histamine release by acting on IgG-IgE complexes bound to IgE receptors, *J. Immunol.*, 148, 3929, 1992.

91. Hamilton, R.G., Molecular engineering: applications to the clinical laboratory, *Clin. Chem.*, 39, 1988, 1993.

92. Mestecky, J., Hamilton, R.G., Magnusson, C.G.M., Jefferis, R., Vaerman, J.P., Goodall, M., de Lange, G.G., Moro, I., Aucouturier, P., Radl, J., Cambiaso, C., Silvain, C., Preud'homme, J.L., Kusama, K., Carlone, G.M., Biewenga, J., Kobaysashi, K., and Reimer, G.B., Evaluation of monoclonal antibodies with specificity for human IgA, IgA subclasses and allotypes and secretory component. Results of an IUIS/WHO collaborative study, *J. Immunol. Methods*, 193(2), 103, 1996.

Chapter 4

IMMUNOLOGIC DIAGNOSIS OF AUTOIMMUNITY

Noel R. Rose

CONTENTS

0-8493-0134-3/97/$0.00+$.50
© 1997 by CRC Press LLC

I. AUTOIMMUNE RESPONSE VS. AUTOIMMUNE DISEASE

Autoimmunity is defined as the immune response to antigens of the host itself. This **autoimmune response** can be demonstrated by the presence of circulating autoantibodies or T lymphocytes reactive with host antigens. A great deal of basic research has been dedicated to unraveling the mechanisms responsible for the body's ability to distinguish its own molecules from foreign molecules (see Chapter 2). Nevertheless, exceptions to the rules governing self/nonself discrimination are well known. Most autoimmune responses do not result in disease. When a response occurs, the pathological consequence of the autoimmune response is called **autoimmune disease**, which is now recognized as an important cause or contributor to human disease. The immunologic diagnosis of autoimmune disease relies mainly on the demonstration of autoantibodies in the patient's serum. This chapter describes the general approach, emphasizing both the uses and abuses of most widely used test procedures.

In undertaking immunologic diagnosis based on the presence of autoantibodies, it is essential to recognize that autoantibodies are normally present. Most of these autoantibodies are members of the IgM isotype and have relatively low affinity for their corresponding antigen (see Chapter 3). They are polyreactive and, consequently, highly interconnected. It has even been suggested that naturally occurring autoantibodies have a physiological function. They may be involved in removing effete or damaged cell products that enter the bloodstream. Equally plausible is the suggestion that naturally occurring autoantibodies may represent an early mechanism of defense against pathogenic microorganisms. For that reason, their high degree of cross-reactivity may provide a substantial advantage in being able to bind a number of invading pathogens. Although of low affinity, IgM autoantibodies are capable of activating the complement cascade, resulting in lysis or opsonization of the pathogens.

The origin of the naturally occurring autoantibodies is still uncertain. It would appear, however, that a relatively large proportion of the B cell repertoire is devoted to producing self-reactive antibodies. In support of this view, many myeloma proteins bind self-antigens.[1] In addition, hybridomas made from B cells of normal individuals frequently produce monoclonal autoantibodies. Often, these antibodies are directed to the cytoskeletal, matrix, or similar large proteins, such as laminin, vimentin, fibronectin, actin, myosin, and collagen.[2] This observation, however, may be biased by the fact that such autoantibodies are relatively easy to demonstrate. More extensive study shows that naturally occurring autoantibodies also react with soluble cell products, such as insulin or thyroglobulin, or intranuclear constituents, such as DNA or topoisomerase.[3,4] Therefore, the presence of these natural autoantibodies sometimes complicates the demonstration of disease-associated autoimmune responses.

Although autoantibodies are common in all human sera, their prevalence is associated with age and sex. The presence and titer of autoantibodies generally increases with age.[5] Since immune responses generally wane with age, this dichotomy causes a striking immunologic paradox; that is, the increase in autoantibodies in the face of a general decrease in immune responses to exogenous antigens.[6] In addition to age, the prevalence of naturally occurring autoantibodies is associated with sex. Natural autoantibodies are more prevalent in women than men. This observation is intriguing because most autoimmune diseases are more frequent in women. The basis of the sex difference in autoimmunity has not been explained. Although elevated estrogen or progesterone levels are frequently cited as the cause for female bias, this hormonal explanation is inadequate, since many autoantibodies continue to rise in women after menopause.[7]

In most test procedures, it is not the presence or absence of an autoantibody that conveys diagnostic significance, but rather its titer and isotype. Most, but not all, disease-associated autoantibodies are present in high titer and are IgG isotype, whereas most, but not all, naturally occurring autoantibodies are low titer IgMs. Exceptions to these general guidelines are sufficiently common that the immunologist must always be alert to the complicating presence of naturally occurring autoantibodies in the diagnostic situation. For that reason, a great deal of current research is devoted to delineating the precise specificity of naturally occurring autoantibodies and contrasting them with the specificity of disease-associated autoantibodies. In autoimmune thyroid disease, for example, our group has shown that the natural autoantibodies are generally directed to those conserved epitopes on the thyroglobulin molecule, which are shared by many different species. In contrast, disease-associated autoantibodies bind primarily the species-limited epitopes of thyroglobulin.[8] We believe that similar instances of defined specificity at the molecular level will improve the laboratory diagnosis of autoimmune disease.

II. CRITERIA OF AUTOIMMUNE DISEASE

Autoimmune disease has been defined as the pathological consequence of an autoimmune response. The mere presence of autoantibodies is insufficient to establish a diagnosis of autoimmune disease, which requires additional clinical and laboratory evidence before reaching such a diagnosis. Recently, we reviewed the steps necessary to establish a human disease as autoimmune.[9] The types of evidence can conveniently be considered as direct, indirect, or circumstantial.

Direct evidence that a human disease is caused by autoimmunity can be obtained in those instances where the pathological injury is due to an autoantibody. Although it is not ethical to reproduce a disease in humans by deliberate serum transfer, nature has provided us with a number of examples of maternal-to-fetal transfer. In this way, it was possible to show that myasthenia gravis is caused by an antibody to the acetylcholine receptor and Graves' disease produced by antibody to the thyrotropin receptor.[10,11] In other instances, transfer of patient's serum to experimental animals successfully reproduces the characteristic pathological changes. Pemphigus vulgaris and bullous pemphigoid have been reproduced by transfer of serum to newborn mice.[12] Sometimes autoantibodies can produce characteristic changes *in vitro* that mimic the disease process, as seen in some forms of hemolytic anemia.[13] Many autoimmune diseases, however, are not caused by the circulating antibody, but rather by cellular immunity. Transfer of such diseases is not yet feasible. Some efforts have been made to utilize immunodeficient SCID mice as *"in vivo"* test tubes, so that both key lymphocytes and target organ of a possible autoimmune disease can be placed in juxtaposition to produce the characteristic lesions.[14] This approach, however, is still in its infancy.

Because of the logistical and ethical restraints involved in assembling direct evidence for the autoimmune etiology of a human disease, most investigations depend upon **indirect evidence** gleaned from experimental animals. Two approaches are widely used. The first requires that the disease be reproduced by experimental immunization, and the second utilizes spontaneously occurring genetic models to replicate the human disease. Each approach has its advantages and shortcomings.

Reproduction of a human disease in an experimental animal requires first that the requisite antigen be identified in human patients. In practical terms, this generally means employing the autoantibody in order to delineate the antigen. An intrinsic problem arises when the antigen recognized by antibody is not the one responsible for initiating a pathogenic autoimmune response. Despite this pitfall, the approach has proved to be highly successful in defining the pathogenic antigens involved in such diseases as chronic thyroiditis, uveitis, and myasthenia gravis.[15-17] The strategy usually employed is to isolate the corresponding antigen from an animal source, inject it into a syngeneic recipient (often accompanied by a potent adjuvant, such as complete Freund's adjuvant or bacterial lipopolysaccharide), and demonstrate that such immunization results in the production of autoantibodies and the appearance of characteristic lesions. A major problem in this strategy is identifying a susceptible experimental animal. Generally, autoimmune responses, particularly pathogenic ones, are genetically limited and, therefore, a number of different species and strains may need to be tested before successful reproduction of a disease can be accomplished. Mice are used most frequently because of the large number of genetically diverse strains available. Moreover, the experimental disease in an animal may not exactly replicate its human analog. Since human autoimmune diseases often involve several antigens, there is a special problem in reproducing the disease with a single, purified antigen. This limitation applies to almost all of the induced models described to date. Experimental immunization, therefore, rarely gives a full and complete picture of a human disease.

The alternative to experimental reproduction of a human disease in animals is to seek out a spontaneous model. Outstanding examples are seen in the murine models of lupus, such as (NZB × NZW)F_1 hybrids, MRL/lpr-lpr, and BXSB.[18] While none of these mouse models can be regarded as a full analog of human lupus, each has contributed substantially to our understanding of the pathogenesis and genetics of the human disorder. Insulin-dependent diabetes is another human autoimmune disease that has not yet been reproduced by experimental immunization. Two spontaneous models, however, are presently available in the NOD mouse and the BB/W rat.[19,20] These models have also contributed greatly to our understanding of this disease. Autoimmune thyroiditis is somewhat unique because both an induced form of disease by experimental immunization with thyroglobulin and spontaneous models present in the OS chicken, the BUF rat, and the NOD H-2^{h-4} mouse are available for investigation.[21]

Although they are not exact replicas of human disease, the experimentally induced and spontaneous models have been essential for establishing the autoimmune etiology of the disorder. In animals, it is possible not only to carry out antibody transfer experiments, but to adoptively immunize recipients with T lymphocytes. In this way, it has been possible to show that the disease is caused by the autoimmune response rather than being the consequence of the disease.

In the case of most human diseases classified as autoimmune, we depend primarily on **circumstantial evidence**. Many autoimmune diseases tend to cluster, either in the same individual or in members of the same family. A patient with autoimmune thyroiditis has a high probability of demonstrating a second or third autoimmune endocrinopathy, such as adrenalitis or diabetes.[22] Relatives of a patient with lupus have a higher than expected prevalence of lupus or related autoimmune diseases, such as rheumatoid arthritis or scleroderma.[23] These clinical observations have given rise to the concept of an autoimmune diathesis; that is, a genetic predisposition to developing autoimmunity. It is still not clear whether this is a single, general predisposition or differs with the different groups of autoimmune diseases. In any case, many diseases of unknown origin, such as scleroderma, are commonly classified as autoimmune because of their affinity for better established autoimmune diseases, such as lupus. The presence of an autoimmune diathesis is best explained by the inheritance of a number of diverse genetic traits. No autoimmune disease has yet been shown to be attributable to a single genetic locus. In most cases, however, the strongest single genetic signal comes from genes of the major histocompatibility complex (MHC), particularly class II MHC (see Chapter 1).[24] In the human, the associations are usually found with the HLA-DP and -DQ markers. Indeed, the presence of a strong HLA association by itself is sometimes cited as circumstantial evidence for an autoimmune etiology, as in the case of ankylosing spondylitis. Moreover, as MHC typing has become refined, the association of particular HLA alleles with disease has increased greatly. It is not out of line to suggest that HLA may be a major predictor or risk factor for the later development of autoimmune disease. If early intervention is reasonable, the subjects may be best defined by their HLA genotype. The search for other genes that contribute to the "autoimmune diathesis" will certainly continue, however, and will strengthen the predictability of autoimmune disease.

The association of particular HLA haplotypes with autoimmune disease suggests that the diversity of molecular epitopes responsible for initiating disease is restricted. Correspondingly, there are a number of diseases where the use of T-cell receptor variable genes early in the course of the disease process appears to be quite limited (see Chapter 14).[25] Either MHC class II V_α or V_β genes may be implicated, although the latter are more often associated with human autoimmune disorders. Indeed, the presence of V_β restriction has, by itself, become an important piece of circumstantial evidence of an autoimmune disease.

Often the clinical identification of a human disease as autoimmune depends mainly upon its response to treatment. A number of drugs capable of suppressing immunity have been successfully employed to treat autoimmune conditions, although the risks of such drugs are obvious. Unless proved otherwise, the effect of the drug should be considered more anti-inflammatory than immunosuppressive, since the dosages given are often insufficient to blunt an autoimmune response.

III. CLASSIFICATION OF AUTOIMMUNE DISEASES

Autoimmune diseases can affect virtually any organ or tissue of the body and, therefore, the clinical manifestations are highly variable. The site of pathology depends primarily upon the distribution and availability of the requisite antigen. Antigens that are widely distributed throughout the body are associated with systemic disease, whereas those confined to a particular tissue or organ are involved in organ-localized autoimmune disease. A convenient classification of autoimmune disease is based on the tissue distribution of pathology. For details of each of these diseases, the reader is referred to Reference 26.

A. Connective Tissue and Rheumatologic Diseases

The most prevalent group of autoimmune diseases attacks the connective tissues or related structures of the body (see Chapter 2). Systemic lupus erythematosus is the prototype of a multiorgan disease. A number of nuclear and cytoplasmic antigens as well as cell surface molecules are targeted by autoimmune responses in lupus, especially native or denatured DNA. The disease is due to the formation of immune complexes, especially DNA–anti-DNA, and characteristically affects multiple tissues and organs. It may involve the skin, the cardiovascular system, the nervous system, the gastrointestinal system, or the renal glomeruli. It is often kidney damage that is the most life-threatening injury in this disease. Although rheumatoid arthritis is thought of primarily as a disease of the joints, it is a systemic condition accompanied by vasculitis caused by immune complexes consisting of rheumatoid factor and its immunoglobulin antigen. Scleroderma affects the connective tissue of the skin, but it is often the esophagus that is the site of the major pathology. Polymyositis/dermatomyositis involve both the skin and the muscles, whereas polymyalgia rheumatica appears to be an autoimmune response primarily involving muscle. One of the most interesting diseases in the connective tissue group is Sjøgren's syndrome (sicca syndrome) with its manifestations of dry eyes and dry mouth. Although the disease clusters with rheumatoid arthritis or lupus, the major pathology involves the lacrimal and salivary glands. Not infrequently such patients also have manifestations of endocrine autoimmunity.

B. Renal Disease

Autoimmune diseases of the kidney fall into two major types. Immune complexes deposited in the glomeruli induce an inflammatory response, resulting in glomerular sclerosis and renal failure. Although any immune complex can, in principle, localize in the kidney, frequent candidates are immune complexes involving autoantigens, such as seen in lupus. A second form of glomerulonephritis involves the production of autoantibodies to the glomerular or tubular basement membranes. These antibodies may follow infection, for example, by β-hemolytic streptococci or exposure to toxins, such as chlorinated hydrocarbons or heavy metals.

C. Skin Disease

A number of important skin diseases are associated with autoimmunity. Pemphigus vulgaris is caused by antibody to the intraepithelial desmosomes, whereas bullous pemphigoid antibodies are directed to antigens of the epithelial basement membrane. A characteristic finding of dermatitis herpetiformis is the presence of deposits of IgA immunoglobulin in the dermis.

D. Nervous System Disease

Myasthenia gravis is one of the best-characterized autoimmune diseases. Autoantibodies to the acetylcholine receptor are present in almost every case. They block the function of the receptor, interrupting neuromuscular signaling and resulting in progressive weakness. Multiple sclerosis, characterized by plaques of demyelinization in the brain and spinal fluid, is associated with an autoimmune response to myelin antigens. A possible experimental analog of this disease is found in the form of allergic encephalomyelitis, one of the best characterized of the experimentally induced autoimmune diseases. The role of autoimmunity in peripheral neuropathies, including Guillain-Barré syndrome, is often cited, although firm evidence is still lacking.

E. Cardiovascular Disease

The classic example of an autoimmune disease associated with microbial infection is rheumatic heart disease, a sequela of infection by *Streptococcus pyogenes*. The mechanism is believed to be molecular mimicry, that is, the presence on the streptococcal membrane of an antigen that resembles a constituent of the heart. Recent evidence suggests that myosin may be that antigen, although the disease has not yet been reproduced experimentally. In the U.S., rheumatic heart disease has become rare, although it is still highly prevalent in many of the developing countries. A more common form of myocarditis in the U.S. follows infection with Coxsackievirus. This disease is characterized by production of multiple antibodies to heart antigens. The disease has been reproduced by experimental immunization of mice with purified myosin, making myosin the leading candidate as initiating antigen. Many vasculitides, such as Wegener's granulomatosis and nephrosclerosis, are associated with autoimmune responses, especially to antineutrophil cytoplasmic antigens (ANCA).

Antiphospholipid syndrome is associated with clotting problems, thrombosis, spontaneous abortion, and stroke, and derives its name from the presence of antibodies to anionic phospholipids and a cofactor β_2 glycoprotein-1.

F. Gastrointestinal Disease

Two important diseases of the liver are associated with characteristic autoimmune responses. In some cases of chronic active hepatitis, antibodies are found to smooth muscle cells where the major antigen has been identified as actin. Sometimes these patients also have antinuclear antibodies. In primary biliary cirrhosis, antibodies to mitochondria can be demonstrated; one antigen is the enzyme, pyruvic oxidase. The inflammatory bowel diseases, Crohn's disease and ulcerative colitis, are often cited as autoimmune disorders, although the antigens have not been identified and no immunological tests are available.

G. Endocrine Disease

Autoimmune thyroiditis has become the prototypic organ-localized disease. The primary antigen, thyroglobulin, is capable of inducing the disease experimentally. Other antigens, such as thyroid peroxidase, however, are useful indicators of clinical activity. In Graves' disease, antibodies to the thyrotropin receptor are responsible for the induction of hyperthyroidism. Insulin-dependent diabetes has emerged as one of the most debilitating of the autoimmune diseases. It is characterized by the presence of autoantibodies to glutamic acid decarboxylase, insulin, and several other beta cell constituents, but the initiating antigen has not yet been established with certainty. The result, however, is the immunological destruction of the beta cells of the pancreatic islets. Other endocrine disorders, such as adrenalitis, hypoparathyroidism, or hypophysitis are associated with production of autoantibodies to the particular organ.

Pernicious anemia is caused by antibodies to the gastric secretion, intrinsic factor, which facilitates absorption of vitamin B12. Antibodies to gastric mucosa are frequently present. This disease is often associated with the autoimmune endocrinopathies, such as chronic thyroiditis.

H. Hematologic Disease

Acquired hemolytic anemia represents the classic example of an autoimmune response to a circulating red blood cell. IgM antibodies are associated primarily with cold-reactive anemias, in which the blood cells are injured if the temperature falls to subnormal levels. However, warm hemolytic anemias certainly can result in sequestration of the IgG antibody-coated red blood cells in spleen and other reticuloendothelial tissues. Other blood cells are also susceptible to antibody-mediated destruction seen in the form of leukopenias or thrombocytopenias. However, the demonstration of antibodies to these cells is difficult because of spontaneous absorption of immunoglobulin. Finally, one of the most important emerging autoimmune diseases is seen in the form of an autoimmune response to clotting factors. This antiphospholipid syndrome may result in bleeding tendencies (the lupus anticoagulant), increased clotting as a cause of stroke, or spontaneous abortion.

IV. METHODS FOR DETECTING AUTOANTIBODIES

A. Precipitation and Agglutination

The appropriate method for demonstrating autoantibodies is determined by the position and properties of the antigen and the level of sensitivity desired. Precipitation and agglutination were the first methods employed for demonstrating autoantibodies in human sera. Precipitation of cardiolipin has long served as a method for supporting the diagnosis of syphilis. Immunoprecipitation, using radioisotope-labeled antigen, is a more sensitive method for detecting antibodies, and nephalometric or turbidimetric analyses have replaced precipitation in larger laboratories. Precipitation in agar remains a good method for the precise recognition of the cellular antigens involved in lupus and related connective tissue diseases. The classic Ouchterlony test is still used for verifying antibodies to Sm or other nuclear antigens. Agglutination reactions are highly sensitive methods for demonstrating antibody. Indirect, or conditioned, hemagglutination requires that a soluble antigen be attached to a particle, such as a red blood cell or latex. Latex agglutination is a widely used test for the measurement of rheumatoid factor, whereas agglutination of red blood cells treated with chromic chloride or tannic acid is the most sensitive procedure for demonstrating antibodies to thyroglobulin. The direct Coombs' anti-globulin test for immunoglobulin on the surface of red blood cells is the cornerstone for the diagnosis of autoimmune hemolytic anemia.

B. Immunofluorescence

A commonly used test for the detection of antibodies to tissue antigens is indirect immunofluorescence. The great versatility of this test is due to the fact that the antigen need not be precisely characterized or purified. In fact, multiple tissue substrates can be used and antibodies to a number of tissues recognized. The most common test for antinuclear antibodies utilizes either tissue slices or tissue culture cells. Antibodies to smooth muscle or mitochondria as seen in hepatic diseases, such as chronic active hepatitis or primary biliary cirrhosis, are readily measured on composite blocks of several different tissues. ANCA utilizes fixed or treated neutrophils as substrate. In some instances, peroxidase is preferable to fluorescein as a tag. The tissue architecture is more readily recognized, and permanent preparations can be obtained. However, endogenous peroxidases can cause false positive results.

C. Immunoassays

Immunoassays have long been employed to detect autoantibodies in a very sensitive manner. The requisite antigen can be attached directly to the plastic vessel or "captured" by a first layer of antibody. Patient serum is then added and immunoglobulin measured by means of a radioisotope enzymatic or fluorescent marker. At this time, the enzyme-linked immunosorbent assay (ELISA) is the most widely used test for measuring autoantibodies to tissue antigens. It is most appropriate when the antigen is available in purified form.

D. Western Immunoblots

An important addition to the immunological armamentarium has been the Western immunoblot. This procedure does not require that the antigen be pure, but only that it be present in a relatively high concentration in a tissue preparation. The antigen mixture is first separated by electrophoresis, transferred to nitrocellulose membrane, and reacted with the patient serum. The location of the antibody is identified by secondary antibodies conjugated to an enzyme that will develop a color when a chromogenic substance is added. The method is often used to verify or characterize reactions to complex antigens.

E. Functional Tests

The final group is represented by a group of bioassays and receptor assays. They are often employed in demonstrating antibodies to cell receptors; for example, antibody to the thyrotropin receptor present in Graves' disease can be demonstrated either by direct binding to the thyrotropin receptor or by measuring the increase in cAMP production by cultured thyroid cells.

Detailed descriptions of the many tests available for demonstration of autoantibodies are presented in recent publications.[27,28] The reader is directed to these references for details of the methodology as well as discussions of the appropriate interpretation involved in the procedures.

REFERENCES

1. Yativ, N., Buskila, D., Blank, M., Burek, C. L., Rose, N. R., and Shoenfeld, Y., The detection of antithyroglobulin activity in human serum monoclonal immunoglobulins (monoclonal gammopathies), *Immunol. Res.*, 12, 330, 1993.
2. Dighiero, G., Guilbert, B., Fernand, J. P., Lymberi, P., Danon, F., and Avrameas, S., Thirty-six human monoclonal immunoglobulins with antibody activity against cytoskeleton proteins, thyroglobulin, and native DNA: immunologic studies and clinical correlations, *Blood*, 62, 264, 1983.
3. Bresler, H. S., Burek, C. L., Hoffman, W. H., and Rose, N. R., Autoantigenic determinants on human thyroglobulin. II. Determinants recognized by autoantibodies from patients with chronic autoimmune thyroiditis compared to autoantibodies from healthy subjects, *Clin. Immunol. Immunopathol.*, 54, 76, 1990.
4. Grabar, P., Autoantibodies and the physiological role of immunoglobulins, *Immunol. Today*, 4, 337, 1983.
5. Bottazzo, G. F. and Doniach, D., Autoimmune thyroid disease, *Annu. Rev. Med.*, 37, 217, 1986.
6. Talor, E. and Rose, N. R., Hypothesis: the aging paradox and autoimmune disease, *Autoimmunity*, 8, 245, 1991.
7. Rose, N. R., Thymus function, aging and autoimmunity, *Immunol. Lett.*, 40, 225, 1994.
8. Caturegli, P., Mariotti, S., Kuppers, R. C., Burek, C. L., Pinchera, A., and Rose, N. R., Epitopes on thyroglobulin: a study of patients with thyroid disease, *Autoimmunity*, 18, 41, 1994.
9. Rose, N. R. and Bona C., Defining criteria for autoimmune diseases (Witebsky's postulates revisited), *Immunol. Today*, 14, 426, 1993.
10. Lefvert, A. K., Anti-indiotype antibodies in myasthenia gravis, *Biological Applications of Antiidiotypes*, Bona, C., Ed., CRC Press, Boca Raton, FL, 1988, 22.
11. Davies, T. and DeBernardo, E., Thyroid autoantibodies and diseases, *An Overview in Autoimmune Endocrine Disease*, Davies, T., Ed., J. Wiley & Sons, New York, 1983, 127.
12. Anhalt, G. J., Labib, R. S., Voorhees, J. J., Beals, T. F., and Diaz, L. A., Induction of pemphigus in neonatal mice by passive transfer of IgG from patients with the disease, *N. Engl. J. Med.*, 306, 1189, 1982.
13. Donath, J., and Landsteiner, K., Ueber paroxysmale Hämoglobinurie, *Muench. Med. Wochenschr.*, 51, 1590, 1904.
14. Volpé, R., Kasuga, Y., Akasu, F., Morita, T., Yoshikawa, N., Resetkova, E., and Arreaza, G., The use of the severe combined immunodeficient mouse and the athymic "nude" mouse as models for the study of human autoimmune thyroid disease, *Clin. Immunol. Immunopathol.*, 67, 93, 1993.
15. Witebsky, E., Rose, N. R., Terplan, K., Paine, J. R., and Egan, R. W., Chronic thyroiditis and autoimmunization, *J. Am. Med. Assoc.*, 164, 1439, 1957.
16. Gery, I. and Streilein, J. W., Autoimmunity in the eye and its regulation, *Curr. Opinion Immunol.*, 6, 938, 1994.
17. Gomez, C. M. and Richman, D. P., Chronic experimental autoimmune myasthenia gravis induced by monoclonal antibody to acetylcholine receptor: biochemical and electrophysiological criteria, *J. Immunol.*, 139, 73, 1987.
18. Theofilopoulos, A. N. and Dixon, F. J., Murine models of systemic lupus erythematosus, *Adv. Immunol.*, 37, 269, 1985.
19. Makino, S., Kunimoto, Y., Muraoka, Y., Mizushima, Y., Katagiri, K., and Tochino, Y., Breeding of a non-obese, diabetic strain of mice, *Exp. Anim. (Jikken Dobutsu)*, 29, 1, 1980.

20. Nakhooda, A. F., Like, A. A., Chappel, C. I., Murray, F. T., and Marliss, E. B., The spontaneous diabetic Wistar rat: metabolic and morphologic studies, *Diabetes*, 26, 100, 1977.

21. Kuppers, R. C., Neu, N., and Rose, N. R., Animal models of autoimmune thyroid disease, *Immunogenetics of Endocrine Disorders*, Farid, N. R., Ed., Alan R. Liss, New York, 1988, 111.

22. Hall, R., Dingle, P. R., and Roberts, D. F., Thyroid antibodies: a study of first degree relatives, *Clin. Genet.*, 3, 319, 1972.

23. Rose, N. R., The spectrum of autoimmunity: mechanisms of organ-specific and nonorgan-specific diseases, *Immunopathol. Immunotherapy Lett.*, 3, 8, 1988.

24. Rose, N. R. and Burek, C. L., The interaction of basic science and population-based research: Autoimmune thyroiditis as a case history, *Am. J. Epidemiol.*, 134, 1073, 1991.

25. Baroldi, G., Corallo, S., Moroni, M., Repossini, A., Mutinelli, M. R., Lazzarin, A., Antonacci, C. M., Cristina, S., and Negri, C., Focal lymphocytic myocarditis in acquired immunodeficiency virus (AIDS): a correlative morphologic and clinical study in 26 consecutive fatal cases, *J. Am. Coll. Cardiol.*, 12, 463, 1988.

26. Rose, N. R. and Mackay, I. R., *The Autoimmune Diseases*, 3rd ed., Academic Press, Orlando, FL, (in press).

27. Rose, N. R., et al., *Manual of Clinical Laboratory Immunology*, 5th ed., ASM Press, Washington, D.C., (in press).

28. Peter, J. B. and Shoenfeld, Y., *Autoantibodies*, Elsevier, Amsterdam, 1996.

Chapter 5

INFECTIOUS DISEASE SEROLOGY

Kimberly L. Kane and James D. Folds

CONTENTS

0-8493-0134-3/97/$0.00+$.50
© 1997 by CRC Press LLC

I. INTRODUCTION

A. General Principles

The concept that extrinsically derived disease may exist inside humans and animals and may be transmitted from one individual to another has been discussed for at least 4 centuries and has been the basis for studying infectious diseases. By speculating upon the way hosts fight infectious diseases, we have broadened our understanding of the immune system as well. As we comprehend the function of the immune system, we learn not only how to prevent disease, but also how to diagnose it accurately. While our techniques for diagnosing infectious diseases have changed over the years, our strategies have not. By taking advantage of the memory and specificity of the immune system, we can precisely define those challenges to the integrity of the whole system.

The purpose of this chapter is to highlight some of the most important historical, current, and prospective techniques that may be useful in the laboratory diagnosis of infectious diseases. The advantages, disadvantages, and proposed improvements of each methodology are discussed in the context of clinical diagnosis. Additionally, the caveats of immunologic testing will be included where appropriate within discussions of diagnosis, treatment, and prognosis.

The primary reason for performing serological studies in the diagnosis of infectious diseases is to identify the cause of an ongoing infection when cultures of the pathogen are unsuccessful or impractical. While culture of the causative agent would provide the definitive answer, many organisms are too difficult or dangerous to culture or have a long incubation period, making microbiological testing less useful to the clinician who is treating the patient. In many cases, serology allows the clinician to identify the causative agent and to evaluate the status of the patient's immune response against the causative agent rapidly. The outcome of the assay very often reveals the pathogen and may help identify the stage of the patient's infection. Serology may offer a faster, less labor intensive alternative to culture that is not dependent on specimen quality or viability of the microorganisms. It is applicable to the identification of bacteria, fungi, viruses, and parasites. However, serology is more dependent on the quality of the patient's immune response and the timing of specimen collection with respect to the onset of symptoms and the course of the disease. Additionally, serologic results may be more difficult to interpret than are cultures because of the large number of variables that may affect the immune response to a given pathogen. Nevertheless, serological studies have become a foundation for laboratory diagnosis of bacterial, viral, fungal, and parasitic infections.

The principle behind all serologic assays is the specificity of an antibody for a defined and unique epitope on an antigen and the strong noncovalent interactions that make the interaction stable. The epitope of the antigen is that portion of the antigen which is recognized and bound by the antibody. Likewise, the paratope is the portion of the antibody which recognizes and binds to the antigen. This interaction, because of its specificity and stability, allows for the binding and detection of antigens present in very small quantities. The memory of the immune system is also crucial for the use of serologic tests. The ability of the host's immune response to remember those pathogens it has seen before and to mount a faster response with a larger production of IgG compared to IgM permits the distinction between primary and secondary responses. The nature of the antigen–antibody interaction is based upon the polymorphic region of the antibody molecule that binds strongly to the epitope (antigenic determinant) on the antigen for which the antibody is specific. In other words, the paratope of the antibody binds to the epitope of the antigen, leading to a strong and specific interaction that can be easily measured in the laboratory. Although different antigens or pathogens may possess cross-reactive or similar epitopes, this interaction is considered to be very specific. Thus, when positive identification of an organism by culture is not possible, serology provides an alternative analysis of the patient's infection status.

There must be a means to visualize or measure the binding interaction in order to use the formation of antigen–antibody complexes for the identification of pathogens. There are a variety of techniques by which these complexes can be detected. When antigen–antibody complexes (immune complexes) form, they become less soluble in liquid or agar; therefore, the degree of precipitation should be proportional to the number of complexes formed. Alternatively, either the antigen or the antibody may be tagged with a label that can be followed; for example, a radioactive molecule or a fluorescent compound could be used. Then the label (i.e., the radioactivity or the fluorescence) can be traced. Another method involves fixing the antigen or the antibody to a solid matrix, like a microtiter plate, so that molecules which bind will be captured and can be quantitated. This method requires a secondary step to measure the amount of antigen or antibody that has bound to the immobilized antigen or antibody.

Alternatively, if the antigen or antibody is attached to latex beads, then combining patient serum with the labeled beads will allow cross-linking to occur. When cross-linking between multiple molecules of antigen and antibody occurs, the latex beads will agglutinate forming an observable clump in the reaction cell. One last method that will allow visualization of antigen–antibody complex formation involves antigens that are bound to the surface of a cell. Red blood cells are used because of the ease with which they can be coated with antigen and the ease with which they may be seen due to the presence of the hemoglobin. After antibody binds to the antigen on the surface of the red blood cells, heterogeneous complement is added and will lyse the red blood cells to which antibody is bound. Then, the absence of intact red blood cells indicates the presence of antigen–antibody complex formation.

B. Limitations

A caveat for the interpretation of serological techniques is that they rely upon the appropriate production of antibody by the host. Thus, serologic methods will only detect the presence of disease when the patient produces antibodies against the pathogen. This point must be remembered in evaluating immunosuppressed or immunodeficient patients who may not produce sufficient or appropriately specific antibodies. Furthermore, qualitative differences in humoral responses may be crucial in the serological identification of microorganisms. Because serologic techniques are used for more than just identification of causative agents, it is important to understand the role of other characteristics of the immune response. As the immune response progresses, the level of specific antibodies, or titer, present in the peripheral blood should increase until the causative agent has been cleared. Once the agent is eliminated, the titer generally begins to fall. Therefore, changes in titer can be used to predict the disease course. Similarly, the isotype may switch during infection in a normal host. However, immunosuppressed or immunodeficient patients may not exhibit some or all of these characteristics. For example, a child with an immunodeficiency may not make detectable levels of specific antibodies against organisms in a vaccine preparation, and consequently, increases in antibody titers following immunization will be absent. Even cellular immunodeficiencies may show a decreased specific antibody response because helper T lymphocytes are unable to provide cytokines to drive B-cell proliferation, differentiation, and isotype switching. Some immunoglobulin class deficiencies may also interfere with the diagnosis of infectious diseases by serology because the distinction between primary and secondary immune responses is based upon the switch from IgM to other immunoglobulin isotypes.

   Clearly, infection with the human immunodeficiency virus 1 (HIV) leads to decreased numbers of CD4+ T cells and, along with many other cellular disorders, may produce clinical symptoms of acquired immunodeficiency syndrome (AIDS). This infection may prevent efficient use of serologic tests because the infected patients become immunocompromised.[1] HIV-infected individuals produce especially weak IgM responses during primary infections. Additionally, they may not demonstrate a significant rise in IgG titer upon reexposure to a known antigen. Because HIV infections inactivate the helper T-lymphocyte population, T cells are unable to stimulate antibody production or isotype switching. These changes in antibody production are essential to accurate determination of the patient's infectious disease status.

   Similar to the prerequisite for a functional immune response, there is an obligation for appropriate patient serum sampling to accurately identify the timing and disease course. Specimens taken very early after disease onset may not show measurable antibody levels because there has not been adequate time for the development of a complete antibody response. For accurate interpretation, most infectious disease serologic tests require both acute and convalescent samples. These samples should be taken 2 to 3 weeks apart. The purpose of more than one sample is to identify changing titers of each of the isotypes of antibodies. Under certain circumstances, a single very high titer antibody response may be indicative of an active or very recent infection. During a primary response, IgM titers usually rise first, followed by increasing IgG titers. If sampling occurs too early in the course of the disease, the serum may not reflect yet the rise in IgG; rises in both IgM and IgG may indicate primary infections. Additionally, different patients have different background titers against different antigens, and therefore, one patient's background IgG titer may be similar to an increased titer in another patient. To distinguish a new or recent infection from a past infection, a second sample must be analyzed to detect any changes in the titer with respect to the first sample. Generally, a fourfold change in titer is considered diagnostic of current infection; whether the titer rises or falls will depend upon when during the course of infection the samples were taken.[2] Rarely, very high IgM levels against specific pathogens have been used to presumptively diagnose ongoing infection in the absence of a second serum sample. However, this conclusion should still be confirmed with a follow-up specimen.

   Again, infections, such as those with HIV, can confound the analysis of acute and convalescent serum pairing in disease diagnosis. Patients with compromised immune responses will not always show large (i.e., fourfold changes) differences in immunoglobulin titers when exposed to a new antigenic challenge. Additionally, they may not show an anamnestic response during a recurrence of an old infection. HIV patients usually show overall diminished IgM responses that may be completely absent late in the disease course. Care should be taken when monitoring any immunocompromised patient by serology because of the possibly inaccurate interpretations that may be made from serologic results. An example of an illness that merits special attention is toxoplasmosis, which frequently occurs in HIV-infected patients; during this disease, patients sometimes make very little antibody against specific antigens, and specific antibody titers may not rise in spite of the presence of causative organisms.[2] Therefore, the absence of a specific antibody under these circumstances should not be used to definitively rule out infection if the clinical picture suggests that toxoplasmosis may be in the differential diagnosis.

C. Prospective Developments

Several new techniques have recently been applied to the diagnosis of infectious diseases. One of the best improvements is the added ability to test directly for the antigen in question, rather than testing for the presence of the pathogen indirectly by measuring an antibody response against the pathogen. These tests for antigen eliminate the dependence upon the immune response. Because these tests do not measure antibody production, they are effective even in patients who are immunocompromised or immunodeficient. This approach also eliminates false positive reactions due to cross-reactive epitopes. Antibodies that are specific for similar or cross-reactive epitopes will not be detected by a test that examines antigen directly.

In addition to direct antigen detection, the diagnosis of infectious diseases has benefited from technical advances in enzyme immunoassays. A major development based on enzyme-linked technology has been the IgM capture assay. Enzyme-linked immunosorbant assays (ELISA) or enzyme immunoassays are based on the specificity of antibody for antigenic epitopes resulting in a stable bond that can withstand washing. These assays are further discussed in Section II.

Anti-immunoglobulin reagents have been useful in serologic diagnosis and flow cytometry. Production of anti-immunoglobulin is based on the principle that an antibody can be an antigen for another antibody. Use of anti-immunoglobulin results in amplification of the detection signal. Labeled anti-immunoglobulin reagents, as secondary or tertiary antibodies specific for the original detection antibody, increases the number of enzymatic, radioactive, luminescent, or fluorescent tags. By increasing the tag to antigen ratio, the signal will be stronger, allowing better discrimination between positive and negative samples. Alternatively, one may use the biotin–avidin amplification cascade.[3] These two reagents bind strongly to each other with multiple binding sites per molecule. By attaching a tag to one of these compounds and attaching the other compound to the detection antibody, the signal from the tag in a positive sample is enhanced. Anti-complement antibodies can also be used to detect antigen–antibody complexes if complement is allowed to interact with the complexes in the reaction well.[3] The complement recognizes and binds to the immune complex, and anti-complement antibodies that are labeled will bind to the attached complement. The anti-complement antibodies can be labeled with a detectable tag, and then the presence of the tag indicates immune complex formation has occurred and that antigen-specific antibody has been produced by the patient.

One last concept to remember is that serologic techniques can be used in multiple combinations. Tests for antigen and antibody can be used simultaneously to increase sensitivity and specificity of testing procedures. This will be discussed in more detail later in this chapter. This is most often useful in fluorescence assay systems. Additionally, many different detection systems can be used with any available antigen-specific test. Therefore, serologic techniques can be tailored to provide the best sensitivity and specificity for each application. This enhances the ability of the immunology laboratory to provide reliable and accurate results.

II. SEROLOGICAL METHODS

Table 1 lists the most common traditional techniques applied in the clinical immunology laboratory for infectious disease diagnosis. While only one example of an application of each test is given in Table 1, all of these techniques can be used in many different detection systems. Certain of these techniques have been replaced by other techniques that are more sensitive or specific.

A. Double Diffusion

Double diffusion in agar, developed by Ouchterlony, is a classical method that is used to determine the presence or absence of specific antibodies and antigens.[1-3] In this assay, wells in an agar plate are filled with known antigens and antibodies. These antigen or antibody proteins will diffuse across the agar, and when they meet, if they are specific for each other, they will form a precipitation line of immune complexes. When two adjacent specimens contain the same antigen or antibody, a characteristic line will appear where these two meet with their respective antigen or antibody. The classic patterns which form allow the identification of the antigen present in the patient specimen. In this way, antigen-specific antibodies can be identified by subclass or

TABLE 1

Classical Methods and Their Applications in Infectious
Disease Serology

Method	Application
Double diffusion in agar	Fungal serology
Counterimmunoelectrophoresis	Bacterial antigen detection
Hemagglutination	MHA-TP for *T. pallidum*
Hemagglutination inhibition	Viral serology
Latex agglutination	Bacterial antigen detection
Coagglutination	Bacterial antigen detection
Complement fixation	Bacterial and viral serologies
Neutralization assay	Antibodies to bacterial toxins
Immunofluorescence assay	
Direct	Bacterial and viral serologies
Indirect	Bacterial and viral serologies
Immunoassay	
Radioimmunoassay	Viral serologies
Enzyme-linked immunoassay	Bacterial and viral serologies

antigenic components can be distinguished. This test has been used for
fungal and parasitic serologies, including histoplasmosis, aspergillosis,
amebiasis, echinococcosis, trichinosis, and trypanosomiasis.

B. Counterimmunoelectrophoresis

Counterimmunoelectrophoresis is another technique that has been
used for the detection of bacterial antigens from *Neisseria meningitidis*,
Hemophilus influenza type b, *Streptococcus pneumoniae*, and group B
Streptococcus.[1] It is very similar to double diffusion, except that an
electric current is applied to increase the rate of protein traveling
through the agar. This improvement shortens the time required from
over 24 h to less than 1 h. It also increases the sensitivity of the assay
many fold over simple immunodiffusion. This method was widely
used for the detection of bacterial antigens in the cerebrospinal fluid
or urine from children suspected of having bacterial meningitis. More
recently, this method has been replaced by latex agglutination, which
is more sensitive and easier to perform.

C. Hemagglutination

Hemagglutination is a method that visualizes the antigen–antibody
interaction by using red blood cells previously coated with the antigen
under investigation.[3] Using a variety of different methods, specific
soluble antigens can be coupled to red blood cells. Then, when the
patient's serum is added, the antibody present binds the antigen on

the cell surface, cross-links different cells together, and causes the cells to agglutinate. By examining the cells under the microscope or by examining the cell pellet, it is possible to determine if agglutination has occurred. This method has been standardized for many bacterial and protozoan antigens. An example of one of the assays currently using this technique is the microhemagglutination–*Treponema pallidum* (MHA-TP) that detects the presence of antibodies against *Treponema pallidum* in patients suspected of having syphilis. One disadvantage to agglutination tests is that especially high titers of antibody may interfere with the formation of a lattice, leading to a false negative result because of the prozone phenomenon. The prozone occurs when the concentration of antigen is low and the concentration of antibody is high. Under these conditions, antigen–antibody complex formation is reduced since antigen concentration is limiting, thereby resulting in falsely negative results. However, this test can detect even low levels of IgM directed against the specific antigen because IgM is 750 times more efficient at cross-linking red blood cells than is IgG.[2] This is a very sensitive method that is used in many clinical laboratories today as well as a number of state public health laboratories.

D. Hemagglutination Inhibition

A variation of the hemagglutination assay is the hemagglutination inhibition assay. Because certain viruses spontaneously agglutinate animal red blood cells, this assay can be used to quantitate antiviral antibodies present by their ability to block the spontanteous agglutination after binding to the viral particles. Therefore, the amount of hemagglutination is inversely proportional to the amount of antiviral specific antibodies in the patient sample.

E. Latex Agglutination

Latex agglutination is similar to hemagglutination because it is dependent on the formation of antigen–antibody complexes which cross-link the solid phase of the reaction which, in this case, is a latex bead. This assay can be adapted for the measurement of antigen or antibody in the specimen, which can be serum, cerebrospinal fluid, urine, or other body fluids. It has been used for quantitating capsular polysaccharide from microorganisms like *Cryptococcus neoformans* and heterophile antibody during Epstein-Barr viral infections.[2,4] Latex agglutination is widely accepted as the method of detection for bacterial antigens in suspected cases of bacterial meningitis in young children. Urine is an excellent specimen for these studies and the antigenic polysaccharide may be excreted in urine for days after the infection.

F. Coagglutination

Coagglutination is very similar to latex agglutination. The primary difference is that, instead of coating latex beads with antibody specific for the antigen being tested for, the antibody is bound to certain strains of *Staphylococcus aureus*.[3] This is achieved by protein A, a surface component of certain staphylococcal strains that has a natural affinity for the Fc portion of IgG. It is used primarily for the detection of bacterial antigens in a specimen. The advantage of this method is the ease with which antibody of any specificity can be conjugated to a solid substrate.

G. Complement Fixation

Complement fixation is a test that is still widely used today for many bacterial, viral, and chlamydial infections.[1,3] The principle of the assay is competition for a limited amount of complement between immune complexes from a known indicator system and complexes formed by antibodies in patient samples specific for the antigen under study. The first step of the assay allows the patient specimen and the appropriate antigen or antibody to interact with each other and with complement components. The complement will interact with any antigen–antibody complexes that form with the patient sample and will not be free to interact during the second step of the assay. In the second step, the indicator system, antibody-coated red blood cells, is mixed with any remaining complement components. The amount of red cell lysis observed is inversely proportional to the amount of immune complex formation during the first step. Therefore, if a patient has, for example, a mycoplasmal infection, then, the presence in the patient of *Mycoplasma*-derived antigens will be identified by their interaction with known anti-mycoplasma antibodies. The amount of red cell lysis in this case would be very low because the majority of the complement would have bound the *Mycoplasma*-specific immune complexes and would not be available to lyse the red blood cells. The complement fixation test (CF) is useful for the confirmation of the laboratory diagnosis of Rocky Mountain spotted fever. Although CF antibodies appear very late in the infection, the test has a high specificity and is useful for epidemiologic purposes.

H. Neutralization Assays

Neutralization assays take advantage of the ability of antibodies to bind to and inhibit the toxicity of bacterial toxins, the adherence of bacterial cells, and the internalization of intracellular pathogens.[1,2] These assays are sometimes used clinically for the detection of antibodies directed against viruses. However, these assays are labor intensive and require several days to 1 week to complete and are being replaced in many cases by ELISA assays. Neutralization is accomplished by mixing the patient's sera with a toxin or virus culture. This combination is then injected into an animal in the case of the toxin assay or incubated on a susceptible cell line for several days in the case of a virus. If the injected animal becomes ill, then the toxin was not bound by antibody. If the animal remains healthy, then the toxin was neutralized by the presence of toxin-specific antibodies from the patient's serum. Alternatively, the appearance of viral growth or the formation of viral plaques in culture indicates that no specific antibodies were present in the serum. If antibodies are present, they will bind to the virus and inhibit its infectivity and plaques will not appear. This method can be used to titer the serum antibody concentration and may be used with paired sera to identify ongoing or recent past infection.

I. Direct and Indirect Immunofluorescence

Immunofluorescence assays are widely used in immunology laboratories for many infectious diseases of viral and bacterial origin.[1] In the indirect assay, antigens derived from the organism are adhered to a plastic or glass solid phase. The patient's serum is added to the well or bead or other solid phase, and if specific antibodies are present, they will bind to the antigen. The last step involves the addition of a fluorescently labeled antihuman immunoglobulin. The presence of specific antibody in the patient specimen can then be detected by the presence of fluorescent staining of the microbial antigen. This general procedure can be modified for the identification of antigen present in the serum, as discussed in more detail later. Indirect immunofluorescence is especially useful for determining the presence of antibody directed against viruses. Depending on the specificity of the secondary anti-immunoglobulin conjugate, IgM and IgG can be distinguished from each other.[1] It is also used for determining the presence of antitreponemal antibodies in the fluorescence treponemal antibody absorption (FTA-ABS) assay for syphilis.

Immunofluorescence is also used for detecting microorganisms directly by using fluorescently labeled antibodies specific for various pathogens. Slides made from the patient specimen are incubated with the fluorescently labeled antibodies directed against the pathogen itself, not against immunoglobulin. Using fluorescent microscopy, the presence of organisms can be confirmed both by positive fluorescent staining and by morphology. Unfortunately, this method cannot be automated, and must be read by highly trained technologists. It is subjective, rather than objective, in analysis, but it is a very sensitive test. Amplification methods using secondary immunoglobulin conjugates (specific for other immunoglobulin) can make the fluorescent signal more intense and clearly distinguishable from any background staining. While highly specific, direct immunofluorescence may not yield definitive results in many cases because of difficulties in obtaining suitable specimens or because of low concentrations of antigen.

J.   Radioimmunoassay

Another method for detecting antibodies against bacterial or viral pathogens takes advantage of radioisotopes that can be used to label or tag molecules involved in an antigen–antibody interaction. Radioimmunoassays (RIA) employ radioactively labeled antibodies that can be quantitated by gamma emission counters.[1,5] The amplification afforded by the isotopic labeling makes this assay extremely sensitive. RIAs can accurately measure picogram amounts of antigen and antibody, and they have been adapted for measuring many different hormones and metabolites as well. Quantitative analysis can be performed by generating a standard curve using known amounts of antigen or antibody. Competition between the known amount of radioactively labeled antigen or antibody and the unknown amount in the patient sample provides for very accurate determinations of antigen or antibody in the sample. Hepatitis serologies were performed by RIA before ELISA assays were available, and RIA proved to be a highly sensitive method for measuring antibody concentrations. The major drawback of this assay is that it requires working with radioactivity and its concomitant hazards, disposal requirements, and regulations.

K.   Enzyme Immunoassay

The ELISA, an alternate method of detecting antigen–antibody complexes, uses enzymatic activity to produce a colored product that is proportional to the number of enzyme molecules in the assay.[1] First, an antibody or antigen is adhered to a plastic plate, bead, or well. Natural electrostatic and van derWaals interactions cause proteins to bind to polystyrene or similar plastics tightly enough to withstand forceful washing with a buffer. The serum is added to the plate, and if antibody specific for the antigen on the plate or antigen recognized by the antibody on the plate is present, then it will bind and remain with the solid phase. A secondary antibody that is linked covalently to an enzyme and is specific either for immunoglobulin (if antibody is being detected) or antigen (if antigen in the serum is being detected) is added. A colorless substrate for the enzyme, which forms a colored product after hydrolysis, provides the basis for detection of the antigen–antibody complexes. If the serum component was present and the secondary antibody bound to it, then the enzyme remains with the solid phase and will convert the substrate. The production of the colored product is directly proportional to the amount of enzyme-linked antibody present in the plate. The amount of color can be determined by spectrophotometry, and a conversion will allow the determination of the amount of serum component present, either antigen or antibody.

The capture assays are similar in principle, but they include another step to "capture" the IgM in the microtiter plate well before the other reagents are added.[6] Then the antigen and secondary detection antibodies are added. In this way, the problem of competition between antigen-specific IgG and antigen-specific IgM is eliminated since only IgM remains in the plate to be examined for antigen specificity. This will enhance the sensitivity of IgM ELISA assays because IgM antibodies are usually present in low concentration and the small quantities of IgM do not have to compete for binding to antigen with large quantities of antigen-specific IgG.

These assays can be used to detect antigen or antibody in the patient specimen. If antibody production is being tested, then plastic wells coated with antigen are incubated with the patient's serum. A secondary reagent, enzyme-linked anti-immunoglobulin is added to the well, followed by a substrate. If patient antibodies are present, then the secondary reagent will be bound and will interact with the substrate. The substrate is converted to a colored product by the enzyme, and the amount of color change can be measured spectrophotometrically. If the presence of antigen is being determined, then a sandwich method may be used with enzyme-linked immunoassay technology. In this assay, an antibody specific for the antigen is coated on the plastic well. Then, the patient sample is added to the well, and any antigen in the sample will be bound by the antibody. A second antibody specific for the antigen, usually different from the first antibody and enzyme conjugated, is added with a substrate. If antigen is present in the specimen, then the second antibody will bind and will change the substrate to a colored product. Again, the amount of color change can be quantitated by a spectrophotometer. ELISA assays are usually slightly less sensitive than RIA assays, but they are more accurate than many of the other assays that can be employed for bacterial and viral serologies. ELISA assays can be as sensitive as 10^{-12} to 10^{-13} mol/l, while RIA technology can detect 10^{-14} mol/l.[2] Additionally, ELISAs maintain the potential for automation and can be performed in large groups because of the application of 96 well plates to ELISA technology. Plate readers and multichannel pipettes are already available to increase the speed and efficiency of ELISA techniques.

ELISA assays can also be adapted for the detection of antigen from serum and other body sites to increase the sensitivity and specificity of infectious disease testing. Testing for antigen is more direct and less dependent on the immune status of the patient than are assays that measure antibody production. It is also easier to detect the presence of antigen than to culture many organisms. ELISA assays for antigen are especially advantageous for detecting the presence of organisms that are difficult or dangerous to isolate from culture.

One consideration for these assays is the preservation of proteins in an antigenically viable form. If the protein is degraded or unfolded, it may not be recognized by the antibodies used in the detection system. Additionally, some specimens are less than optimum in pH or salt concentration and may need to be washed or further processed before antigen–antibody complexes can be formed and detected. Antigen–antibody interactions are very susceptible to pH and ionic strength in the environment, and therefore, physiologic pH and salt concentrations must be achieved for immunologic assays to be accurate. However, many of the antigens recognized in urine or CSF are polysaccharides derived from the outer membranes and capsules of infectious agents, and polysaccharides are much less susceptible to changes in the pH or osmolarity. For example, antigenically viable *H. influenza b* antigens can be detected in the urine for up to 2 weeks following vaccination. These methods may become very useful as rapid determinations of the patient's infectious disease status that can be confirmed by tests for specific antibody.

Tests for specific antibody are available for some antigens, the most commonly used assays being for diphtheria, tetanus, hepatitis, and influenza. These assays are used to determine the effectiveness of vaccines and the ability of patients to develop a measurably intact immune response. Assays for specific antibody can also be used to determine the patient's immune status regarding chicken pox, rubella, or measles. If patients have an intact and functional immune system, they will form antibodies to organisms following vaccination or natural infection. Those antibodies are detectable in the serum and can be measured by ELISA techniques as described before.

III. EVALUATION OF IMMUNOCOMPETENCE

Specific antibody assays are extremely useful in the evaluation of immunocompetence, particularly those which measure antibodies formed in response to vaccinations which most children normally receive. Because most people have been exposed to these antigens, the absence of antibodies in the serum may help clinicians identify patients who have not yet been exposed to the antigen and those patients with immune defects. Patients with ineffective cellular immune responses will not make good antibody responses because the B lymphocytes will not receive the appropriate costimulation necessary from T lymphocytes. Patients with humoral defects, who fail to make good antibody responses to any antigens, will also have significantly decreased levels of specific antibodies. These patients have defects in antibody synthesis and will not produce sufficient levels of specific antibodies.

Additionally, specific immunodeficiency syndromes may be associated with defined and limited immunologic defects that may predispose patients to particular kinds of infections. Patients with deficiencies of humoral immunity usually suffer from recurrent pyogenic infections, often originating in the respiratory tract. X-linked lymphoproliferative disease appears to be accompanied by IgG subclass deficiencies. Decreases in IgG2 and IgG4 have been linked to recurrent infections and autoimmune diseases. IgG2 deficiencies are most often associated with recurrent sinopulmonary infections and decreased responsiveness to polysaccharide antigens. Examples of IgA deficiencies are also found and may result in increased susceptibility to bacterial infections of the respiratory, gastrointestinal, or genitourinary tracts.

All of these patients can be identified by their inability to respond to infectious diseases with the production of specific antibodies. Thus, infectious disease serologies are even useful for diagnosing illnesses in patients suspected of being immunocompromised.

IV. DISCRIMINATION OF CURRENT AND PAST INFECTIONS

One of the challenges of infectious disease serologies is the distinction between current or recent infections and past infections. It is often clinically relevant to determine whether a patient currently has a particular infection, not just whether the patient has, at some previous time, been exposed to the infective organisms. A principal distinction between primary and secondary responses to antigen is the proportion of IgM to IgG in the response. The primary response is delayed and may contain elevated levels of IgM antibodies because the primary response predates somatic mutation and class switching. The secondary response has a shorter lag time because of the presence of memory B cells and contains primarily subclasses of IgG. The secondary response may result in more efficient clearing of the antigen because affinity maturation has occurred: that is, those antibodies with greater affinity for the antigen are produced in greater abundance late in an immune response or upon rechallenge with the antigen. Thus, the ability to identify the amount of antigen-specific IgM, which is more characteristic of the primary response, is crucial for practical application of infectious disease serologic assays to clinical diagnosis.

There are many caveats to the detection of antigen-specific IgM. For example, the serum concentration of IgM is much lower than the serum concentration of IgG. That makes the detection of specific IgM more difficult because the higher concentration of IgG may mask its detection. Because IgG and IgM antibodies may bind to the same epitopes, it is not possible to distinguish the antigen specific region of an IgG molecule from the antigen-specific region of an IgM molecule. Therefore, binding characteristics cannot be used to separate IgG and IgM responses in total antibody assays. It is sometimes difficult to distinguish the immunoglobulin molecules because of their similarities in structure. However, some separation methods exist which allow the two immunoglobulins to be measured independently.

Most separation techniques take advantage of the differences in molecular weight between the two molecules. IgM exists primarily as a pentamer, while IgG is usually a monomer in serum. Old methods of separation, like ultracentrifugation, separate IgG and IgM by size and molecular weight. Sucrose or other density gradients also separate these two molecules during centrifugation. These techniques are labor intensive and are very time consuming; therefore, they are not practical for use in clinical laboratories for diagnostic purposes. However, there were not other methods available for measuring IgM specifically without separating the IgM from IgG before performing immunologic assays. Newer methods for separation of IgM from IgG have been developed to simplify the process, and they include ion exchange column separation and protein A column separation. Protein A separation works well to separate IgM from IgG because IgG binds with strong affinity to protein A. Subclasses 1, 2, and 4 of IgG bind with much stronger affinity than IgG3 and can be separated easily and rapidly.

Because each of the separation methods has inherent disadvantages, tests that would measure antigen-specific IgM without requiring separation or purification steps have been designed for use in the clinical laboratory. The capture assay represents the best technology developed thus far for identifying antigen-specific IgM. The capture assay, described earlier, allows the IgM response to be measured independently from the IgG response by using μ-chain-specific anti-IgM antibodies.[6] Capture assays focus the detection system only on the antigen-specific IgM because the capture antibodies are specific for the Fc portion of the IgM, making it μ-chain specific. Capture assays are less useful for detecting antigen-specific IgG because the vast majority of serum immunoglobulins are IgG, but very little will be antigen-specific. Thus, the antigen-specific IgG will be hard to detect in the presence of the remaining IgG that also binds to the Fc-specific antibody on the solid phase. On the other hand, in most cases, when IgM is present, it is directed against a single antigen (i.e., a virus). This makes capture assays more useful for IgM-mediated responses where there is much less free IgM in the serum, and most of it is specific for the currently infecting pathogen.

This is especially true in congenital infections where the baby has not been exposed to any other pathogens, except those acquired from the mother. Therefore, IgM capture assays are ideally suited for the detection of antigen-specific IgM in congenital infections where the presence of antigen-specific IgG may not indicate infection or disease in the infant. Antigen-specific IgG may be derived from the mother or the baby because IgG is subject to transplacental transfer to the baby.

Capture assays may be subject to complications. For example, the first step antibody should be polyclonal so that it will bind to the μ chain of IgM from different patients. If monoclonal antibodies are used, some patient IgM may escape detection because of allotypic differences in the Fc portion of the immunoglobulin. Allotypic differences are changes in the conserved region protein sequence or structure between individuals of the same species. Polyclonal antisera will be able to bind to multiple epitopes within the μ chain of IgM, whereas monoclonal sera will bind to a single epitope that may be variously exposed or available to antibody binding in different patients. Therefore, if monoclonal antisera are used, some patients may make antigen-specific IgM that cannot be detected because the one epitope recognized by the solid phase antibody is not available to be bound to the column. Additionally, the presence of rheumatoid factor, constantly a concern in traditional assays for IgM, may contribute to inaccurate results. Rheumatoid factor, IgM that is specific for IgG, may bind to the IgG present on the solid phase and with the secondary reagent that is enzyme linked.[1] Rheumatoid factor can create false positive test results in some assays because the IgM that binds is not antigen specific. The secondary reagent may be bound by the IgM captured by the solid phase antibody, rather than by any antigen bound to the IgM. Alternatively, other tests for IgM may be complicated by competition for antigen with IgG. In other words, antigen-specific IgG binds to the antigen and competes with IgM for binding and detection by the secondary reagent. Competition with IgG may yield false-negative results, but capture assays prevent or greatly reduce the possibility that IgG will compete with IgM for binding to antigen. Despite possible complications, capture assays are widely used for the accurate detection of antigen specific IgM. These assays are especially useful and likely to become most often the test of choice for detecting primary viral infections in newborns.

V. CAVEATS OF SEROLOGIC EVALUATION

As mentioned earlier, one of the problems that must be addressed by serologic techniques is the low concentration in serum of antigen-specific antibody compared with the total serum immunoglobulin concentration. This is an especially significant problem with immunofluorescence techniques that require distinctions of subtle degrees of fluorescent staining by a technologist. Because technologists must evaluate the results of immunofluorescence assays subjectively, it is very crucial that distinctions between negative and slightly positive samples be clear. There are several amplification techniques that have been used to increase the signal that will be detected when antigen-specific antibody is present in any of the assays described thus far. Immunoglobulin amplification can be accomplished by the use of secondary and tertiary reagents specific for other immunoglobulins. Antibodies, because they have two antigen combining sites, can bind to more than one antigen at once. It is also true that when immunoglobulin is the antigen there are multiple sites that can be bound by other antibodies. This allows for a several-fold amplification of the signal when anti-immunoglobulin reagents are used.

Signal amplification is especially important in fluorescent assays where there may be relatively high background staining. Amplification of the signal may help distinguish specific staining from background staining. Other methods of amplification include complement–anti-complement cascades. In this method, complement is bound to antibodies specific for the test component. The secondary reagent is specific for the complement from the first step. Again, the principle is that there are multiple binding sites that allow for increasing the tag to original antigen ratio. As the number of tag molecules per original antigen increases, the signal will increase in intensity.

VI. NEWER METHODS AND EMERGING APPLICATIONS

A. Immunoblotting

A relatively new method that is becoming important in infectious disease serologic testing is immunoblotting.[1,2] Table 2 gives the important components of immunoblotting or Western blotting protocols. Briefly, antigens derived from the pathogen studied are electrophoretically separated on a polyacrylamide gel on the basis of molecular weight and complexity. The proteins are transferred to a nitrocellulose membrane by electrophoretic transfer using an electric current at a 90° angle from the original current applied to the gel. The nitrocellulose

TABLE 2

Principal Components of Immunoblotting

1. Sample preparation and electrophoretic separation
2. Transfer to nitrocellulose membrane
3. Blocking of the residual capacity of the membrane
4. Incubation with primary antibody
5. Detection of binding of the antibody–antigen with a secondary labeled reagent

antigen distribution, which is of a known configuration exactly like the distribution on a polyacrylamide gel, can be stained with a variety of primary antibodies with specificities for the antigens present just like an ELISA. The secondary labeled antibody will detect the presence of bound primary antibody. Usually, the primary antibodies used in the assay are those present in the patient serum. If the patient has been exposed to the pathogen and formed specific antibodies, these antibodies will bind to the antigen on the nitrocellulose filter.

The fundamental advantage is that the antigen that is bound by the antibody is actually visualized on the blot by an enzyme reaction. This allows for the distinction between antigen specificities and allows a partial characterization of the immune response. This antigenic pattern displayed by the patient's sera may also allow comparison with the response of other patients, and causative organisms may be compared as well. Cross-reactive antibodies present in the serum are less likely to bind to specific bands on the blot, while specific antibodies may only bind to one particular antigen on the blot. Cross-reactive antibodies may bind to cell culture components or to similar proteins that are present in other organisms. Because the antigens eliciting specific antibodies can be identified, this technique has become a standard confirmatory assay for other serologic screening assays. Antigens derived from many pathogens can be identified by this method, and some of them are mentioned in Table 3.

One possible disadvantage of immunoblotting is occasional, nonspecific staining patterns. An example of this is reaction with cell culture components. For example, HIV virus is grown in an H-9/HTLV-IIIB T-lymphocyte cell line. Culture components may be partially purified with the virus and may also be present on the nitrocellulose. Culture component-specific antibodies may bind to the blot as well, but they usually result in a nonspecific staining pattern. The primary antigenic stimulus from culture is fetal calf serum used in tissue culture of the cells used to grow the pathogen. This was a problem when immunoblotting was originally used as a confirmatory assay for HIV infection. More recent protein purification techniques and more sensitive and specific assay protocols have greatly reduced this complication in the current clinical laboratory.

TABLE 3

Infectious Microorganisms Detected by Antibodies and Immunoblotting

Bacteria	Viruses	Fungi	Protozoa
Borrelia	BK viruses	*Aspergillus fumigatus*	*Entamoeba*
Brucella	Blue tongue virus	*Candida albicans*	*Leishmania*
Campylobacter	Bursal disease virus	*Coccidioides immitis*	*Giardia*
Chlamydia	Cauliflower mosaic virus	*Paracoccidioides brasilliensis*	*Plasmodium*
Clostridium	Corona virus	*Blastomyces dermatitidis*	*Pneumocystis*
Gonococcus	Cytomegaloviruses		*Toxoplasma*
Hemophilus	Epstein-Barr virus		
Leptospira	Hepatitis virus		
Meningococcus	Herpes virus		
Micropolyspora	HIV-1		
Mycobacteria	HIV-2		
Mycoplasma	HTLV1		
Rickettsia	Japanese encephalitis virus		
Streptococcus	Parvovirus		
Treponema	Pseudorabies virus		
Yersinia	RSV		
	Rotavirus		
	SV-40		

In practice, many serologic techniques incorporate a combination of the different technologies discussed so far. In other words, principles from different kinds of ELISAs or different kinds of agglutination reactions may be combined into a single assay. Because the clinical laboratory continues to respond to the needs of clinicians when diagnosing patient illnesses, new techniques and combinations of techniques are continually being tested. Initial testing of patient specimens may be performed using screening assays that should be rapid and highly sensitive and able to detect all possible positive results. Screening assays should result in very few false negative results; false positive results are preferable at this stage of testing. These assays are usually less expensive and require minimal time and work by the technologist. Confirmatory assays are frequently more labor intensive and must be highly specific, as well as being sensitive. These assays are usually much more expensive and should distinguish false-positive from true-positive results by being very specific for a particular antigen. These assays often require more technical expertise and may not be suited to large numbers of patient samples. ELISA and latex agglutination techniques are favorite screening assays because of their simplicity and sensitivity. Blotting techniques, immunofluorescence, and hemagglutination have become the mainstay of confirmatory assays because they allow visualization of the specific antigen–antibody interaction. Two classic examples of a screening and confirmatory pair are the rapid plasma reagin (RPR) and FTA-ABS for *Treponema pallidum* and the

ELISA and Western blot for detecting antibodies to HIV. The RPR is a rapid simple nonspecific assay to detect the presence of antibodies to cholesterol, lecithin, and cardiolipin and is very predictive of infections with *T. pallidum*. The FTA-ABS is a specific immunofluorescence test that detects the presence of antibodies specific for *T. pallidum*. The HIV ELISA is very sensitive and quantitative, while the Western blot has been used to establish specific diagnostic criteria for the laboratory diagnosis of HIV infection. A patient must have a specific antibody for at least two of these three proteins: p24, gp41, and gp160/120 in order to fulfill the criteria for seroreactivity. Proteins are named by their molecular weight and posttranslational modification. Therefore, p24 is a protein of 24 kDa; gp41 is a glycoprotein of 41 kDa; and gp160/120 is a glycoprotein of 160 kDa with a breakdown product of 120 kDa. A similar approach is being used for the laboratory diagnosis of Lyme disease, where an ELISA serves as the screening test, and immunoblotting is used for confirmation.[7] The Lyme Western blot is newer and is still the subject of extensive testing to determine the best diagnostic criteria for interpretation. One manufacturer suggests a combination of bands, which must include proteins with the following molecular weights: p41 and at least one of p30, p31, p34, p39, or p66 for IgM-specific responses. The IgG response is similar. However, Steere[8] proposes a different set of criteria, but this is still somewhat developmental. Lyme disease diagnosis is very complicated and difficult to confirm in the clinical laboratory.

The diagnosis of syphilis presents a complex diagnostic problem and requires a unique combination of techniques for laboratory diagnosis. In adults, the RPR assay is used as a screening test, and the FTA-ABS, an indirect immunofluorescence assay, or the MHA-TP, a hemagglutination assay, is used for confirmation. The laboratory diagnosis of congenital syphilis is much more complex and requires a combination of clinical observations and laboratory techniques. It would be helpful if techniques were available to detect *T. pallidum*-specific infant IgM because neonatal serum may contain IgG antibodies that are of maternal origin. Maternal and fetal IgG antibodies are not easily distinguishable in clinical laboratories. Therefore, an accurate test for infection of the newborn is dependent on the detection of the presence of IgM in the newborn since maternal IgM does not cross the placenta. Several investigators have attempted to use immunoblotting in the laboratory diagnosis of congenital syphilis.[9-11] It is vital to diagnose congenital syphilis, especially in asymptomatic infants, so appropriate antibiotic therapy can be given. Figure 1 shows an example of the immunoblotting technique which successfully differentiates neonatally and maternally derived antibodies. This technique shows significant promise but is still under development. Other congenital infections which require

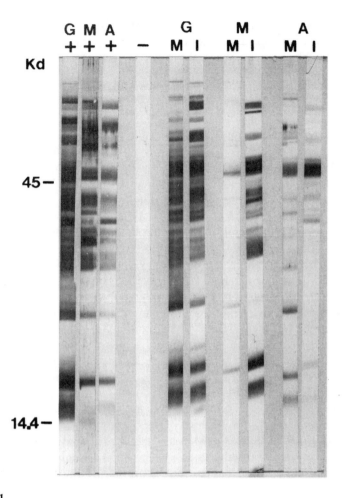

Figure 1

Immunoblotting for the detection of *T. pallidum* antibodies in congenital syphilis. In this figure, serum from a mother infected with *Treponema pallidum* was collected and tested by immunoblotting techniques in parallel with the serum of her infant, who was suspected of being congenitally infected with *T. pallidum*. Lanes labeled "M" were tested using serum from the mother; lanes labeled "I" were tested using serum from the infant. G, M, and A refer to the immunoglobulin isotype detected by the secondary antibody conjugate. The first three lanes contain positive control sera, and the fourth lane contained nonimmune sera and was probed with all the secondary conjugates. It is possible to identify many *T. pallidum*-derived bands on the nitrocellulose membrane, but the primary antigens with immunodominance are the 47 kDa, 15 kDa, and 17 kDa proteins. Both the mother and the infant serum specimens contain IgG specific for *T. pallidum*. However, some bands are present only in the infant or are present in higher abundance in the infant. These observations suggest that the infant is also producing *T. pallidum*-specific IgG antibodies that are not present in the maternal serum nor present due to transplacental transfer. In the IgM and IgA specific blots, several bands identified by the infant's serum are not identified by maternal serum. Therefore, this blot suggests that the infant tested was congenitally infected with syphilis and was making anti-*T. pallidum*-specific antibodies.

careful discrimination of neonatal and maternal antibody include tox-oplasmosis, rubella infections, cytomegalovirus (CMV) and herpes viral infections, and HIV. Tests for neonatal IgM have been useful to this point, but improvements in detection techniques for these infections may be clinically useful.

Newer methods are continually being studied and tested in the clinical setting to determine their accuracy, sensitivity, and specificity. Still, many assays remain to be improved for use in the immunology laboratory. Assays for antigen, rather than for antibody, are always useful because an increasing number of infectious disease patients are immunocompromised by infections or immunosuppressive therapy. Any assay for antigen will remove the dependence on an intact immune response that is present in any assay which relies on the presence of antibody against a pathogen.

Assays that are less dependent on the intact immune response will also become crucial for the evaluation of transplantation patients. These patients are typically immunosuppressed by cyclosporine or steroid antirejection therapy. As a result, these patients do not develop effective immune responses against pathogens they encounter. Additionally, because they are immunocompromised, the rapid diagnosis of their infectious disease is especially important. It is currently quite difficult to provide an accurate laboratory diagnosis for patients on immuno-suppressive therapy. This category should also include patients with autoimmune diseases that lead to autoreactive antibodies that interfere with serologic diagnosis and who are also frequently treated with immunosuppressive therapies.

The accurate diagnosis of viral diseases by serology is a prevailing trend because of the time required to culture viruses from patient specimens. Some viruses, like CMV, hepatitis viruses, and Epstein-Barr virus, are especially difficult to culture, as well, making serologic techniques of even greater demand. Therefore, attempts to improve the speed and accuracy of viral serologic diagnosis are common. The diagnosis of hepatitis represents another area where an improved immunological or molecular technique would be useful since culture techniques are not adequate for clinical diagnosis of hepatic viral illnesses. Serologic techniques have been applied to the identification of immunoglobulin responses against viral hepatitis entities, but these assays are insufficient for diagnosis in all cases. Hepatitis C, for example, does not stimulate a strong antibody response following exposure. Most people do not reach peak antibody titers until at least 6 months after exposure and onset of the viral infection. Because the specific antibody response is delayed, the detection of antibodies in the serum is not satisfactory at the onset of the illness. Thus, additional molecular or immunological techniques are needed for improved diagnosis of hepatitis C viral infections.

There is increasing interest in identifying a serologic counterpart for tuberculosis. *Mycobacterium tuberculosis* is very difficult to identify by smear or culture with low sensitivity by both techniques. It is an extremely slow growing organism, requiring several weeks of culture and laboratory time. With the growing numbers of HIV-infected patients, tuberculosis is again rising in prevalence and is becoming a major public health concern. Unfortunately, the population most at risk is not capable of mounting effective cellular or humoral immune responses. It is also true that patients with mycobacterial infections can be immunosuppressed as a result of the mycobacterial infection itself. A complicating feature of this illness is that antibody-driven responses are relatively ineffective in clearing the microorganisms from the host, and cellular responses to tuberculoid antigens are the same with active tuberculosis and inactive tuberculosis. Thus, ongoing infection cannot be determined by the use of cellular immune response measurement by the tuberculin skin test which takes 48 to 72 h and is only qualitative in nature. Current ELISA tests being developed for tuberculoid antigens are not very specific and are inaccurate because of the relatively high contamination of the environment with other mycobacteria.

It is worth repeating that an improved method to distinguish maternal and neonatal immunoglobulin is needed for the diagnosis of congenitally acquired infections. Most congenital infections require immediate therapy to prevent or reduce long term sequelae, and thus, rapid laboratory diagnosis is crucial.[12,13] Some IgG subclasses cross the placenta, and lymphocytes of maternal origin have been found in neonatal circulation. IgM and IgA do not cross the placenta in significant concentrations to influence the outcome of IgM- or IgA-specific serologic assays. Recent work with congenital syphilis promises more accurate and rapid laboratory confirmed diagnosis. IgM-, IgA-, and IgG-specific Western blots aid in the distinction of maternal and neonatal antibodies that specifically bind treponemal antigens. Figure 1 shows an example of an immunoblot assay for congenital syphilis. The maternal serum shows the antibodies derived from the mother, while the infant serum contains unique specificities not present in the maternal serum.

VII. INTERPRETATION

It is not surprising that interpreting serologic assays might be confusing or difficult because so many variables can influence the outcome of a patient's immune response in addition to technical limitations of the assays. Therefore, the use of serologic results should always be within the context of the clinical evaluation. If the patient's symptoms and history are consistent with the serologic results, then the results may be used as confirmation of the clinical diagnosis. On the other hand, if the clinical diagnosis and the laboratory diagnosis do not agree, then the physician must act first on the clinical diagnosis.

Among those factors which interfere with laboratory diagnosis of infectious disease are the timing of sampling during the disease course, the pairing of serum samples, the distinction between a primary and a secondary response, and the actual test sensitivities and specificities. First, the timing of samples during the disease course is critical because early in a primary immune response very little specific antibody may be detected. For some infections it may take 4 to 6 weeks to reach peak antibody levels during a primary response. Additionally, antibiotics or other therapies can result in low levels of antibodies being detected or, in some cases, may ablate the immune response completely. This is especially important in the serologic diagnosis of Lyme disease and may be implicated for diagnosis of primary syphilis. Alternatively, late in the disease course, IgM antibodies decrease and may not be detected by IgM-specific serologic tests. Under those conditions where antibody may be difficult to detect, tests for antigen become especially important. Antigen detection methods can be successful during acute illness when the antibody response may not have been stimulated sufficiently to detect circulating antibodies. Antigen may also be present during therapy when antibody levels are artificially low.

Paired serum samples are useful for determining changes in specific antibody titers during the course of disease and can provide serologic confirmation. Paired sera are considered more reliably accurate than are individual samples which may be subject to the sampling problems mentioned above. By taking two serum samples 2 to 3 weeks apart, most of the sampling problems are avoided, and increasing or decreasing titers are captured. Certainly, therapy should not be withheld pending the results of paired serum samples. In some disease states like acute toxoplasmosis, a single sample with a very high titer may be considered presumptively diagnostic and warrant treatment.

Primary and secondary immune responses may be distinguished by the ratio of antigen-specific IgM to IgG which is higher during a primary response. However, as mentioned previously, tests for antigen-specific IgM may be unreliable. It must be remembered that patients infected with HIV, and sometimes other viruses like CMV and Epstein-Barr virus, may have diminished cellular and humoral responses. As a result, the levels of IgM they make in response to a primary challenge with an antigen may be exceedingly low and difficult to detect. In such cases, detection of pathogens by serology may be nearly impossible, and determining whether the response is primary or secondary even more difficult. On the other hand, early during HIV infection, increased polyclonal antibody secretion may result in false positive serologic results. This polyclonal stimulation may lead to antibody production in a nonantigen-driven fashion, thereby confusing accurate diagnosis of autoimmune and infectious diseases. Alternatively, the secondary response is often impaired in HIV-infected individuals, which will limit the distinction between primary infection and reactivation of infection and which may affect treatment decisions.

Lastly, the inherent characteristics of the test performed may interfere with the interpretation of the laboratory results. Some assays are inherently less sensitive than others and may yield a negative result in contrast to a more sensitive technique. Knowing which tests are most sensitive may be helpful in ranking the importance of different test results. For example, a patient with a negative Rocky Mountain spotted fever latex agglutination reaction and a positive RMSF immunofluorescence result should be considered positive for RMSF because the IFA is more sensitive than the latex test. The specificity of the assay may also interfere with the interpretation of serologic results. For example, patients with autoimmune diseases frequently have cross-reactive antibodies that may give false positive results in a serologic assay. Some of the screening tests are especially susceptible to cross-reactive antibodies, making the results of the confirmatory assays more relevant. An example where the specificity of the test is crucial is when a patient has a positive RPR and a negative FTA-ABS. In this case, the FTA represents the more specific assay and should be weighted more heavily in the clinical decision than the RPR.

All of these factors may play a role in the interpretation of serologic results, and in deciding which further tests are performed. Because of the difficulties encountered when interpreting infectious disease serologies, it is imperative for clinicians and laboratorians to collaborate in the diagnosis of a patient's illness. This cooperation may prevent discrepancies between laboratory and clinical diagnoses.

VIII. FUTURE PERSPECTIVES IN MOLECULAR DIAGNOSIS

There are many changes on the forefront of immunology that may substantially affect how infectious diseases are diagnosed. Many of the enzyme-linked assays are being automated so that the results are completely objective and less susceptible to technical error. This automation increases the speed and efficiency of the immunology laboratory, as well, which is crucial for clinical settings. With the spread of HIV, the number of patients with secondary infections is increasing, and these improvements in technology will better meet this demand.

Molecular diagnosis is the latest improvement in the diagnosis of infectious diseases. Molecular biological techniques are being applied to the clinical setting for the purpose of identifying the causative agents of difficult-to-diagnose diseases.[14-16] The polymerase chain reaction

(PCR) and *in situ* hybridization are being used successfully to identify the DNA of pathogens in human samples directly. These methods do not rely upon the function of an intact immune system, making them more useful techniques in immunocompromised patients. These techniques are very sensitive and often have resolution 10- to 1000-fold beyond currently available techniques. PCR is being applied to syphilis, tuberculosis, obscure and common viral illnesses, rickettsial illnesses, HIV, and chlamydial infections. Details of molecular techniques and their applications in infectious diseases are thoroughly discussed in Chapter 6.

Molecular techniques also facilitate epidemiological studies. Bacterial strains and isolates can be characterized and compared at the genomic level, often providing a new understanding of how infections are communicated. With this knowledge, modes of transmission may be identified and controlled. Eventually, it is likely that molecular techniques may allow diagnosis of infection without any serologic assays. As the technology permits a more direct examination of the patient, the ability of the clinical immunology laboratory to quickly and accurately diagnose the illness will expand.

REFERENCES

1. *Manual of Clinical Laboratory Immunology*, 4th ed., Rose, N.R., de Macario, E.C., Fahey, J.L., Friedman, H., and Penn, G.M., Eds., American Society for Microbiology, Washington, D.C., 1992.
2. Stites, D.P. and Terr, A.I., *Basic and Clinical Immunology*, 7th ed., Appleton & Lange, Norwalk, CT, 1991.
3. James, K., Immunoserology of infectious diseases, *Clin. Microbiol. Rev.*, 3(2), 132, 1990.
4. Terpstra, W.J., Serodiagnosis of bacterial diseases: problems and developments, *Scand. J. Immunol.*, 36, Suppl.(11), 91, 1992.
5. Hyde, R.M., *Immunology*, 2nd ed., National Medical Series, from Williams & Wilkins, Harwal Publishing, Malvern, PA, 1992.
6. Wilson, A. J., Sant, H., Van Duser, P.K., and Wentz, M., Enzyme-based methods for IgM serology: standard indirect ELISA vs. antibody-capture ELISA, *Lab. Med.*, 23(4), 259, 1992.
7. Duffy, J., Lyme disease, *Ann. Allergy*, 65, 1, 1990.
8. Dressler, F., Whalen, J.A., Reinhardt, B.N., and Steere, A.C., Western blotting in the serodiagnosis of Lyme disease, *J. Infect. Dis.*, 167, 392, 1993.
9. Meyer, M.P., Eddy, T., and Baughn, R.E., Analysis of western blotting (immunoblotting) technique in diagnosis of congenital syphilis, *J. Clin. Microbiol.*, 32(3), 629, 1994.
10. Sanchez, P.J., McCracken, G.H., Wendel, G.D., Olsen, K., Threlkeld, M., and Norgard, M.V., Molecular analysis of the fetal IgM response to *Treponema pallidum* antigens: implications for improved serodiagnosis of congenital syphilis, *J. Infect. Dis.*, 159(3), 508, 1989.

11. Schmitz, J.L., Gertis, K.S., Mauney, C., Stamm, L.V., and Folds, J.D., Laboratory diagnosis of congenital syphilis by immunoglobulin M (IgM) and IgA immuno-blotting, *Clin. Diag. Lab. Immunol.*, 1(1), 32, 1994.

12. Sison, A.V. and Campos, J.M., Laboratory methods for early detection of human immunodeficiency virus type I in newborns and infants, *Clin. Microbiol. Rev.*, 5(3), 238, 1992.

13. Albert, J., Biberfeld, G., Borkowsky, W., Caniglia, M., DeRossi, A., Elia, L., Fundaro, C., Giaquinto, C., Henrard, D., Hoff, R., Jansson, M., Lombardi, V., Marchisio, P., Pahwa, S., Plebani, A., Rogers, M., Rossi, P., Rouzious, C., Scarlatti, G., Scott, G., Tamashiro, H., Thongcharoen, P., van der Groen, G., Verani, P., Wahren, B., and Wolinsky, S., Report of a consensus workshop, Siena, Italy, January 17–18, 1992: Early diagnosis of HIV infection in infants, *J. Acq. Immune Def. Syndromes*, 5(11), 1169, 1992.

14. Desselberger, U. and Collingham, K., Reviews of molecular biology of sexually transmitted diseases: molecular techniques in the diagnosis of human infectious diseases, *Genitourin. Med.* 66, 313, 1990.

15. Krech, T., New techniques in rapid viral diagnosis, *FEMS Microbiol. Immunol.*, 89, 299, 1992.

16. Tompkins, L.S., The use of molecular methods in infectious diseases, *N. Engl. J. Med.*, 327(18), 1290, 1992.

Chapter 6

MOLECULAR TECHNIQUES APPLIED TO INFECTIOUS DISEASES

Preeti Pancholi and David H. Persing

CONTENTS

0-8493-0134-3/97/$0.00+$.50
© 1997 by CRC Press LLC

I. INTRODUCTION

Definitive identification of the disease-causing microorganism is the first and most important goal in infection control and prevention. Culture techniques have traditionally been considered as the "gold standard" for identification of microorganisms. Although adequate for most circumstances, there are many situations in which culture may be suboptimal. For example, the microorganism may be present in small numbers, may take a long time to grow, or may lack a system for *in vitro* cultivation. Recognition of these problems and the tremendous progress made in the field of molecular diagnostics has led to the development of molecular techniques for detection of nucleic acids (DNA or RNA) of a pathogen as a means of identifying the infectious agent. Since nucleic acid amplification methods, utilizing the polymerase chain reaction (PCR), can amplify nucleic acid target sequences from infectious organisms several million-fold, these methods can be used to detect the presence of low numbers of a pathogen in a variety of clinical specimens. Nucleic acid-based techniques have been developed for the rapid diagnosis of diseases caused by a large number of viruses, bacteria, fungi, spirochetes, rickettsia, and other infectious agents.[1,2] Nucleic acid probes have also been designed that distinguish point mutations and other genetic alterations in the genomes of microorganisms. "Broad-range" reagents have also been developed for investigation of diseases with unknown causative agents or etiologies.[3]

There are several reasons why diagnostic laboratories might want to employ nucleic acid amplification assays in the diagnosis of infectious diseases. First, these assays provide the potential for culture-independent detection and identification of infectious agents directly from specimens. This is especially useful in situations where the infectious organism grows either slowly or not at all. Probes can also be used to provide molecular fingerprints of different organisms as aids in defining their epidemiology and pathogenesis. In some cases, detection of antimicrobial resistance genes offers the potential for simultaneous detection of an infectious agent and determination of its antimicrobial resistance profile directly from the patient specimen.

The purpose of this chapter is to provide information on nucleic acid-based detection systems for identification of infectious organisms and to review their potential advantages and disadvantages in the overall context of disease.

II. CONVENTIONAL (NONAMPLIFIED) PROBE-BASED DETECTION

The first application of molecular diagnostics for detection of infectious organisms in clinical specimens was by the use of conventional (nonamplified) nucleic acid probes. Nucleic acid probes are segments of DNA or RNA (twenty to several thousand bases long) that bind with high specificity to complementary sequences of nucleic acid targets under appropriate conditions of pH, temperature and ionic strength. The hybridization reaction consists of the **probe** (complimentary oligonucleotide) to which a **reporter molecule** is attached and, the **target** DNA. Typically, the probe molecule is a sequence of DNA or RNA, complementary to the target sequence that has been labeled with a

TABLE 1

Some Applications of Nucleic Acid Probes
in Infectious Diseases

Direct detection
Identification and culture confirmation
Subspecies identification via genetic fingerprinting
Epidemiology — molecular typing
Antimicrobial resistance

"reporter group." Nucleic acid probes by virtue of their relative simplicity and broad applicability in the diagnosis of infectious diseases have achieved utility in many clinical laboratories. Table 1 lists some applications of conventional probes.

Although less sensitive than nucleic acid amplification techniques, nucleic acid hybridization assays have provided for culture-independent detection and identification of infectious agents directly in clinical specimens and/or for culture confirmation. DNA probes have proved useful for identification of enterotoxin-producing strains of *Escherichia coli* that are otherwise biochemically identical to nonenterotoxin producing *E. coli*. Availability of some culture confirmation probes in kit form have allowed smaller laboratories to perform on-site testing for certain organisms (for, e.g., Streptococcus group A), and to avoid the cost of sending these specimens to reference laboratories. Numerous DNA probes now commercially available for culture confirmation of several bacteria and fungi[1] and appear to be particularly well suited for the identification of fastidious or slow growing organisms such as *Mycobacterium tuberculosis*, pathogenic dimorphic fungi or for viruses such as human papillomavirus for which no culture system is available. Some examples of the uses of such probes are provided here.

A. Diagnosis of Slow Growing Microorganisms

1. Mycobacteria

Because of the recent resurgence of tuberculosis, the Centers for Disease Control and Prevention (CDC) has advised using the latest technologies available for the rapid identification of *Mycobacterium tuberculosis* from clinical specimens.[4] Chemiluminescent DNA probes based on microbe-specific ribosomal RNA (rRNA) sequences are in widespread use and allow identification of *Mycobacterium* species (Table 2) weeks before identification by conventional biochemical reactions is possible. Mycobacteria-specific DNA probes (Accu Probe; Gen Probe Inc.; San Diego, CA) have proven to be highly sensitive and

TABLE 2

Commercially Available Nucleic Acid Probes
Frequently Used for Culture Confirmation of
Slow-Growing Micoorganisms

Bacteria

Mycobacterium tuberculosis complex
Mycobacterium avium
Mycobacterium intracellulare
Mycobacterium gordonae
Mycobacterium kansasii

Fungi

Histoplasma capsulatum
Blastomyces dermatitidis
Coccidioides immitis
Cryptococcus neoformans

specific. Discrepant results[5] are rare. Probes also have been used to identify organisms directly from BACTEC or other broth media, or from solid media. In these cases, results are obtained within hours. Detection is, however, limited to only a few species of mycobacteria for which probes are available, and cannot be performed directly on clinical specimens.

2. Fungi

As for mycobacterial infections, fungal infections are more prevalent due to the increasing numbers of patients who are immunocompromised. A considerable level of experience is currently required for the laboratory diagnosis of fungal isolates, based on recovery of fungi and direct exam of clinical isolates. Serological assays, although helpful in some instances, are limited in sensitivity and specificity. Presently, there are chemiluminescent-labeled nucleic acid probes, based on fungal-specific ribosomal RNA sequences, available commercially (Gen Probe, Inc, San Diego, CA) for confirmation of a limited number of medically important fungi (Table 2). These include the dimorphic fungi *Blastomyces dermatiditis*, *Histoplasma capsulatum*, *Cryptococcus neoformans*, and *Coccidiodes immitis*. These fungi typically require several weeks for definitive identification by the older methods. Although highly specific, these probes are not yet sensitive enough for direct specimen detection. Therefore, initial culture is required prior to detection. After culturing, even a single small colony of a yeast or filamentous form of the fungi is sufficient for testing.

B. Diagnosis of Infections in Normally Sterile Body Sites

Commercially available chemiluminescent DNA probes have been used to detect the ribosomal ribonucleic acid (rRNA) of blood-borne organisms including *Staphylococcus aureus*, *Streptococcus pneumoniae*, *E. coli*, *Haemophilus influenzae*, *Enterococcus* sp., and *Streptococcus agalactiae*. Specific identification is usually performed on specimens taken from positive blood culture bottles.[6] Gram stains are typically performed prior to testing in order to indicate which probes would be most appropriate. *Salmonella typhi* was similarly identified from isolator blood culture systems using DNA probes.[7]

Rapid and accurate detection of infectious organisms is also of high priority in treating bacterial meningitis. The currently available immunological tests and latex agglutination tests often do not offer sufficient sensitivity and specificity. A combination of PCR amplification using a universal bacterial primer, coupled with specific probes, has been described for the detection and identification of multiple species of bacteria that cause meningitis.[8]

C. Diagnosis of Sexually Transmitted Diseases

Sexually transmitted diseases (STD) are one of the most important public health problems among adolescents and young adults in the U.S. and contribute to significant morbidity and health care costs.[9] Because the currently available methods (culture, biochemicals, enzyme immunoassays, coagglutination, and fluorescent antibody techniques) for diagnosis of STDs have certain limitations, there has been a considerable interest in the development of molecular diagnostic techniques.

Various nucleic acid assay formats have been used for identification of STD pathogens (Table 3). Probe-based kits for the detection of *Chlamydia trachomatis* and *Neisseria gonorrheae* (GC) are commercially available. The kit assay utilizes an acridinium ester-labeled DNA probe targeted to a 16S rRNA of the target organism. Detection of hybridized probe-target rRNA complexes is performed via a chemiluminiscent probe system called the hybridization protection assay (see below).

Probes for GC come in two formats: (1) for culture confirmation (GC Accuprobe assay) and (2) for direct detection of organisms from endocervical or urethral swabs (PACE II assay). The PACE II and the AccuProbe assays for GC, which are Food and Drug Administration (FDA) certified, have been found to be excellent assays for the diagnosis and culture confirmation of GC.[10] Both the methods were rapid, equivalent or superior to the currently available assay systems (culture, carbohydrate utilization, fluorescent-antibody staining tests).

TABLE 3

Genitourinary Pathogens and Their Detection Formats

Organism	Assay (Source)
Bacterial	
Neisseria gonorrhoeae	DNA hybridization (Gen-Probe; Accu-Probe)
Chlaymydia trachomatis	PCR (Roche Molecular Diagnostics, Fairlawn, NJ)
	DNA hybridization (Gen-Probe)
Trichomonas vaginalis	DNA hybridization (MicroProbe; Bothell, WA)
Gardnerella vaginalis	DNA hybridization (MicroProbe; Bothell, WA)
Viral	
Human papillomaviruses	DNA hybridization (Digene Diag, Inc. Beltsville, MD)

The PACE II probe test kits for *C. trachomatis* are for direct detection of the organisms in urethral and/or endocervical sources.[11] The kits have undergone extensive testing in (1) male vs. female populations, (2) asymptomatic vs. symptomatic individuals, and (3) low vs. high *Chlamydia* prevalence populations. Overall, most evaluations found the PACE II assay equivalent to culture for detection of *Chlamydia* in the populations tested.[10] In addition, Gen-Probe now offers direct testing of both GC and *C. trachomatis* on material obtained from a single swab. This hybridization assay has also been cleared by the FDA.

Pertinent to this discussion, it should be mentioned that even higher sensitivity of detection of *C. trachomatis* has been achieved by the recently FDA approved Roche Amplicor™ commercial PCR-ELISA kit. The kit uses biotinylated primer pairs from cryptic plasmid (inclusive of all serological variants) for amplification of *C. trachomatis* from patient endocervical specimen. Following amplification, the biotinylated PCR products are hybridized to an immobilized oligonucleotide capture probe on a microtiter plate and detected via an avidin–enzyme conjugate.[12-14] A uracil N-glycosylase (dUTP) amplicon carryover prevention system minimizes false positive results. The ease of obtaining urine specimens instead of uretheral specimens in males has prompted investigation of urine for the detection of chlamydial urethritis. Preliminary data have shown PCR to be more sensitive than either culture or antigen detection.[10,15]

DNA probe test kits are also available for the detection of *Gardnerella vaginalis*[10] and *Trichomonas vaginalis*,[16] which are associated with bacterial vaginosis and vaginitis, respectively. However, because these organisms may reflect normal flora in the vaginal tract of asymptomatic women, the use of these tests should be limited to women with symptoms.

Since no culture system currently exists for human papillomavirus (HPV) a DNA hybridization test kit (Vira Pap®) (Table 3) that detects HPV infections directly in clinical specimens has been widely used.

TABLE 4

Molecular Detection of Drug Resistance

Advantages

Detection of a wide variety of resistance genes
Useful for subtyping resistance determinants
Detection of point mutations ("oligotyping")
Resolving indeterminate susceptibility results
Increased sensitivity and specificity
Does not require subculturing
Decreased detection time
Epidemiologic typing of isolates during outbreaks

Disadvantages

Silent loci may lead to false positive results
Difficult to determine the specific origin of the resistant gene in mixed flora

Because of the limited number of probes available for typing HPV, however, a negative Vira Pap® test does not rule out the presence of other HPV types. While HPV DNA detection may improve the specificity of histological diagnosis of HPV-related lesions, the identification of defined risk factors either of viral or host origin, might further increase the diagnostic utility of HPV testing. These factors may include certain alleles of the major histocompatibility complex [17] (MHC) and/or *p53* viral mutation.[18]

D. Diagnosis of Antimicrobial Drug Resistance

Drug resistance among common microorganisms is increasing worldwide. The clinical implications of drug resistance depend on the timely recognition of the problem, so that appropriate therapy can be initiated. The cloning and sequencing of many resistance genes has provided an impetus for the development of rapid nucleic acid techniques to detect drug-resistant organisms. Table 4 lists some of the advantages and disadvantages of nucleic acid-based detection of drug resistance.

While nucleic acid-based detection methods are available for a variety of microorganisms (Table 5), the choice to implement these procedures must take into account the potential benefits and disadvantages of the new techniques. For example, rapid and reliable identification of an isolate of methicillin-resistant *Staphylococcus aureus* (MRSA) is important for determination of appropriate therapy and proper isolation of the patient to prevent nosocomial spread. Routine susceptibility

TABLE 5

Detection of Antimicrobial Resistance Genes by Nucleic Acid Techniques

Antimicrobial Agent	Target	Organism Group	Method
Beta-Lactams	blaTEM	*Enterobacteriaceae*	Probe, PCR
		Haemophilus spp.	Probe
		Neisseria spp.	Probe
	blaSHV	*Enterobacteriaceae*	Probe
	blaCARB	Pseudomonads	Probe
	mec	Staphylococci	Probe, PCR
Aminoglycosides	aph-type	gnr, gpc	Probe, PCR
	ant-type	gnr, gpc	Probe, PCR
	aac-type	gnr, gpc	Probe, PCR
Erythromycin	erm	gpc	Probe, PCR
	ere	gpc, gnr	Probe
Quinolones	gyrA	Staphylococci	Sequencing
Sulfonamides	sulI	gnr	Probe
	sulII	gnr	Probe
Trimethoprim	DHFRI	gnr	Probe
	DHFRII	gnr	Probe
	DHFRIII	gnr	Probe
	DHFRV	gnr	Probe
Chloramphenicol	cat	gnr	Probe
		Staphylococci	Probe
	cmr	*Haemophilus ducrei*	Probe
		Clostridium difficile	Probe
Tetracycline	tet(A-E)	gnr	Probe
	tet(M)	Streptococci	Probe, PCR
		Mycoplasma spp.	Probe
		Bacteroides spp.	Probe
		Ureaplasma spp.	Probe
	tet(O)	Streptococci	Probe
		Campylobacter spp.	Probe
	tet(Q)	*Bacteroides* spp.	Probe
Vancomycin	van(A,B,C)	Enterococci	Probe,PCR
Rifampin	rpoB	*M. tuberculosis*	PCR
Ziduvodine	Reverse transcriptase	HIV	PCR

From Tenover, F. C., Popovic, T., and Olsvik, O., *Clin. Microbiol. Newslett.*, 15, 177, 1993. With permission.

testing may often be unreliable due to the frequently encountered "heterogeneous expression" of methicillin resistance in clinical isolates of *staphylococci*,[19,20] wherein strains expressing very low levels of methicillin resistance may fail to be recognized. At present there is no universal agreement on the choice of either an optimal procedure or minimum inhibitory concentration (MIC) breakpoints for the identification of methicillin resistance.[21,22] It has been consistently shown that most cases of methicillin resistance in *staphyloccci* are due to the acquisition of the mec A gene (that encodes a low affinity penicillin-binding protein) (PBP2a), and that all methicillin susceptible strains lack this gene. Detection of mec gene by DNA hybridization and PCR assays has proved useful for identification of MRSA.[23-27] They also provide a useful tool for the evaluation of procedures based on phenotypic expression of resistance.[28]

Nucleic acid-based methods have also proved useful for the detection of high level aminoglycoside resistance in enterococci. DNA hybridization studies using nine DNA probes and PCR methods[29,30] that use primer sets specific for the genes encoding aminoglycoside enzymes have been designed that can detect up to four aminoglycoside-modifying genes in a single strain of enterococci.[31] Determination of aminoglycoside resistance patterns has also been found to be useful epidemiologically for characterization of isolates from hospital outbreaks.[32,33]

Application of nucleic acid-based detection will be particularly useful for the direct detection of drug resistant *M. tuberculosis* (MTB) in patient specimens. Amplification of the RNA polymerase (rpo B) gene segment has been used to detect rifampin resistance (Rif[r]).[35] Rif[r] in turn provides a useful marker for the detection of multidrug-resistant TB. A more detailed discussion of this approach is presented below.

The use of molecular methods for the timely detection of drug resistance in organisms such as *S. aureus* and MTB is expected to lead to quicker patient isolation, a more informed choice of patient therapy, and a decrease in the time the patient is infectious. However, there are potential limitations of this technology as listed in Table 4.

III. HYBRIDIZATION FORMAT

There are three basic hybridization formats commonly employed for DNA probe assays: (1) filter or solid support hybridization, (2) solution (homogeneous) hybridization, and (3) *in situ* hybridization.[36]

Solid phase, or filter hybridization, is usually performed as a dot or Southern blots. In the dot blot, the intact cells are lysed and the DNA is denatured and fixed onto nylon membranes. The bound nucleic acid is then hybridized with DNA probes in solution. After washing away unbound probe, the membrane is developed. Variations of the standard dot blot have been proposed to decrease nonspecific background interferences. These include the sandwich hybridization and reversible target capture formats.[37] Commercially available, solid phase assays are currently available for screening and typing several strains of human papillomavirus.

The Southern hybridization assay is a specialized technique that requires purified sample DNA of high molecular weight. DNA is digested with a restriction endonuclease, and the fragments are separated by gel electrophoresis. The nucleic acids are then transferred to a nylon membrane for hybridization with a specific probe. Although this technique is used extensively for the detection and typing of human papillomavirus infections, because of its complexity and requirement of a large quantity of sample, it remains mostly a research tool and has limited clinical utility.

With the solution phase hybridization format, the target nucleic acid hybridizes with the probe in solution or liquid phase. The probe must be single stranded and incapable of self-annealing. The hybridization product is detected by one of three methods: binding to hydroxyapatite columns after digestion with S1 nuclease; detection of labeled sandwich hybrids in polyacrylamide gels; or more popularly, by a "hybridization protection" assay.[38,39] In the latter, a chemiluminescent acridinium ester-bound probe is subjected to alkaline hydrolysis after the hybridization reaction. The double-stranded nucleic acid protects the chemiluminescent ester from hydrolysis, while the unbound probe is degraded. Hybridized product can then be quantitated with a luminometer. Many commercially available DNA probe kits are based upon solution phase hybridization.

A variation of solid phase hybridization, namely, *in situ* hybridization (ISH) is a powerful technique useful for localizing genes or gene expression to individual cells or cell populations. In ISH, the target nucleic acid is liberated from its cellular surroundings and made available for hybridization with probes (Figure 1). It allows the simultaneous analysis of tissue morphology, host response, and the presence of the infectious agent. Information can also be derived with regard to latent or active infection. Probes (DNA or RNA) in general must be relatively small to favor tissue penetration. The *in situ* hybridization technique has been successfully applied for the detection of Epstein-Barr virus (EBV),[40,41] human immunodeficiency virus,[42,43] human papillomavirus,[44,45] JC virus, and bacterial and fungal pathogens.[1]

More recently, double labeling studies that combine immunohistology and *in situ* hybridization have been used to study EBV[41] and HPV[17] infections. Double labeling with radiolabeled EBV-specific RNA probes, in combination with immunostaining with monoclonal antibodies specific for TCR-beta, CD45RO (T cell antigens), CD20 (B cell antigens), CD68 (macrophage; histiocytic antigens), and CD30 (activation antigen), have revealed that EBV-associated T cell (and not B cell) proliferation is a primary feature of EBV-associated hemophagocytic syndrome (EBV-AHS). These findings may have direct implications on treatment strategies for EBV-AHS.[46]

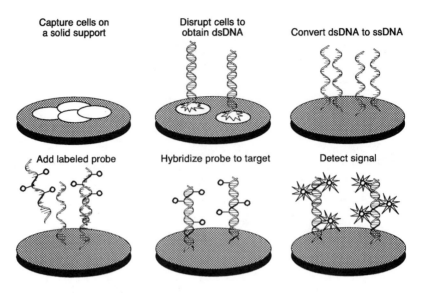

Figure 1

In situ hybridization. Basic steps in a DNA probe hybridization assay. The sample containing cells is captured (or blotted) on a solid support such as a nitrocellulose filter disk. The cells are then lysed to release the DNA, which binds to the solid support. Usually the filter is washed, and unreacted sites on the filter are blocked. A labeled probe is then added and allowed to hybridize to the sample DNA. Unbound probe is washed away, and the hybridized probe is detected. (From Pfaller, M. X., *Infect. Control Hosp. Epidemiol.*, 11, 661, 1990. With permission.)

IV. REPORTER GROUPS FOR DETECTION OF NUCLEIC ACID HYBRIDIZATION

Nucleic acid probes used in hybridization assays may be labeled isotopically or nonisotopically. Radioactive isotope labels (^{32}P, ^{35}S, ^{3}H, and ^{125}I) have been commonly used in the past. These require detection by autoradiography or beta scintillation counters. Although they are exquisitely sensitive, the radioactive isotope detection systems may not be practical for most clinical laboratories. Disadvantages include limited shelf life (based upon the half-life of the isotope), radiation hazards, daunting safety regulations that must be complied with, and problems with radioactive disposal. Nonradioactive detection systems have recently been developed that are more amenable to clinical settings and that lack the disadvantages of handling radioisotopes.

The current nonradioactive detection systems employ labels such as biotin, chemiluminescence substances (e.g., isoluminol), digoxigenin, and enzymes (e.g., horseradish peroxidase [HRP], alkaline phosphatase [AP]). Biotin and digoxigenin can be detected with antibody or avidin reagent coupled to a signal-generating compound. Various signal-generating systems may be used for the same reporter moiety. For example, with a biotinylated probe, avidin may be tagged with a fluorescent reporter group or coupled to an enzyme, such as AP or HRP. Detection of these reporter molecules can be performed either chromogenically (colorimetric substrate detection of HRP, AP) or by chemiluminescence (via luminometer that measures light released by chemiluminescent reporters after hybridization is complete). Procedures for labeling DNA or RNA probes are now available in the form of commercially available kits, complete with chromogenic or chemiluminescent substrates. Sensitivities of chemiluminescent and enzymatic assays in many instances approach or exceed those of ^{32}P-labeled probes.

For *in situ* hybridization, radioactive probes can be detected by autoradiography of specimen slides overlayed with silver emulsion, or by the nonradioactive methods. The number of exposed silver grains is often proportional to the number of target copies. Biotin or digoxigenin, which form a colored precipitate over the hybridization site after incubation with enzyme substrate, has recently been used for detecting human papillomavirus in human cervical specimens.

Despite the popularity of conventional probes in certain clinical settings, the use of such probes for direct detection of microbes in clinical specimens has been limited. Nucleic acid amplification techniques have been developed to impart greater sensitivity.

V. NUCLEIC ACID AMPLIFICATION TECHNIQUES

In vitro nucleic acid amplification, results in the enzymatic duplication and amplification of species specific nucleic acid sequences. Unlike conventional culture techniques, nucleic acid amplification techniques are not limited by the ability of the organism to grow. As noted above, since infectious agents are often present in clinical specimens in only small numbers, nucleic acid amplification methods have been employed for their direct detection. Infectious agents that either cannot be cultured or that require long periods for culture are attractive candidates for *in vitro* amplification techniques. The latter methods have been divided into three major categories based on the method of amplification (Table 6).

A. Target Amplification

Common to all target amplification methods is the utilization of *in vitro* enzymatic replication of a target molecule such that it can be

TABLE 6

Amplification Techniques

Target amplification

Polymerase chain reaction (PCR)
Transcription-based amplification system (TAS)
Strand displacement reaction (SDA)

Probe amplification

QB replicase amplification
Ligase chain reaction (LCR)

Signal amplification

Compound probes
Branched DNA probes

readily detected. The final amplification product thus contains target-specific information that can be further characterized.

1. Polymerase Chain Reaction

In 1985, scientists at the Cetus Corporation described an *in vitro* genetic amplification technique known as the polymerase chain reaction (PCR). PCR has revolutionarized many aspects of the basic and applied sciences. Its inventor, Kary Mullis, won the 1993 Nobel prize in chemistry. PCR uses repeated cycles of oligonucleotide-directed DNA synthesis to carry out *in vitro* replication of target nucleic acid sequences (Figure 2). The oligonucleotides used in a given reaction are synthesized to be complimentary to their annealing sites within the two different strands (the sense and nonsense strand) of a target sequence, from 150 to 3000 nucleotide bases apart.

Each cycle of PCR consists of three steps: (1) a denaturing step, in which the target DNA is incubated at high temperature so that the target strands are separated and thus made accessible to the excess primers in the reaction buffer; (2) an annealing step, in which the reaction mixture is cooled to allow the primers to anneal to their complementary sequences on the target sequence; and (3) an extension reaction, usually carried out at an intermediate temperature, in which the primers are extended on the DNA template by a DNA polymerase. Each time a cycle is completed, there is a theoretical doubling of the target sequence. However, while this doubling no doubt occurs in the initial cycles, in later cycles amplification becomes less efficient due to effective dilution of the polymerase and other reaction components by the large number of available DNA templates. Nevertheless, repeating

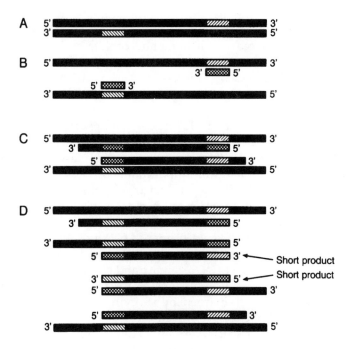

Figure 2

The PCR. In the first cycle, a double-stranded target sequence is used as a template, with the primer-binding sites indicated by hatched lines (A). These two strands are separated by heat denaturation, and the two synthetic oligonucleotide primers (cross-hatched lines) anneal to their respective recognition sequences in the 5′ -to- 3′ orientation (B). Note that the 3′ ends of each primer are facing each other. A thermostable DNA polymerase initiates synthesis at the 3′ ends of each primer (C). Extension of the primer via DNA synthesis results in new primer-binding sites. The net result after one round of synthesis is two "ragged" copies of the original target DNA molecule. In the second cycle, each of the four DNA strands shown in panel C anneals to primers (present in excess) to initiate a new round of DNA synthesis (D). Of the eight single-stranded products, two are of a length defined by the distance between and including the primer-annealing sites; this "short product" accumulates exponentially in subsequent cycles. (From Persing, D. H., in *Diagnostic Molecular Microbiology: Principles and Applications,* Persing, D. H., Smith, T. F., Tenover, F. C., and White, T. J., Eds., American Society for Microbiology, Washington, D.C., 1993, chap. 3. With permission of the Mayo Foundation.)

this cycle from 20 to 60 times often results in amplification of the target sequence over a millionfold.

Two recent technical innovations have simultaneously simplified and greatly increased the power of PCR. Since temperature requirements for each of the steps of PCR differ, the discovery that the thermostable DNA polymerase (*Taq* polymerase), isolated from the thermophilic bacterium *Thermus aquaticus,* is able to withstand repeated cycles of heating to 95°C has made it possible to carry out PCR without reopening tubes and adding fresh polymerase after each denaturing step. A second innovation is the development of the programmable thermal cycler. The thermal cycler, essentially a programmable heating block, is capable of carrying out successive heating and cooling cycles unattended and eliminates the tedious task of transferring reaction tubes between water baths or heating blocks. This has fostered partial automation and simplification so that PCR can now be performed in a diagnostic laboratory.

Many adaptations of the PCR process that are relevant to clinical diagnostics have been described.[47] Those more frequently used include **nested PCR, multiplex PCR**, and **reverse transcriptase PCR**. Nested PCR generally uses two sets of amplification primers — one set targeted within the amplification product of the other set — and two rounds of amplification, in order to amplify specific target DNA.[48,49] This procedure is designed to increase the sensitivity of PCR by directly reamplifying the product from a primary PCR via a second reaction. Nested PCR offers an extremely sensitive method of direct detection of target molecule by direct DNA staining and elimination of the steps in additional the postamplification hybridization using a labeled probe. Enhanced sensititivity is achieved by verifying the specificity of the first product. Nested PCR is, however, prone to contamination. Open transfer of first round products can lead to contamination by the second PCR reaction, since the first round products cannot be inactivated. In multiplex PCR, multiple primer pairs specific for different targets are included in the same amplification reaction.[50] For example, a multiplex PCR reaction that employed one set of primers specific for the mec A gene and the second primer pair that amplified the 16S rDNA ubiquitous among *S. aureus* has been described.[27] Besides providing internal controls for amplifiability of the sample, cost–effective panels of tests for multiple pathogens from a single specimen can also be developed.[51] An exciting application of multiplex PCR is for screening of drug resistance determinants along with the detection and identification of the pathogen.[52]

While initially developed for amplification of DNA targets, PCR has had a major impact on detection of RNA targets such as ribosomal RNA, messenger RNA, and viral nucleic acids (hepatitis C, influenza virus, picornavirus). Detection of RNA templates requires three steps: (1) a RNA reverse transcription (where the extracted RNA is first converted to cDNA by using a retroviral reverse transcriptase), (2) a DNA primer extension, and (3) a polymerase chain reaction. This process has been simplified recently with the discovery of a new thermostable DNA polymerase (Tth) isolated from *Thermus thermophilus*.[53] This single enzyme is capable of converting RNA to cDNA at 72°C in the presence of manganese (Mn^{2+}). A simple change in buffer conditions by the addition of magnesium and ethylene glycol tetraacetic acid (EGTA) switches the template specificity of the *T. thermophilus* polymerase from

RNA to DNA. In addition, Tth may be more resistant to blood components that inhibit *Taq* DNA polymerase.

Because the reverse transcription methods can detect messenger RNA, their results provide information on the expression of different genes. Consequently, specific detection of RNA targets may discriminate dormant from actively growing pathogens and may be useful in monitoring antimicrobial therapy. The ability of PCR to quantify mRNA will be particularly useful for the study of chronic and reactivation diseases such as tuberculosis, HIV, cervical cancer, and CMV. An intriguing approach for the detection of viable but noncultivable organisms in tissues has recently been demonstrated in *Mycobacterium leprae*.[54] In this approach, the authors employed a cDNA-linked PCR amplification of the 71-kDa heat shock protein (hsp) mRNA as a target for determining viability of *M. leprae*. The assay is based on the proposition that due to short half-life (about 2 min) of prokaryotic mRNA, dead bacilli will have either no mRNA or much reduced levels as compared to viable bacilli. This approach may also be applied for detecting drug resistance to antileprosy compounds, and may prove to be superior in ease, speed, and sensitivity than the mouse foot-pad models currently used for this purpose. Effectiveness of new antileprosy compounds for therapy can also be potentially monitored.

Efficient detection of PCR products in clinical diagnostic laboratories require formats that are (1) sensitive and specific, (2) nonisotopic, and (3) amenable to automation. Choice of appropriate detection method depends on several factors, such as the level of specificity of the amplification and the need for high sensitivity of detection. The earliest description of PCR used radioactively labeled probes for the detection of amplified products.[55] This was followed by visualization of amplified DNA by using ethidium bromide-stained gels.[56] A combination of both these techniques (Southern blots, dot blots, oligomer hybridization analysis) have been used extensively for many PCR protocols. These methods provide excellent sensitivy and specificity. Although radioactive probes can now be replaced with chemiluminescent probes, these methods are generally time consuming and labor intensive and require special training of laboratory personnel.

Because probes provide additional sensitivity and specificity for detection of the amplified product, methods that combine PCR amplification with nonisotopic detection such as dot blots,[57] reverse dot blots,[58] the colorimetric microtiter plate assay,[12] and the hybridization protection assay[59] have been developed for the detection of PCR products. The reverse dot blot is a novel detection format. In this format, sequence-specific capture probes immobilized on a solid support (such as nylon strips) are used to hybridize products (e.g., DNA double-stranded products for PCR) obtained after amplification. If biotinylated primers are used in amplification, the bound target can be visualized using a strepavidin-horseradish peroxidase enzyme conjugate. While this detection method can be both sensitive and specific and is convenient for analyzing a large number of samples, it is not easily adapted to laboratory automation because membrane strips must be individually processed and the results visually recorded.

Other assays have been developed that employ 96-well microtiter plate detection formats.[60,61] The latter take advantage of existing laboratory technology for plate handling and quantification of results. In the "sandwich hybridization" format (which is similar in concept to the reverse dot blot), amplification of target DNA occurs in the presence of biotinylated primers.[60] The amplified DNA with its 5' biotinylated end is then specifically captured via capture probes bound to the wells of a 96-well microtiter plate. After washing away the unbound DNA, a chromogenic substrate is added to detect the amplified DNA colorimetrically (Figure 3). Similar assays have been described for the detection of *Chlamydia trachomatis*,[12] and for human immunodeficiency virus.[62]

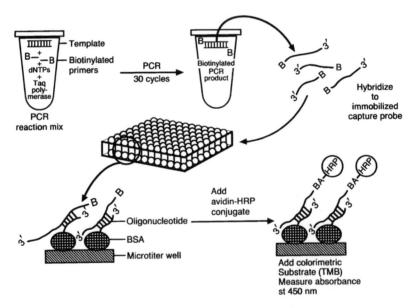

Figure 3

Microtiter plate-based colorimetric detection of PCR amplification products. An oligonucleotide probe specific for the amplified target sequence is bound to wells of the plate. Biotinylated amplified target DNA is hybridized to the wells and then washed and detected with avidin-horseradish peroxidase (HRP) and a chromogenic substrate. B, biotin; BSA, bovine serum albumin; BA, biotin-avidin complex; TMB, tetramethylbenzidine; dTNP, deoxynucleoside triphosphate. (From Persing, D. H., *J. Clin. Micro.*, 29, 1281, 1991. With permission.)

Detection of rare sequence variants within the amplification products presents additional challenges. The most sensitive method for detecting single nucleotide variants is the "allele-specific" PCR. One such system is single-strand conformation polymorphism analysis (PCR-SSCP). In PCR-SSCP, the target sequence in genomic DNA or cDNA is simultaneously amplified and labeled by using radioactive-labeled primers or nucleotides. The amplified product is then denatured to a single-stranded form and subjected to nondenaturing polyacrylamide gel electrophoresis. Bands of the single-stranded DNA at different positions in the autoradiogram indicate the presence of mutations.[63] PCR-SSCP has been used successfully for the detection of rifampin-resistant tuberculosis bacilli.[64] Detection of single base pair mutations has also been applied to the study of resistance of viruses to azidothymidine, zalcitabine (ddc), and didanosine (ddi).

In addition to the above-mentioned techniques, direct sequencing of PCR products has been shown to be extremely useful for detecting more extensive sequence variations at a single nucleotide level. For example, direct sequencing of PCR-amplified products obtained by the "broad range primer" approach (that targets the 16S ribosomal RNA) has been used for genotypic identification of novel and uncultured pathogens (Section VII). Sequence determination has also been useful for detecting nucleotide sequence alterations in pathogens such as hepatitis B virus that may be associated with fulminant hepatic necrosis, or in delineating hepatitis C virus genotypes, which may vary in their virulence or response to alpha-interferon therapy.[65]

While Roche's PCR technology currently dominates the field of DNA amplification, several other firms are preparing their own versions for target and probe amplification (Table 7). These and other signal amplification techniques that do not require thermal cycling (for example branched DNA detection) will be described.

2. Transcription-Based Application: TAS and 3SR

A transcription-based amplification systems (TAS) was first described in 1989 as a non-PCR alternative for target amplification.[66] Jointly developed by SISKA Diagnostics and the Salk Institute, TAS can also use DNA or RNA as starting material. TAS consists of a cDNA synthesis step, followed by an *in vitro* transcription step, using the cDNA as template to generate multiple copies of RNA. TAS efficiency amplified target sequence 2 to 5×10^6-fold after completion of 4 cycles. This method was applied to the detection of the *vif* region of the HIV-1 RNA genome, where it was determined that fewer than one HIV-1 infected cell could be detected in a population of 10^6 uninfected cells.[66] A major drawback to TAS was that heat was needed to denature the RNA–DNA intermediates formed during each cycle of the reaction.

TABLE 7

A Comparison of Enzyme-Catalyzed Amplification Methods

Method	Type of Amplification	No. Target sp. Primers or Probes Required	No. Enzymes Required	Reaction Time (h)	Thermocycling Required	Potential Uses	Patent Rights
PCR	Target	2	1	2–4	Yes	Target detection, cloning, sequencing	Roche Molecular Systems
LCR	Target	4	1	≤2	Yes	Target detection; drug resistance typing	Abbott Diagnostics (Abbott Park, IL)
3SR	Target	2	3	<1	No (Isothermal)	Target detection, cloning, sequencing	Baxter Diagnostics (McGaw Park, IL)
Q β replicase	Probe	1	1	≤1	No (Isothermal)	Target detection	Gene Track Systems (Framingham, MA)
SDA	Target	4	2	2–3	No (Isothermal)	Target detection	Becton Dickinson Instrument System (Sparks, MD)

Heating inactivated the enzymes used in TAS, requiring their replacement at the end of each cycle.

A refinement of the TAS technique was made after the discovery that addition of the enzyme *Escherichia coli* RNase H eliminated the need for heat denaturation of RNA–DNA duplexes. Addition of this enzyme allowed development of an isothermal amplification technique that exploited simultaneous activity of three enzymes — RNase H, avian myeloblastosis virus reverse transcriptase, and T7 polymerase.[67-69] This process was termed **self-sustaining sequence replication** (3SR) or **nucleic acid sequence-based amplification** (NASBA) (Figure 4). The initial steps in the reaction involve the formation of cDNAs from the target RNA by using oligonucleotide primers containing a T7 polymerase binding site. The RNase in the reaction degrades the initial strands of target RNA in the RNA–DNA hybrids after they have served as templates for the first primer. The second primer binds to the newly formed cDNA and is extended, resulting in the formation of double-stranded cDNAs with one or both strands serving as transcription templates for T7 RNA polymerase.[67-69] A well-established property of T7 RNA polymerase is the ability to produce many molecules of RNA from each molecule of template, often exceeding a 3- to 40-fold ratio of product to template. This feature of T7 polymerase has been exploited in order to provide a potent amplification step; the newly synthesised cDNA serves as a template for the synthesis by T7 polymerase of a large molar excess of RNA, which then serves as the substrate for the next cycle. In many respects, 3SR mimics *in vitro* the natural process of replication of the RNA genome of retroviruses. It has been reported that up to 10^8-fold amplification can be achieved in 30 min.[69]

Because reaction conditions with 3SR do not extensively denature DNA, the 3SR is well suited to selective amplification of single-stranded RNA targets. Pretreatment of samples for purification of RNA with DNase prior to amplification (as in PCR) is not required.[47] The single-stranded RNA products of the 3SR reaction have facilitated the detection and characterization of both nucleoside- and nonnucleoside drug-resistant strains of HIV[70-72] and in detecting HIV-1 RNA in the plasma of pediatric patients.[73] 3SR has also been used successfully in the detection of *Chlamydia trachomatis*[74] and human papillomavirus infection.[75]

3. Strand Displacement Amplification

Strand displacement amplification (SDA) is a recently described *in vitro* target amplification method that is based on the ability of DNA polymerases to initiate DNA synthesis at a single-stranded nick within a DNA target molecule.[76] This is followed by displacement of nicked strand during DNA synthesis. Displaced single-stranded molecules

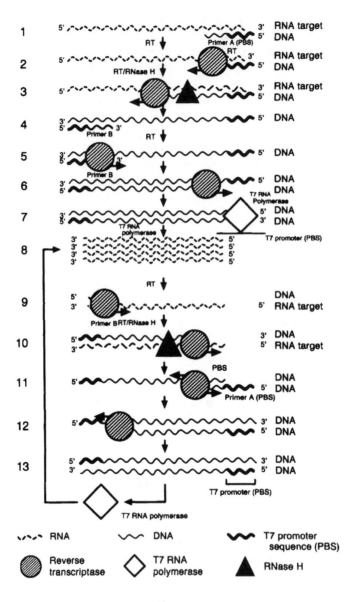

Figure 4

then serve as substrates for additional simultaneous nicking and displacement reactions (Figure 5). The key technology behind SDA is generation of site-specific nicks by a restriction endonuclease prior to amplification.

For amplification, the target DNA sample is heat denatured in the presence of primers and other reagents, after which Hinc II and exo⁻

Klenow fragments of DNA polymerase are added, and the sample is incubated at 37°C. Greater than 10^7-fold amplification of a genomic sequence from MTB was achieved in 2 hours, even in the presence of as much as 10 μg of human DNA. Like 3SR, reactions of SDA are isothermal and simultaneous. Recent modification of SDA eliminates the need for prior restriction endonuclease digestion, and the new target generation scheme uses four primers in a concerted series of DNA polymerase extension and displacement reactions.[77] SDA has been used to amplify a 47-base pair target of the insertion sequence IS6110 from *M. tuberculosis* and *M. bovis*.[78] Recently, a sensitive and rapid chemiluminescent SDA assay was described that could detect as few as 1 to 25 initial IS6110 targets in five species of the MTB complex.[79] Negative results were obtained with 8 other mycobacteria species and 32 nonmycobacterial species.

B. Probe Amplification Techniques

Unlike target amplification methods, amplification of the probe molecules does not result in the incorporation of target information beyond what is originally present in the specimen. Instead, the amplification process occurs by enzymatic duplication of the probe molecules present in the reaction at the outset. Probe-based amplification techniques can be employed for the detection of a signature (target specific) nucleotide sequence within a pathogen.

Figure 4

Nucleic acid amplification by 3SR. 3SR is a continuous series of reverse transcription and transcription that replicates RNA target sequences by means of cDNA intermediates. The initial step in the reaction involves the formation of cDNA from the target RNA using oligonucleotide primers with a T7 binding site (steps 1, 2). The RNase H in the reaction degrades the initial strands of target RNA in the RNA–DNA hybrids after they have served as templates for the initial primer (step 3). The second T7 containing primer then primes the initial single-stranded cDNA, resulting in the formation of double-stranded cDNA with one strand capable of serving as the transcription template for T7 RNA polymerase (steps 4–7). This results in the synthesis of numerous copies of antisense RNA (step 8). These antisense RNAs serve as templates for one of the T7-containing oliginucleotide primers. After a round of priming, the steps of DNA polymerization by reverse transcriptase, RNase H degradation of the RNA–DNA hybrid, and priming and extension of the newly formed cDNA are repeated (steps 9–12). At this stage of the reaction both strands of the cDNA are capable of serving as transcription templates for T7 polymerase (step 13). These cDNAs can yield either sense or antisense RNAs, which then reenter the cycle of priming and extension of the newly formed cDNA strand by the other T7-containing oligonucleotide primer with the subsequent formation of additional double-stranded cDNAs that can serve as templates for either sense or antisense RNA synthesis. (From Persing, D. H., in *Diagnostic Molecular Microbiology: Principles and Applications,* Persing, D. H., Smith, T. F., Tenover, F. C., and White, T. J., Eds., American Society for Microbiology, Washington, D.C., 1993, chap. 3. With permission of the Mayo Foundation.)

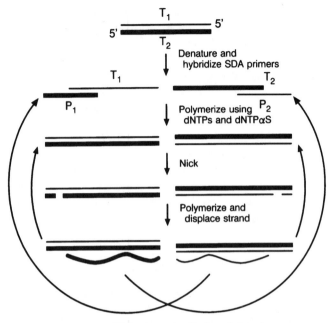

Hybridize SDA primers to displaced strands

Figure 5
SDA reaction. After restriction enzyme digestion and denaturation of a double-stranded target fragment, primers P_1 and P_2 bind to single-strand target fragments T_1 and T_2. The primers contain recognition sites at their 5′ ends for a restriction enzyme. DNA replication with three deoxynucleoside triphosphates (dNTPs) and one dNTP (αS) produces double-stranded primer-target complexes with hemiphosphorothioate recognition sites, which are subsequently nicked by the appropriate restriction enzyme. A DNA polymerase lacking 5′-to-3′ exonuclease activity extends the 3′ end at the nick and displaces the downstream strand. Nicking and polymerization/displacement steps cycle continuously because of regeneration of a nickable recognition site. Exponential amplification occurs because strands displaced from the P_1–T_1 complex serve as target for primer P_2 and strands displaced from the P_2T_2 complex serve as target for primer P_1. (From Persing, D. H., in *Diagnostic Molecular Microbiology: Principles and Applications*, Persing, D. H., Smith, T. F., Tenover, F. C., and White, T. J., Eds., American Society for Microbiology, Washington, D.C., 1993, chap. 3. With permission of the Mayo Foundation.)

One such system is the QB replicase amplification of RNA probe molecules (Figure 6). Named after the major enzyme responsible for the replication of genomic RNA of the QB bacteriophage, QB replicase is a 215-kDa RNA-directed RNA polymerase that is assembled in *E. coli* during infection by QB bacteriophage.[80] The enzyme specifically recognizes a unique folded RNA structure formed by intramolecular base pairing of the QB RNA genome. Application of the QB replicase for nucleic acid amplification arose from the finding that some substrates of QB such as the midvariant (MDV) RNAs, can tolerate short probe inserts and still serve as template for QB replicase. This modified MDV-1

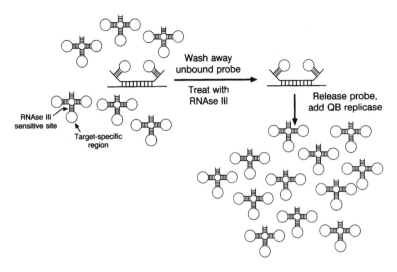

Figure 6

QB replicase. A QB replicase substrate which contains both a target-specific probe region and an endonuclease cleavage site formed by intramolecular base pairing of the probe is produced. When the molecule is annealed to the target sequence, it is RNase III resistant. Unbound probe is treated with RNase and then washed from the reaction mixture by target cycling.[276] QB replicase is then added to the washed target–probe complex, and the reaction is incubated at 37°C, resulting in amplification of the probe. (From Persing, D. H., in *Diagnostic Molecular Microbiology: Principles and Applications*, Persing, D. H., Smith, T. F., Tenover, F. C., and White, T. J., Eds., American Society for Microbiology, Washington, D.C., 1993, chap. 3. With permission of the Mayo Foundation.)

is then used as a hybridization probe. After the probe has annealed specifically to its target and the unbound probe is washed away, the probe is enzymatically replicated *in vitro* by QB replicase to levels that can be readily detected.[81-83] Novel procedures that utilize capture DNA probes have been utilized to decrease nonspecific hybridization signals, which appear to be a formidable problem in QB replicase amplification system.[83] The advantages offered by the QB replicase system include speed and sensitivity (10^7- to 10^9-fold target amplification), and the lack of a requirement for thermal cycling. Microorganisms such as *C. trachomatis*, *Plasmodium falciparum*, HIV-1, CMV, and *Neisseria gonorrheae*[84] have been detected by the QB amplification system.

An alternative probe amplification technique that does not depend on polymerases to copy genetic information *in vitro* is the **ligase chain reaction** (LCR). Developed by Abbott Laboratories, this method employs a thermal stable DNA ligase to join two pairs of complementary oligonucleotide probes after they have bound to a target sequence *in vitro*.[85] The newly ligated product now mimics one strand of the original target sequence and can serve as template for ligation of complementary oligonucleotides. A repetitive cycle of heating and cooling

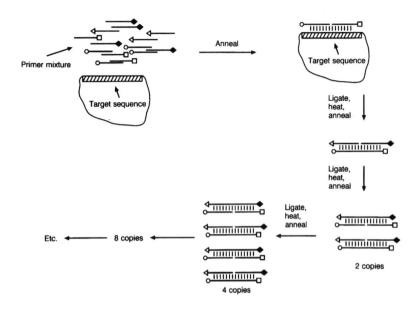

Figure 7

LCR. Oligonucleotide probes are annealed to template molecules in a head-to-tail fashion, with the 3' end of one probe abutting the 5' end of the second. DNA ligase joins the adjacent 3' and 5' ends to form a duplicate of one strand of the target. A second primer set, complementary to the first, then uses this duplicated strand (as well as the original target) as a template for ligation. Repeating the process results in a logarithmic accumulation of ligation products, which can be detected via the functional groups attached to the oligonucleotides. (From Persing, D. H., in *Diagnostic Molecular Microbiology: Principles and Applications,* Persing, D. H., Smith, T. F., Tenover, F. C., and White, T. J., Eds., American Society for Microbiology, Washington, D.C., 1993, chap. 3. With permission of the Mayo Foundation.)

allows denaturation and annealing in the presence of thermal-stable ligase and excess probes so that exponential amplification of the number of specific target sequences is achieved (Figure 7). Since a single base pair mismatch prevents ligation and amplification, the sensitivity and specificity of LCR is generated during the amplification process. The specificity of hybridization of the oligonucleotide probes to the target governs the overall specificity of amplification.

Because of its sensitivity, the LCR assay is compatible with nonradioactive detection and has the potential for automation. Detection of LCR products can be accomplished in a variety of ways.[86,87] Sandwich immunoassays can be devised where the distal terminus of one probe is labeled with a hapten such as fluorescein, and its adjacent partner carries a different hapten such as biotin. After ligation, only the ligated LCR product will display both haptens on the same molecule. Product detection formats have been devised in which antifluorescein-coated microparticles are used to capture the fluorescein-labeled end of the ligation product; an antibiotin:alkaline phosphatase conjugate is used to detect the biotin-labeled end of the ligation product. These formats are compatible with IMX® analyzers (Abbott Laboratories) that are already in place in many laboratories throughout the world.

Performance of LCR was recently compared with that of PCR for the detection of *C. trachomatis* and for HIV, and was found to be equivalent in sensitivity and specificity.[86] Application of LCR have also been documented for a number of other infectious agents,[87] including *N. gonorrheae, Borrelia burgdorferi*, mycobacteria, and human papillomavirus. LCR can also be used to detect point mutations[85] because a mismatched base pair at the point of ligation can prevent ligation of the oligonucleotides. A summary and comparison of the enzyme–catalyzed amplification techniques is presented in Table 7.

C. Signal Amplification Techniques

Unlike target nucleic acid amplification or probe amplification methods, signal amplification methods are designed to increase the signal generated from the probe molecule itself. The nonisotopically labeled probes generally employ horseradish peroxidase or alkaline phosphatase for signal generation (Section IV). Signal amplification procedures do not involve nucleic acid target or probe amplification and may therefore be less prone to contamination problems that are of concern in enzyme-catalyzed amplification techniques. Their overall sensitivity, however, is lower than that of nucleic acid target or probe amplification procedures.

Several signal amplification procedures have been designed to increase the sensitivity of signal generation.[88,89] One such system — the branched DNA (bDNA) is arguably the most powerful. Developed by Chiron Corporation,[90,91] this system employs two types of probes simultaneously: (1) a "primary" probe, recognizing the target sequence and containing multiple binding sites for "secondary" probes, and (2) the secondary probes themselves, each of which contains a reporter group (Figure 8). Incubation of these components with target DNA sequences results in the formation of a "Christmas tree" probe network, in which the primary probe is bound to its target via its target-specific region, leaving the unbound sequence available for binding by the reporter-bearing secondary probes. Depending upon the type of reporter probe used, up to 3000 reporter molecules can be incorporated onto each target sequence. The probe trees thus generated can assume a variety of shapes, depending on whether the primary and secondary probes are linear or circular; but the net result is the same: the signal-generating capability of the probe is significantly increased. bDNA probe systems offer the advantages of excellent specificity and provide quantification

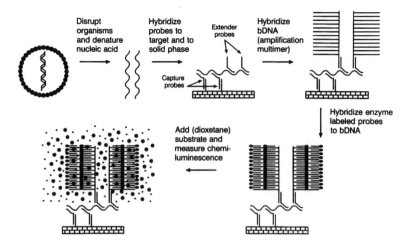

Figure 8

bDNA-based signal amplification. Target nucleic acid is released by disruption and capture to a solid surface via multiple contiguous capture probes. Contiguous extender probes hybridize with adjacent target sequences and contain additional sequences homologous to the branched amplification multimer. Enzyme-labeled oligonucleotides bind to the bDNA by homologous base pairing, and the enzyme–probe complex is measured by detection of chemiluminescence. All hybridization reactions occur simultaneously. (From Persing, D. H., in *Diagnostic Molecular Microbiology: Principles and Applications*, Persing, D. H., Smith, T. F., Tenover, F. C., and White, T. J., Eds., American Society for Microbiology, Washington, D.C., 1993, chap. 3. With permission of the Mayo Foundation.)

ability over a range of several orders of magnitude. bDNA systems are currently being developed for several viruses such as hepatitis B and C viruses,[91-93] cytomegalovirus[94] (CMV), and HIV,[95] and may prove useful for monitoring antiviral therapy.

The fact that several different capture and target-binding probes can be incorporated into a single test system provides another advantage to bDNA probe systems. Although some viruses like HCV and HIV may depict significant sequence heterogeneity, and some capture and target probes may fail to hybridize, the signal production is not completely lost because of the presence of several remaining probe complexes.

VI. SPECIFIC APPLICATIONS

A. Diagnosis of Bacterial Infections

A wide range of bacterial pathogens can be detected by nucleic acid amplification techniques. Pertinent examples are given in Table 8.

TABLE 8

Bacterial Pathogens Detected by Nucleic Acid Amplification

Mycobacterium sp.	*Staphylococcus aureus*
Mycobacterium tuberculosis	*Staphylococcus aureus* toxins
Mycobacterium leprae	Bacterial meningitis pathogens
Mycobacterium avium-intracellulare	Whipple's disease-associated bacillus
Mycobacterium genavense	*Yersinia pestis*
Chlamydia trachomatis	*Yersinia enterocolitica*
Borrelia burgdorferi	*Helicobacter pylori*
Mycoplasma pneumoniae	*Aeromonas hydrophila*[96]
Mycoplasma sp.	Bacillary angiomatosis agent (*Rochalimaea* sp.)
Mycoplasma fermentens	*Listeria monocytogenes*
Salmonella typhimurium	*Comamonas* sp.
Bordetella pertussis	*Bacillus anthracis*
Legionella pneumophila	Coliform bacteria
Clostridium difficile	*Ureaplasma urealyticum*
Trepenoma pallidium	*Neisseria meningitidis*
Enterotoxigenic *E.coli*	*Neisseria gonorrhoeae*
Enterohemorragic *E.coli*	*Mycoplasma genitalium*
Vibrio cholerae	*Campylobacter* sp.
Shigella sp.	*Corynebacterium diphtheriae*
Rickettsia sp.	*Actinobacillus pleuropneumoniae*
Ehrlichia sp.	*Leptospira* sp.
Chlamydia pneumoniae	*Haemophilus influenzae*

Adapted from Persing, D. H., in *Diagnostic Molecular Microbiology: Principles and Applications*, Persing, D. H., Smith, T. F., Tenover, F. C., and White, T. J., Eds., American Society for Microbiology, Washington, D.C., 1993, chap. 3. With permission of the Mayo Foundation.

1. Detection of Mycobacterium tuberculosis

New tools for the rapid detection and speciation of mycobacteria will have a definite impact in the laboratory diagnosis of mycobacterial infections because of the (1) increased frequency of isolation of mycobacterial species (including presence of fastidious and/or rarely encountered species) in immunocompromised hosts and (2) increased frequency of coinfections among HIV-infected individuals.[97] Various approaches[4,98] have been applied for the detection of MTB from clinical specimens (Table 9). While conventional techniques may take 4 to 8 weeks, more rapid techniques are now available such as the BACTEC® system (Becton Dickinson, Towson, MD), which is based on the measurement of carbon dioxide released by bacteria during metabolism of radioactive palmitate in liquid medium,[99] and the Gen-Probe® identification system based on hybridization of chemiluminescent probes to 16S rRNA sequences. Although these techniques reduce the identification time, they still require at least a 1-week period for cultivation. Theoretically, even more rapid detection of the organism is possible with amplification methods.

TABLE 9

A Comparison of the Different Methods Available for Mycobacteria Testing

Method	Use Directly on Specimen	ID of Culture Isolates	Range of Mycobacteria Detected/ID	Yields Isolates for Susceptibility Testing	Usual Turnaround Time	Commercial Availability
Conventional culture and biochem ID	Yes	Yes	Wide range	Yes	4–10 weeks	Yes
HPLC[112]	No	Yes	Wide range	No	1 day after growth	Yes
BACTEC culture[99]	Yes	No	Wide range det.	Yes	7–15 days	Yes
DNA probes	No	Yes	Limited	No	1 day after growth	Yes
Microtiter DNA hybridization[113]	No	Yes	Wide range	No	1–2 days after growth	No
RFLP and DNA fingerprinting[108,114]	No	Strain ID for epidemiology	Strain ID only	No	1–5 days after growth	Some reagents available
PCR[100-107]	Yes	Yes	Wide range	No	1–2 days	No (Roche); in evaluation
PCR-SSCP[64]	Yes	Yes	Limited ?	No	1–2 days	No
MTD[110,111]	Yes	TB complex only	Wide range	No	1 day	No (Gen Probe); in evaluation
SDA[79] (chemiluminescence)	No	TB complex only	Limited	No	<2 h	No
LCR[109]	Yes	M. TB complex only	Limited	No	1–2 days	No

Note: ID: identification; HPLC: high performance liquid chromatography; PCR: polymerase chain reaction; RFLP: restriction fragment length polymorphism; MTD: amplified *Mycobacterium tuberculosis* direct test; PCR-SSCP: polymerase chain reaction–single-stranded conformation polymorphism; SDA: strand displacement amplification; LCR: ligase chain reaction.

Various amplification techniques (Table 9) have been devised to speed up detection of MTB, with the PCR being the most extensively studied. A number of different target genes have been suggested for the PCR-based detection of MTB. Key mycobacterial targets have included the insertion sequence IS6110,[100,101] 65-kDa heat shock protein,[102] MBP 64 protein, 38 kDa protein, and ribosomal RNA.[103,104] IS6110, a mobile genetic element, is a particularly attractive target because of its specificity and presence in high copy numbers (1 to 20) in most strains of MTB complex (MTB, *M. bovis*, *M. bovis* BCG, *M. africanum*, *M. microti*), and its apparent absence in other species of mycobacteria. Amplification of a 123-bp sequence in IS6110 in sputum and respiratory samples from patients with suspected TB has revealed this to be a clinically sensitive and specific assay with a turn-around-time of 48 h.[105]

Researchers from Roche Molecular Systems, Branchburg, NJ, have reported on a PCR (Amplicor) for the direct detection of MTB in sputum specimens.[106] The assay utilizes biotinylated primers specific for the 16S rRNA gene that amplify a 584 bp product. Specificity of the amplified product is verified by hybridization to a MTB specific probe in a colorimetric microtiter plate format via an avidin-HRP conjugate and substrate system. Besides MTB/*M. bovis* detection, microwell plates with probes specific for other mycobacterial species can be employed. The assay also incorporates a uracil N-glycosylase (UNG) product inactivation protocol to prevent the problems of false positive PCR. Performance of this assay with sputum has shown that the PCR can be used as (1) a rapid diagnostic test for MTB and *M. avium-intracellulare* infections and (2) as an adjunct to AFB smear in identifying patients with pulmonary tuberculosis. Commercialization of the test kit is pending FDA clearance.

Nested PCR has been found to enhance the sensitivity of detection of MTB in clinical specimens. Using a two-tube nested procedure with primer sets specific for the 38-kDa protein gene sequence of MTB complex, Miyazaki et al.[107] found that while the detection limit for the first PCR was 10^2 cfu for MTB, the sensitivity increased to approximately 1000-fold to 0.1 cfu following second PCR. The exquisite sensitivity of the nested PCR was hypothesized to be due to detection of target DNA sequences in dead mycobacterial cells or incomplete DNA fragments in culture medium. Routine use of the nested PCR is not recommended, however, since it is prone to PCR-product carryover contamination that can yield false positives.

A rapid procedure for the identification of cultured mycobacterial isolates based on the combination of enzymatic amplification and restriction analysis of the PCR amplicon has been reported to differentiate closely related species of mycobacteria. In one study, PCR amplification of the 16S rRNA gene followed by restriction analysis of amplified rDNA with restriction enzymes *CfoI, MboI,* and *RsaI* could differentiate 99 strains belonging to 18 different species of the genus *Mycobacterium.*[108]

Besides PCR, other sensitive and rapid diagnostic systems employing ligase chain reaction (LCR) assay[109] and/or strand displacement amplification (SDA) assay[79] have been reported recently. Microtiter plate formats have been described for ease in incorporation in a clinical diagnostic laboratory. In the SDA assay, for example, amplified IS6110 products from MTB complex were detected using a nonisotopic biotinylated oligo deoxynucleotide "capture" probe and an alkaline phosphatase conjugated oligo deoxynucleotide "detection" probe that employs dioxetane substrate for detection. Eight other mycobacterial species and 32 nonmycobacterial species were not detected.[79]

While amplification of the MTB-specific targets by PCR, SDA, and/or LCR hold considerable promise for future commercial availability, the first nucleic acid amplification test to be developed for use in the clinical lab is the Gen-Probe® Amplified MTB direct test[110] (MTD). Currently undergoing clinical trials, and pending FDA clearance, the amplified MTD test comprises transcription-mediated (isothermal) amplification of mRNA via DNA intermediates; and a hybridization protection assay employed in the conventional Gen-Probe tests for detection. Since rRNA is present in a level of about 2000 copies per cell as compared to other target sequences, this test offers advantages of enhanced sensitivity.[111] Detailed studies are, however, warranted because of the ability to detect small numbers of nonviable MTB. Although amplification of PCR targets detects and identifies mycobacteria in clinical specimens quickly, most protocols do not detect susceptibilities or resistance to antimicrobial drugs. Recently, PCR has been used for amplifying and probing for genes that code for resistance.

2. Rifampin Resistance in Mycobacteria

A new development in the wake of the AIDS epidemic has been an alarming increase in the incidence of tuberculosis as well as the development of multidrug resistance strains of TB (MDR-TB). Because of the serious threat of MDR-TB to public health, quick and sensitive detection of MDR-TB is vital. Current methods require 4 to 10 weeks for detection of MDR-TB.

Rifampin is a front line drug used for short term treatment of TB.[115] Resistance to rifampin (Rif[r]) is often present in MDR-TB.[116] Rifampin interferes with transcription and RNA elongation in mycobacteria by binding to the beta subunit (rpo B) of the RNA polymerase. Telenti et al.[35] described 15 distinct mutations present in the rpoB gene in 64-Rif[r] organisms. Most mutations follow single-nucleotide substitutions of a limited number of highly conserved codons which confers

TABLE 10

Analysis of Drug Resistance in *Mycobacterium tuberculosis*

Rifampin Resistance as a Surrogate Marker for Multidrug-Resistant Tuberculosis

Almost all MDR-TB strains are rifampin resistant
Spontaneous, isolated Rif[r] is infrequent
Likelihood of MDR increases with rifampin resistance

Fine Structure Analysis of rpoB of Mycobacterium tuberculosis

Mutations clustered in small area
Most mutations occur at two amino acid positions
Amenable to automated sequencing or reverse dot-blotting

Molecular Detection of Rifampin-Resistance Directly from Specimens

Short turnaround time (1–2 days)
Able to identify organisms to species level based on signature sequences
Potentially useful for epidemiologic exposure studies

"single step" high level resistance of MTB and *M. leprae*[117] to rifampin.
These mutations were absent in 56 susceptible organisms. Additional
rare mutant rpoB alleles, with evidence of geographical variation in
the frequency of occurrence, have recently been described using automated DNA sequencing of the rpoB gene.[118] Besides direct sequencing
of PCR- amplified products, mutants have also been identified via PCR-
SSCP, which detects single base changes in PCR products by generating
different electrophoretic mobility of single-stranded DNA strands of
the PCR products. The applicability of PCR-SSCP in detecting Rif[r]
rapidly was recently shown for minimally grown MTB cultures (Bactec
12B medium with a growth index <100), and for direct screening of 3[+]
to 4[+] acid-fast smear-positive patients.[64] PCR-SSCP implementation
may yield a net time gain of several weeks over conventional testing.
To make PCR-SSCP more suitable to clinical application, fluorescein
instead of radioactivity was employed by these authors.

A genotypic approach that incorporates specific signature sequence
of mycobacteria in tuberculosis that allows determination of resistant
genotype *and* direct identification of mutants has been proposed by
Hunt et al.[52] In their evaluation of Rif[r] by semiautomated DNA
sequencing of the rpoB gene, a "signature sequence" of MTB in the
328-base pair rpoB amplification product was identified. Bacterial species other than MTB did not yield PCR product comprising these
sequences. Table 10 summarizes the key features of Rif[r] in MTB. Other
potential targets for detection of MDR-TB are genes encoding iso-
niazid, streptomycin, pyrazinamide, and ciprofloxacin/quinolone
drug resistance.

B. Lyme Disease

Lyme disease is the most common tick-borne disease in the U.S and is caused by the spirochete *Borrelia burgdorferi*. The majority of the cases have occurred in the northeastern, northwestern, and upper midwestern states.[119] Establishing a clinical diagnosis is often difficult because Lyme borreliosis presents itself as a multisystem disorder with dermatologic, neurologic, and musculoskeletal components. The hallmark of Lyme disease is erythema migrans (EM), an expanding erythematous skin lesion that occurs at the site of the tick bite in 60% of the patients, and which is often accompanied with other nonspecific flu-like symptoms.[120,121]

Lyme disease has typically been defined by clinical evidence supported by serological test results. In spite of significant advances in immunologic assays, accurate diagnosis of Lyme borreliosis remains problematic.[122] As many as 5 to 10% of normal asymtomatic individuals may be seropositive by some assays. The enzyme-linked immunosorbent test (ELISA) which is frequently ordered to screen for antibodies to *B. burgdorferi* has not been standardized, and Western immunoblotting is often needed to clarify questionable ELISA results.[123] Lyme disease may be an overdiagnosed disease because false-positive ELISA test results for *B. burgdorferi* can occur in various inflammatory conditions, including rheumatoid arthritis, systemic lupus erythematosis, syphilis, and nonspirochetal infections such as malaria, Epstein-Barr virus infection, and subacute bacterial endocarditis.[124] In addition, variability in host immune responses in which antibody production may be suppressed or delayed because of antibiotic treatment,[125] along with antigenic complexity of *B. burgdorferi*,[122] may all be responsible in part for the problems associated with serodiagnostic testing.

Culture has been used as an alternative means of laboratory confirmation. While *B. burgdorferi* is a cultivable spirochete and can be cultured from the skin lesions of EM,[126] it is difficult to isolate with any degree of regularity from blood, joint fluid, or CSF. Moreover, culture is neither rapid nor widely available.

More recently, PCR and DNA hybridization techniques have been used to amplify and detect *B. burgdorferi* DNA in cultured spirochetes,[127] Ixodes *dammini/scapularis* ticks,[128,129] infected animals,[130] and patients with Lyme disease in whom culture was negative for the Lyme spirochete.[131] Different target sequences have been utilized for examining the diagnostic potential of PCR in tissues and body fluids from patients with Lyme disease.[132-135] Target sequences for the extrachromosomal gene encoding an outer surface membrane protein (OSP A and OSP B) were found much more frequently than was a genomic 16S rRNA target in synovial fluid specimens.[135]

TABLE 11

Potential Advantages of PCR Testing of Lyme Disease

Rapid turnaround time (2 days as compared with 6–8 weeks) for culture techniques
Serological analysis lacks high positive and negative predictive value
PCR extends the range of specimens that can be tested ("dead" specimens considered
  unsuitable for analysis by conventional means)
For detecting *B. burgdorferi* in patients with possible seronegative or early Lyme disease
To differentiate persistent infection from postinfective immune-mediated phenomenon
  in synovial fluid
For detection of other pathogens within the same specimen, e.g., *B. burgdorferi* and *Babesia
  microti* that share the vector *I. dammini*[138]

The shedding of membrane vesicles containing extrachromosomal DNA (OSP A) from the surface of *B. burgdorferi* and its persistence in synovium long after the organism has been eliminated have raised concern that this persistence of spirochetal DNA may result in false positive PCR results. However, a recent study by Nocton et al.[136] has shown PCR detection of *B. burgdorferi* OSP A DNA to be a highly sensitive and specific indicator of the presence of the spirochete. Their studies indicated that OSP A DNA could be detected in 75 of 88 patients with Lyme arthritis and in none of the 64 control patients. The OSP A DNA was detected primarily in untreated patients with clinically active disease. Following antibiotic treatment, PCR results were usually negative. The authors also addressed another key issue, namely, the persistent arthritis in patients despite multiple courses of antibiotics. In such patients, the crucial question is how long should antibiotic therapy be continued. The authors found that PCR testing could differentiate whether persistent arthritis in patients after treatment was due to active infection vs. a postinfective, immune-mediated phenomenon that persisted after eradication of viable spirochete. PCR may, therefore, aid in therapeutic decisions for patients with persistent Lyme arthritis (Table 11).

Data on the diagnosis of neuroborreliosis by PCR is less clear. Like chronic Lyme arthritis, chronic neurologic Lyme disease, if untreated, can persist. Intrathecal antibody production against *B. burgdorferi* is commonly seen. PCR amplification of *B. burgdorferi* flagellin gene in CSF was shown to be useful in diagnosis of neuroborreliosis in patients in whom serological markers and/or culture were negative.[132] Recently, nested PCR in CSF and urine was studied in children and was found to be a useful adjunct to, but not a substitute for, clinical judgment.[137] Some of the studies in neuroborreliosis to date have been performed in a prospective blinded fashion: given the problems of false positivity of PCR, much of the data in retrospective analysis may be open to question.

C. Detection of Viral Pathogens

A large number of viral pathogens can be readily detected by the use of nucleic acid amplification technology (Table 12). The clinical application of these methods will be specially useful for detecting viruses that grow slowly or not at all (HPV, EBV, HIV, hepatitis virus) or, for specimen sources (cerebrospinal fluid [CSF], formalin-fixed, or parafin-embedded tissue) in which it is difficult to recover viruses like HSV, EBV, JCV by conventional techniques. Detection by PCR of herpes simplex virus from CSF of patients compatible with clinical features of HSV encephalitis/meningitis are particularly valuable because of its sensitivity[141-143] and noninvasiveness as compared to a brain biopsy for identification. HSV-specific sequences have also been successfully amplified from formalin-fixed paraffin-embedded skin biopsies of lesions of erythema multiforme by PCR.[142] PCR was found to be very specific, and no cross-reaction was observed among individuals with various dermatological problems. An important application of nucleic acid technology has been in the amplification of EBV sequences from tissue samples from immunosuppressed patients with lymphoproliferative disorders, AIDS, or transplant-related lymphomas.[144] In these studies, PCR confirmed prior EBNA immunostaining and *in situ* hybridization.[145]

Another important pathogen in immunocompromised patients and infants exposed to congenital infections is CMV. Active CMV infection occurs in 20 to 60% of recipients of all types of allografts. Although many specimens, including urine and saliva, may be cultured for CMV, detection of CMV in these specimens may represent asymptomatic shedding and may not be clinically relevant. Isolation of CMV in blood (viremia), on the other hand, is considered to be a marker of disseminated CMV infection and correlates well with significant disease.[146,147] Diagnosis is important since antiviral drugs such as gancyclovir and foscarnet have become available for treatment of severe CMV disease.

Although culture of CMV on human fibroblast is considered the "gold standard" identification of virus in culture, it may take several days to several weeks. The use of shell vial viral culture procedure, in conjunction with monoclonal antibodies (Mabs) directed at immediate-early CMV antigens, has made it possible to detect CMV within 24 hours.[148] In addition, CMV viremia can be detected directly in white blood cells by the CMV 65-kDa lower matrix phosphoprotein (pp65) antigenaemia assay (CMV-vue; INCSTAR Corp.; Stillwater, MN) within hours.[149] It has been proposed that the latter test may also be used to monitor disease activity and its response to chemotherapy by quantitating the number of circulating leukocytes expressing CMV antigens.[150] In addition, antigenemia has been reported to appear 3 to 9

TABLE 12

Viral Pathogens Detected by Nucleic Acid Amplification

Herpesviridae

    Herpes simplex virus types I and II
    Epstein-Barr virus
    Cytomegalovirus
    Varicella-zoster virus
    Human herpesviruses 6 and 7

Papovaviridae

    Human JC virus
    Human papillomavirus

Flaviviridae

    Hepatitis C virus
    Enteroviruses

Hepadnaviridae

    Hepatitis B virus
    Hepatitis D virus

Retroviridae

    HIV- 1 and HIV-2
    HTLV-I and HTLV-II
    HBLV

Orthomyxoviridae

    Influenza virus
    Parvoviridae
    Human parvovirus B19

Adenoviridae

    Human adenovirus

Togaviridae

    Rubella virus

Picornaviridae

    Rhinovirus
    Hepatitis A virus

Calciviridae

    Hepatitis E virus

Bunyaviridae

    Hantavirus[139,140]

Adapted from Persing, D. H., in *Diagnostic Molecular Microbiology: Principles and Applications*, Persing, D. H., Smith, T. F., Tenover, F. C., and White, T. J., Eds., American Society for Microbiology, Washington, D.C., 1993, chap. 3. With permission of the Mayo Foundation.

days before the onset of viremia (as detected by shell vial) and 1 to 2 weeks before an antibody response.

Several studies have evaluated the use of PCR detection of CMV DNA in blood specimens. A general finding has been that although excellent sensitivities have been obtained, CMV DNA detection has not in all cases been shown to be specific for detection of clinically relevant infections. To make more meaningful statements about symptomatic disease, assays that specifically quantify CMV DNA and/or detect CMV mRNA are being developed. Drouet et al.[151] used a semiquantitative PCR to study the development of CMV retinitis during progression of AIDS by measuring CMV levels in blood. Known amounts of purified CMV DNA in concentrations equivalent to 0.8 to 80,000 CMV genomic copies were included as internal reference standards. They found a strong correlation between high PCR signal and clinical symptoms. A high risk of relapse was noted in these patients if an absence of PCR reactivity was not achieved after antiviral therapy. Detection of CMV mRNA in blood has likewise been used as a marker closely related to active stages of CMV infection. Velzing et al.[152] analyzed peripheral blood leukocytes from 36 immunocompromised patients, for the presence of CMV immediate early antigen (IEA) DNA and CMV IEA mRNA. Primers were derived from the intron–exon structure of the IEA gene that allowed discrimination between amplified DNA originating from mRNA and DNA. A serial fold dilution of plasmid-derived RNA transcript containing the major IEA gene of CMV was incorporated as a control for sensitivity of cDNA synthesis and subsequent PCR. The assay had a detection sensitivity of 10 to 100 RNA molecules. No correlation was found by these authors between serology and the presence of CMV IEA DNA. A close correlation was found between results of CMV mRNA and pp65 antigen detection assay that also correlated with clinical findings.

Storch et al.[153] recently compared detection of CMV infections in blood leukocytes from solid organ transplant patients by PCR, antigenemia, and quantitative shell vial assays. While PCR was the most sensitive of the three for detection of viruses, the commercial pp65 antigenemia assay and quantitative shell vial assay were of equivalent sensitivity for the recognition of CMV infections. Besides blood leukocytes, detection of CMV DNA in plasma or serum has been proposed for indicating clinically significant infections. A strong correlation has been observed between CMV DNA detection in plasma and isolation of CMV from corresponding blood leukocytes,[154] thus supporting the view that besides cell-to-cell contact, virus dissemination might occur by cell-free virus.

Nucleic acid detection techniques are also important for direct assessment of tissue invasive disease for which antiviral therapy might be considered. As compared to *in situ* hybridization assays which may

TABLE 13

PCR Testing for Diagnosis of CMV Disease

Advantages

Detects CMV disease much earlier after transplant than does culture or antigenemia
Strong correlation between viremia and high PCR signal
Quantitative detection of CMV aids determination of symptomatic vs. asymptomatic
  infection
Allows monitoring of patients on antiviral therapy
Useful for assessment of tissue invasive disease

Disadvantages

May detect latent infection
Poor predictive value in immunosuppressed patients

be somewhat less sensitive than a histopathological diagnosis,[155] the detection of genomic CMV DNA by PCR has been found to be extremely useful for (1) confirming histologically proven CMV disease, and more importantly (2) for predicting development of disease in tissues that are culturally and histologically negative for CMV. Wolff et al.[156] showed that CMV-PCR performed on liver biopsy tissues from orthotopic liver transplant patients correctly identified the development of CMV hepatitis 1 to 2 weeks earlier than histological diagnosis.

Because immunocompromised patients might be productively infected with CMV without evidence of clinical disease, a quantitative evaluation of CMV DNA in lung tissue was assesssed by Shibata et al.[157] for the diagnosis of CMV pneumonitis. Using a plasmid DNA containing the immediate early gene 1 of CMV as a PCR standard, they found the copy number of CMV genome in the lung tissue of CMV pneumonitis patients to be 1000-fold more than that of the patients without CMV disease. Strong PCR signals correlated well with virus isolation and CMV-specific histology.

Table 13 summarizes the advantages and disadvantages of PCR testing for the assessment of CMV disease.

D. Retroviruses

The worldwide epidemic spread of human immunodeficiency virus (HIV-1) has stimulated the creation of immunological assays (Table 14 A) for diagnosing the presence of HIV-1 infection, protecting the blood supply, predicting progression to AIDS, and monitoring the effect of antiviral drug therapy. There are, however, several situations (Table 15) where quicker and more sensitive molecular assays (Table 14 B) are desirable. For example, although exposure to HIV nearly always

TABLE 14

Techniques Available for HIV Detection

A. Antibody-Based Detection Systems

Enzyme immuno assay (EIA)
Western blot
Latex agglutination
Radioimmunoprecipitation
Immunofluorescence

B. Molecular Detection Systems

Oligomer solution hybridization (OSP)
DNA probes (hybridization protection assay)
In situ hybridization
Polymerase chain reaction
Self-sustained sequence replication
Ligase chain reaction

TABLE 15

Potential Applications of Nucleic Acid Amplification Techniques
for HIV Detection in:

High risk seronegative individuals
Resolving HIV indeterminate Western blot
Differentiation of HIV-1 from HIV-2[158]
Detection of both HIV-1 proviral DNA and HIV-1 RNA
Detection of HIV-1 point mutations associated with zidovudine resistance *in vitro*[159]
Diagnosis of HIV-1 infection in infants born to sero-positive mothers
Determining efficacy of experimental anti-HIV-1 drugs and vaccines
Diagnosis of neurological involvement

results in the production of diagnostic antibodies, these may not be detected for months to over 1 year.[160,161] Unless the individual is exposed to large quantities of the virus, as is the case with blood transfusions, viral antigens are not detected until the virus has had a chance to replicate into substantial numbers. Establishing the diagnosis of HIV infection can thus be difficult in seronegative persons with acute infection and in neonates born to HIV-positive mothers (see below). Polymerase chain reaction, viral culture, or antigen detection may be useful tests in these settings.

The polymerase chain reaction has been used extensively for diagnosis of human HIV-1 infection. Amplification techniques have been combined with product detection systems to achieve high sensitivity. Two such systems are currently available commercially. The Gen-Probe Corp (San Diego, CA) kit makes use of nonisotopic solution phase acridinium ester-labeled probes for the detection of amplified HIV-1 *gag* PCR products.[59,162] Another nonisotopic detection technique developed by Roche Molecular Systems (Branchburg, NJ), uses *gag* biotinylated primers to generate biotinylated amplicons for detection in a colorimetric assay.[162,163] The kit contains all reagents necessary for sample preparation, amplification, and detection of HIV-1 proviral DNA. Uracil N-glycosylase sterilization (Section IX. E) has been incorporated to avoid potential contamination with amplicons that result in false positive reactions. Other PCR applications have been described that include nested PCR and/or RT-PCR that detects several HIV-specifc mRNAs — including *gag*, *env*, and *tat/rev* in patient peripheral blood mononuclear cells (PBMC) and/or CSF.[164]

Diagnostic retrovirology and immunodiagnosis for early detection of HIV in young children has progressed considerably. Preliminary studies indicate that HIV-1 DNA PCR assays can detect HIV-1 sequences in the peripheral blood mononuclear cells of approximately 50% of infected newborns within the first week of life[165] and in greater than 90% of infected infants after 1 month of age.[166,167] Besides enhanced detection sensitivity, a considerable faster turnaround time (1 day) was achieved as compared to about 4 weeks for HIV-1 cultures. IgA antibody tests and p24 antigen tests have also proved useful, although they are not as sensitive in newborn infants.[168,169] The diagnosis of HIV-1 infection in infants born to seropositive mothers is especially difficult as maternal antibody has been reported to persist for up to 18 months.[170] In all cases, careful interpretation of PCR test results and close correlation with patient risk factors are vital to establish the proper diagnosis.[171]

Various quantitative/semiquantitative HIV-1 PCR assays have been described that measure the proviral load in the DNA sample, or the amount of genomic HIV-1 RNA in plasma samples.[172,173] The hybridization protection assay, under conditions using only a few rounds of amplification to stay within the linear portion of the curve, and rapid solution hybridization kinetics using high levels of the probe, have been used for quantitative detection of proviral DNA.[59]

A microparticle capture method that binds plasma virions on microparticles coated with monoclonal antibodies to external and membrane proteins of HIV-1 was recently described to measure plasma viremia. This method was found to be highly sensitive in detecting genomic HIV-1 RNA in both seropositive and seronegative patient specimens.[174] Quantitation of viral RNA after RT-PCR amplification was determined by comparing the intensity of the signal against a standard dilution series of HIV-1 RNA standards that are amplified and detected concurrently. PCR-based measurement of plasma RNA levels after dideoxynucleoside therapy was found to be useful for analysis of disease stage and progression as well as for monitoring of drug efficacy. While quantification of viral infections *in vivo* is a coveted goal,

TABLE 16

Limitations of the Polymerase Chain Reaction in Retroviral Diagnosis

False-negative results (nucleotide variation in target sequence — need for multiple primer pairs)
Level of detection = <5 copies/2×10^5 cells may not be detected
Poor sample preparation
Lack of standardized protocols for HIV-1 quantification
False positives (product "carry over")

issues relating to variability of reverse transcriptase step and RNA stability during specimen processing and storage need to be addressed before clinical application can be achieved.

Some limitations of PCR in retroviral diagnosis are listed in Table 16. False negative reactions may result for a variety of reasons.[175] Given the heterogeneity of the viral genome, nucleotide variation in the target sequence complementary to the primer pair can result in poor amplification efficiency. To minimize this likelihood, primers are selected from highly conserved sequences of the viral genome. In addition, very low copy numbers of target sequence (less than five copies per 2×10^5 cells) may fail to be detected. Other limitations include the presence of intrinsic inhibitors in some clinical specimens and false positive reaction tests due to contamination of samples and reagents with amplified products. Methods to overcome these limitations are discussed in a following section. Besides PCR, other amplification techniques like self-sustained sequence replication of viral RNA and the ligase chain reaction are under development and offer sensitivity and the potential for automation.[176,177]

E. Viral Hepatitis

Serological markers for clinical diagnosis of viral hepatitis, particularly for hepatitis B virus (HBV) infection, have been well characterized. Acute HBV infection is typically distinguished from chronic disease by a positive IgM, antihepatitis B core antigen (anti-HBc) test. Conversely, patients with chronic hepatitis B remain hepatitis B surface antigen (HBsAg) positive, often with raised serum alanine aminotransferase (ALT) enzymes for more than 6 months.

Antibody-based detection is now complemented by newer molecular biological techniques. HBV DNA is considered to be the most sensitive marker of viral replication and infectivity. The degree of infectivity was previously related to the presence of hepatitis Be antigen in serum and hepatitis B core antigen in liver cells. Hybridization assays (dot blot, liquid phase, Southern blot) have been used as a means of determining both the presence of viral genomes and the response to

TABLE 17

Advantages of PCR in the Diagnosis of Viral Hepatitis

Demonstration of active viremia
Identification of HBV-DNA and HCV-RNA in seronegative patients due to delayed
  seroconversion in acute infection; seronegative chronic carriers; liver transplant patients
  on immunosuppressive therapy
Studies of mother-to-child transmission
Monitoring of antiviral treatment
Analysis of genetic variability and its implications

antiviral treatment.[178] Low levels of hepatitis B viremia are, however, more efficiently detected by the PCR. Because of enhanced detection of small amounts of viral DNA, PCR has markedly improved the diagnostic sensitivity of HBV detection. Thus the study of HBV DNA has become a valuable part of the management of chronic hepatitis B, providing a more reliable evaluation of virus replication and infectivity, and facilitating more precise statements about course and prognosis of the disease (Table 17).

Diagnosis of acute hepatitis C virus (HCV) infection, on the other hand, has remained largely dependent on patient history and the exclusion of non-A, non-B hepatitis. Second generation ELISA tests that utilize recombinant antigens from the core and nonstructural (NS-3) regions of HCV have been developed to detect anti-HCV antibodies in chronic infections. Since patients with autoimmune hepatitis have high levels of gamma globulin, false-positive results can occur with the ELISA assays. A recombinant immunoblot assay (RIBA II) has been developed for confirmation in these cases. Although it is has been estimated that 10 to 30% more HCV antibody positive individuals are detected using the second generation assays. The main value of RIBA has been in excluding false-positive EIA-2 results. In addition, anti-HCV antibodies may appear late (lag times of several weeks to several months) or not at all, although anti-HCV RNA may be detectable on PCR reaction within days of infection (Figure 9). While over 90% of RIBA-positive specimens are also RT-PCR positive,[179] RT-PCR has been found to be useful in identifying viral RNA (viraemia) in serum or plasma during chronic disease in the absence of antibody.[180]

PCR is also a highly sensitive technique for the detection of hepatitis C virus-RNA in liver tissue and peripheral blood cells. For PCR, most laboratories use primers from the 5′ untranslated region of the molecule because it is the most conserved. It is not necessary to use a two-stage "nested" PCR to achieve the greater sensitivity for the HCV genome because significant contamination problems may occur.[179] The sensitivity and specificity of PCR product can be confirmed with labeled HCV-specific probe.

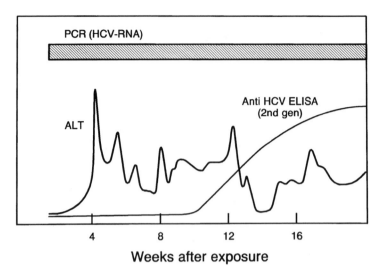

Figure 9
Timing of serologic diagnostic markers of hepatitis C virus (HCV) infection. A characteristic feature of chronic HCV infection is the fluctuation of the aspartate aminotransferase (AST, SGOT) and alanine aminotransferase (ALT, SGPT) levels. It is, however, difficult to correlate symptoms and transaminase levels with the severity of hepatic inflammation. Detection of HCV-RNA by PCR may be useful during early infection. Seropositivity as detected by the second generation anti-HCV ELISA appears weeks to months after infection.

Based on sequence similarities of complete genomic sequences of fragments amplified by PCR, HCV has been classified into at least six major genotypes. The study of genotypes is important for the following reasons: (1) major differences have been observed in the geographical distributions of HCV variants;[181] (2) certain genotypes (such as type 1b) are associated with a higher rate of chronic hepatitis or cirrhosis than are genotypes 2, 3, or 4;[182] (3) a proportion of donors with divergent HCV genotypes may elicit restricted serological responses so as to be undetectable by current blood donor screening methods; and (4) response to treatment with alpha interferon (IFN) may vary for different genotypes (i.e., type 1 may exhibit poorer response to treatment than do types 2 and 3).[65,183,184]

Although therapy with alpha-IFN has been approved by the U.S. FDA, less than half of HCV-infected persons respond to treatment, and only about 10% of patients experience a long-term remission. Since relapse occurs in about half of all patients that respond to alpha-IFN, PCR has been used to monitor both antiviral treatment and reinfection, especially after liver transplantion.[184,185] The antiviral effects of alpha-IFN on chronic HCV infections has been estimated by determining quantitative changes in serum[186] and peripheral blood mononuclear cell HCV-RNA levels.[187]

TABLE 18

Applications of Polymerase Chain Reaction in Transfusion Medicine for
Diagnosis of Infectious Diseases

Confirmation of donors with indeterminate serologies
Screening of blood/blood products for virus during seronegative stages of disease
Simultaneous detection of viruses in one assay
Diagnosis of acute infection caused by passively transferred antibody
Screening of transfusion-related bacteremias using universal probe system

Quantitation of HCV RNA has also been performed with the branched DNA signal amplification technique (Quantiplex™ HCV-RNA assay, Chiron Corporation). The quantitative studies have suggested the mode of acquisition to be an important determinant of viremia, which in turn determines the response to IFN therapy. Significant higher titers of HCV RNA have been observed in patients with concurrent HIV infections as compared to titers in patients with HCV alone.[188]

F. Applications of PCR in Transfusion Medicine

The first application of PCR in transfusion medicine (Table 18) will probably be for confirmation testing of donors who have indeterminate viral serologic results. The polymerase chain reaction can be applied to the study of the entire range of transfusion-transmitted infections. RNA viruses can be analyzed if a DNA copy is made from the viral RNA by treatment with reverse transcriptase. The retroviruses, including HIV-1, HIV-2, HTLV-I, HTLV-II, CMV, HCV, and HBV,[189] have been extensively studied by PCR. The potential to carry simultaneous screening for a number of viruses in one PCR assay may eventually broaden the scope of PCR testing beyond confirmatory testing.

The advantages of PCR also include detection of virus during the "window period" or seronegative stages of infections and during viremia. PCR assays may also be beneficial in detecting contaminants in blood components derived from large pools of plasma. With the development of automation, it has been proposed to use PCR as a routine screening test to identify infected donors who may have no detectable antibody response. However, substantial decreases in costs will have to be achieved before this occurs. PCR can also help overcome the inhibition of diagnosis of acute infection caused by the presence of passively transferred antibody. In addition to viral pathogens, bacteremia due to *Yersinia enterocolitica* and other organisms may be problematic in transfusion medicine.[190,191] Although infrequent, these organisms may be detected by a "universal primer" system (Section VII). This system incorporates a series of primer sequences common to all bacteria and yeasts.[192]

TABLE 19

Protozoal and Helminth Infections
Detectable by Nucleic Acid Techniques

Babesia bigemina
Babesia bovis
Babesia microti
Brugia malayi[193]
Echinococcus multilocularis; E. granulosus[194]
Entamoeba histolytica
Giardia lambia
Leishmania sp.
Naegleria fowleri
Onchocerca volvulus[195]
Plasmodium sp.
Taenia saginata
Toxoplasma gondii
Trichomonas vaginalis
Trypanosoma sp.
Trichinella spirales

Adapted from Persing, D. H., in *Diagnostic Molecular Microbiology: Principles and Applications*, Persing, D. H., Smith, T. F., Tenover, F. C., and White, T. J., Eds., American Society for Microbiology, Washington, D.C., 1993, chap. 3. With permission of the Mayo Foundation.

G. Detection of Parasitic Pathogens

Detection of varous blood and tissue parasites have been described by PCR (Table 19). Babesiosis is a malaria-like illness that is caused by a protozoan parasite, *Babesia*, that invades erythrocytes.[196] The genus *Babesia* comprises more than 100 species of tick-transmitted protozoal pathogens that infect a wide variety of vertebrate hosts.[197] Two species *B. microti* (in the U.S.), and *B. divergens* (in Europe) appear to be responsible for virtually all known cases of babesiosis. *B. microti* shares both a vertebrate host reservoir, *Peromyscus leucopus*, and tick vector (*I.dammini/I.scapularis; I. pacificus*) with *Borrelia burgdorferi*. In endemic areas, therefore, it might be expected that the case load for human babesiosis will parallel the rise in the number of cases of Lyme disease.[198,199] Clinical diagnosis is difficult, especially during the early stages in which nonspecific symptoms may mimic symptoms of other diseases such as Lyme disease or influenza.

Definitive laboratory diagnosis of babesiosis depends on the demonstration of either a *B. microti* specific antibody response,[200] or characteristic intraerythrocytic inclusions on Giemsa-stained thin blood films. The relative scarcity of the parasites in blood and its resemblance to early ring-form trophozoites of *Plasmodium falciparum* render the latter test relatively insensitive.[197,201] Other methods, such as inoculation of patient blood into hamsters, serve to amplify the parasitemia, but require several weeks for confirmation.[202]

Recently, isolation and sequence analysis of a *B. microti*-specific fragment from a gene encoding the nuclear small-subunit ribosomal RNA (ss RNA) has been used to design PCR primers capable of detecting approximately 5 to 10 merozoites in human blood.[203] PCR-based amplification may prove helpful in identifying the "chronic carrier" state in patients with persistent symptoms weeks to months after acute infection, where parasitemia is decreased and organisms cannot be visualized on smears of peripheral blood.[204] In addition, PCR may be helpful to determine the risk of transfusion acquired babesiosis, and to study synergistic pathogenic effects of infection with multiple tick-transmitted pathogens,[138,205,206]

Toxoplasmosis caused by *Toxoplasma gondii* is a significant complication in immunocompromised hosts and pregnant women. Current serological methods test for antitoxoplasma IgG and IgM by indirect immunofluorescent assays. These tests are limited because of the high prevalence of antitoxoplasma antibodies in the general population and by the inability of some immunocompromised patients to mount an antibody response. Cell culture of CSF, amniotic fluid or blood in fibroblast cell lines,[207] mouse inoculation,[208] and gene amplification[209,210] have been used as alternatives to detect parasitemias in infected animal models. Gene amplification by PCR is more sensitive than cell culture,[211] and may become available in clinical laboratories as techniques are refined and automated.

Several laboratory procedures, including microscopic examination of blood smears and immunological assays, already exist for identification of *Plasmodium* species. Recently, development of both genus and species specific primers derived from sequences of the ss rRNA have become available for the detection of *Plasmodium* species[212] (*P. falciparum; P. vivax, P. malariae,* and *P. ovale*) and provide additional information not offered by conventional methods. For example, PCR has been used to detect mixed *Plasmodium* infections[213] in individuals from highly endemic areas. PCR detection and quantification of *P. vivax* circumsporozoite (CS) gene have also been found to be a useful means to monitor the response to chloroquine therapy.[214] In this study, the 15 patients with *P. vivax* infections were negative for *P. vivax* CS DNA by day 4 after initiation of therapy. Because *Plasmodium* strains vary considerably in their response to chemotherapy, PCR-based methods may be of value in predicting chloroquine treatment failure in *P. vivax* infections. Filter paper samples, which are easy to collect and transport and which provide a simple and practical method for detecting, typing, quantitating, and monitoring drug resistance in field settings may provide yet another advantage.[215]

TABLE 20

Some Newly Described Pathogens Detected by PCR

Pathogen	Culture Technique Available
Mycobacterium genovense	Yes
Tropheyma whippelii	No
Erlichia chaffensis	No
Rochalimaea henselae; R. quintana	Yes
Mycoplasma fermentens	Yes
Mycobacterium paratuberculosis	No
Human herpesvirus 6	No
Hantavirus	Yes

Other situations where PCR may prove useful are for the distinction of pathogenic *Entamoeba histolytica* from morphologically similar commensal *E. dispar*. Riboprinting and PCR-amplification of ss rDNA followed by digestion of product with restriction enzymes has been used as a means to distinguish pathogenic *E. histolytica* from other *Entamoeba* species.[216]

VII. DETECTION OF NEWLY DESCRIBED PATHOGENS BY NUCLEIC ACID AMPLIFICATION

In recent years, PCR has provided the means for detecting and identifying many new organisms for which culture techniques may or may not exist (Table 20). *Mycoplasma fermentens,* for example, has recently been identified as a possible pathogen in humans.[217] Lack of reliable serological assays and generally low yields in culture make *M. fermentens* amenable to PCR diagnosis. Similarly, *Mycobacterium paratuberculosis*, a specific intestinal pathogen, has recently been identified in inflamed intestinal tissue of a majority of people with Crohn's disease.[218] Insertion sequence (IS) like elements that occur in multiple copies of the *M. fermentens* and *M. paratuberculosis* genome[219,220] have been employed as targets for amplification. This has provided the means for the development of a highly specific and sensitive tests.[217] The association of *M. paratuberculosis* with Crohn's disease however, is still controversial.[220]

PCR amplification has recently been used for the detection of human herpesvirus 6 (HHV-6). HHV-6, a T lymphotropic virus, is the etiologic agent of exanthem subitum. It is also the cause of 30% of Epstein-Barr virus and human CMV-negative cases of infectious mononucleosis.[221] The latency of herpesviruses has somewhat limited the diagnostic utility of PCR, however. HHV can be reactivated in cultures of healthy adult peripheral blood mononuclear cells,[222] thus making interpretation of a positive PCR result difficult. Quantitative PCR or reverse transcriptase PCR that specifically amplifies viral mRNA[223] may help in the resolution of true from a false positive result. Until then, diagnosis of acute illness with HHV-6 will likely rely on serological conversion.

A particularly promising application of target amplification is the future identification of a wide range of microorganisms using the so called **universal primers**. This technique is based on common sequence elements such as those in the large- and small-subunit rRNA 23S and 16S genes of prokaryotes and eukaryotes. Because of the crucial structural constraints of the 16S rRNA molecules, certain conserved regions of these sequences are found among all members of the bacterial kingdom, while other regions are unique to a particular genus.[224] Species-specific oligonucleotides for identification of many nonviral species of clinical importance can be deduced from published or newly derived 16S rRNA sequences.[225] Amplification of target using broad range primers, followed by the determination of the nucleotide sequence flanked by these primers, allows direct comparisons of one organism with another. Advances in DNA sequencing technology and computer-assisted database search facilities allows the detection of old as well as new emerging pathogens (Figure 10).

A universal primer amplification to bacterial 16S rRNA genes was used to recover and characterize a wide range of mycobacterial species. Using a system for genus-specific amplification of the same 16S gene target, Kirschner et al. have recently identified a novel uncultured species, *Mycobacterium genovense* from the liver of AIDS patients with disseminated mycobacterial infection.[226] Relman et al.,[227,228] using a similar approach, recovered unique bacterial DNA sequences specific for the agents of bacillary angiomatosis and Whipple's disease (*Tropheryma whippelli*). Sequence determination of amplified DNA products has been used to design specific PCR primers that allow direct detection of the disease bacillus in tissues that may be contaminated with other microorganisms.[229]

Recently, a tick-borne disease, ehrlichiosis, has similarly been identified in blood specimens obtained from patients with acute phase of infection using the 16S rRNA phylogenetic approach.[230] Clinically, ehrlichiosis presents itself very similar in symptomology to Rocky Mountain spotted fever and responds well to tetracycline or chloramphenicol.[231,232] Laboratory diagnosis of ehrlichiosis is currently based on the presence of a four-fold rise or fall in antibody titer in acute and convalescent phase serum.[233] The diagnosis is therefore usually retrospective. In addition, there is the problem of specificity in antibody-based detection due to cross-reactivity with other rickettsial diseases.[234] Furthermore, since cases of ehrlichiosis are now being reported with

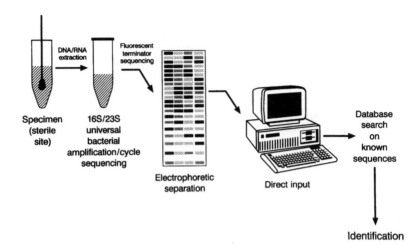

Figure 10

Nucleic acid sequence-based microbial identification. Broad-range (universal) primers are used in a target amplification protocol for amplification of 16S or 23S ribosomal DNA sequences. An automated sequencer determines the composition of the intervening nucleotides and directly enters sequence data into a computerized work station. Data base analysis creates a hierachical cluster of related sequences and then generates a list of identical organisms. (From Persing, D. H., in *Diagnostic Molecular Microbiology: Principles and Applications,* Persing, D. H., Smith, T. F., Tenover, F. C., and White, T. J., Eds., American Society for Microbiology, Washington, D.C., 1993, chap. 3. With permission of the Mayo Foundation.)

greater frequency,[235-238] PCR assay may therefore be a good means both for preventing misdiagnosis and for determining the need for early treatment with appropriate antibiotics.

A serious limitation in the wide application of the "broad range" eubacterial primer approach for identification of unknown microorganisms is the presence of inherent contamination of *Taq* polymerase and PCR reagents with bacterial DNA.[239] While more purified reagents are awaited, this approach is currently applicable to either sterile biopsy specimens that microscopically show the organism of interest and no other organism, or to specimens that have a large number of the microorganism of interest. It has been estimated that a 100-fold excess of input DNA over unwanted contaminating DNA will ensure that the input DNA will be preferentially amplified. In addition, the discovery of a single thermostable enzyme that can function as a reverse transcriptase and as a DNA polymerase will allow amplification and sequencing directly from 16S rRNA targets that are present in a thousand or more copies per bacterial cell, facilitating reverse transcriptase, DNA amplification, and nucleic acid sequencing-based identification of microorganisms directly from clinical specimens.[53]

TABLE 21

Uses of Molecular Typing Methods

Follow-up of the longitudinal course of infections in the individual patient
Monitoring of the spread of bacterial pathogens during epidemics
Elucidation of the modes of nosocomial transmission during outbreaks of infection at
  hospitals or local communities
Control of the efficacy of hygeine measures

Other conditions for which suspected infectious causes are yet unidentified include Wegener's granulomatosis, multiple sclerosis, sarcoidosis, rheumatoid arthritis, juvenile onset diabetes, idiopathic lymphoproliferative disorders, thrombotic thrombocytopenic purpura, Kawasaki's disease, and Brainard diarrhea, to name a few. Perhaps the application of broad-range application techniques will lead to the identification of etiolologic agents for some of these diseases.

VIII. INFECTION EPIDEMIOLOGY

The changing microbiological spectra of infectious disease, particularly those seen in immunocompromised hosts and in nosocomial outbreaks, have underscored the need for new epidemiological methods. Microbiology laboratories provide two services essential to hospital epidemiologists in recognizing and investigating clusters of common-source or cross-infection: identification of organisms to the genus/species level and subspecies-level typing to differentiate strains within a species (Table 21).

Many typing methods have been proposed for comparing strains of bacteria to distinguish between endogenous microrganisms and nosocomial epidemics among simultaneous or successive cases in the same area. Phenotypic markers — including biochemical profiles, serological, phage susceptibility, and antibiotic resistance, while useful in certain instances,[240,241] are often poorly discriminatory. Additional genotypic methods have been developed to increase the discriminatory power of epidemiological investigations. Two additional major considerations for typing methods are reproducibility and specificity.

Numerous DNA-based methods (Table 22) have been developed for typing bacterial agents since the latter cause the most nosocomial infections. Data from the National Nosocomial Infection Surveillance System (NNIS), suggests that coagulase negative *Staphylococcus* (CNS) play an important role in nosocomial infections, particularly in blood stream infections.[242] Several methods have been utilized for typing CNS. "Antibiogram" analysis that utilize combined results of antimicrobial susceptibility and biochemical profiles, multilocus enzyme

TABLE 22

Nucleic Acid-Based Typing Methods

Technique	Comments
DNA sequencing	Universally applicable; allows direct comparison of genomic sequences
Chromosomal DNA	Universally applicable; generates restriction profiles complex profile of entire genome
Plasmid analysis	Not universally applicable; plasmid instability limits usefulness
DNA hybridization	Requires specific DNA probes; not universally applicable
Pulsed field gel electrophoresis (PFGE)	Excellent discriminating capacity; universally applicable
PCR-RFLP	Universally applicable; quick; less expensive
Arbitrarily primed PCR (AP-PCR)	Simple; requires single primer with no prior sequence information
Ribotyping	Not universally applicable; targets 16S ribosomal operon; stability

electrophoresis, cellular fatty acid analysis, phage typing, plasmid profiling, and DNA fingerprinting have been employed.[243] While each system offers some advantage, no entirely satisfactory typing system currently exists for CNS.

Chromosomal DNA restriction DNA profiles (RFLP) have been successfully applied to the diagnosis of many bacterial species, particularly streptococci[244] and *Clostridium difficile*.[245] With this technique, a number of DNA fragments of varying size are generated after digestion of DNA with a restriction endonuclease. Variations in the size of the restriction fragment generally result from point mutations, from deletions, or from rearrangements of the chromosome that alter restriction enzyme sites. A drawback of this technique is that complex profiles may be generated that are hard to interpret.

To decrease the complexity of chromosomal DNA restriction analysis, Southern blotting of restriction endonuclease-generated DNA is carried out. Hybridization is then performed with DNA or RNA probes directed to specific bacterial targets. Probes have been derived from genes coding for putative virulence factors, insertion sequences,[246] antibiotic resistance, bacteriophage DNA, and ribosomal RNA.[247] For example, probes for genes encoding exotoxin A were found to be useful for subtyping *Pseudomonas aeroginosa* isolates from cystic fibrosis patients.[248] The use of this procedure may be limited to larger medical centers because of the addition of the probing step in the Southern blots and the limited availability of many probes.

Ribotyping, in comparison, is a powerful typing technique, in which hybridization of restriction fragments of chromosomal fragments is performed with a probe specific to rRNA (16S and 23S).[249] An *E. coli* "universal" rRNA probe is commercially available for this purpose (Boehringer Mannheim Biochemicals, Indianapolis, IN; Sigma Chemical Co., St. Louis, MO). For adaptibility in the clinical lab, sensitive nonradioactive detection systems using biotin, digoxigenin, or chemiluminescence have been devised.[250] Ribotyping relies on the principle that genes coding for rRNA are highly conserved and most bacteria contain multiple ribosomal operons (*rrn* loci). Ribotyping has been found useful for subtyping diverse bacteria, including species of the family Enterobacteriaceae, *Haemophilus*, *Neisseria meningitidis*, *Listeria monocytogenes*, *Camyplobacter*, *Salmonella*, and *Staphylococcus*.[251] Some bacteria like *Mycobacterium* and *Mycoplasma* species, which contain only one or two *rrn* loci, are however not suitable for ribotyping since only 1 to 2 bands are generated to be discriminatory value. An attractive feature of ribotyping is its extreme stability for long term follow-up of strains for epidemiological purpose.

An excellent example of a typing system based on a unique genetic element is that using the MTB insertion sequence element IS6110. The heterogeneity in the RFLP pattern of IS6110 that reflects both the copy number and sites of insertion is useful in typing MTB strains implicated in nosocomial transmission of TB among HIV+ individuals and in tracing outbreaks of MTB.[252] The fingerprint patterns of IS6110 RFLP remained almost identical in spite of changes in drug resistance profiles during long term follow-up of TB patients.[253] This is in sharp contrast to plasmid profiling, which is more useful for short-duration outbreaks and isolates that have not been subcultured extensively. It is well recognized that plasmids (autonomous, self-replicating extrachromosomal DNA elements which may encode virulence factors or antimicrobial resistance genes) can readily be lost or gained *in vivo* and/or *in vitro*. In spite of this potential limitation, plasmid profiling has been found to be useful for subtyping several bacterial species.[254] Plasmid profiling was also useful in the investigation of a large food-borne *Salmonella* outbreak that occurred in Illinois in 1985.[255] However, plasmid typing cannot be used for organisms such as *Xanthomonas maltophilia*, *Serratia marcescens*, and some *Acinetobacter* that are frequently implicated in outbreaks of nosocomial infections and are devoid of plasmids.[256]

Microbial typing by pulsed field gel electrophoresis (PFGE) has proved to be highly discriminatory and in many instances superior to other available techniques. PFGE is a variation of agarose gel electrophoresis that generates large restriction fragments such that the entire genome can be resolved as distinct fragments (10 to 2000 kb) in a single gel. PFGE has been applied to subtyping several Gram-negative and Gram-positive bacteria. Particularly impressive results have been obtained with *Listeria monocytogenes*,[257] *E. coli*,[258] and *M. avium*.[259]

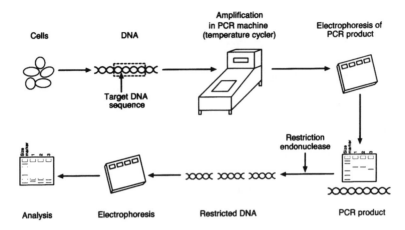

Figure 11
Schematic illustration of PCR-RFLP. (From Swaminathan, B. and Matar, G. M., in *Diagnostic Molecular Microbiology: Principles and Applications, Persing*, D. H., Smith, T. F., Tenover, F. C., and White, T. J., Eds., American Society for Microbiology Washington, D.C., 1993, chap. 2. With permission.)

Molecular methods that employ restriction enzymes require large quantities of DNA for digestion, which can be a drawback when the number of microorganisms is limiting. Amplification methods using the PCR have been devised to allow analysis of DNA from a very small number of cells. PCR-based methods that amplify a known or a random (AP-PCR) sequence followed by cleavage of amplified products with restriction endonuclease and gel electrophoresis may gain prominence, since no Southern blotting or probing is necessary (Figure 11). Virulence genes, outer membrane protein genes, and 16S rRNA genes have been targeted for PCR-RFLP subtyping for *L. monocytogenes, Chlamydia trachomatis,* and *Neisseria meningitidis,* respectively.[254] DNA sequence analysis of short segments of DNA from variable segments of the gene of interest has also been used reliably to determine if two strains are similar or different. This approach was utilized for determining transmission of human HIV from a dentist to his patients in Florida.[260]

Because of the diversity of the techniques available, the decision to choose one method over another will depend on the needs of the hospital epidemiologist and the level of expertise available. While methods for genotypic analysis using plasmid profiles and restriction endonuclease analysis of similar-sized plasmids are ready for application in moderate and large-sized laboratories, further computer-generated identification systems that employ epidemiology software need to be developed for wider applications.

IX. OPTIMIZATION OF AMPLIFICATION REACTIONS

Consideration of multiple factors is required for successful amplification of a pathogen by nucleic acid amplification. Since PCR amplification currently dominates other amplification techniques, the following section will pertain to optimization of PCR reactions. This discussion includes specimen selection and sample handling; sample preparation; target selection; primer selection; reaction optimization; and amplification product inactivation methods. More detailed discussion on each of these aspects is available in other reviews.[2,261]

A. Specimen Selection and Sample Preparation

A variety of specimen types may be encountered in a diagnostic laboratory. While individual procedures for processing samples may vary, in general the procedure must be able to release nucleic acids from target organisms; prevent degradation of free nucleic acids; concentrate the nucleic acid into a small volume; remove any substances that may inhibit the nucleic acid amplification or hybridization; and place the nucleic acids in amplification or hybridization buffer. These and other considerations have been discussed in depth elsewhere.[262] Specimen consideration and sample preparation is an important first step for the presentation of target nucleic acid sequences for amplification (Table 23). Examples of the types of specimens required for different classes of pathogens are illustrated in Table 24.

B. Target Selection

The vast variety of organisms in the microbial world and the resultant diversity in their nucleic acids complicates the development of hard and fast rules for target selection (Table 25). Genetic stability of a target (for example, a highly conserved ribosomal sequence) is perhaps the most important consideration, because loss or alteration of the target sequence may result in loss of reactivity. In many situations, target sequences present on a potentially unstable genetic element, such as a plasmid or transposon sequence, can provide adequate sensitivity and specificity if the element is associated with virulence. Detection of virulence-associated genetic elements have in fact been shown to be very useful in distinguishing pathogenic from nonpathogenic organisms. Exotoxin-producing strains of *Staphylococcus aureus*,[263] verotoxin-producing strains of *Escherichia coli*,[264] and the invasin gene of *Yersinia enterocolitica*[265] have been used.

TABLE 23

Considerations Necessary to Select Appropriate Sample Preparation Method

Specimen Considerations

Specimen type (blood, plasma, serum, sputum, CSF, urine etc.)
Processing of specimen during or after collection (collection of blood in tubes containing
  anticoagulants; liquefaction of sputum, etc.
Volume of sample to be processed (larger volumes are required for nucleic acid
  hybridization as compared to nucleic acid amplification procedures)
Level of extraneous nucleic acid (serous vs. purulent fluid; whole blood vs. plasma or
  serum)
Physical properties of specimen (swab, fluid, tissue, viscosity, etc.)
Presence of amplification inhibitors (urine, CSF specimens, for example, are particularly
  problematic)

Organism Considerations

Bacterial load within specimens (the number of pathogenic organisms per volume of
  specimen)
Durability of cell wall against lysis (difficulty in lysing fungi and *Mycobacterium* species)
Tendency of organisms to lyse spontaneously (*Mycoplasma* species)
Desire to sterilize the specimen during sample preparation (*Mycobacterium* species, HCV,
  HIV, etc.)

Nucleic Target Characteristics

RNA vs. DNA (RNA is more labile than DNA and needs special handling)
Double-stranded vs. single-stranded
Requirement of isolation of RNA without contaminating DNA (i.e., in quantifying HIV
  without amplifying the provirus)

Adapted from Greenfield, L. and White, T. J., in *Diagnostic Molecular Microbiology: Principles and Applications,* Persing, D. H., Smith, T. F., Tenover, F. C., and White, T. J., Eds.,
American Society for Micribiology, Washington, D.C., 1993, chap. 4. With permission of
the Mayo Foundation.

The presence of multiple target copies present in an microorganism
may further aid in enhancing sensitivity of an assay. This has been
accomplished by various ways: (1) pretreatment of DNA with DNase
I to dissociate repeat sequences; or (2) use of rRNA sequences which
may be present in a few thousand copies per bacterial cell in comparison with DNA target sequences. If RNA detection is desired, a reverse
transcription step is required to convert RNA into DNA.

Another important consideration is the length of the target
sequence. Targets slightly larger than 200 base pairs in length are optimal since longer PCR products are more efficiently inactivated using
current inactivation protocols (Section IX.E).

TABLE 24

Types of Specimens Required for Different Classes of Pathogens

Specimen	Examples of Pathogens Detected	Comments
Blood/blood fractions	*Babesia, Ehrlichia, Plasmodium, T. pallidum*	Heme/porphyrin inhibit Taq DNA polymerase; EDTA or citrate are preferred anticoagulants
Plasma/serum	Hepatitis B virus (DNA); HCV (RNA); HIV (RNA)	Specimen of choice when target organism found in cell-free fraction; RNA targets more labile than DNA targets
Urine	*C. trachomatis* (male); CMV; *Leptospira; Gonococcus*	Urinary inhibitors vary widely
Cerebrospinal fluid	HSV; CMV; Enterovirus; *B. burgdorferi; T. pallidum;* bacteria that cause meningitis	CSF occasionally contains uncharacterized inhibitors of DNA polymerases
Endocervical swab	*Chlamydia trachomatis;* human papillomavirus	Dacron swabs recommended; inhibition noted in some specimens collected with cytobrush
Sputum	*M. tuberculosis; Legionella pneumophila*	Acidic mucopolysaccharides are known inhibitors of DNA polymerasaes
Feces	Enteric bacteria: *E. coli, Vibrio, Shigella, Salmonella*	Difficult to remove inhibitors; inhibitor substances often coextracted with DNA

TABLE 25

Some Factors that Affect Target Selection

Genetic stability of target
Target copy number
Genetic linkage to target sequences
Sequence stability
DNA vs. RNA
Sequence conservation
Target size

C. Primer Selection

Primer selection plays a critical role in determining the successful outcome of an amplification process. Numerous factors must be considered for the design of efficient primers (Table 26). The nature of the genetic target has a direct bearing on primer selection. For PCR protocols, target-specific primer length ranges from 15 to 30 bp. Typically, if the target displays high sequence conservation, the size of the oligonucleotide is less restricted, while for amplification of polymorphic sequences, size of primers and primer-binding sites that display sufficient

TABLE 26

Primer Design Considerations

Oligonucleotide length
Melting temperature
Sequence composition
Physical characteristics (self annealing)
Primer–primer interactions
Target length
Location on the target sequence

---

conservation must be considered. Oligonucleotide design also takes into consideration the melting temperature (Tm) of individual primers along with prediction of self-complementary and interprimer annealing. Tm is the melting temperature at which 50% of the strands of an oligonucleotide bound to its target nucleic acid separate in solution. Tm is dependent on the oligonucleotide concentration, the sequence composition, and the composition of the solvent. For optimal PCR, the calculated Tm of both primers used in the amplification should be as close as possible (generally in the range of 55°C to 65°C. These conditions impart greater target specificity and aid in the choice of amplification inactivation protocols.

Computer-assisted selection of oligonucleotides for amplification protocols are available. While these programs are very good at performing several important functions of oligonucleotide design, no single program considers all factors important to primer selection.

D. Reaction Optimization

Factors that enhance analytical sensitivity of PCR have been listed in Table 27. Controversy exists, however, over which components of the reaction to optimize first. An important consideration in any protocol is whether or not human genomic DNA will copurify with that of the agent. Dilutions of target DNA should be added to a constant amount of human DNA to determine optimal concentrations. Other factors that may affect the efficiency of PCR are the presence of reactionspecific inhibitors intrinsic to the specimen or acquired as a result of highly competitive primer artifacts that accumulate in the laboratory.

The use of the enzyme *Taq* DNA polymerase isolated from the thermophilic bacterium *Thermus aquaticus* deserves special mention. The availability of a thermostable enzyme has simplified the procedure for PCR in terms of automation. Amplification by PCR is now carried out in a single tube at higher temperatures that enhance the specificity for primer annealing. The so called "hot start" procedures may lead to greater yield of the amplification product and reduced nonspecific

TABLE 27

Reaction Optimization Parameters for PCR

Annealing temperature
Magnesium ion concentration
Deoxynucleoside triphosphate
Enzyme concentration
Primer concentration
Cosolvents
Product inactivation protocols
"Hot start" protocols

amplification that result from "primer-dimer" formation. The latter refers to the formation of a double-stranded PCR product consisting of the two primers and their complementary sequences.

E. Amplification Product Inactivation Methods

The routine application of DNA/RNA amplification for clinical laboratory identification of infectious organisms must include adequate precautions to avoid contamination. The very attribute that makes PCR a powerful amplification technique also makes it prone to contamination by tiny amounts of DNA or RNA targets that may lead to false positive results. Nucleic acid contamination which may occur from a variety of sources such as: (1) clinical specimens containing large numbers of target molecules, and resulting in cross-contamination between specimens; or (2) organisms grown in culture (or cloned DNA from such organisms) is another cause of wide spread contamination. Furthermore, because PCR can generate trillions of DNA copies, repeated amplification of the same target sequence inevitably leads to accumulation of amplification products. In the case of PCR, ligase chain reaction, and strand displacement amplification, DNA products will accumulate, whereas in protocols involving self-sustaining sequence replication or QB replicase, RNA products will predominate. Several methods have now been described for PCR that may be very useful for helping to avoid false-positives due to amplification product "buildup." Some of these have been listed in Table 28. These methods, however, vary in their efficiency. A direct comparison of three of these methods has been published recently.[266,267] The common theme in all these approaches is the ability to prevent amplification products from serving as templates if carried over into a subsequent reaction — without compromising their detection.

In the enzymatic method, dUTP is substituted for TTP in all amplification reaction mixtures, resulting in incorporation of U in place of T in the amplified product. Prior to amplification, the bacterial enzyme

TABLE 28

Amplification Product Inactivation Methods

Preamplification Sterilization

Enzymatic inactivation by uracil N-glycosylase[268,269]

Postamplification Sterilization

Photochemical inactivation with furocoumarins[269,270]
Chemical inactivation by primer hydrolysis[271] or hydroxylamine treatment[272]

Topical Inactivation Methods[269]

UV light irradiation
Sodium hypochlorite (bleach)

UNG is added to the reaction mix and briefly incubated at room temperature (~25°C) to inactivate (cleave) the uracil-containing DNA strands that are carried over from previous amplification. UNG-degraded amplicons can no longer serve as templates for further amplification. The UNG itself is then inactivated by heating to 94°C. Because naturally occurring target DNA does not contain large numbers of uracil residues, this method distinguishes between U-containing amplicons carried over from previous reactions and the T-containing DNA from an organism in a clinical specimen. Thus, the UNG protocol allows "live" amplicons to accumulate in the laboratory, but a pre-PCR sterilization step selectively eliminates them prior to amplification (Figure 12).

In the post-PCR method, on the other hand, a psoralen derivative (such as isopsoralen) is added to the PCR mixture prior to amplification. This compound does not substantially interfere with primer annealing or *Taq* polymerase activity and is thermally stable. After PCR amplification, but before the reaction tubes are opened, the tubes are exposed to long-wave UV light, which penetrates them and photochemically inactivates the isopsoralen to form cyclobutane adducts with pyrimidine residues on the amplified DNA. This step blocks *Taq* polymerase from catalyzing subsequent amplification.

While successfull inactivation of amplicons greater than 200 to 300 bp in length (with roughly 50% G + C content) can be achieved by these procedures, they can introduce additional problems. Residual UNG activity can decrease the sensitivity of PCR, and high concentrations of isopsoralen can inhibit PCR. Moreover, neither of the methods described above can be used as as a quick solution for an existing amplicon contamination problem.

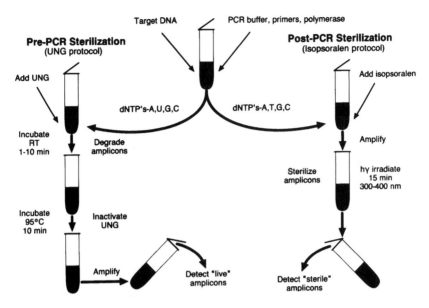

Figure 12
Pre-PCR and post-PCR sterilization methods. In the pre-PCR (enzymatic) method, previously amplified DNA (containing U in place of T) is selectively degraded prior to amplification. In the post-PCR (photochemical) protocol, an isopsoralen compound is included prior to PCR. After amplification, but before the products are removed for analysis, the tubes are exposed to long-wave UV light, resulting in cross-linking of amplified DNA. RT, room temperature; h; dNTP, deoxynucleoside triphosphate.

Besides amplification product inactivation methods, there is a need for topical methods that can be used to clean spills of amplification mixtures and for cleaning working surfaces as part of a routine quality control program. The most effective method to date is a dilute solution (10%) of sodium hypochloride (bleach). Bleach produces oxidative damage to DNA so that it cannot be amplified. It is, however, important to rinse bleach-treated surfaces with ethanol and/or water after treatment since bleach also attacks finishes and metal surfaces. Since no sterilization method is likely to be 100% efficient, these methods should not be used as a replacement for good laboratory techniques. Strict separation of pre- and post-amplification procedures should be maintained[273] and quality control measures incorporated for successful implementation of diagnostic PCR.[274] Inactivation of short amplification products associated with LCR or SDA may be more challenging. These methods are currently under development. A photochemical sterilization method for inactivating 3SR products using isopsoralen has been published recently.[275]

TABLE 29

Current Limitations of Nucleic Acid Amplification Systems

Prone to contamination
Limited availability of many probes
Lack of expertise in most dignostic laboratories
Limited automation
Lack of quantitative test results
High cost of test
Interpretation of test results: oversensitivity
Monitoring therapy in patients

F. Procedural Standardization and Quality Control

The National Commmittee for Clinical Laboratory Standard (NCCLS) has recently prepared draft guidelines for the implementation of nucleic acid amplification-based tests in the clinical microbiology laboratory. Included in the guidelines are recommendations for reaction optimization, reagent and sample preparation, amplification product inactivation, and quality control. The adoption of these guidelines by clinical laboratories performing PCR and other nucleic acid amplification methods will go far towards improving the reliability of these methods for clinical laboratory testing. In addition, proficiency testing panels are now in development within several professional organizations such as the College of American Pathologists (CAP) and NCCLS.

X. LIMITATIONS OF NUCLEIC ACID AMPLIFICATION TECHNOLOGY

DNA hybridization and PCR techniques are currently the most often used nucleic acid techniques for the detection of microorganisms from clinical specimens. The preceding sections have discussed the utility of these and other amplification techniques. While PCR assays offer many advantages for the laboratory diagnosis of infectious diseases, there are some major limitations of this technology which should be kept in mind (Table 29).

PCR, because of its exquisite sensitivity, is extremely prone to contamination with even small traces of extraneous nucleic acids. Any contamination can lead to false positive results. Incorporation of appropriate product inactivation protocols, combined with physical separation of pre- and post-PCR areas, must be a part of every laboratory protocol. Internal controls should be incorporated to determine both the amplifiability and the potential contamination that may occur in amplification reactions. In fact, the greatest challenge in bringing PCR in routine clinical use will be to develop assays without burdening the system with so many controls so as to make the tests impractical and cost-prohibitive.

Interlaboratory procedural standardizaion, especially for tests unavailable in kit form, is a formidable challenge. Through cumulative efforts, protocols are being developed for better sample preparation methods to remove intrinsic inhibitors which effect the efficiency of PCR. Professional organizations such as NCCLS and CAP will play a major role in the development of laboratory standards and external proficiency testing programs to monitor interlaboratory variability.

In most of its current formats, PCR provides only a positive or a negative test result. The extreme sensitivity of PCR may potentially allow detection of (1) incidental pathogens, the presence of which in small numbers (for example CMV and HPV) does not lead to disease and (2) potential problems in following therapy because of the ability to detect nonviable organisms. Test results need to be interpreted in collaboration with clinicians to assess their clinical significance.

At present, the cost of direct identification is slightly greater by molecular assays than by conventional methods. Advances that simplify and automate amplification procedures are expected to overcome this drawback. Moreover, the increased costs may be justified by savings in antibiotic therapy, shortened hospital stays, and saved lives.

The greatest challenge for the introduction of nucleic acid detection methods in clinical laboratories may be in the area of education. Training programs for medical technologists, clinical microbiology fellows, and pathology residents must now incorporate training in the molecular technology — to provide an in-depth understanding of these diagnostic procedures along with the power and pitfalls of molecular techniques. Such an education will provide a smooth transition from more conventional methods to future technologies.

XI. SUMMARY

Technological advancement in the field of molecular biology has truly revolutionalized the diagnosis of infectious diseases. We have witnessed the evolution of the PCR test from a useful research tool to its application in the detection of disease where culture is not practical. Currently, nucleic acid amplification-based tests are labor intensive and expensive, requiring both dedicated personnel and space for implementation. PCR test services for infectious diseases are currently only available from reference laboratories. Through the combined efforts of researchers, laboratory professionals, and test developers, amplification techniques are being developed into formats suitable for commercial distribution. Moreover, other probe and signal amplification techniques will likely be developed to supplement PCR assays.

It should be realized that DNA probes and nucleic acid amplification techniques are not meant to replace conventional assays that provide cost-effective, rapid, and sensitive results. Nucleic acid analysis is the method of choice if: (1) the nucleic acid is the only available target; (2) sufficient sensitivity is not obtained by other conventional assays; (3) an assay is required for poorly or slowly growing organisms; and (4) a high level of specificity is needed for microbial typing and molecular epidemiology. It should be borne in mind that most nucleic acid amplification protocols do not provide information on antibiotic susceptibility of the organism, and cultures are therefore still required.

In addition to its obvious role in detection and characterization of infectious agents, PCR can be extremely valuable in studying the natural history of infectious diseases, the mechanisms by which dormant infections are reactivated, and the establishment of threshold levels of microbial transcription and translation needed for the clinical symptoms. Microbial taxonomy has been revolutionized by the analysis of ribosomal nucleic acids.

Decisions to utilize molecular diagnostic procedures should consider the overall impact on clinical practice and patient management. In today's cost-containment era, it may be advantageous to restrict molecular techniques to pathogens that lack a practical culture system or to drug-resistant organisms, so that quicker isolation and appropriate therapy choices can be initiated.

REFERENCES

1. Tenover, F. C. and Unger, E. R., Nucleic acid probes for detection and identification of infectious agents, in *Diagnostic Molecular Microbiology: Principles and Applications*, Persing, D. H., Smith, T. F., Tenover, F. C., and White, T. J., Eds., American Society for Microbiology, Washington, D.C., 1993, chap. 1.
2. White, T.J., Madej, R., and Persing, D. H., The polymerase chain reaction: clinical applications, in *Adv. Clin. Chem.*, 29, 161, 1992.
3. Wilson, K. H., New vistas for bacteriologists, *ASM News*, 58, 318, 1992.
4. Huebner, R. E., Good, R. C., and Tokars, J. I., Current practices in mycobacteriology: results of a survey of state public health laboratories, *J. Clin. Microbiol.*, 31, 771, 1993.
5. Butler, W. R., O'Connor, S. P., Yakrus, M. A., and Gross, W. M., Cross-reactivity of genetic probe for detection of *Mycobacterium tuberculosis* with newly described species *Mycobacterium celatum*, *J. Clin. Microbiol.*, 32, 536, 1994.
6. Davis, T. E. and Fuller, D. D., Direct identification of bacterial isolates in blood cultures by using a DNA probe, *J. Clin. Microbiol.*, 29, 2193, 1991.

7. Rubin, F. A., McWhirter, P. D., Punjabi, N. H., Lane, E., Sudarmono, P., Pulungsih, S. P., Lesmana, M., Kumala, S., Kopecko, D. J., and Hoffman, S. L., Use of a DNA probe to detect *Salmonella typhi* in the blood of patients with typhoid fever, *J. Clin. Microbiol.*, 27, 1112, 1989.

8. Leong, D. U. and Greisen, K. S., PCR detection of bacteria found in cerebrospinal fluid, in *Diagnostic Molecular Microbiology: Principles and Applications*, Persing, D. H., Smith, T. F., Tenover, F. C., and White, T. J., Eds., American Society for Microbiology, Washington, D.C., 1993, chap. 1.21.

9. Centers for Disease Control (CDC), Annual report from Division of STD/HIV Prevention, U.S. Department of Health and Human Services, CDC, Atlanta, p. 13, 1991.

10. Chaplin-Robertson, K., Use of molecular diagnostics in sexually transmitted diseases, *Diagn. Microbiol. Infect. Dis.*, 16, 173, 1993.

11. Kluytmans, J. A., Niesters, H. G., Mouton, J. W., Quint, W.G., Ijpelar, J.A., Van Rijsoort-Vos J.H., Habbena, L., Stolz, E., Michel, M.F., and Wagenvoort, J.H., Performance of a nonisotopic DNA probe for detection of *Chlamydia trachomatis* in urogenital specimens, *J. Clin. Microbiol.*, 29, 2685, 1991.

12. Loeffelholz, M. J., Lewinski, C. A., Silver, S. R., Purohit, A. P., Herman, S. A., Buonagurio, D. A., and Dragon, E. A., Detection of *Chlamydia trachomatis* in endocervical specimens by polymerase chain reaction, *J. Clin. Microbiol.*, 30, 2847, 1992.

13. Bass, C. A., Jungkind, D. L., Silverman, N. S., and Bond, J. M., Clinical evaluation of a new polymerase chain reaction assay for detection of *Chlamydia trachomatis* in endocervical specimens, *J. Clin. Microbiol.*, 31, 2648, 1993.

14. Bauwens, J. E., Clark, A. M., and Stamm, W. E., Diagnosis of *Chlamydia trachomatis* endocervical infection by a commercial polymerase chain reaction assay, *J. Clin. Microbiol.*, 31, 3023, 1993.

15. Rasmussen, S. J., Smith-Vaughan, H., Nelson, M., Chan, S.-W., Timms, P., and Capon, A. G., Detection of *Chlamydia trachomatis* in urine using enzyme immunoassay and DNA amplification, *Mol. Cell. Probes*, 7, 425, 1993.

16. Muresu, R., Rubino, S., Rizzu, P., Baldini, A., Colombo, M., and Cappucinelli, P., A new method for identification of *Trichomonas vaginalis* by fluorescent DNA *in situ* hybridization, *J. Clin. Microbiol.*, 32, 1018, 1994.

17. Cromme, F. V., Snijders, P. J. F., Van den Brule, A. J. C., Kenemans, P., Meijer, C. J. L. M., and Walboomers, J. M. M., MHC class I expression in HPV 16 positive cervical carcinomas is post-transcriptionally controlled and independent from c-myc overexpression, *Oncogene*, 8, 2969, 1993.

18. Tervahauta, A. I., Syrjänen, S. M., Väyrynen, M., Saastamoinen, J., and Syrjänen, K. J., Expression of p53 protein related to the presence of human papillomavirus (HPV) DNA in genital carcinomas and precancer lesions, *Anticancer Res.*, 13, 1107, 1993.

19. Chambers, H. F., Methicillin-resistant staphylococci, *Clin. Microbiol. Rev.*, 1, 173, 1988.

20. Tomaz, A., Nachman, S., and Leaf, H., Stable classes of phenotypic expression in methicillin-resistant clinical isolates of staphylococci, *Antimicrob. Agents Chemother.*, 35, 124, 1991.

21. Ryffel, C., Kayser, F. H., Berger-Bachi, B., Correlation between regulation of mecA transcription and expression of methicillin resistance in staphylococci, *Antimicrob. Agents Chemother.*, 36, 25, 1992.

22. Ünal, S., Weiner, K., Degirolami, P., Barsanti, F., and Eliopoulos, G., Comparison of tests for detection of methicillin-resistant *Staphylococcus aureus* in a clinical microbiology laboratory, *Antimicrob. Agents Chemother.*, 38, 345, 1994.

23. Ligozzi, M., Rossolini, G. M., Tonin, E. A., and Fontana, R., Nonradioactive DNA probe for detection of gene for methicillin resistance in *Staphylococcus aureus*, *Antimicrob. Agents Chemother.*, 35, 575, 1991.

24. Youmans, G. R., Davis, T. E., and Fuller, D. D., Use of chemiluminescent DNA probes in the rapid detection of oxacillin resistance in clinically isolated strains of *Staphylococcus aureus*, *Diag. Microbiol. Infect. Dis.*, 16, 99, 1993.

25. Predari, S. C., Ligozzi, M., and Fontana, R., Genotypic identification of methicillin-resistant coagulase-negative staphylococci by polymerase chain reaction, *Antimicrob. Agents Chemother.*, 35, 2568, 1991.

26. Ubukata, K., Nakagami, S., Nitta, A., Yamane, A., Kawakami, S., Sugiura, M., and Konno, M., Rapid detection of the mecA gene in methicillin-resistant staphylococci by enzymatic detection of polymerase chain reaction products, *J. Clin. Microbiol.*, 30, 1728, 1992.

27. Geha, D. J., Uhl, J. R., Gustaferro, C. A., and Persing, D. H., Multiplex PCR for identification of methicillin-resistant staphylococci in the clinical laboratory, *J. Clin. Microbiol.*, 32, 1768, 1994.

28. Pascale, R., Meyran, M., Carpentier, E., Thabaut, A., and Drugeon, H. B., Comparison of phenotypic methods and DNA hybridization for detection of methicillin-resistant *Staphylococcus aureus*, *J. Clin. Microbiol.*, 32, 613, 1994.

29. Shaw, K. J., Hare, R. S., Sabatelli, F. J., Rizzo, M., Cranier, C. A., Naples, L., Kocsi, S., Munayyer, H., Mann, P., Miller, G. H. et al., Correlation between aminoglycoside resistance profiles and DNA hybridization of clinical isolates, *Antimicrob. Agents Chemother.*, 35, 2253, 1991.

30. Flamm, R. K., Phillips, K. L., Tenover, F. C., and Plorde, J. J., A survey of clinical isolates of Enterobacteriaceae using a series of DNA probes for aminoglycoside resistance genes, *Mol. Cell. Probes*, 7, 139, 1993.

31. van de Klundert, J. A. M. and Vliegenthart, J. S., PCR detection of genes coding for aminoglycoside-modifying enzymes, in *Diagnostic Molecular Microbiology: Principles and Applications*, Persing, D. H., Smith, T. F., Tenover, F. C., and White, T. J., Eds., American Society for Microbiology, Washington, D.C., 1993, chap. 6.6.

32. Licitra, C. M., Brooks, R. G., Terry, P. M., Shaw, K. J., and Hare, R. S., Use of plasmid analysis and determination of aminoglycoside-modifying enzymes to characterize isolates from an outbreak of methicillin-resistant *Staphylococcus aureus*, *J. Clin. Microbiol.*, 27, 2535, 1989.

33. Weems, J. J. Jr., Lowrance, J. H., Baddour, L. M., and Simpson, W. A., Molecular epidemiology of nosocomial, multiply aminoglycoside resistant *Enterococcus faecalis*, *J. Antimicrob. Chemother.*, 24, 121, 1989.

34. Tenover, F. C., Popovic, T., and Olsvik, O., Using molecular methods to detect antimicrobial resistance genes, *Clin. Microbiol. Newslett.*, 15, 177, 1993.

35. Telenti, A., Imboden, P., Marchesi, F., Lowrie, D., Cole, S., Colston, M. J., Matter, L., Schopfer, K., and Bodmer, T., Detection of rifampicin-resistance mutations in *Mycobacterium tuberculosis*, *Lancet*, 341, 647, 1993.

36. Pfaller, M. A., Diagnostic applications of DNA probes, *Infect. Control Hosp. Epidemiol.*, 11, 661, 1990.

37. Wolcott, M. J., Advances in nucleic acid-based detection methods, *Clin. Microbiol. Rev.*, 5, 370, 1992.

38. Arnold, L. J., Hammond, P. W. Jr., Wiese, W. A., and Nelson, N. C., Assay formats involving acridinium-ester-labeled DNA probes, *Clin. Chem.*, 35, 1588, 1989.

39. Nelson, N. C. and Kacian, D. L., Chemiluminescent DNA probes: a comparison of the acridinium ester and dioxetane detection systems and their use in clinical diagnostic assays, *Clin. Chim. Acta.*, 194, 73, 1990.

40. Montone, K. T., Friedman, H., Hodinka, R. L., Hicks, D. G., Kant, J. A., and Tomaszewski, J. E., *In situ* hybridization for Epstein-Barr virus *Not*I repeats in post-transplant lymphoproliferative disorder, *Mod. Pathol.*, 5, 292, 1992.

41. Mizutani, S., Kawaguchi, H., Toshiyuki, M., Herbst, H., Niedobitek, G., Asada, M., Tsuchida, M., Hanada, R., Kinoshita, A., Sakura, M, and Kobayashi, N., Analysis of the target cell for Epstein-Barr virus infection in Epstein-Barr virus associated hemophagocytic syndrome (EBV-AHS), *Leukemia*, 7, 593, 1993.

42. Singer, R. H., Byron, K. S., Lawrence, J. B., and Sullivan, J. L., Detection of HIV-1-infected cells from patients using nonisotopic *in situ* hybridization, *Blood*, 74, 2295, 1989.

43. Unger, E. R., Budgeon, L. R., Myerson, M. L., Ou, C.-Y., Warfield, D. T., and Feorino, P. M., Demonstration of human immunodeficiency virus by colorimetric *in situ* hybridization: a rapid technique for formalin-fixed paraffin-embedded material, *Mod. Pathol.*, 2, 200, 1989.

44. Amortegui, A. J. and Meyer, M. P., *In-situ* hybridization for the diagnosis and typing of human papillomavirus, *Clin. Biochem.*, 23, 301, 1990.

45. Iwasawa, A., Kumamoto, Y., and Fujinaga, K., Detection of human papillomavirus deoxynucleic acid in penile carcinoma by polymerase chain reaction and *in situ* hybridization, *J. Urol.*, 149, 59, 1993.

46. Kawaguchi, H., Miyashita, T., Herbst, H., Neidobitek, G., Asada, M., Tsuchida, M., Hanada, R., Kinoshita, A., Sakurai, M., Kobayashi, N, and Mizutani, S., Epstein-Barr virus-infected T lymphocytes in Epstein-Barr virus-associated hemophagocytic syndrome, *J. Clin. Invest.*, 92, 1444, 1993.

47. Persing, D. H., *In vitro* nucleic acid amplification techniques, in *Diagnostic Molecular Microbiology: Principles and Applications*, Persing, D. H., Smith, T. F., Tenover, F. C., and White, T. J., Eds., American Society for Microbiology, Washington, D.C., 1993, chap. 3.

48. Erlich, H. A., Gelfand, D., and Sninsky, J. J., Recent advances in the polymerase chain reaction, *Science*, 252, 1643, 1991.

49. Feray, C., Samuel, D., Thiers, V., Gigou, M., Pichon, F., Bismuth, A., Reynes, M., Maisonneuve, P., Bismuth, H., and Brechot, C., Reinfection of liver graft by hepatitis C after liver transplantation, *J. Clin. Invest.*, 89, 1361, 1992.

50. Chamberlain, J. S., Gibbs, R. A., Rainier, J. E., and Caskey, C. T., Multiplex PCR for the diagnosis of Duchenne muscular dystrophy, in *PCR Protocols: A Guide to Methods and Applications*, Innis, M. A., Gelfand, D. H., Sninsky, J. J., and White, T. J., Eds., Academic Press, San Diego, CA, 1990, 272.

51. Bej, A. K., Mahbubani, M. H., Miller, R., Dicesare, J. L., Haff, L., and Atlas, R. M., Multiplex PCR amplification and immobilized capture probes for detection of bacterial pathogens and indicators in water, *Mol. Cell. Probes*, 4, 353, 1990.

52. Hunt, J. M., Roberts, G. D., Stockman, L., Felmlee, T. A., and Persing, D. H., Detection of a genetic locus encoding resistance to rifampin in mycobacterial cultures and in clinical specimens, *Diag. Microbiol. Infect. Dis.*, 18, 219, 1994.

53. Myers, T. W. and Gelfand, D. H., Reverse transcription and DNA amplification by a *Thermus thermophilus* DNA polymerase, *Biochemistry*, 30, 7861, 1991.

54. Patel, B. K. R., Banerjee, D. K., and Butcher, P. D., Determination of *Mycobacterium leprae* viability by polymerase chain reaction amplification of 71-kDa heat shock protein mRNA, *J. Infect. Dis.*, 168, 799, 1993.

55. Mullis, K. B. and Faloona, F. A., Specific synthesis of DNA *in vitro* via a polymerase-catalyzed chain reaction, *Methods Enzymol.*, 155, 335, 1987.

56. Saiki, R. K., Scharf, S., Faloona, F., Mullis, K. B., Horn, G. T., Erlich, H. A., and Arnheim, N., Enzymatic amplification of β-globin genomic sequences and restriction site analysis for diagnosis of sickle cell anemia, *Science*, 230, 1350, 1985.

57. Bugawan, T. L., Saiki, R. K., Levenson, C. H., Watson, R. M., and Erlich, H. A., The use of non-radioactive oligonucleotide probes to analyze enzymatically amplified DNA for prenatal diagnosis and forensic HLA typing, *Biotechnology*, 6, 943, 1988.

58. Saiki, R. K., Walsh, P. S., Levenson, C. H., and Erlich, H. A., Genetic analysis of amplified DNA with immobilized sequence-specific oligonucleotide probes, *Proc. Natl. Acad. Sci. U.S.A.*, 86, 6230, 1989.

59. Ou, C. Y., McDonough, S. H., Cabanas, D., Ryder, T. B., Harper, M., Moore, J., and Schochetman, G., Rapid and quantitative detection of enzymatically amplified HIV-1 DNA using chemiluminescent oligonucleotide probes, *AIDS Res. Hum. Retroviruses*, 6, 1323, 1990.

60. Keller, G. H., Huang, D.-P., Shih, J. W.-K., and Manak, M. M., Detection of hepatitis C virus DNA in serum by polymerase chain reaction amplification and microtiter sandwich hybridization, *J. Clin. Microbiol.*, 28, 1411, 1990.

61. Wahlberg, J., Lundeberg, J., Hultman, T., and Uhlén, M., General colorimetric method for DNA diagnostics allowing direct solid-phase genomic sequencing of the positive samples, *Proc. Natl. Acad. Sci. U.S.A.*, 87, 6569, 1990.

62. Keller, G. H., Huang, D.-P., and Manak, M. M., A sensitive nonisotopic hybridization assay for HIV-1 DNA, *Anal. Biochem.*, 177, 27, 1989.

63. Hayashi, K., PCR-SSCP: a method for detection of mutations, *GATA*, 9, 73, 1992.

64. Telenti, A., Imboden, P., Marchesi, F., Schmidheini, T., and Bodmer, T., Direct, automated detection of rifampin-resistant *Mycobacterium tuberculosis* by polymerase chain reaction and single-strand conformation polymorphism analysis, *Antimicrob. Agents Chemother.*, 37, 2054, 1993.

65. Kanai, K., Kako, M., and Okamoto, H., HCV genotypes in chronic hepatitis C and response to interferon, *Lancet*, 339, 1543, 1992.

66. Kwoh, D. Y., Davis, G. R., Whitfield, K. M., Chappelle, H. L., and Gingeras, T., Transcription-based amplification system and detection of amplified human immunodeficiency virus type 1 with a bead-based sandwich hybridization format, *Proc. Natl. Acad. Sci. U.S.A.*, 86, 1173, 1989.

67. Compton, J., Nucleic acid sequence-based amplification, *Nature* (London), 350, 91, 1991.

68. Fahy, E., Kwoh, D. Y., and Gingeras, T. R., Self-sustained sequence replication (3SR): an isothermal transcription-based amplification system alternative to PCR, *PCR Methods Applic.*, 1, 25, 1991.

69. Gingeras, T. R. and Kwoh, D. Y., *In vitro* nucleic acid target amplification techniques: issues and benefits, *Praxis Biotechnol.*, 4, 403, 1992.

70. Guatelli, J. C., Gingeras, T. R., and Richman, D. D., Nucleic acid amplification *in vitro*: detection of sequences with low copy numbers and application to diagnosis of human immunodeficiency virus type 1 infection, *Clin. Microbiol. Rev.*, 2, 217, 1989.

71. Gingeras, T. R., Prodanovich, P., Latimer, T., Guatelli, J. C., Richman, D. D., Barringer, K. J., Use of self-sustained replication amplification reaction to analyze and detect mutations in zidovudine-resistant human immunodeficiency virus, *J. Infect. Dis.*, 164, 1066, 1991.

72. Gingeras, T., Novel amplification targets for 3SR, *Clin. Chem.*, 39, 726, 1993.

73. Bush, C. E., Donovan, R. M., Peterson, W. U., Jennings, M. B., Bolton, V., Sherman, D. G., vanden Brink, K. M., Beninsig, L. A., and Godsey, J. H., Detection of human immunodeficiency virus type 1 RNA in plasma samples from high-risk pediatric patients by using the self-sustained sequence replication reaction, *J. Clin. Microbiol.*, 30, 281, 1992.

74. Haydock, P. V. and Kochik, S. A., 3SR detection of *Chlamydia trachomatis*, in *Diagnostic Molecular Microbiology: Principles and Applications*, Persing, D. H., Smith, T. F., Tenover, F. C., and White, T. J., Eds., American Society for Microbiology, Washington, D.C., 1993, chap. 1.10.

75. Brown, J. T. and Wortman, A. T., Rapid amplification of human papillomavirus type 16 and 18 E6 and E7 mRNA by 3SR, in *Diagnostic Molecular Microbiology: Principles and Applications*, Persing, D. H., Smith, T. F., Tenover, F. C., and White, T. J., Eds., American Society for Microbiology, Washington, D.C., 1993, chap. 2.18.

76. Walker, G. T., Fraiser, M. S., Schram, J. L., Little, M. C., Nadeau, J. G., and Mali-nowski, D. P., Strand displacement amplification — an isothermal, *in vitro* DNA amplification technique, *Nucleic Acids Res.*, 20, 1691, 1992.
77. Walker, G. T., Empirical aspects of strand displacement amplification, *PCR Meth. Applic.*, 3, 1, 1993.
78. Walker, G. T., Little, M. C., Nadeau, J. G., and Shank, D. D., Isothermal *in vitro* amplification of DNA by a restriction enzyme/DNA polymerase system, *Proc. Natl. Acad. Sci. U.S.A.*, 89, 392, 1992.
79. Spargo, C. A., Haaland, P. D., Jurgensen, S. R., Shank, D. D., and Walker, G. T., Chemiluminescent detection of strand displacement amplified DNA from species comprising the *Mycobacterium tuberculosis* complex, *Mol. Cell. Probes*, 7, 395, 1993.
80. Eoyang, L. and August, J., Q beta RNA polymerase from phase 2 beta infected *E. coli*, in *Procedures in Nucleic Acid Research*, Cantoni, G. L. and Davis, D. R., Eds., Harper and Row, New York, NY, 1971, 829.
81. Lizardi, P. M., Guerra, C. E., Lomeli, H., Tussie-Luna, I., and Kramer, F. R., Expo-nential amplification of recombinant-RNA hybridization probes, *Clin. Chem.*, 35, 1826, 1988.
82. Lomeli, H., Tyagi, S., Pritchard, C. G., Licardi, P. M., and Kramer, F. R., Quantita-tive assays based on the use of replicatable hybridization probes, *Clin. Chem.*, 35, 1826, 1989.
83. Pritchard, C. G. and Stefano, J. E., Amplified detection of viral nucleic acid at subattomole levels using Q beta replicase, *Ann. Biol. Chem.*, (Paris) 48, 492, 1990.
84. Klinger, J. D. and Pritchard, C. G., Amplified probe-based assays — possibilities and challenges in clinical microbiology, *Clin. Microbiol. News*, 12, 189, 1990.
85. Barany, F., Genetic disease detection and DNA amplification using cloned ther-mostable ligase, *Proc. Natl. Acad. Sci. U.S.A.*, 88, 189, 1991.
86. Laffler, T. G., Carrino, J. J., and Marshall, R. L., The ligase chain reaction in DNA-based diagnosis, *Ann. Biol. Clin.*, 50, 821, 1993.
87. Lee, H., Infectious disease testing by ligase chain reaction, *Clin. Chem.*, 39, 729, 1993.
88. Fahrlander, P. D. and Klausner, A., Amplifying DNA probe signals: a "Christmas tree" approach, *Biotechnology*, 6, 1165, 1988.
89. Wiedbrauk, D. L., Molecular methods for virus detection, *Lab. Med.*, 23, 737, 1992.
90. Sanchez-Pescador, R., Stempien, M. S., and Urdea, M. S., Rapid chemiluminescent nucleic acid assays for detection of TEM-1 β-lactamase-mediated penicillin resis-tance in *Neisseria gonorrhoeae* and other bacteria, *J. Clin. Microbiol.*, 26, 1934, 1988.
91. Urdea, M. S., Fultz, T., Anderson, T. J., Running, M., Haniren, J. A., Ahle, S., and Chang, C. A., Branched amplification multimers for the sensitive, direct detection of human hepatitis viruses, *Nucleic Acids Symp. Ser.*, 24, 197, 1991.
92. Sanchez-Pescador, R., Sheridan, P. J., Detmer, J. J., Hunt, W. P., Chan, C.S., Wright, T., Okano, A., Wilber, J. C., Newoard, P. D., and Urdea, M. S., Quantitative detec-tion of HCV RNA in human sera using a chemiluminescence signal amplification oligonucleotide probe assay, *Hepatology*, 16, 588, 1992.
93. Lau, J. Y. N., Davis, G. Y., Kniffen, J., Qian, K.-P., Urdea, M. S., Chan, C. S., Mizo-kanu, U., Neuwald, P. D., and Wilber, J. C., Significance of serum hepatitis C virus RNA levels in chronic hepatitis C, *Lancet*, 341, 1501, 1993.
94. Shen, L. P., Kolberg, J. A., Spaete, R. R., Miner, R., and Drew, W. L., A quantitative detection method for detection of human cytomegalovirus DNA using a branched DNA enhanced label amplification assay [Abstr.], 92nd General Meeting of the American Society for Microbiology, Washington, D.C., p. 408, 1992.
95. Panchl, C. A., Kern, D. G., Sheridan, P. J., Stempien, M. M., Todd, J. A., Zhu, Y. S., Gong, Y., Cimino, G. D., Wilber, J. C., Urdea, M. S., and Neuwald, P. D., Quanti-tative detection of HIV RNA in plasma using a signal amplification probe assay [Abstr.], 32nd Interscience Conference on Antimicrobial Agents and Chemother-apy, American Society for Microbiology, Washington, D.C., Abst. #1247, 1992.

96. Lior, H. and Johnson, W. M., Application of the polymerase chain reaction (PCR) to detection of the aerolysin gene in whole cell cultures of beta-hemolytic *Aeromonas hydrophila*, *Experentia*, 47, 421, 1991.

97. Kirschner, P., Vogel, U., Hein, R., and Böttger, E. C., Bias of culture techniques for diagnosing mixed *Mycobacterium genavense* and *Mycobacterium avium* infection in AIDS, *J. Clin. Microbiol.*, 32, 828, 1994.

98. Witebsky, F. G. and Conville, P. S., The laboratory diagnosis of mycobacterial disease, *Infect. Dis. Clin. N. Am.*, 7, 359, 1993.

99. Abe, C., Hosojima, S., Fukasawa, Y., Takahashi, M., Hirano, K., and Mori, T., Comparison of MB-check, BACTEC, and egg-based media for recovery of mycobacteria, *J. Clin. Microbiol.*, 30, 878, 1992.

100. Eisenach, K. D., Cave, M. D., Bates, J. H., and Crawford, J. T., Polymerase chain reaction amplification of a repetitive DNA sequence specific for *Mycobacterium tuberculosis*, *J. Infect. Dis.*, 161, 977, 1990.

101. Thierry, D., Brisson-Nöel, A., Lévy-Frébault, V., Nguyen, G., Guesdon, J., and Gicquel, B., Characterization of a *Mycobacterium tuberculosis* insertion sequence, IS6110, and its application in diagnostics, *J. Clin. Microbiol.*, 28, 2668, 1990.

102. Brisson-Nöel, A., Azner, C., Chureau, C., Nguyen, S., Pierre, C., Bartoli, M., Bonete, R., Pialoux, G., Gicquel, B., and Garrigue, G., Diagnosis of tuberculosis by DNA amplification in clinical practice evaluation, *Lancet*, 338, 364, 1991.

103. Böddinghaus, B., Rogall, T., Flohr, T., Blocker, H., and Bottger, E.C., Detection and identification of Mycobacteria by amplification of rRNA, *J. Clin. Microbiol.*, 28, 1751, 1990.

104. Jonas, V., Alden, M. J., Curry, J.-I., Kamisango, K., Knott, C. A., Lankford, R., Wolfe, J. M., and Morre, D. G., Detection and identification of *Mycobacterium tuberculosis* directly from sputum sediments by amplification of rRNA, *J. Clin. Microbiol.*, 31, 2410, 1993.

105. Eisenach, K. D., Sifford, M. D., Cave, M. D., Bates, J. H., and Crawford, J. T., Detection of *Mycobacterium tuberculosis* in sputum samples using a polymerase chain reaction, *Am. Rev. Resp. Dis.*, 144, 1160, 1991.

106. TB Weekly, September 13, 1993, p 9.

107. Miyazaki, Y., Koga, H., Kohno, S., and Kaku, M., Nested polymerase chain reaction for tuberculosis in clinical samples, *J. Clin. Microbiol.*, 31, 2228, 1993.

108. Vaneechoutte, M., DeBeenhouwer, H., Claeys, G., Verschraegen, G., and De Rouck, A., Identification of *Mycobacterium* species by using amplified ribosomal DNA restriction analysis, *J. Clin. Microbiol.*, 31, 2061, 1993.

109. Winn-Dean, E. S., Batt, C. A., and Wiedmann, M., Non-radioactive detection of *Mycobacterium tuberculosis* LCR products in a microtitre plate format, *Mol. Cell. Probes*, 7, 179, 1993.

110. Abe, C., Hirano, K., Wade, M., Kazumi, Y., Takahashi, M., Fukasawa, Y., Yoshimura, T., Miyagi, C., and Goto, S., Detection of *Mycobacterium tuberculosis* in clinical specimens by polymerase chain reaction and Gen-Probe amplified *Mycobacterium tuberculosis* direct test, *J. Clin. Microbiol.*, 31, 3270, 1993.

111. Pfyffer, G. E., Kissling, P., Wirth, R., and Weber, R., Direct detection of *Mycobacterium tuberculosis* complex in respiratory specimens by a target-amplified test system, *J. Clin. Microbiol.*, 32, 918, 1994.

112. Butler, W. R., Ahearn, D. G., and Kilburn, J. O., High-performance liquid chromatography of mycolic acids as a tool in the identification of *Corynebacterium, Nocardia, Rhodococcus*, and *Mycobacterium* species, *J. Clin. Microbiol.*, 23, 182, 1986.

113. Kusunoki, S., Ezaki, S., Tamesada, M., Hatanaka, Y., Asano, K., Hashimoto, Y., and Yabuuchi, E., Application of colorimetric microdilution plate hybridization for rapid genetic identification of 22 *Mycobacterium* species, *J. Clin. Microbiol.*, 29, 1596, 1991.

114. Telenti, A., Marchesi, F., Batz, M., Bally, F, Böttger, E., and Bodmer, T., Rapid differentiation of Mycobacteria to the species level by polymerase chain reaction and restriction enzyme analysis, *J. Clin. Microbiol.*, 31, 175, 1993.

115. Centers for Disease Control and Prevention, National action plan to combat multidrug-resistant tuberculosis, *Morbid. Mortal. Weekly Rep.*, 41, 1, 1992.

116. Al-Drainer, F., Drug resistance in tuberculosis, *J. Chemother.*, 2, 147, 1990.

117. Honoré, N. and Cole, S., The molecular basis of rifampin resistance in *Mycobacterium leprae*, *Antimicrob. Agents Chemother.*, 37, 414, 1993.

118. Kapur, V., Ling-Ling, L. I., Iordanescu, S., Hamrick, M. R., Wanger, A., Kreiswirth, B. N., and Musser, J. M., Characterization by automated DNA sequencing of mutations, in the gene (rpoB) encoding the RNA polymerase β subunit in rifampin-resistance *Mycobacterium tuberculosis* strains from New York City and Texas, *J. Clin. Microbiol.*, 32, 1095, 1994.

119. Centers for Disease Control, Lyme disease — United States, 1987 and 1988, *Morbid. Mortal. Weekly Rep.*, 38, 668, 1989.

120. Abele, D. C. and Anders, K. H., The many faces and phases of borreliosis I — Lyme disease, *J. Am. Acad. Dermatol.*, 23, 167, 1990.

121. Kazmierczak, J. J. and Davis, J. P., Lyme disease: ecology, epidemiology, clinical spectrum, and management, *Adv. Pediatr.*, 39, 207, 1992.

122. Michelle, P. D., Lyme borreliosis: a persisting diagnostic dilemma, *Clin. Microbiol. Newslett.*, 15, 57, 1993.

123. Holt, D. A., Pattani, N. J., Sinnott, J. T., and Bradley, E., Lyme borreliosis, *Infect. Control Hosp. Epidemiol.*, 12, 493, 1991.

124. Sigal, L.H., The polymerase chain reaction assay for *Borrelia burgdorferi* in the diagnosis of Lyme disease, *Ann. Intern. Med.*, 120, 520, 1994.

125. Fraser, D. D., Kong, L. I., and Miller, F. W., Molecular detection of persistent *Borrelia burgdorferi* in a man with dermatomyositis, *Clin. Exp. Rheumatol.*, 10, 387, 1992.

126. Berger, B. W., Johnson, R. C., Kodner, C., and Coleman, L., Cultivation of *Borrelia burgdorferi* from erythema migrans lesions from perilesional skin, *J. Clin. Microbiol.*, 30, 359, 1992.

127. Schwartz, T., Bittker, S., Bowen, S. L., Cooper, D., Pavia, C., and Wormser, C. P., Polymerase chain reaction amplification of culture supernatants for rapid detection of *Borrelia burgdorferi*, *Eur. J. Clin. Microbiol. Infect. Dis.*, 12, 879, 1993.

128. Persing, D. H., Telford, S. R. III, Spielman, A., and Barthold, S. W., Detection of *Borrelia burgdorferi* infection in *Ixodes dammini* ticks with the polymerase chain reaction, *J. Clin. Microbiol.*, 28, 566, 1990.

129. Persing, D. H., Telford, S. R. III, Rys, P. N., Dodge, D. E., White, T. J., Malawista, S. E., and Spielman, A., Detection of *Borrelia burgdorferi* DNA in museum specimens of *Ixodes dammini* ticks, *Science*, 249, 1420, 1990.

130. Hofmeister, E. K., Markham, R. B., Childs, J. E., and Arthur, R. R., Comparison of polymerase chain reaction and culture for detection of *Borrelia burgdorferi* in naturally infected *Peromyscus leucopus* and experimentally infected C.B-17 *scid/scid* mice, *J. Clin. Microbiol.*, 30, 2625, 1992.

131. Schwartz, I., Wormser, G. P., Schwartz, J. J., Cooper, D., Weissensee, P., Gazumyan, A., Zimmermann, E., Goldberg, N. S., Bittker, S., Campbell, G. L., and Paula, C. S., Diagnosis of early Lyme disease by polymerase chain reaction amplification and culture of skin biopsies from erythema migrans lesions, *J. Clin. Microbiol.*, 30, 3082, 1992.

132. Kruger, W. H. and Pulz, M., Detection of *Borrelia burgdorferi* in cerebrospinal fluid by the polymerase chain reaction, *J. Med. Microbiol.*, 35, 98, 1991.

133. McGuire, B. S., Chandler, F. W., Felz, M. W., Huey, L. O., and Field, R. S., Detection of *Borrelia burgdorferi* in human blood and urine using the polymerase chain reaction, *Pathobiology*, 60, 163, 1992.

134. Liebling, M. R., Nishio, M. J., Rodriguez, A., Sigal, L. H., Jin, T., and Louie, J. S., The polymerase chain reaction for the detection of *Borrelia burgdorferi* in human body fluids, *Arthritis Rheum.*, 36, 665, 1993.
135. Persing, D. H., Rutledge, B. J., Rys, P. N., Podzorski, D. S., Mitchell, P. D., Reed, K. D., Liu, B., Fikrig, E., and Malawista, S. E., Target imbalance: disparity of *Borrelia burgdorferi* genetic material in synovial fluid from Lyme arthritis patients, *J. Infect. Dis.*, 169, 668, 1994.
136. Nocton, J. J., Dressler, F., Rutledge, B. J., Rys, P. N., Persing, D. H., and Steere, A. C., Detection of *Borrelia burgdorferi* DNA by polymerase chain reaction in synovial fluid from patients with Lyme arthritis, *N. Engl. J. Med.*, 330, 229, 1994.
137. Huppertz, H. I., Schmidt, H., and Karch, H., Detection of *Borrelia burgdorferi* by nested polymerase chain reaction in cerebrospinal fluid and urine of children with neuroborreliosis, *Eur. J. Pediatr.*, 152, 414, 1993.
138. Piesman, J., Mather, T. N., Dammin G. J., Telford, S. R. III, Lastavica, C. C., and Spielman, A., Seasonal variation of transmission risk of Lyme disease and human babesiosis, *Am. J. Epidemiol.*, 126, 1187, 1987.
139. Puthavathana, P., Lee, H. W., and Kang, C. Y., Typing of hantaviruses from five continents by polymerase chain reaction, *Virus Res.*, 26, 1, 1992.
140. Xiao, S. Y., Chu, Y. K., Knauert, F. K., Lofts, R., Dalrymple, J. M., and LeDuc, J. W., Comparison of hantavirus isolates using a genus-reactive primer pair polymerase chain reaction, *J. Gen. Virol.*, 73, 567, 1992.
141. Aslanzadeh, J., Osmon, D. R., Wilhelm, M. P., Epsy, M.J., and Smith, T.F., A prospective study of the polymerase chain reaction for detection of herpes simplex virus in cerebrospinal fluid submitted to the clinical microbiology laboratory, *Mol. Cell. Probes*, 6, 367, 1992.
142. Aslanzadeh, J., Helm, K. F., Espy, M. J., Muller, S. A., and Smith, T. F., Detection of HSV-specific DNA in biopsy tissue of patients with erythema multiforme by polymerase chain reaction, *Brit. J. Dermatol.*, 126, 19, 1992.
143. Aslanzadeh, J., Garner, J. G., Feder, H. M., and Ryan, R. W., Use of polymerase chain reaction for laboratory diagnosis of herpes simplex virus encephalitis, *Ann. Clin. Lab. Sci.*, 23, 196, 1993.
144. Purtilo, D. T., Strobach, R. S., Okano, M., and Davis, J. R., Epstein-Barr virus-associated lymphoproliferative disorders, *Lab. Invest.*, 67, 5, 1992.
145. Telenti, A., Marshall, W. F., and Smith, T. F., Detection of Epstein-Barr virus by polymerase chain reaction, *J. Clin. Microbiol.*, 28, 2187, 1990.
146. Myers, J. D., Ljungman, P., and Fisher, L. D., Cytomegalovirus excretion as a predictor of cytomegalovirus disease after marrow transplantation: importance of cytomegalovirus viremia, *J. Infect. Dis.*, 162, 373, 1990.
147. Salmon, D., Lacassin, F., Harzic, M., Leport, C., Perronue, C., Bricaire, F., Brun-Vezinet, F., and Wilde, J. L., Predictive value of cytomegalovirus viremia for the occurrence of CMV organ involvement in AIDS, *J. Med. Virol.*, 32, 160, 1990.
148. Gleaves, C. A., Smith, T. F., Shuster, E. A., and Pearson, G. R., Comparison of standard tube and shell vial cell culture techniques for the detection of cytomegalovirus in clinical specimens, *J. Clin. Microbiol.*, 21, 217, 1985.
149. The, T. H., Vander Bij, W., Vanden Berg, A. P., van der Giessen, M., Weits, J., Sprenger, H. G., and van Son, W. J., Cytomegalovirus antigenemia, *Rev. Infect. Dis.*, 12(Suppl. 7), S734, 1990.
150. Mazzulli, T., Improved diagnosis of cytomegalovirus infection by detection of antigenemia or use of PCR methods, *Clin. Microbiol. Newslett.*, 15, 97, 1993.
151. Drouet, E., Boibieux, A., Michelson, S., Ecochard, R., Biron, F., Peyramond, D., Colimon, R., and Denoyel, G., Polymerase chain reaction detection of cytomegalovirus DNA in peripheral blood leukocytes as a predictor of cytomegalovirus disease in HIV-infected patients, *AIDS*, 7, 665, 1993.

152. Velzing, J., Rothbarth, P. H., Kroes, A. C. M., and Quint, W. G. V., Detection of cytomegalovirus mRNA and DNA encoding the immediate early gene in pheripheral blood leukocytes from immunocompromised patients, *J. Med. Virol.*, 42, 164, 1994.

153. Storch, G. A., Buller, R. S., Bailey, T. C., Ettinger, N. A., Langlois, T., Gaudreault-Keener, M., and Welby, P. L., Comparison of PCR and pp65 antigenemia assay with quantitative shell vial culture for detection of cytomegalovirus in blood leukocytes from solid-organ transplant recipients, *J. Clin. Microbiol.*, 32, 997, 1994.

154. Spector, S. A., Merril, R., Wolf, D., and Danker, W., Detection of human cytomegalovirus in plasma of AIDS patients during acute visceral disease and DNA amplifcation, *J. Clin. Microbiol.*, 30, 2359, 1992.

155. Espy, M. J., Paya, C. V., Holley, K. E., Ludwig, J., Hermans, P. F., Wiesner, R. H., Krom, R. A. F., and Smith, T. F., Diagnosis of cytomegalovirus hepatitis by histopathology and *in situ* hybridization in liver transplantation, *Diagn. Microbiol. Infect. Dis.*, 14, 293, 1991.

156. Wolff, M. A., Rand, K. H., Houck, H. J., Brunson, M. E., Howard, R. J., Langham, M. R., Davis, G. L., Mailliard, M. E., Myers, B. M., Andres, J., Novak, D. A., Haiman, S., and Parris, C. J., Realtionship of the polymerase chain reaction for cytomegalovirus to the development of hepatitis in liver transplant recipients, *Transplantation*, 56, 572, 1993.

157. Shibata, M., Terashima, M., Kimura, H., Kuzushima, K., Yoshida, J., Horibe, K., and Morishima, T., Quantitation of cytomegalovirus DNA in lung tissue of bone marrow transplant recipients, *Human Pathol.*, 23, 911, 1992.

158. Peeters, M., Gershy-Damet, G.-M., Fransen, K., Koffi, K., Coulibaly, M., Delaporte, E., Piot, P., and van derGroen, G., Virological and polymerase chain reaction studies of HIV-1/HIV-2 dual infection in cote d'Ivoire, *Lancet*, 340, 339, 1992.

159. Richman, D., Guatelli, J. C., Grimes, J., Tsiatis, A., and Gingeras, T., Detection of mutations with zidovudine resistance in human immunodeficiency virus by use of polymerase chain reaction, *J. Infect. Dis.*, 164, 1075, 1991.

160. Wolinsky, S. M., Rinaldo, C. R., and Kwok, S., Human immunodeficiency virus type I (HIV-1) infection a median of 18 months before a diagnostic Western blot, *Ann. Intern. Med.*, 111, 961, 1989.

161. Figuero, M. E. and Rasheed, S., Molecular pathology and diagnosis of infectious diseases, *Am. J. Clin. Pathol.*, 95, S8, 1991.

162. Whetsell, A. J., Drew, J. B., Milman, G., Hoff, R., Dragon, E. A., Alder, K., Hui, J., Otto, P., Gusta, P., Farzadegan, H., and Wolinsky, S. M., Comparison of three nonradioisotopic polymerase chain reaction-based methods for detection of human immunodeficiency virus type 1, *J. Clin. Microbiol.*, 30, 845, 1992.

163. Jackson, J. B., Ndugwa, C., Miro, F. et al., Nonisotopic polymerase chain reaction methods for the detection of HIV-1 in Ugandan mothers and infants, *AIDS*, 5, 1463, 1989.

164. Goswami, K. K., Miller, R. F., Harrison, M. J., Hamel, D. J., Daniels, R. S., and Tedder, R. S., Expression of HIV-1 in the cerebrospinal fluid detected by the polymerase chain reaction and its correlation with central nervous system disease, *AIDS*, 5, 797, 1991.

165. Comeau, A. M., Hsu, H. W., Schwerzler, M., Mushinsky, G., and Grady, G. F., Detection of HIV in specimens from newborn screening programs, *N. Engl. J. Med.*, 326, 1703, 1992.

166. Anonymous, Report of a consensus workshop, Siena, Italy, January 17–18, 1992. Early diagnosis of HIV infection in infants (review), *J. Acquired Immun. Def. Syndr.*, 5, 1169, 1992.

167. Krivine, A., Firtion, G., Cao, L., Francoual, C., Henrion, R., and Lebon, P., HIV replication during the first weeks of life, *Lancet*, 339, 1187, 1992.

168. Sison, A. V. and Campos, J. M., Laboratory methods for early detection of human immunodeficiency virus type 1 in newborns and infants, *Clin. Microbiol. Rev.*, 5, 238, 1992.

169. Kline, M. W., Lewis, D. E., Hollinger, F. B., Reuben, J. M., Hanson, I. C., Kozinetz, C. A., Hanson, I. C., Dimitrov, D. H., Rosenblatt, H. M., and Shearer, W. T., A comparative study of human immunodeficiency virus culture, polymerase chain reaction and anti-human immunodeficiency virus immunoglobulin A antibody detection in the diagnosis during early infancy of vertically acquired human immunodeficiency virus infection, *Pediatr. Infect. Dis. J.*, 13, 90, 1994.

170. Anonymous., Mother-to-child transmission of HIV infection. The European collaborative study, *Lancet*, 2, 1039, 1988.

171. Bylund, D. J., Ziegner, H. H., and Hooper, D. G., Review of testing for human immunodeficiency virus, *Clin. Lab. Med.*, 12, 305, 1992.

172. Arens, M., Use of probes and amplification techniques for the diagnosis and prognosis of human immunodeficiency virus (HIV-1) infections, *Diagn. Microbiol. Infect. Dis.*, 16, 165, 1993.

173. Jackson, J. B., Detection and quantitation of human immunodeficiency virus type 1 using molecular DNA/RNA technology, *Arch. Pathol. Lab. Med.*, 117, 473, 1993.

174. Henrard, D. R., Mehaffey, W. F., and Allain, J. P., A sensitive viral capture assay for detection of plasma viremia in HIV-infected individuals, *AIDS Res. Human Retroviruses*, 8, 47, 1992.

175. Kwok, S., and Sninsky, J. J., PCR detection of human immunodeficiency virus type 1, in *Diagnostic Molecular Microbiology: Principles and Applications*, Persing, D. H., Smith, T. F., Tenover, F. C., and White, T. J., Eds., American Society for Microbiology, Washington, D.C., 1993, chap. 2.1.

176. Bush, C. E., Donovan, R. M., Peterson, W. R., Jennings, M. B., Bolton, V., Sherman, D. G., Vanden Brink, K. M., Beninsig, L. A., and Godsey, J. H. Detection of human immunodeficiency virus type 1 RNA in plasma samples from high-risk pediatric patients by using the self-sustained sequence replication reaction, *J. Clin. Microbiol.*, 30, 281, 1992.

177. Gingeras, T. R., Prodanovich, P., Latimer, T., Guatelli, J. C., Richman, D. D., and Barringer, K. J., Use of self-sustained sequence replication amplification reaction to analyze and detect mutations in zidovudine-resistant human immunodeficiency virus, *J. Infect. Dis.*, 164, 1066, 1991.

178. Schmilovitz-Weiss, H., Levy, M., Thompson, V., and Dusheiko, G., Viral markers in the treatment of hepatitis B and C, *Gut*, 34, S26, 1993.

179. Wilber, J. C., Development and use of laboratory tests for hepatitis C infection: a review, *J. Clin. Immunoassay*, 16, 204, 1993.

180. Bréchot, C., Polymerase chain reaction for the diagnosis of viral hepatitis B and C, *Gut*, 34, S39, 1993.

181. McOmish, F., Yap, P. L., Dow, B. C., Follett, E. A. C., Seed, C., Keller, A. J., Cobain, T. J., Krusius, T., Kalho, E., Naukkarinen, R., Lin, C., Lai, C., Leong, S., Medgyesi, G. A., Héjjas, M., Kitokawa, H., Fukada, K., Cuypers, T., Saeed, A. A., Al-Rasheed, A. M., Lin, M., and Simmonds, P., Geographical distribution of hepatitis C virus genotypes in blood donors: an international collaborative survey *J. Clin. Microbiol.*, 32, 884, 1994.

182. Dusheiko, G., Schmilovitz-Weiss, H., Brown, D., McOmish, F., Yap, P. L., Sherlock, S., McIntyre, N., and Simmonds, P., Hepatitis C virus genotypes. An investigation of type-specific differences in geographic origin and disease, *Hepatology*, in press.

183. Yoshioka, K., Kakumu, S., Wakita, T., Ishikawa, T., Itoh, Y., Takayanagi, Y., Higashi, Y., Shibata, M., and Morishima, T., Detection of hepatitis C virus by polymerase chain reaction and response to interferon-α therapy: relation to genotypes of hepatitis C virus, *Hepatology*, 16, 293, 1992.

184. Okada, S., Akahane, Y., Suzuki, H., Okamoto, H., and Mishiro, S., The degree of variability in the amino terminal region of the E2/NS1 protein of hepatitis C virus correlates with responsiveness to interferon therapy in viremic patients, *Hepatology*, 16, 619, 1992.

185. Cha, T. A., Beall, E., Irvine, B., Kolberg, J., Chien, D., Kuo, G., and Urdea, M. S., At least five related, but distinct, hepatitis C viral genotypes exist, *Proc. Natl. Acad. Sci. U.S.A.*, 89, 7144, 1992.

186. Watanabe, S., Kobayashi, Y., Konishi, M., Yokoi, M., Kakehashi, R., Kaito, M., and Suzuki, S., Appropriate interferon-alpha therapy for chronic hepatitis-C — an assessment by quantitative changes in serum hepatitis-C virus-RNA, *Intern. Med.*, 32, 523, 1993.

187. Okuda, M., HCV-RNA assay in peripheral blood mononuclear cells in relation to IFN therapy, *Gastroenterol. Jpn.*, 28, 535, 1993.

188. Sherman, K. E., O'Brien, J., Gutierrez, A. G., Harrison, S., Urdea, M., Neuwald, P., and Wilber, J., Quantitative evaluation of hepatitis C virus RNA in patients with concurrent human immunodeficiency virus infections, *J. Clin. Microbiol.*, 31, 2679, 1993.

189. Jackson, J. B., The polymerase chain reaction in transfusion medicine, *Transfusion*, 30, 51, 1990.

190. Tipple, M. A., Bland, L. A., Murphy, J. J., Arduino, M. J., Pantibo, A. L., Farmer, J. J., III, Tourault, M. A., Macpherson, C. R., Menitove, J. E., Grindon, A. J., Johnson, P. S., Strauss, R. G., Bufill, J. A., Ritch, P. S., Archer, J. R., Tablan, O. C., and Jarvis, W. R., Sepsis associated with transfusion of red cells contaminated with *Yersinia enterocolitica*, *Transfusion*, 30, 207, 1990.

191. Halpin, T. J., Kilker, S., Epstein, J., and Tourault, M., Bacterial contamination of platelet pools — Ohio, 1991, *Morbid. Mortal. Weekly Rep.*, 41, 36, 1992.

192. Piper, K., Brecher, M. E., Bland, L., and Persing, D. H., Use of a chemiluminescent universal bacterial probe for pretransfusion screening of blood products [Abstr.], 92nd General Meeting of the American Society for Microbiology, Washington, D.C., p. 116, 1992.

193. Sim, B. K., Mak, J. W., Cheong, W. H., Sutanto, I., Kwiniawan, L., Marwoto, H. A., Franke, E., Campbell, J. R., Wirth, D. F., and Piessens, W. F., Identification of *Brugia malayi* in vectors with a species-specific DNA probe, *Am. J. Trop. Med. Hyg.*, 35, 559, 1986.

194. Gottstein, B., Molecular and immunological diagnosis of echinococcosis, *Clin. Microbiol. Rev.*, 5, 248, 1992.

195. Zimmerman, P. A., Guderian, R. H., Aruajo, E., Elson, L., Phadke, P., Kubofcik, J., and Nutman, T. B., Polymerase chain reaction-based diagnosis of *Onchocera valvulus* infection: improved detection of patients with Onchocerciasis, *J. Infect. Dis.*, 169, 686, 1994.

196. Spach, D. H., Liles, W. C., Campbell, G. L., Quick, R. E., Anderson, D. E., and Fritsche, T. R., Tick-borne diseases in the United. States, *N. Engl. J. Med.*, 329, 936, 1993.

197. Telford, S. R., III, Gorenflot, A., III, Brasseur, P., and Spielman, A., Babesial infections in man and wildlife, in *Parasitic Protozoa*, Kreie, J. P. and Baker, J. R., Eds., Academic Press, New York, 1992, chap. 1.

198. Dammin, G. J., Spielman, A., Benach, J. L., and Piesman, J., The rising incidence of clinical *Babesia microti* infection, *Human Pathol.*, 12, 398, 1981.

199. Anderson, J. F., Mintz, E. D., Gadbau, J. J., and Magnarelli, L. A., *Babesia microti*, human babesiosis, and *Borrelia burgdorferi* in Connecticut, *J. Clin. Microbiol.*, 29, 2779, 1991.

200. Chisholm, E. S., Ruebush, T. K. III, Sulzer, A. J., and Healy, G. R., *Babesia microti* infection in man: evaluation of an indirect immunofluorescent antibody test, *Am. J. Trop. Med. Hyg.*, 27, 14, 1978.

201. Bradt, A. B., Weinstein, W. M., and Cohen, S., Treatment of babesiosis in asplenic patients, *J. Am. Med. Assoc.*, 245, 1938, 1981.
202. Ekkind, P., Piesman, J., Ruebush, T. K., III, Spielman, A., and Juranek, D. D., Methods for detection of *Babesia microti* infection in wild rodents, *J. Parasitol.*, 66, 107, 1980.
203. Persing, D. H., PCR detection of *Babesia microti*, in *Diagnostic Molecular Microbiology: Principles and Applications*, Persing, D. H., Smith, T. F., Tenover, F. C., and White, T. J., Eds., American Society for Microbiology, Washington, D.C., 1993, chap. 4.5.
204. Krause, P., Sikand, V. J., Boco, L., Christianson, D., Cartter, M., Magera, J., and Persing, D. H., PCR diagnosis of *Babesia microti* infection in humans [Abstr.], 33rd Interscience Conference on Antimicrobial Agents and Chemotherapy, New Orleans, LA, p. 322, 1993.
205. Piesman, J., Mather, T. N., Telford, S. R., III, and Spielman, A., Concurrent *Borrelia burgdorferi* and *Babesia microti* infection in nymphal *Ixodes dammini*, *J. Clin. Microbiol.*, 24, 446, 1986.
206. Persing, D. H., Mathiesen, D., Marshall, W. F., Telford, S. R., III, Spielman, A., Thomford, J. W., and Conrad, P. A., Detection of *Babesia microti* by polymerase chain reaction, *J. Clin. Microbiol.*, 30, 2097, 1992.
207. Shepp, D. H., Hackmann, R. C., Conley, F. K., Anderson, J. B., and Meyers, J. D., *Toxoplasma gondii* reactivation identified by detection of parasitemia in tissue culture, *Ann. Intern. Med.*, 103, 218, 1985.
208. Tirard, V., Hackman, R.C., Conley, F.K., Anderson, J.B., and Meyers, J.D., Toxoplasma gondii reactivation identified by detection of parasitemia in tissue culture, *Ann. Intern. Med.*, 103, 218, 1985.
209. Weiss, L. M., Udem, S. A., Salgo, U., Tanowitz, H. B., and Wittner, M., Sensitive and specific detection of toxoplasma DNA in an experimental murine model: use of *Toxoplasma gondii*-specific cDNA and the polymerase chain reaction, *J. Infect. Dis.*, 163, 180, 1991.
210. Johnson, J. D., Holliman, R. E., and Sarva, D., Detection of *Toxoplasma gondii* using the polymerase chain reaction, *Biochem. Soc. Trans.*, 18, 665, 1990.
211. Hilt, J. A. and Filice, G. A., Detection of *Toxoplasma gondii* parasitemia by gene amplification, cell culture, and mouse inoculation, *J. Clin. Microbiol.*, 30, 3181, 1992.
212. Mathiopoulos, K., Bouaré, M., McConkey, G., and McCutchan, T., PCR detection of *Plasmodium* species in blood and mosquitoes, in *Diagnostic Molecular Microbiology: Principles and Applications*, Persing, D. H., Smith, T. F., Tenover, F. C., and White, T. J., Eds., American Society for Microbiology, Washington, D.C., 1993, chap. 4.3.
213. Brown, A. E., Kain, K. C., Pipithkul, J., and Webster, H. K., Demonstration by the polymerase chain reaction of mixed *Plasmodium falciparum* and *P. vivax* infections undetected by conventional microscopy, *Trans. Royal Soc. Trop. Med. Hyg.*, 86, 609, 1992.
214. Kain, K. C., Brown, A. E., Lanar, D. F., Ballou, W. R., and Webster, H. K., Response of *Plasmodium vivax* variants to chloroquine as determined by microscopy and quantitative polymerase chain reaction, *Am. J. Trop. Med. Hyg.*, 49, 478, 1993.
215. Kain, K. C., Brown, A. E., Mirabeli, L., and Webster, H. K., Detection of *Plasmodium vivax* by polymerase chain reaction in a field study, *J. Infect. Dis.*, 168, 1323, 1993.
216. Clark, C. G., PCR detection of pathogenic *Entamoeba histolytica* and differentiation from other intestinal protozoa by ripoprinting, in *Diagnostic Molecular Microbiology: Principles and Applications*, Persing, D. H., Smith, T. F., Tenover, F. C., and White, T. J., Eds., American Society for Microbiology, Washington, D.C., 1993, chap. 4.4.

217. Wang, R. Y.-H. and Lo, S.-C., PCR detection of *Mycoplasma fermentens* infection in blood and urine, in *Diagnostic Molecular Microbiology: Principles and Applications*, Persing, D. H., Smith, T. F., Tenover, F. C., and White, T. J., Eds., American Society for Microbiology, Washington, D.C., 1993, chap. 5.4.

218. Sanderson, J. D. and Hermon-Taylor, J., Mycobacterial diseases of the gut: some impact from molecular biology, *Gut*, 33, 145, 1992.

219. Hu, W. S., Wang, R.Y.H., Liou, R.S., Shih, W.K., and Lo, S.C., Identification of an insertion-sequence-like genetic element in the newly recognized human pathogen *Mycoplasma incognitus, Gene*, 93, 67, 1990.

220. Cartun, R. W., Van Kruiningen, H. J., Pedersen, C. A., and Berman, M. M., An immunocytochemical search for infectious agents in Crohn's disease, *Modern Pathol.*, 6, 212, 1993.

221. Ablashi, D. V., Krueger, G. R. F., and Salahuddin, S. Z., Human herpesvirus-6: epidemiology, molecular biology and clinical pathology, in *Perspectives in Medical Virology*, Vol. 4, Elsevier Science Publishers, Amsterdam.

222. Frenkel, N., Schirmer, E. C., Wyatt, L. S., Katsafanas, G., Roffman, E., Danovich, R. M., and June, C. H., Isolation of a new herpesvirus from human CD4+ T cells, *Proc. Natl. Acad. Sci. U.S.A.*, 87, 748, 1990.

223. Klotman, M. E., Lusso, P., Bacchus, D., Corbellino, M., Jarrett, R. F., and Berneman, Z. N., Detection of human herpesvirus 6 and human herpesvirus 7 by PCR amplification, in *Diagnostic Molecular Microbiology: Principles and Applications*, Persing, D. H., Smith, T. F., Tenover, F. C., and White, T. J., Eds., American Society for Microbiology, Washington, D.C., 1993, chap. 5.3.

224. Woese, C. R., Bacterial evolution, *Microbiol. Rev.*, 51, 221, 1987.

225. Relman, D. A., The identification of uncultured microbial pathogens, *J. Infect. Dis.*, 168, 1, 1993.

226. Kirschner, P., Meier, A., and Böttger, E. C., Genotypic identification and detection of Mycobacteria facing novel and uncultured pathogens, in *Diagnostic Molecular Microbiology Principles and Applications*, Persing, D. H., Smith, T. F., Tenover, F. C., and White, T. J., Eds., American Society for Microbiology, Washington, D.C., 1993.

227. Relman, D. A., Loutit, J. S., Schmidt, T. M., Falkow, S., and Tompkin, L. S., The agent of bacillary angiomatosis: an approach to the identification of uncultured pathogens, *N. Engl. J. Med.*, 323, 1573, 1990.

228. Relman, D. A., Schmidt, T. M., MacDermott, R. P., and Falkow, S., Identification of the uncultured bacillus of Whipple's disease, *N. Engl. J. Med.*, 327, 293, 1992.

229. Relman, D. A., PCR based detection of the uncultured bacillus of Whipple's disease, in *Diagnostic Molecular Microbiology Principles and Applications*, Persing, D. H., Smith, T. F., Tenover, F. C., and White, T. J., Eds., American Society for Microbiology, Washington, D.C., 1993, chap. 5.2.

230. Anderson, B. E., Dawson, J. E., Jones, D. C., and Wilson, K. H., *Ehrlichia chaffeensis*, a new species associated with human ehrlichiosis, *J. Clin. Microbiol.*, 29, 2838, 1991.

231. Harkness, J. R., Ehrlichiosis, *Infect. Dis. Clin. N. Am.*, 5, 37, 1991.

232. Anderson, B. E., PCR detection of *Rickettsia rickettsii* and *Ehrlichia chaffeensis*, in *Diagnostic Molecular Microbiology Principles and Applications*, Persing, D. H., Smith, T. F., Tenover, F. C., and White, T. J., Eds., American Society for Microbiology, Washington, D.C., 1993, chap. 1.3.

233. Goldman, D. P., Artenstein, A. W., and Bolan, C. D., Human ehrlichiosis: a newly recognized tick-borne disease, *Am. Fam. Phys.*, 46, 199, 1992.

234. Dawson, J. E., Fishbein, D. B., Eng, T. R., Redus, M. A., and Greene, N. R., Diagnosis of human ehrlichiosis with the indirect fluorescent antibody test: kinetics and specificity, *J. Infect. Dis.*, 162, 91, 1990.

235. McDade, J. E., Ehrlichiosis — A disease of animals and humans, *J. Infect. Dis.*, 161, 609, 1990.

236. Anderson, B. E., Sumner, J. W., Dawson, J. E., Tzianabos, T., Greene, C. R., Olson, J. G., Fishbein, D. B., Olsen-Rasmussen, M., Holloway, B. P., George, E. H., and Azad, A. F., Detection of the etiologic agent of human Ehrlichiosis by polymerase chain reaction, *J. Clin. Microbiol.*, 30, 775, 1991.

237. Dunn, B. E., Monson, T. P., Dumler, J. S., Morris, C. C., Westbrook, A. B., Duncan, J. L., Dawson, J. E., Sims, K. G., Anderson, B. E., Identification of *Ehrlichia chaffeensis* morulae in cerebrospinal fluid mononuclear cells, *J. Clin. Microbiol.*, 30, 2207, 1992.

238. Dumler, J. S., Sutter, W. L., and Walker, D. H., Persistent infection with *Ehrlichia chaffeensis*, *Clin. Infect. Dis.*, 17, 903, 1993.

239. Meier, A., Persing, D. H., Finken, M., and Böttger, E. C., Elimination of contaminating DNA within PCR reagents implications for a general approach to detect uncultured pathogens, *J. Clin. Microbiol.*, 31, 646, 1993.

240. Maki, D. G., Rhame, F. S., Mackel, D. C., and Bennett, J. V., Nationwide epidemic of septicemia caused by contaminated intravenous products. I. Epidemiologic and clinical features, *Am. J. Med.*, 60, 471, 1976.

241. Goetz, M. B., Mulligan, M. E., Kwok, R., O'Brien, H., Coballes, C., and Garcia, J. P., Management and epidemiologic analysis of an outbreak due to methicillin-resistant *Staphylococcus aureus*, *Am. J. Med.*, 92, 607, 1992.

242. Jarvis, W. R., Nosocomial outbreaks: the Centers for Disease Contro's Hospital Infections Program experience 1980–1990, *Am. J. Med.*, 91(Suppl. 3B), 1015, 1991.

243. Birnbaum, D., Kelly, M., and Chow, A. W., Epidemiologic typing systems for coagulase-negative Staphylococci, *Infect. Control Hosp. Epidemiol.*, 12, 319, 1991.

244. Seppälä, H., Vuopio-Varikila, J., Österblad, M., Jahkola, M., Rummukainen, M., Holm, S. E., and Huovinen, P., Evaluation of methods for epidemiologic typing of group A Streptococci, *J. Infect. Dis.*, 169, 519, 1994.

245. Clabots, C. R., Johnson, S., Olson, M. M., Peterson, L. R., and Gerding, D. V., Acquisition of *Clostridium difficile* by hospitalized patients: evidence for colonized new admissions as a source of infection, *J. Infect. Dis.*, 166, 561, 1992.

246. van Soolingen, D., Hermans, P. W. M., de Haas, P. E. W., Soll, D. R., and van Embden, J. D. A., Occurrence and stability of insertion sequences in *Mycobacterium tuberculosis* complex strains: evaluation of an insertion sequence-dependent DNA polymorphism as a tool in the epidemiology of tuberculosis, *J. Clin. Microbiol.*, 29, 2578, 1991.

247. Owen, R. J., Chromosomal DNA fingerprinting — a new method of species and strain identification applicable to microbial pathogens, *J. Med. Microbiol.*, 30, 89, 1989.

248. Loutit, J. S. and Tompkins, L. S., Restriction enzyme and Southern hybridization analyses of *Pseudomonas aeruginosa* strains from patients with cystic fibrosis, *J. Clin. Microbiol.*, 29, 2897, 1991.

249. Stull, T. L., LiPuma, J. J., and Edlind, T. D., A broad-spectrum probe for molecular epidemiology of bacteria: ribosomal RNA, *J. Infect. Dis.*, 157, 280, 1988.

250. Gustaferro, C. A. and Persing, D. H., Chemiluminescent universal probe for bacterial ribotyping, *J. Clin. Microbiol.*, 30, 1039, 1992.

251. Maslow, J. V., Mulligan, M. E., and Arbeit, R. D., Molecular epidemiology: applications of contemporary techniques to the typing of microorganisms, *Clin. Infect. Dis.*, 17, 153, 1993.

252. Crawford, J. T., Applications of molecular methods to epidemiology of tuberculosis, *Res. Microbiol.*, 144, 111, 1993.

253. Cave, M. D., Eisenach, K. D., Templeton, G., Salfinger, M., Mazurek, G., Bates, J. H., and Crawford, J. T., Stability of DNA fingerprint pattern produced with IS6110 in strains of *Mycobacterium tuberculosis*, *J. Clin. Microbiol.*, 32, 262, 1994.

254. Swaminathan, B. and Matar, G. M., Molecular typing methods, in *Diagnostic Molecular Microbiology: Principles and Applications*, Persing, D. H., Smith, T. F., Tenover, F. C., and White, T. J., Eds., American Society for Microbiology, Washington, D.C., 1993, chap. 2.

255. Mayer, L. W., Use of plasmid profiles in epidemiologic surveillance of disease outbreaks and in tracing the transmission of antibiotic resistance, *Clin. Microbiol. Rev.*, 1, 228, 1988.

256. Miller, J. M., Molecular technology for hospital epidemiology, *Diagn. Microbiol. Infect. Dis.*, 16, 153, 1992.

257. Brosch, R., Buchrieser, C., and Rocourt, J., Subtyping of *Listeria monocytogenes* serovar 4b by use of low frequency-cleavage restriction endonucleases and pulsed-field gel electrophoresis, *Res. Microbiol.*, 142, 667, 1991.

258. Arbeit, R. D., Arthur, M., Dunn, R., Kim, C., Selander, R. K., and Goldstein, R., Resolution of recent evolutionary divergence among *Escherichia coli* from releated lineages: the application of pulsed field electrophoresis to molecular epidemiology, *J. Infect. Dis.*, 161, 230, 1990.

259. Arbeit, R. D., Slutsky, A., Barber, T. W., Maslon, J. N., Niem Czyk, S., Falkinham, Jo'zd., O'Conner, G. T., and von Reyn, G. F., Genetic diversity among strains of *Mycobacterium avium* causing monoclonal and polyclonal bacteremia in patients with AIDS, *J. Infect. Dis.*, 167, 1384, 1993.

260. Centers for Disease Control and Prevention Update: transmission of HIV infection during an invasive dental procedure — Florida, *Morbid. Mortal. Weekly Rep.*, 40, 21, 1991.

261. Persing, D. H., Target selection and optimization of amplification reactions, in *Diagnostic Molecular Microbiology: Principles and Applications*, Persing, D. H., Smith, T. F., Tenover, F. C., and White, T. J., Eds., American Society for Microbiology, Washington, D.C., 1993, chap. 4.

262. Greenfield, L. and White, T. J., Sample preparation methods, in *Diagnostic Molecular Microbiology: Principles and Applications*, Persing, D. H., Smith, T. F., Tenover, F. C., and White, T. J., Eds., American Society for Microbiology, Washington, D.C., 1993, chap. 6.

263. Johnson, W. M. and Tyler, S. D., PCR detection of genes for enterotoxins, exfoliative toxins, and toxic shock syndrome toxin-1 in *Staphylococcus aureus*, in *Diagnostic Molecular Microbiology: Principles and Applications*, Persing, D. H., Smith, T. F., Tenover, F. C., and White, T. J., Eds., American Society for Microbiology, Washington, D.C., 1993, chap. 1.20.

264. Olsvik, O. and Strockbine, N. A., PCR detection of heat-stable, heat-labile, and Shiga-like toxin genes in *Escherichia coli*, in *Diagnostic Molecular Microbiology: Principles and Applications*, Persing, D. H., Smith, T. F., Tenover, F. C., and White, T. J., Eds., American Society for Microbiology, Washington, D.C., 1993, chap. 1.16.

265. Ibrahim, A., Liesack, W., and Stackebrandt, E., Polymerase chain reaction — gene probe detection system specific for pathogenic strains of *Yersinia enterocolitica*, *J. Clin. Microbiol.*, 30, 1942, 1992.

266. Espy, M. J., Smith, T. F., and Persing, D. H., Dependence of polymerase chain reaction product inactivation protocols on amplicon length and sequence composition, *J. Clin. Microbiol.*, 31, 2361, 1993.

267. Rys, P. N. and Persing, D. H., Preventing false positives: quantitative evaluation of three protocols for inactivation of polymerase chain reaction amplification products, *J. Clin. Microbiol.*, 31, 2356, 1993.

268. Longo, M. C., Berninger, M. S., and Hartley, J. L., Use of uracil DNA glycosylase to control carry-over contamination in polymerase chain reaction, *Gene*, 93, 125, 1990.

269. Persing, D. H. and Cimino, G. D., Amplification product inactivation methods, in *Diagnostic Molecular Microbiology: Principles and Applications*, Persing, D. H., Smith, T. F., Tenover, F. C., and White, T. J., Eds., American Society for Microbiology, Washington, D.C., 1993, chap. 5.

270. Cimino, G. D., Metchette, K., Tessman, J. W., Hearst, J. E., and Isaacs, S. T., Post-PCR sterilization: a method to control carryover contamination for the polymerase chain reaction, *Nucleic Acids Res.*, 19, 99, 1991.

271. Walder, R. Y., Hayeb, J. R., and Walder, J. A., Use of PCR primers containing a 3'-terminal ribose residue to prevent cross-contamination of amplified sequences, *Nucleic Acids Res.*, 21, 4339, 1993.

272. Aslanzadeh, J., Application of hydroxylamine hydrochloride for post-polymerase chain reaction sterilization, *Ann. Clin. Lab. Sci.*, 22, 280, 1992.

273. McCreedy, B. J. and Callaway, T. H., Laboratory design and work flow, in *Diagnostic Molecular Microbiology: Principles and Applications*, Persing, D. H., Smith, T. F., Tenover, F. C., and White, T. J., Eds., American Society for Microbiology, Washington, D.C., 1993, chap. 8.

274. Dieffenbach, C. W. and Dreksler, G. S., Setting up a PCR laboratory, *PCR Meth. Applic.*, 3, S2, 1993.

275. Versailles, J., Berckhan, K., Ghosh, S. S., and Fahy, E., Photochemical sterilization of 3SR reactions, *PCR Methods Applic.*, 3, 151, 1993.

276. Hunsaker, W.R., Badri, H., Lombardo, M., and Collins, M.L., Nucleic acid hybridization assays employing dA-tailed capture probes. II. Advanced multiple capture methods, *Anal. Biochem.*, 181, 360, 1989.

277. Persing, D.H., Polymerase chain reaction: trenches to benches, *J. Clin. Microbiol.*, 29, 1281, 1991.

Chapter 7

CYTOKINES IN HUMAN IMMUNOLOGY

Barbara Detrick and John J. Hooks

CONTENTS

0-8493-0134-3/97/$0.00+$.50

I. INTRODUCTION: OVERVIEW OF CYTOKINES

Biomedical researchers have tried to isolate and characterize selected molecules associated with specific biological activities and disease states. However, years of investigation have led to the description of mediators with a diverse range of actions on a variety of cell types. Today, we recognize that cytokines are multifunctional proteins whose biological properties suggest a key role in hematopoiesis, immunity, infectious disease, tumorgenesis, homeostasis, tissue repair, and cellular development and growth. [1,2]

Dramatic advances in recombinant DNA and monoclonal antibody technology have greatly enhanced our knowledge of cytokines, their interactive role in health and disease, their activities in animal models, and their clinical utility. Because of their major participatory role in nearly all pathophysiologic processes and their therapeutic potential, there is a need to identify and measure cytokines. In the clinical laboratory, cytokine assessment has been used to monitor disease progression and activity. For example, the proinflammatory cytokines, tumor necrosis factor (TNF), interleukin-1 (IL-1) and interleukin-6 (IL-6) are frequently detected in the sera of patients with septic shock. These cytokines appear to play a critical role in the development of septic shock, and tracking their presence may be of prognostic value in severe sepsis. In addition, the increasing use of cytokines and cytokine antagonists as therapeutic modalities requires the measurement of cytokine levels to determine the pharmacokinetics of the administered molecule. In the research laboratory, the measurement of cytokine gene expression is currently being explored with the hope that this approach will offer clues to better define the mechanisms of cytokine action in disease processes. For example, targeted disruption of the mouse TGF-β1* gene generates "knockout" mice defective in TGF-β1 production. Multifocal inflammatory disease develops in these animals and suggests a critical immunosuppressive role for TGF-β1.[3] As a consequence of these

---

* TGF-β = transforming growth factor-β.

expanding applications, the future use of cytokine monitoring in both the clinical and research setting will undoubtedly increase.

The aim of this chapter is to identify the production and activities of cytokines and their receptors, to identify those cytokines with current or potential therapeutic application, and finally, to highlight ways to measure cytokines. In this chapter we will not attempt to identify all of the described cytokines and effector molecules. Rather, we have selected those cytokines which may have relevance in terms of clinical immunologic monitoring and which may be directed toward therapeutic strategies. Due to the rapid developments in this area, this cytokine list will continually require updating. For more detailed descriptions of this diverse topic, the reader is directed to recent reviews in the literature.[1,2,4]

II. CYTOKINES: PRODUCTION AND ACTIVITIES

Before we enter into a description of the cytokines, there are certain general considerations which should be noted. First, the names used to describe the factors are frequently erroneous, since the biological activities of the cytokine extend beyond the named activity. For example, interferon gamma (IFN-γ) interferes in or inhibits virus replication, but it also acts as a potent immunoregulatory molecule. Moreover, the interleukins not only initiate communication among immune cells, but they can also induce profound effects on nonimmune cells. In many cases, cytokines have been rediscovered and given a new name reflecting the newly described function. Therefore, we have included Table 1, which lists the cytokines and some of their synonyms and actions.

Second, cytokines usually act as signaling molecules by binding to their own glycoprotein receptors on cell membranes.[5] This initial interaction is followed by a relay of the signal to the cell nucleus. Signal transduction is mediated as in many hormone-receptor systems via kinase-mediated phosphorylation of cytoplasmic proteins. In fact, tyrosine kinase activity is intrinsic to many cytokine receptors. For the purpose of this discussion we will highlight two aspects of the receptor system: the production of soluble receptors and the potential role of receptor antagonists. Even when separated from the intact molecule, the receptor polypeptide domains can retain function. Receptors, for instance, released into the serum can bind to their ligand. This can impact upon the interpretation of cytokine assays and cytokine therapy. Since receptor expression can be activated in a variety of disease states, approaches to block this activation and/or block the specific cytokine–receptor interaction is actively under investigation and will be discussed in the section on cytokine analysis in clinical immunology.

TABLE 1

Cytokine Synonyms

Present Designation	Former Name
Interferons (IFN)	
IFN-α	Leukocyte (Le) IFN, Type 1 IFN
IFN-β	Fibroblast IFN, Type 1 IFN
IFN-γ	Immune IFN, Type II IFN
Tumor necrosis factor (TNF)	
TNF-α	Cachectin
TNF-β	Lymphotoxin
Interleukins	
IL-1	Lymphocyte-activating factor (LAF), endogenous pyrogen (EP), mitogenic protein (mp), helper peak-1 (HP-1), T-cell replacing factor III (TRFIII), B-cell activating factor (BAF), B-cell differentiating factor (BDF), osteoclast activating factor, hemopoietin-1, melanoma growth inhibitory factor, tumor inhibitory factor-2
IL-2	T-cell growth factor (TCGF)
IL-3	Colony-forming unit-stimulatory factor (CFU-SA), multicolony growth factor, P-cell-stimulating factor, burst-promoting activity, Thy-1-inducing factor, WEHI-3 growth factor
IL-4	B-cell growth factor (BCGF1), B-cell stimulatory factor (BSF1), B-cell differentiation factor (BCDF)
IL-5	T-cell replacing factor (TRF-1), B-cell growth factor (BCGFII), T-cell-derived eosinophil differentiation factor (EDF), IgA-enhancing factor (IgA-EF), eosinophil colony-stimulating factor (EO-CSF), B-cell growth and differentiation factor (BGDF)
IL-6	Interferon β2, 26 kDa protein, B-cell stimulatory factor-2 (BSF-2), hybridoma/plasmacytoma growth factor, hepatocyte-stimulating factor, cytotoxic T-cell differentiating factor, monocyte-derived human B-cell growth factor
IL-7	Lymphopoietin-1 (LP-1)
IL-8	Neutrophil attractant/activating protein (NAP-1), monocyte-derived neutrophil chemotactic factor (MDNCF), neutrophil-activating factor (NAF), T-lymphocyte chemotactic factor (TCF), leukocyte adhesion inhibitor (LA1)
IL-10	Cytokine synthesis inhibitory factor
IL-12	NK cell stimulating factor
Colony stimulating factors (CSF)	
GM-CSF	CSF-2, macrophage-granulocyte inducer
G-CSF	Pluripoietin, GM-CSF-b, macrophage/granulocyte inducer type 1 (MG-1G)
M-CSF	CSF-1
Stem cell factor	Kit-ligand (KL), steel factor, mast cell growth factor

Third, cytokine activity can be overlapping or redundant, and interactions among cytokines can occur through a cascading effect. Cytokines are potent regulatory molecules which modify inflammation, cell growth, and differentiation. The advent of cDNA cloning techniques has generated recombinant molecules which are pure preparations of individual cytokines. Studies with these recombinant molecules and with transgenic and knockout mice have underscored the redundant and cascading or cyclic nature of these cytokine systems. It is now clear that cytokines share similar activities, and cytokines induce or augment the actions of other cytokines. An appreciation of these tenets has enriched our knowledge of the potential clinical applications of cytokines.

Production of cytokines by Th1* and Th2 subsets of T cells is an example of cytokine interactions or cross-regulation.[6] Activation of the Th1 subset of T cells results in the production of IL-2, IFN-γ, and IL-12, which stimulates predominantly cell-mediated immune responses mediated by cytotoxic T cells, macrophages, and natural killer (NK) cells. In contrast, activation of Th2 subset of T cells results in the production of IL-4, IL-5, IL-6, and IL-10, which stimulates predominantly humoral immune responses mediated by antibodies. Opposing effects of cytokines are seen with IL-10 and IL-12. IFN-γ production is up-regulated by IL-12 and down-regulated by IL-10. An appreciation of the cytokine interactions is creating an impetus for investigators to try to modify pathologic responses by manipulating cytokine interactions within a particular tissue.

The rapid emergence of new cytokines and the identification of new activities for established cytokines make a comprehensive comment on each individual cytokine difficult. Therefore, only selected cytokines will be highlighted. For the purpose of discussion we have grouped the cytokines into four groups: interferons, TNF, interleukins, and growth factors. Listings of the cytokines and their actions can be found in Tables 2 and 3.

A. Interferons

Although the interferons (IFNs) were first identified in 1957 as antiviral proteins, they are now also recognized as immunoregulatory proteins capable of altering a variety of cellular processes, such as cell growth, differentiation, gene transcription, and translation.[7-10] There are three general types of IFNs: IFN-α, -β, and -γ.[8] The cell making the IFN and the substance triggering its production are important factors in determining the type of IFN produced (Table 2). IFN-α is produced by leukocytes in response to a variety of IFN inducers, such as viruses,

---

* Th = T helper lymphocyte; Th1 = T helper, subset 1; Th2 = T helper, subset 2.

TABLE 2

Cytokine Production and Action

Cytokine Family	Producer[a]	Effects
Interferons		
Alpha	Leukocytes	Antiviral, immunoregulatory, antiproliferative (enhance MHC class I, NK cell activity)
Beta	Fibroblasts	Antiviral, immunoregulatory, antiproliferative
Gamma	T cells, NK cells	Antiviral, immunoregulatory, antiproliferative (enhance MHC class I and II, macrophage activation)
TNF		
Alpha	Macrophage, lymphocytes	Activate macrophages and cytotoxic cells; induce cachexia, acute phase proteins, cytokines (IL-1, IL-6)
Beta	T cells	Activate macrophages; induces cytokines (IL-1, IL-6)
Colony-stimulating factors		
M-CSF	Monocytes	Proliferation of macrophage precursors
G-CSF	Macrophages	Proliferation, differentiation, activation of neutrophilic granulocyte lineage
GM-CSF	T cells, macrophages	Proliferation of granulocytes and macrophages precursors
Stem cell factor	bm stromal cells, fibroblasts, fetal liver cells	Proliferation and differentiation of early myeloid and lymphoid cells (synergizes with other cytokines)

[a] This list is not inclusive; primary cells have been identified.

bacterial products, polynucleotides, tumor cells, and allogeneic cells. The cell types responsible for synthesizing IFN-α include B cells, T cells, macrophages, NK, and large granular cells. If any of these inducers should interact with fibroblasts, epithelial cells, or to a lesser extent, leukocytes, IFN-β is produced. As an integral part of the immune response, T cells (either CD4 or CD8) are capable of manufacturing IFN-γ. The interaction of sensitized T cells with antigens or specific antigen–antibody complexes results in the production of IFN-γ. The NK cell has also been shown to produce IFN-γ. Moreover, the cytokine IL-2, which is produced by T lymphocytes, can also stimulate T cells to produce IFN-γ.

The IFNs can positively or negatively regulate cellular actions. These potent molecules act by modulating gene expression which can result in the production of cytoplasmic proteins. These IFN-induced proteins may then function in a number of ways: they may inhibit virus replication, regulate immune reactivity, suppress cell proliferation and oncogene expression, and alter cell differentiation. The antiviral actions of the IFNs are not based on their direct interaction with virions.

Instead, the IFNs act by binding to cell surface receptors which consequently affect transmembrane signaling and protein synthesis. Over 25 IFN-induced proteins which can participate in inducing the antiviral state have been identified. Most of the attention has been directed at three of these proteins, which include protein kinase (eIF-2a protein kinase), 2'5'-oligo-A synthetase, and Mx protein. Their major mode of action is the inhibition of translation of the viral genome into virus-specific proteins.

All of the IFNs can augment or depress a wide variety of immune reactions. The types of immune cells and functions that can be modified by the IFN system are shown in Table 2. IFN proteins can modify immune reactivity by acting at the level of B cells, T cells, NK cells, macrophages, basophils, or bone marrow stem cells.[7,8] Immune responses altered by such interactions include antibody production, T-cell cytotoxicity, graft-vs.-host reactions, mitogen and/or antigen stimulation, delayed-type hypersensitivity, NK cell cytotoxicity, various macrophage functions, immunoglobulin E (IgE)-mediated histamine release, and bone marrow stem cell maturation. It is possible that the actions of the IFNs on these cell types and the altered immune reactivity may be important in the pathophysiology of autoimmunity, immune deficiency, malignancy, and infectious diseases.

One of the more intriguing aspects of the IFN system is the ability of the IFNs to act as regulators of cell surface antigens and receptor expression. The IFNs can enhance the expression of cell surface proteins or receptors on a variety of animal and human cells. All of the IFNs can enhance the expression of the major histocompatibility complex (MHC) class I antigens, T-cell antigens, β_2-microglobulin, immunoglobulin-Fc receptors, and tumor-associated antigens.[7,8] However, only IFN-γ is capable of enhancing the synthesis and expression of the MHC class II antigens. Since T helper cells recognize exogenous antigen in association with class II antigens on the antigen-presenting cell (APC), IFN induction of these molecules may be a basic mechanism in the initiation and perpetuation of the immune response.

These potent actions of the IFNs and the advances in biotechnology are the underlying factors which have identified the clinical relevance of the IFNs. In fact, they are now Food and Drug Administration (FDA)-approved for a number of diseases ranging from infections to chronic granulomatous disease.

B. Tumor Necrosis Factor

Tumor necrosis factors are cytokines with inflammatory and anti-tumor activity which are presently identified as TNF-α and TNF-β. TNF-α was originally found in the circulation of mice. Endotoxin-treated mice contained a cytokine, cachectin, which produced a wasting syndrome in mice. [11] Another group of investigators was evaluating ways in which LPS-treated mice produced a serum factor which induced tumor necrosis.[12] Cachectin and TNF are both identified as TNF-α. TNF-β, on the other hand, was first isolated from activated T cells and was called lymphotoxin.[13,14] TNF-α and -β are structurally related, bind to the same cellular receptors and produce similar biological changes in a variety of cells. While TNF-α is produced by neutrophils, activated lymphocytes, macrophages, NK cells, and some nonlymphoid cells, such as astrocytes, endothelial cells, smooth muscle cells, and some transformed cells, TNF-β appears to be solely produced by T cells.

Both the TNFs and the IFNs are highly pleiotropic factors (Table 2). In fact, TNF has been shown to induce or suppress the expression of a variety of genes resulting in the production of growth factors, other cytokines, inflammatory mediators, and acute phase proteins.[11] TNF was originally studied for its ability to kill tumor cells. However, its potent inflammatory properties have become the primary focus of attention. TNF modulates both lymphoid and nonlymphoid cells to synthesize and release other immunostimulatory cytokines, such as IL-1 and IL-6. Furthermore, TNF induces fever, PGE2 and collagenase synthesis, bone and cartilage resorption, inhibition of lipoprotein lipase, and an increase in hepatic acute-phase proteins and complement components. Experimental administration of TNF can result in hypotension, leukopenia, local tissue necrosis, and shock.

Because of its promising role as an antiproliferative agent, TNF is continuing to be evaluated as a possible therapeutic strategy in cancer. However, the potent inflammatory properties of TNF may offer even more avenues for clinical application. Numerous clinical investigations have been initiated to evaluate agents that block TNF activity, particularly in septic shock and severe rheumatoid arthritis.

C. Interleukins

This name was originally coined in 1981 to describe the leukocyte-derived molecules which also acted upon leukocytes. We now know the interleukins can be made by and interact with a variety of cell types. The various interleukins (IL-1 through IL-13), the cells which produce these cytokines, and their diverse biological activities are listed in Table 3.[1,2,15-48] We will address IL-1, IL-2, IL-4, IL-6, IL-10, and IL-12.

1. Interleukin-1

IL-1 is recognized as IL-1α or IL-1β, which are different gene products utilizing the same cellular receptors. Both IL-1α and IL-1β are

TABLE 3

Cytokine (Interleukin) Production and Action

Cytokine Family	Producer	Inducers	Effects	Ref.
IL-1	Many cells (macrophages)	LPS, endotoxin, infectious agents, TNF, GM-CSF	Stimulates T cells and antigen-presenting cells (APC), induces TNF, IL-2, IL-6, IL-8, CSFs	1, 2, 15, 16, 71
IL-2	T cells (CD4+)	TCR complex on APC, IL-1	Up-regulates expression of IL-2R; induces proliferation and maturation of T cells; enhances production of IL-2, IFN-γ	1, 2, 23, 24, 25, 88
IL-3	T cells, thymic epithelial	Antigen stimulation	Growth factor for hematopoietic cells	1, 2, 52, 53
IL-4	T cells	Antigen stimulation	Growth factor for B cells, isotype switching to IgE, FcRII expression, expansion of Th2 subset	1, 2, 6, 26, 27, 29
IL-5	T cells	Antigen stimulation	Differentiation and proliferation of eosinophils, B-cell growth factor	1, 2, 31
IL-6	Many cells	LPS, endotoxin, IL-1,TNF, IFN-γ	B-cell stimulation — antibody production, plasmacytoma growth factor, hepatocyte-stimulating factor, acute phase protein synthesis	1, 2, 32, 33
IL-7	Stromal cells of thymus and bone marrow	Constitutively expressed	Promotes B- and T-cell development and growth	1, 2, 35, 36
IL-8	Many cells (macrophages)	LPS, IL-1, TNF, viruses	Neutrophil chemoattractant	1, 2, 37
IL-9	T cells	T cell mitogens	Helper T-cell factor, enhances erythroid colony formation, stimulates megakaryoblastic leukemia cells	1, 2, 38
IL-10	T cells Monocytes	Antigen stimulation	Inhibits IFN-γ and IL-12 production, suppresses cellular immunity, inhibits Th1 activities, promotes antibody secretion by B cells	1, 2, 6, 41, 42
IL-11	Bone marrow stromal cells		Synergistic effects on hematopoiesis and thrombopoiesis	1, 2, 43
IL-12	Monocytes, B cells	Antigen stimulation	Enhances IFN-γ production, activates T and NK cells, promotes cellular immunity, expands Th1 subset activities	1, 2, 6, 45, 46, 47
IL-13	T cells		IL-4 like effects, suppresses macrophage cytotoxicity and suppresses production of proinflammatory cytokines (TNF-α, IL-1, IL-6, IL-8, IL-12)	1, 2, 49, 50

produced by macrophages and a variety of other cell types in response to immunostimulatory factors, such as lipopolysacchardie (LPS), endotoxin, infectious agents, and TNF.[15,16]

The biological activities of the IL-1 molecules are varied and important for immune reactivity. IL-1 can induce cells to synthesize more of itself and other cytokines, such as TNF and IL-6. In fact, IL-1, IL-6, and TNF are all proinflammatory cytokines with overlapping biological properties. Another critical function of IL-1 is the activation of T cells. As a consequence of this activation, IL-2, IL-4, and granulocyte-macrophage CSF (GM-CSF) are produced and the expression of IL-2 receptors (IL-2R) is up-regulated.[17] IL-1 also triggers numerous activities in nonlymphoid cells. Endothelial cells and smooth muscle cells respond by producing prostaglandin, while synovial cells produce collagenase.[18] Moreover, IL-1 has been shown to initiate an acute phase response in the liver and initiate insulin production. These basic and varied inflammatory and cytotoxic responses of the IL-1 proteins have led investigators to consider this molecule as a potent contributor to inflammation and autoimmunity. Strategies aimed at blocking the pathologic effects associated with IL-1 are being identified and evaluated in clinical trials.

2. Interleukin-2

IL-2 was originally isolated and identified as T-cell growth factor.[19,20] These initial studies led directly to the isolation of the first human retrovirus, human T-cell leukemia virus (HTLV).[21] It is now known that IL-2 is synthesized and secreted primarily by $CD4^+$ T lymphocytes. The release of IL-2 by the T cell probably represents a commitment to T-cell activation. The T cell is activated by mitogens or by antigen-specific interactions between the CD3 T-cell receptor complex (TCR) plus CD4 and the MHC molecules on the surface of the antigen–presenting cell.[22] This activation of $CD4^+$ T cells results in the production and release of IL-2, the expression of IL-2 receptors, and the clonal expansion of antigen specific T cells. This series of events is critical to immune reactivity.

Biological activities of IL-2 are dependent upon the molecule interacting with specific TCRs.[23] There are at least three components of the IL-2 receptor, IL-2Rα, IL-2Rβ, and IL-2Rγ chains. A 45-kDa cleavage product of IL-2Rα is the soluble IL-2R, which is released from the surface of the T cell and is recognized by anti-Tac monoclonal antibody. The identification of sIL-2R may have clinical significance, and its presence is being evaluated as a marker for T-cell involvement or activation in a number of diseases. [23]

It is of interest to note that IL-2Rβ and IL-2Rγ are members of the hematopoietin receptor superfamily which also includes receptors for

IL-3, IL-4, IL-6, IL-7, GM-CSF, granulocyte-CSF (G-CSF), and erythropoietin. Recent studies have identified the potential importance of cytokine receptor systems. The primary defect in X-linked severe combined immunodeficiency (XSCID) is in the IL-2Rγ chain. A loss of IL-2 receptor activity alone was not sufficient to account for the devastation of the immune system in XSCID. However, the IL-2Rγ chain is shared by IL-2, IL-4, and IL-7.[24,25] A defect in IL-2Rγ chain affects IL-2, IL-4, and IL-7, which are critical factors needed to boost different stages in the growth and development of T and B cells. Thus, a defect in a single cytokine receptor protein resulted in an inactivation of multiple cytokine systems.

The importance of cellular function in tumor immunity was appreciated when studies demonstrated that the cytotoxic activity of NK cells could be up-regulated and amplified both *in vitro* and *in vivo* by addition of IL-2 and IFN-γ. In fact, these findings serve as the basis for ongoing adoptive cellular immunotherapy approaches now being applied to human tumors. This topic is discussed in Section III.

3. Interleukin-4

IL-4 is a T cell-derived cytokine which was initially recognized as a B-cell growth factor, (B-cell stimulating factor (BSF-1)).[26,27] In the mouse, IL-4 gene expression may be limited to a specific subset of T cells, Th2 cells.[28] The biological activity of IL-4 is not restricted to the B cell or B-cell growth factor actions.[29,22] Rather this cytokine may also induce FcRII (CD23) on the surface of B cells, act as a switching factor for IgE and IgG1 expression during B-cell differentiation, and enhance the generation of cytotoxic T cells that are sensitized to a specific antigen.

4. Interleukin-6

IL-6 is another potent pleiotropic cytokine which is produced by a variety of lymphoid and nonlymphoid cells.[30,32,33] The cellular production of IL-6 can be positively or negatively regulated by a number of signals. For example, mitogen- or antigen-specific stimulation of lymphocytes can induce IL-6 production. Alternatively, the bacterial product, LPS, and viruses can modulate IL-6 production. Finally, other cytokines, particularly IL-1 and TNF, are both potent inducers of IL-6 production in a variety of cell types.

IL-6 can affect cells in many different ways (Table 3). When IL-6 binds to its receptor on B cells, the cells are stimulated to differentiate and secrete antibody.[32] IL-6 will also act as a growth factor for myelomas, hybridomas, and plasmacytoma and may function as an autocrine growth factor in multiple myeloma. Moreover, IL-6 has colony-stimulating activity on hepatopoietic stem cells. This molecule stimulates hepatocytes which are capable of inducing the production of acute phase proteins.[34] In fact, in the liver, IL-6 enhances the production of fibrinogen, C-reactive protein, haptoglobin, and serum amyloid A. These activities indicate that IL-6 production, during infection or injury, may contribute to inflammatory and immune responses.

Presently, we know IL-6 can contribute to pathologic processes in inflammatory diseases and in selected malignancies. Based on these observations, current therapeutic strategies are aimed at abrogating IL-6 production and action.

5. Interleukin-10

IL-10 was recently identified as a mouse Th2 cell product which has the ability to inhibit Th1 cell production of IFN-γ.[39] This cytokine is also produced by B cells and monocytes and can enhance the proliferation of murine thymocytes in response to IL-2 and IL-4.[40] Since this cytokine inhibits IFN-γ production, it also inhibits antigen presentation and consequently suppresses the IFN-γ–induced cytokines, TNF-α, IL-1, IL-6, IL-8, and GM-CSF. Recent studies also indicate that IFN-γ inhibits IL-10 production. Thus IFN-γ and IL-10 antagonize the production and function of each other.[41] The *in vivo* relevance of these apparently contradictory responses remains to be resolved. However, studies indicate that administration of IL-10 to mice protects them from lethal endotoxemia.[42]

6. Interleukin-12

IL-12 is produced by monocytes and B cells and has multiple effects on T and NK cell function .[44,45] This cytokine appears to have a crucial role in initiating the Th1 cell response and has been described to induce IFN-γ production.[46] In addition, IL-10 inhibits IFN-γ production by suppression of IL-12 synthesis.[47] Recent studies show that administration of IL-12 to mice initiates Th1 cell responses and protective immunity in cutaneous leishmaniasis.[48]

D. Hematopoietic Growth Factors

Before entering into a discussion of the colony–stimulating factors (CSFs), we will first briefly outline stem cells and hematopoiesis. There is a multipotent stem cell which has the capability to reproduce and differentiate along both myeloid and lymphopoietic lineages. Steps of progressive maturation allow the more differentiated cell to develop. For example, the multipotent stem cell may differentiate into a myeloid stem cell, followed by differentiation steps leading to the development of platelets, erythrocytes, neutrophils, monocytes and eosinophils.

Alternatively, the multipotent stem cell may differentiate into pre-T or pre-B cells, which eventually develop into mature T cells and B cells. The regulation of these differentiation steps may be, in part, accomplished by the selective expression of cell surface receptors and the interactions of growth factors with these receptors. Normal hematopoiesis in the adult occurs in the bone marrow.

The term "CSFs" has been used to identify those cytokines which stimulate hematopoietic progenitor cell colony formation in semi-solid media. Presently there are four CSFs described: (1) IL-3, (2) macrophage CSF (M-CSF, CSF-1), (3) granulocyte CSF (G-CSF), and (4) granulocyte-macrophage CSF (GM-CSF).[51] Recently, a protein called stem cell factor has been identified, which is thought to directly stimulate human stem cells (Table 2). All of the CSFs are proving to be valuable tools for clinical use. They are important molecules in the *in vivo* and *ex vivo* expansion of hematopoietic stem and progenitor cells. These expanded cells may then be beneficial in the treatment of bone marrow damage seen in congenital cytopenias or as a consequence of chemotherapy and/or radiation.

1. Interleukin-3

IL-3 is produced by T cells and functions as a CSF which induces the differentiation of hematopoietic cells.[52] IL-3 can promote the growth of many different types of cells, including T and B cells, macrophages, mast cells, granulocytes, megakaryocytes, and erythroid precursors.[53] IL-3 can also be produced by human thymic epithelial cells, murine mast cells, and keratinocytes. Since IL-3 is a potent CSF, it is currently being used in combination with other CSFs as treatment for myelosuppression induced by chemotherapy or bone marrow transplantation.[22]

2. Colony-Stimulating Factor (CSF)

GM-CSF interacts with stem cells, resulting in the production of granulocyte, macrophage, and eosinophil colonies. GM-CSF can be produced by a variety of cells, such as T cells, B cells, macrophages, mast cells, endothelial cells, and fibroblasts in response to immune and inflammatory stimuli.[54,55] In addition to its CSF actions, GM-CSF initiates an array of biological effects. For example, it has been observed to: (1) enhance phagocytosis of neutrophils, eosinophils, and macrophages; (2) enhance antibody-dependent cell-mediated cytotoxicity (ADCC) of neutrophils, eosinophils, and macrophages; and (3) induce the synthesis and release of IL-1 and TNF-α from monocytes.[51,56,57]

G-CSF induces granulocyte colony formation in bone marrow culture and is considered a neutrophil-specific hemopoietin. G-CSF is produced by cells of the macrophage/monocyte lineage and is produced following stimulation with endotoxin, TNF-α or IFN-γ. Moreover, fibroblasts, endothelial cells, and bone marrow stromal cells are capable of producing G-CSF following stimulation with IL-1, TNF, or LPS.[55,58]

M-CSF is a growth factor specific for mononuclear phagocytes, which is produced by numerous cell types including: bone marrow stromal cells, fibroblasts, and epithelial cells of the endometrium. Not only does M-CSF stimulate replication of mononuclear phagocytes, but it also enhances the tumoricidal and antimicrobial actions of these cells. [59-61]

3. Stem Cell Factor

Recently, a new growth factor has been described which acts at an earlier differentiation level than the other known CSFs. This new factor, stem cell factor, acts as a ligand for c-kit receptor.[62,63] The c-kit receptor, encoded by the c-kit proto-oncogene, is a transmembrane receptor with tyrosine kinase activity. The importance of stem cell factor and c-kit receptor in hematopoiesis was first noted in W mutant mice. In this strain of mouse, lesions in the c-kit gene locus are associated with anemia, mast cell deficiency, and low numbers of progenitors for various hemopoietic lineages.

This cytokine has generated enthusiastic support for its potential as an *in vitro* growth factor for primitive hematopoietic progenitors. *In vitro* expansion of early progenitors with stem cell factor appears to provide a rich source of transplantable bone marrow. Moreover, some studies indicate that stem cell factor can synergize with other CSFs, to further augment *in vitro* cell expansion. Recently, Muench et al. [64] have shown that when a combination of IL-1 and stem factor were used to expand bone marrow progenitors, there was an effective production of blood leukocytes, platelets, and erythrocytes in lethally irradiated mice.

E. Growth Factors

In addition to the hematopoietic growth factors, there are numerous additional cytokine growth factors which influence cellular growth and differentiation. One factor that has received widespread attention by both the research and clinical community is TGF-β. TGF-β is a multifunctional cytokine that often demonstrates opposing effects on the development, physiology, and immunologic responses of a variety of cells. This apparently paradoxical cytokine is known to influence cellular differentiation, bone formation, angiogenesis, hematopoiesis, cell cycle progression, cell migration, and extracellular matrix production. Researchers are currently studying this cytokine for its therapeutic promise in wound healing and bone repair, as well as its reported bioactivities as both a proinflammatory and anti-inflammatory mediator.[4]

III. CLINICAL APPLICATIONS OF CYTOKINES

The wide involvement of cytokines in the pathogenesis and therapy of disease has made cytokines valuable in the clinical arena. Table 4 outlines some of the current clinical applications of cytokines. First, the detection of cytokines implicated in the pathogenesis of a number of diseases has broadened our knowledge of cytokine biology. For example, cytokine measurements in certain acute and chronic inflammatory states have been used as indicators of disease progression and activity. Second, the measurement of cytokine production has provided us a useful monitor of immune status. This approach examines the functional capacity of cells and correlates these data with an individual's immunocompetence. Third, the increasing use of cytokines in therapy represents an exciting new class of therapeutic agents. Both *in vivo* and *ex vivo* cytokine therapy are fast becoming a standard part of the therapeutic armature. Transplantation, malignancy, and immunodeficiency are some of the pathologies effectively being treated with cytokines. Fourth, the emergence of cytokine antagonists offers yet another clinical tool for treating a variety of acute and chronic conditions. Anticytokine antibody, antireceptor antibody, soluble cytokine receptors, and receptor antagonists offer promise as selective immunosuppressive agents. Finally, the development of vaccines for infectious diseases and cancer frequently require adjuvants to potentiate immunity. In a number of model systems, cytokines have been shown to be effective immunological adjuvants. The varied clinical applications of cytokines will be addressed in this section which focuses on IFN, TNF, IL-1, IL-6, IL-2, and hematopoietic growth factors.

A. Interferons-Varied Clinical Applications

The IFNs are multifunctional cytokines which have found numerous clinical applications. Identification of the IFNs in sera of patients with a variety of infections and immunoregulatory disorders has recently been reviewed.[7] IFN-α can be identified in viral infections and is frequently the first noted potent response of the host to these infections. Acid-labile forms of IFN-α can also be noted in patients with systemic lupus erythematosis (SLE), vasculitis, and related immunoregulatory disorders.[65,66]

Cytokine therapy has received major impetus from the IFN molecules. The IFNs have proven to be potent antiviral agents, immunomodulators, and antineoplastic agents. In fact, the IFNs are licensed in more than 40 countries for therapeutic indications in infectious, immunologic, and neoplastic diseases (Table 5).[8,67] The U.S. FDA has approved the therapeutic use of the IFNs in hairy-cell leukemia,

TABLE 4

Clinical Applications of Cytokines

Application	Example
I. Detection in diseases	IL-1, IL-2R, IL-6, TNF, IFN-γ in inflammatory and autoimmune diseases, graft rejection, malignancy
II. Monitor immunocompetence	Cytokine (IL-2, IFN-γ) production *in vitro*
III. Cytokine therapy	
a. *Ex vivo*	
1. Stimulation of cells	CSF-treated bone marrow cells for transplantation IL-2-, IFN-γ–treated LAK cells in cancer
2. Gene insertion	TNF in malignancy
b. *In vivo*	IFNs in infectious disease, malignancy, immune dysfunction
	Cytokine combinations in bone marrow transplantation
IV. Modalities for reducing cytokine activity	
a. Anticytokine antibody	Anti-IL-1, TNF, IFN-γ in inflammation and autoimmunity
b. Antireceptor antibody	Anti-IL-1R, anti-IL-2R
c. Soluble receptor	sIL-2R
d. Receptor antagonists	IL-1ra
e. Enzyme inhibition	Inhibition of IL-1 convertases
f. Drugs	CyA, FK506, rapamycin
V. Vaccine therapy cytokine adjuvants	IFN-α,β,γ — infectious disease and tumor vaccines
	IL-2 — infectious disease and tumor vaccines
	IL-7 — infectious disease vaccines (HSV, HIV)
	TNF — cancer vaccines
	IL-12 — parasitic vaccines (malaria)

Kaposi's sarcoma, condyloma acuminatum (genital warts), AIDS, hepatitis B and hepatitis C, and in chronic granulomatous disease.[1,8,67] The varied diseases which have responded positively to IFN therapy are outlined in Table 5.[8,10,68] These therapeutic indications for the IFNs are based on monotherapy approaches. Combinations of IFN-α and -γ and/or combinations of the IFNs with chemotherapeutic agents are surely an integral part of the future of IFN therapy.[69]

The presence of IFN may be determined using either a biological activity assay or an immunologic detection system.[7] For reasons outlined in Section IV, immunologic detection by enzyme-linked immunosorbent assay (ELISA) of the IFNs is the approach of choice for the clinical laboratory. The biological activity assay, which is more sensitive but more labor intensive, is not routinely used in the clinical laboratory. Nevertheless, this bioassay should be performed occasionally to assess the biological activity of the samples tested.

TABLE 5

Disease States Which Respond To IFN Therapy

IFN	Infectious Diseases	Malignancy	Immune Dysfunctions	Vascular Proliferative Disorders
Alfa	Hepatitis B Hepatitis C Genital warts Herpes simplex virus AIDS Laryngeal papillomatosis	Hairy cell leukemia Kaposi's sarcoma Chronic myelogenous leukemia Non-Hodgkins lymphoma Multiple myeloma Cutaneous T-cell lymphoma Malignant melanoma Basal cell carcinoma		Angiomas Subretinal neovascular proliferative disease
Beta			Multiple sclerosis	
Gamma	Intracellular parasites (Leishmaniasis, toxoplasmosis) Leprosy	Myeloid leukemia Cutaneous T-cell lymphoma Metastatic renal cell carcinoma Kaposi's sarcoma Basal cell carcinoma Cervical intraepithelial neoplasia	Chronic granulomatosis disease	

B. Proinflammatory Cytokines — TNF, IL-1, IL-6

The proinflammatory cytokines, IL-1, TNF, and IL-6 have a variety of biological properties in common. Because these cytokines are mediators of inflammation, their presence in body fluids may be a useful indicator of disease activity. As mentioned earlier, IL-1 and TNF exhibit synergism and both induce IL-6 production. IL-1 and TNF are inflammatory cytokines which can induce the deleterious effects of infection and injury. Therefore, blocking TNF with anti-TNF antibodies or soluble TNF receptors and blocking IL-1 with IL-1 receptor (IL-1R) antagonist (IL-1ra), anti-IL-1 antibodies, anti-IL-1R antibodies, or soluble IL-1R can all down-regulate the serious effects of infection and injury (Table 4).

TNF is one of the most abundant products of macrophages and can be readily observed following activation of immune responses to invading bacterial, parasitic, and viral organisms. In fact, TNF may play a critical role in septicemia and septic shock.[70-72] TNF can be identified in the serum and CSF of patients with meningococcal disease, in children with infectious purpura, and in patients with sepsis. In many of these studies, IL-1 and IL-6 were also detected. Recently, Braegger et al.[73] suggested that TNF levels in stool samples may provide a monitor of disease activity in inflammatory bowel disease. TNF production has also been detected in a variety of inflammatory conditions, such as rheumatoid arthritis. Monitoring levels of TNF in serum or synovial fluid has revealed that TNF levels are higher in patients with active disease as compared to patients with low disease activity.

Cytokine therapy with TNF was originally directed toward cancer patients who may benefit from tumor necrosis factor. However, due to severe toxic effects, such as fever, leukopenia, and hypotension, TNF cannot be administered directly.[71,74] An alternative, more promising approach to therapy is to limit TNF production or action. Animal studies in rodents and primates indicate that monoclonal anti-TNF antibodies may limit septic shock and death.[75,76] Human clinical trials have documented that anti-TNF antibody therapy results in improved cardiac function in septic shock patients.[77,78] Clinical trials evaluating the ability of anti-TNF and/or anti-LPS to down-regulate mediators of sepsis are currently under study.[70]

The second proinflammatory cytokine, IL-1, has also been detected in body fluids from a variety of inflammatory conditions, including septic shock, rheumatoid arthritis, and fatal cerebral malaria.[79] Moreover, elevated IL-1 levels in renal transplant patients has been detected 1 to 2 days prior to graft rejection.[80] This augmented cytokine response is a reflection of activated immune reactivity and may not be considered specific for the rejection process. Whether or not this correlation proves to be a useful monitor of graft rejection remains to be determined.

The therapeutic uses of IL-1, although intriguing, are still speculative. In human phase 1 trials, administration of IL-1α and IL-1β indicate that IL-1 produces fever, sleepiness, anorexia, myalgias, and hypotension, with an increase in circulating neutrophils and platelets.[81,82] These factors may be detrimental to the host. In fact, down-regulation of IL-1 production or action may be a more advantageous approach to therapy.[15] Both monoclonal antibodies to IL-1 molecule and the IL-1 receptor antagonist are receiving considerable attention as potential therapies (Table 8).

IL-1ra is a naturally occurring inhibitor of IL-1 function which was purified from the urine of patients with monocytic leukemia. [83] A functionally active recombinant molecule has been synthesized and competes with the binding of IL-1 to its cell surface receptor.[15] IL-1ra is a 17-kDa polypeptide which is usually detected in a 25-kDa glycosylated form. The IL-1ra has been shown to be functionally active both *in vitro* and *in vivo*. Initial animal studies demonstrated that the administration of IL-1ra limits the devastating effects of septic shock. In fact, administration of IL-1ra prevented death in animals receiving lethal doses of LPS or *E. coli.*[15,84]

IL-6 is readily detected in the serum, plasma, synovial fluid, or vitreous during inflammatory diseases. For example, serum IL-6 levels correlate with the presence of infections and may be of prognostic value in severe sepsis.[85] IL-6 is frequently associated with the presence of other proinflammatory cytokines. In septic shock, IL-6 is observed in conjunction with TNF, IL-1, IL-8, and IFN-γ.[86] Therapeutic approaches to down-regulate the proinflammatory cytokines have not extensively focused on IL-6. This is probably due to the fact that IL-6 is a poor inducer of IL-1 and TNF. In contrast, TNF and IL-1 are good inducers of IL-6. Therapeutic strategies concentrating on down-regulating TNF and IL-1, mentioned above, should also depress IL-6 production.

In the clinical immunology laboratory, the ELISA assay is the most convenient method for TNF, IL-1, and IL-6 detection. The bioassays for these cytokines are cytotoxic and differentiation assays are more suited to research investigations.[87]

C. Interleukin-2 and Soluble Interleukin-2 Receptor-Based Therapies

T cells are a critical unit of immune reactivity.[88] When these cells are stimulated by a foreign antigen, they are activated and begin to synthesize IL-2. The transition from resting to activated T cells also results in the expression of high-affinity IL-2 receptors on T cells. T-cell proliferation results when IL-2 interacts with its receptor. This process generates effector T cells which participate in immune responses. IL-2R expression is usually not associated with normal resting cells, but is associated with abnormal or activated cells noted in patients with certain leukemias and autoimmune diseases and in patients undergoing allograft rejection. Monitoring the soluble IL-2R in serum from these patients is an indication of cellular activation.[88]

The clinical applications of IL-2/IL-2 receptor systems can be viewed in two general aspects of immune intervention (Table 4). First, IL-2 has been employed as an immunostimulating molecule, particularly in malignancy.[89,90] Second, immunosuppressive therapies have focused on mechanisms aimed at blocking IL-2 production and IL-2/IL-2 receptor interactions.

Immunostimulation with IL-2 has received considerable attention in the treatment of malignancy.[91] One form of adoptive therapy has focused on the isolation of potentially reactive lymphocytes infiltrating solid tumors, expanding these cells *in vitro* with IL-2, and reinfusing the cells into the patient. Preliminary but encouraging results in human patients have suggested that these T cells can localize to tumor sites and mediate a significant therapeutic effect. Similar studies are underway using NK cells that have been activated *in vitro* with IL-2 and administered back into the patient. Finally, the use of lymphocyte-activated killer (LAK) cells has shown promise in patients with melanoma and renal cell carcinoma. Although much work remains to be done in perfecting this approach to tumor management, studies such as these have created a new enthusiasm for effective treatments against tumor development.

Currently, immunosuppressive therapies are targeted to down-regulate IL-2 production or block the receptor (Table 4). Modalities, such as cyclosporine and FK 506, inhibit IL-2 gene transcription. On the other hand, rapamycin does not affect IL-2 synthesis but does inhibit IL-2/IL-2 receptor-mediated cell proliferation. These drugs have gained wide acceptance in both transplantation and autoimmune diseases.[92] The presence of IL-2 alpha receptor (IL-2Rα) on T cells is noted in certain lymphoid malignancies, autoimmune diseases, and allograft rejection. Recently, numerous therapeutic strategies have focused on preventing the interaction of IL-2 with its receptor. One approach is to block this cytokine-receptor interaction with anti-IL-2R antibody. This technology has expanded and incorporated murine monoclonal antibody against IL-2 receptor; humanized antibodies to IL-2R, and monoclonal antibodies armed with toxins and radionuclides.[88,93,94] The use of humanized antibodies is an attempt to limit the production of antibodies by the patient which neutralize the therapeutic effects of the treatment antibody. Humanized antibodies are combination antibodies consisting of a rodent molecule containing the complementarity-determining regions and a human antibody containing the constant and framework regions. Use of these antibodies holds great hope for the future.

D. Hematopoietic Growth Factors for Transplantation

The administration of hematopoietic growth factors to enhance differentiation and proliferation of hematopoietic stem cells is a rapidly expanding area of treatment in infectious diseases, immunodeficiencies and transplantation.[95,96] *Ex vivo* and *in vivo* administration of cytokines, growth factors, and combinations of these cytokines are finding increased applications in a number of clinical situations. Furthermore, gene therapy, in conjunction with these approaches, promises to provide new avenues of management.[97-99] Hematopoietic growth factors, identified in Table 2, are presently used as differentiating and proliferating factors for bone marrow transplantation. The clinical laboratory will be asked increasingly to monitor these cytokines and the cytokines produced by their *ex vivo* stimulation of bone marrow and peripheral blood cells.

E. Cytokines as Vaccine Adjuvants

The exciting advances introduced by molecular biology and peptide chemistry have revolutionized vaccine research. However, recombinant proteins and synthetic peptides are often weak immunogens that require the addition of adjuvants to potentiate immune reactivity. This need has led to the identification of a variety of potent vaccine adjuvants which can enhance vaccine effectiveness. Some of the new adjuvants include immune stimulating compounds (ISCOMS), muramyl peptides, lipid A derivatives, and liposomes.[100,101] In addition to selecting adjuvants that induce a broad range of cytokines, cytokines themselves are now being used as the adjuvant in a vaccine formulation.[102-105] Several cytokines have been shown to be effective adjuvants in a number of model systems, enhancing protection induced by viral, bacterial, and parasitic vaccines as well as stimulating immunity in tumor models and in clinical trials.

IFN-γ and IL-2, in particular, show promise as effective adjuvants. IFN-γ, for instance, increases class II expression on antigen-presenting cells, augments antibody production, and up-regulates T-cell activity, all properties that would enhance immune reactivity. In animal parasitic or viral vaccine models, IFN-γ has demonstrated significant adjuvanticity. For example, in animals receiving leishmania vaccine preparations containing IFN-γ, both enhanced amnestic responses as well as protection against challenge infection were achieved. IL-2, like IFN-γ, has also been studied extensively as an immune potentiator. Several reports have documented enhanced protection against virus infections, such as rabies virus and herpes simplex virus, when IL-2 was formulated with the viral antigen.[102,103] More recently, the incorporation of cytokine adjuvants into liposomes has been described as a novel and effective delivery system. This slow release system is particularly useful for optimal cytokine stimulation of immunity. IL-2 appears well suited to this vaccine system and has been studied most extensively.[102,104] For example, protection against influenza A was significantly enhanced by administering the vaccine mixed with IL-2 containing liposomes. [104]

Innovative strategies are also being applied to optimize the benefits of cytokine adjuvants. One such aim involves balancing the pleiotropic effects of the cytokines. IL-1, for instance, has been shown to possess potent adjuvant activity. However, IL-1 has numerous side effects associated with its proinflammatory action, and this limits its use as an adjuvant. Recently, a small fragment of IL-1β, peptide 163-171, which is devoid of all proinflammatory activity, but not immunostimulating activity, has been examined in a number of experimental tumor systems.[106,107] Data from these studies indicate that although the peptide induces impressive levels of antitumor immunity, large amounts of this less toxic derivative are required to achieve comparable immune stimulation noted in the natural molecule. This approach is currently being fine-tuned and applied to other cytokines. Such an approach is aimed at enhancing the desired specific immune effect of the cytokine, while minimizing its nonspecific, deleterious effects.

As our understanding of cytokine biology increases and recombinant cytokine technology expands, the opportunity to systematically design vaccines with cytokine adjuvants that direct the immune response in a desired way becomes a reasonable goal. Table 4 identifies some of the more commonly studied cytokine adjuvants. A thorough review of cytokine adjuvants may be found in Ho et al. [102]

IV. OVERVIEW OF CYTOKINE ASSAYS

A. Methods

There are three basic methods available to evaluate cytokines: immunoassays, bioassays, and molecular assays (Table 6). The bioassay is the most sensitive assay. In addition, the bioassay is the only approach that provides information about the bioactivity of the molecule. However, this approach is frequently difficult to perform and is time-consuming and less specific than the immunoassays. For these reasons, the immunoassays are most often used in the clinical laboratory setting to measure cytokine levels.

The immunoassays include the ELISA or the enzyme immunoassay (EIA). These tests can frequently be performed with a commercially available kit consisting of a primary monoclonal antibody which captures the cytokine, a biotinylated monoclonal antibody which detects

TABLE 6

Monitoring Cytokines in the Clinical Immunology Laboratory

Approach	Source	Assay	Interpretation
Cytokine production (*in vitro*)	Peripheral mononuclear cells	Bioassay or immunoassay	Assess immunocompetence
Presence of cytokine	Serum, plasma, vitreous, synovial fluid, CSF	Bioassay or immunoassay	Monitor alterations in infections, malignancy, transplantation, immunodeficiencies and autoimmune disorders; monitor cytokine pharmacokinetics and cytokine therapy
	Tissue	Immunocytochemical assays	
Presence of cytokine mRNA	Tissue	Northern blot, PCR, *in situ* hybridization	Monitor alterations in infections, malignancy, transplantation, immunodeficiencies and immunologically related disorders

the primary reaction, and a color reaction system such as streptavidin–enzyme–enzymatic substrate complex, which provides the detection system. These assays offer several distinct advantages, such as specificity, rapid turnaround time, and ease of performance. However, they are not as sensitive as the bioassay, and these techniques do not distinguish between active and inactive cytokine fragments.

In addition to measuring cytokines in body fluids, cytokines can also be localized in tissues. Immunocytochemical staining is used to identify cytokine proteins in tissue samples.[108] Recently, an innovative approach for detecting minute amounts of cytokine proteins has been developed.[109] Phillips and associates have implemented capillary zone electrophoresis for the detection and measurement of tissue bound cytokines in frozen biopsy specimens.[109]

The bioassays can be grouped into four general types of assays. These assays are listed in Table 7 and include: proliferation, cytotoxicity or cytostasis, differentiation, and antiviral assays. Proliferation assays are characterized by the ability of a cytokine to induce the growth of susceptible target cells. The cytokines most often identified by these assays include IL-1, IL-2, IL-4, IL-5, IL-6, and IL-7. The second category of bioassays consists of cytotoxicity or cytostasis assays. These assays are characterized by the ability of the cytokine to kill or inhibit the growth of susceptible target cells. TNF-α and TNF-β killing of L929

TABLE 7

Bioassays Used to Monitor Cytokine Activity

Assay	Definition	Cytokine Example
Proliferation	Growth of susceptible target cells	IL-1, IL-2, IL-3, IL-4, IL-5, IL-6, IL-7, IL-8, IL-9, IL-10, IL-11
Cytotoxicity	Death or inhibition of growth of susceptible target cells	TNF (L929 cell killing) IL-1 (cytostasis of A375 melanoma)
Differentiation	Induce differentiation of susceptible target cells	CSF, IL-3, stem cell factor (growth on soft agar) IFN-γ (MHC class II expression, increased macrophage phagocytosis) IL-6 (Immunoglobulin secretion by hybridoma cells) IL-8 (chemotactic activity)
Antiviral activity	Induce antiviral state in susceptible target cells (not toxic to cellular function)	IFN-α, IFN-β, IFN-γ

cells and IL-1 induction of cytostasis of A375 melanoma cells are examples of this assay system. Differentiation assays constitute the third group of bioassays. These assays are characterized by the ability of a cytokine to induce differentiation of a target cell. The most popular mediators examined by this technique include: colony stimulating factors (IL-3, CSFs, and stem cell factor) which support the growth of human bone marrow cells on soft agar; IL-6 which induces immunoglobulin secretion by hybridoma cells; IFN-γ which induces MHC class II antigen expression on a variety of cells and enhances macrophage phagocytosis; and IL-8, a chemokine, which enhances neutrophil chemotaxis. The fourth category of bioassays consists of antiviral assays. These assays are characterized by the development of an antiviral state within the cell. IFN-α, IFN-β, and IFN-γ can all be identified with these assays. In this assay, one unit of biological activity is the reciprocal of the highest dilution of sample which inhibits virus replication by 50%. The exact type of IFN present within the sample may be identified by neutralization; i.e., inhibition of antiviral actions with specific monoclonal antibody directed against IFN-α, IFN-β, and IFN-γ.

Molecular techniques, which measure cytokine gene expression, are also used to evaluate cytokines.[110,111] This approach is most frequently employed in a research setting. Analysis of cytokine gene expression basically involves the determination of cytokine mRNA. However, certain general considerations should be noted. The cytokine genes are usually not constitutively expressed. As we have already noted, the transcription of these genes is regulated by the presence of inducer molecules. A second consideration is the fact that cytokine mRNA production is usually transient. Since these mRNAs are present for only a short time period, their detection may be missed. Finally, RNA is rapidly degraded and appropriate isolation precautions are required to retard RNA degradation.

Presently, there are at least three general ways to measure cytokine mRNA. Northern blotting is the simplest method. However, it may not detect cytokine mRNA, due to the low level of cytokine gene expression. Alternatively, the polymerase chain reaction (PCR) is a more sensitive way to detect gene expression. The PCR assay allows for the detection of minute amounts of mRNA, but does not provide the cellular localization. Finally, *in situ* hybridization may be used to identify cytokine mRNA. In this assay, antisense RNA or cDNA probes are used to localize the cellular sites of cytokine gene expression. In summary, Northern blotting allows for the identification of cytokine mRNA if sufficient quantities are present, PCR assays allow for the identification of minute amounts of cytokine mRNA, and *in situ* hybridization assays allow for the tissue and cellular localization of cytokine gene expression.

An overview of the approaches used to monitor cytokines in the clinical immunology laboratory is provided in Table 6. As noted, measuring the presence of the cytokine or its gene expression is helpful in a number of situations, such as monitoring alterations in a variety of disorders and assessing cytokine pharmacokinetics and therapy. However, it is also useful to measure the ability of cells to produce the cytokine. Cytokine production *in vitro* has been shown to be a reliable index of immune status. It can be achieved by incubating peripheral blood mononuclear cells with mitogens, such as conconavalin A, phytohemagglutinin, or LPS, and assaying the secreted cytokine by either the immunoassay or the bioassay. The cytokines most often evaluated with this approach are IFN-γ and IL-2. Their presence is indicative of functional T-cell activation, and suggests that cells may be effective in antigen presentation and lymphocyte proliferation. This information provides a reliable assessment of immune competence.

B. Interpretation and Pitfalls

The advantages and disadvantages of the bioassays and the immunoassays are outlined in Table 8. Most clinical laboratories monitor cytokines with immunoassays. As mentioned above, the availability of commercial kits, the speed of the assay, and its specificity certainly justify rapid screening by these methods. However, it is important that the bioassay be used to spot check the immunoassay to determine the biological function and potency of the cytokines.

TABLE 8

Cytokine Monitoring Assays: Advantages and Disadvantages

Assay	Advantages	Disadvantages
Bioassay	Identifies function and potency Very sensitive (1 pg/ml)	Lengthy (days to weeks) Requires viable cells Multiple cytokines may share same bioactivity Need careful controls (neutralize activity with specific anticytokine antibody) Numerous inhibitors may be present in body fluids
Immunoassay	Easy to perform (kits available) Sensitive (10–50 pg/ml) Timely (few hours) Small sample size (<0.1 ml) Specificity Reproducibility Not affected by other cytokines and inhibitors of bioassays	May be biologically inactive yet maintain immunoreactive epitope Less sensitive than bioassay

There are a number of pitfalls or potential problems that could affect the interpretation of data obtained from cytokine monitoring. Table 9 identifies some of these difficulties. These factors are separated into three components: short cytokine half lives, inhibitory factors in the sera or body fluids, and serum components that interfere with bioassays.

Critical elements for the clinical immunology laboratory are quality assurance and quality control (Table 10). This is especially true for the measurement of cytokines. The laboratory must correlate its data with data generated with reference reagent standards and laboratory standards. Furthermore, the laboratory should establish its own normal ranges. Reference reagent standards should be used to calibrate bioassays and ELISA assays so that the laboratory can report data in biological units or pg/ml in reference to the international standards. The World Health Organization (WHO) has helped to coordinate programs to provide these reference reagent standards. These standards can be obtained from the National Institute for Biological Standards and Control (NIBSC) in Great Britain or from the Biological Response Modifiers Program (BRMP), National Cancer Institute, NIH, Bethesda, MD. Laboratory standards should also be developed by the laboratory. These laboratory standards can be used to assess inter-assay and intra-assay variability. Finally, each laboratory should establish a normal range for

TABLE 9

Pitfalls Which May Influence the Interpretation of Cytokine Assays

Factors	Examples
Cytokine half-lives	Short half-lives in the circulation (due to distribution to tissues, binding to cell receptors, spontaneous degradations, aggregation, etc.)
Inhibitory factors	Serum proteins bind to cytokines (α-macroglobulin, in sera albumin)
	Soluble cytokine receptors
	Autoantibodies to cytokines
	Autoantibodies to cytokine receptors
	Protease activity
	Drugs
Serum components that interfere with bioassays	Steroids, other hormones, prostaglandins
	Presence of other cytokines
	Receptor antagonist

TABLE 10

Quality Assurance and Quality Control of Cytokine Assays

Reference reagent standard	Calibrate the bioassays and ELISA assay determinations with an international standard; use to report units and/or pg/ml
	Obtain from WHO (National Institute for Biological Standards, Great Britain or Biological Response Modifier Program, NCI, NIH, Bethesda, MD)
Laboratory standard	Develop own standards in the laboratory; used to monitor interassay and intraassay variability
Normal ranges	Each laboratory should establish normal ranges for the detection of cytokines in body fluids and for the production of cytokines *in vitro*

the presence of cytokines in body fluids and for the production of cytokines *in vitro*.

V. CONCLUSIONS AND FUTURE DIRECTIONS

Dramatic advances in our knowledge of cytokine biology have progressed steadily during the past two decades. These advances have paralleled the development of an appreciation of the intricacies of maintaining homeostasis and the therapeutic potential of cytokines and cytokine receptors in modifying pathogenic processes. Because of their importance, it is critical to have accurate laboratory tools to identify and monitor cytokines. This review has focused on cytokine assays, their interpretation, and pitfalls.

Initially, cytokines were identified in selected disease states. Assessment of cytokine levels has revealed important parameters in the pathogenic processes and has given impetus to many of the newer clinical strategies. These data have provided a rationale for the direct administration of cytokines to alter disease progression in a variety of conditions such as infections, malignancy, and transplantation. More recent efforts have focused on the therapeutic utility of cytokine receptor antagonists and anticytokine monoclonal antibodies to down-regulate pathogenic responses to cytokine production. Future therapeutic applications of cytokines and cytokine antagonists will advance us toward the goal of manipulating these molecules to optimize their beneficial effects, while mitigating their deleterious effects.

REFERENCES

1. Gallin, J. I., Goldstein, I. M., and Snyderman, R., *Inflammation: Basic Principles and Clinical Correlates*, 2nd ed., Raven Press, New York, 1992.
2. Oppenheim, J. J., Rossio, J. L., and Gearing, A. J. H., *Clinical Applications of Cytokines: Role in Pathogenesis, Diagnosis and Therapy*, Oxford University Press, New York, 1993.
3. Shull M. M., Ormsby, I., Kier, A. B., Pawlowski, S., Diebold, R. J., Yin, M., Allen, R., Sidman, C., Proetzel, G., Calvin D., Annunziata, N., and Doetschman, T., Targeted disruption of the mouse transforming growth factor-β1 gene results in multifocal inflammatory disease, *Nature*, 359, 693, 1992.
4. Sporn, M. B. and Roberts, A. B., *Peptide Growth Factors and Their Receptors I*, Springer-Verlag, New York, 1991.
5. Sadowski, H. B., Shuai, K., Darnell, J. E., and Gilman, M. Z., A common nuclear signal transduction pathway activated by growth factor and cytokine receptors, *Science*, 261, 1739, 1993.
6. Paul, W. E. and Seder, R. A., Lymphocyte responses and cytokines, *Cell*, 76, 241, 1994.
7. Hooks, J. J. and Detrick, B., Evaluation of the interferon system, in *Manual of Clinical Laboratory Immunology*, 4th ed., Rose, N. R., DeMacario, E. V., Fahey, J. L., Friedman, H., and Penn, G. M., Eds., American Society for Microbiology Publications, Washington, D.C., 1992, 240.
8. Baron, S., Tyring, S. K., Fleischmann, W. R., Coppenhaver, D. H., Niesel, D. W., Klimpel, G. R., Stanton, J., and Hughes, T. K., The interferons: mechanisms of action and clinical applications, *JAMA*, 266, 1375, 1991.
9. Borden, E. C., Interferons: pleiotropic cellular modulators, *Clin. Immunol. and Immunopathol.*, 62, S18, 1992.
10. Nathan, C., Interferon and inflammation, in *Inflammation: Basic Principles and Clinical Correlates*, 2nd ed., Gallin, J. I., Goldstein, I. M., and Snyderman, R., Eds., Raven Press, New York, 1992, 265.

11. Cerami, A., Inflammatory cytokines, *Clin. Immunol. Immunopathol.*, 62, S3, 1992.

12. Carswell, E. A., Old, L. J., Kassel, R. L., Green, S., Fiore, N. and Williamson, B., An endotoxin-induced serum factor that causes necrosis of tumors, *Proc. Natl. Acad. Sci. U.S.A.*, 72, 3666, 1975.

13. Williams, T. W. and Granger, G. A., Lymphocyte *in vitro* cytotoxicity: lymphotoxins of several mammalian species, *Nature*, 219, 1076, 1968.

14. Ruddle, N. H. and Waksman, B. H., Cytotocity mediated by soluble antigen and lymphocytes in delayed hypersensitivity. III. Analysis of mechanism, *J. Exp. Med.*, 128, 1267, 1968.

15. Dinarello, C. A., Interleukin-1 and interleukin-1 antagonism, *Blood*, 77, 1627, 1991.

16. Oppenheim, J. J., Kovacs, E. J., Matsushima, K., and Durum, S. K., There is more than one interleukin 1, *Immunol. Today*, 7, 45, 1986.

17. Herrmann, F., Oster, W., Meuer, S. C., Lindemann, A. and Mertelsmann, R. H., Interleukin 1 stimulates T lymphocytes to produce granulocyte-monocyte colony-stimulating factor, *J. Clin. Invest.*, 81, 1415, 1988.

18. Eastgate, J. A., Wood, N. C., Digiovine, F. S., Symons, J. A., Grinlinton, F. M., and Duff, G. W., Correlation of plasma interleukin 1 levels with disease activity in rheumatoid arthritis, *Lancet*, 2, 706, 1988.

19. Morgan, D. A., Ruscetti, F. W., and Gallo, R., Selective *in vitro* growth of T lymphocytes from normal human bone marrow, *Science*, 193, 1007, 1976.

20. Mier, J. W. and Gallo, R. C., Purification and some characteristics of human T-cell growth factor from phytohemagglutinin-stimulated lymphocyte-conditioned media, *Proc. Natl. Acad. Sci. U.S.A.*, 77, 6134, 1980.

21. Poiesz, B. J., Ruscetti, F. W., Gazdar, A. F., Bunn, P. A., Minna, J. D., and Gallo, R. C., Detection and isolation of type C retrovirus particles from fresh and cultured lymphocytes of a patient with cutaneous T-cell lymphoma, *Proc. Natl. Acad. Sci. U.S.A.*, 77, 7415, 1980.

22. Greene, W. C., The interleukins, in *Inflammation: Basic Principles and Clinical Correlates*, 2nd ed., Gallin, J.I., Goldstein, I. M., and Snyderman, R., Eds., Raven Press, New York, 1992, 233.

23. Waldmann, T. A., The interleukin-2 receptor, *J. Biol. Chem.*, 266, 2681, 1991.

24. Noguchi, M., Nakamura, Y., Russell, S.M., Ziegler, S.F., Tsang, M., Cao, X., and Leonard, W.J., Interleukin-2 receptor γ chain: a functional component of the interleukin-7 receptor, *Science*, 262, 1877, 1993.

25. Russel, S.M., Keegan, A.D., Harada, N., Nakamura, Y., Noguchi, M., Leland, P., Friedmann, M.C., Miyajima, A., Puri, R.K., Paul, W.E., Leonard, W.J., Interleukin-2 receptor γ chain: a functional component of the interleukin-4 receptor, *Science*, 262, 1880, 1993.

26. Isakson, P. C., Pure, E., Vitetta, E. S., and Krammer, P. H., T cell-derived B cell differentiation factor(s): effect on isotype switch of murine B cells, *J. Exp. Med.*, 155, 734, 1982.

27. Howard, M., Farrar, J., Hilfiker, M., Johnson, B., Takatsu, K., Hamaoka, T. and Paul, W. E., Identification of a T cell-derived B-cell growth factor distinct from interleukin 2, *J. Exp. Med.*, 155, 914, 1982.

28. Mosmann, T. R. and Coffman, R. L., Two types of mouse helper T-cell clone: Implications for immune regulation, *Immunol. Today*, 8, 223, 1987.

29. Yakota, T., Arai, N., Arai, K. -I., Zlotnik, A., Interleukin-4, in *Peptide Growth Factors and Their Receptors I*, Sporn, M. B. and Roberts, A. B., Eds., Springer-Verlag, New York, 1991, 577.

30. Hirano, T., Yasukawa, K., Harada, H., Taga, T., Watanabe, Y., Matsuda, T., Kashiwamura, S., Nakajima, K., Koyama, K., Iwamatsu, A., Tsunasawa, S., Sakiyama, F., Matsui, H., Takahara, Y., Taniguchi, T., and Kishimoto, T., Complementary DNA for a novel human interleukin (BSF-2) that induces B lymphocytes to produce immunoglobulin, *Nature*, 324, 73, 1986.

31. Schrezenmeier, H., Thome, S.D., Tewald, F., Fleischer, B. and Raghavachar, R., Interleukin-5 is the predominant eosinophilopoietin produced by cloned T lymphocytes in hypereosinophilic syndrome, *Exp. Hematol.*, 21, 358, 1993.

32. Hirano, T., Akira, S., Taga, T., and Kishimoto, T., Biological and clinical aspects of interleukin 6, *Immunol. Today*, 11, 443, 1990.

33. Nagineni, C. N., Detrick, B., and Hooks, J. J., Synergistic effects of gamma interferon on inflammatory mediators that induce interleukin-6 gene expression and secretion by human retinal pigment epithelial cells, *Clin. Diag. Lab. Immunol.*, 1, 569, 1994.

34. Gauldie, J., Richards, C., Harnish, D., Lansdorp, P., and Baumann, H., Interferon β2/B-cell stimulatory factor type 2 shares identity with monocyte-derived hepatocyte-stimulating factor and regulates the major acute phase protein response in liver cells, *Proc. Natl. Acad. Sci. U.S.A.*, 84, 7251, 1987.

35. Goodwin, R. G., Lupton, S., Schmierer, A., Hjerrild, K. J., Jerzy, R., Clevenger, W., Gillis, S., Cosman, D., and Namen, A. E., Human interleukin 7: molecular cloning and growth factor activity on human and murine B-lineage cells, *Proc. Natl. Acad. Sci. U.S.A.*, 86, 302, 1989.

36. Namen, A. E., Lupton, S., Hjerrild, K., Wignall, J., Mochizuki, D. Y., Schmierer, A., Mosley, B., March, C. J., Urdal, D., Gillis, Cosman, D., and Goodwin, R. G., Stimulation of B-cell progenitors by cloned murine interleukin-7, *Nature (London)*, 333, 571, 1988.

37. Oppenheim J. J., Sachariae, C. O. C., Mukaida, N., and Matsushima, K., Properties of the novel proinflammatory supergene "intercrine" cytokine family, *Annu. Rev. Immunol.*, 9, 617, 1991.

38. Uyttenhove, C., Simpson, R. J., and Van Snick, J., Functional and structural characterization of P40, a mouse glycoprotein with T-cell growth factor activity, *Proc. Natl. Acad. Sci. U.S.A.*, 85, 6934, 1988.

39. Fiorentino, D. F., Bond, M. W., and Mosmann, T. R., Two types of mouse T helper cell: IV Th2 clones secrete a factor that inhibits cytokine production by Th1 clones, *J. Exp. Med.*, 170, 2081, 1989.

40. Suda, T., O'Garra, A., MacNiel, I., Fischer, M., Bond, M. W., and Zlotnik, A., Identification of a novel thymocyte growth-promoting factor derived from B cell lymphomas, *Cell. Immunol.*, 129, 228, 1990.

41. Chomarat, D., Rissoan, M. C., Banchereau, J., and Miossec, P., Interferon γ inhibits interleukin 10 production by monocytes, *J. Exp. Med.*, 177, 523, 1993.

42. Howard, M., O'Garra, A., Biological properties of interleukin 10, *Immunol. Today*, 13, 198, 1992.

43. Paul, S. R., Bennett, F., Calvettik J. A., Kelleher, K., Wood, C. R., O'Hara, R. M., Jr., Leary, A. C., Sibley, B., Clark, S. C., Williams, D. A., and Yang, Y. C., Molecular cloning of a cDNA encoding interleukin 11, a stromal cell-derived lymphopoietic and hematopoietic cytokine, *Proc. Natl. Acad. Sci. U.S.A.*, 87, 7512, 1990.

44. Kobayashi, M., Fitz, L., Ryan, M., Hewick, R. M., Clark, S. C., Chan, S., Loudon, R., Sherman, F., Perussia, B., and Trinchieri, B., Identification and purification of natural killer cell stimulatory factor (NKSF), a cytokine with multiple biological effects on human lymphocytes, *J. Exp. Med.*, 170, 827, 1989.

45. Brunda, M.J., Interleukin-12, *J. Leukocyte Biol.*, 55, 280, 1994.

46. D'Andrea, A., Rengaraju, M., Valiante, N. M., Chehimi, J., Kubin, M., Aste, M., Chan, S. H., Kobayashi, M., Young, D., Nickbarg, E., Chizzonite, R., Wolf, S. F., and Trinchieri, G., Production of natural killer cell stimulatory factor (interleukin 12) by peripheral blood mononuclear cells, *J. Exp. Med.*, 176, 1387, 1992.

47. D'Andrea, A., Aste-Amezaga, M., Valiante, N. M., Ma, X., Kubin, M., and Trinchieri, G., Interleukin 10 (IL-10) inhibits human lymphocyte interferon γ-production by suppressing natural killer cell stimulatory factor/IL-12 synthesis in accessory cells, *J. Exp. Med.*, 178, 1041, 1993.

48. Sypek, J. P., Chung, C. L., Mayor, S. E. H., Subramanyam, J. M., Goldman, S. J., Sieburth, D. S., Wolf, S. F., and Schaub, R. G., Resolution of cutaneous leishmaniasis: interleukin 12 initiates a protective T helper immune response, *J. Exp. Med.*, 177, 1797, 1993.

49. Zurawski, G. and deVries, J. E., Interleukin 13, an interleukin 4-like cytokine that acts on monocytes and B cells, but not on T cells, *Immunol. Today*, 15, 19, 1994.

50. Muxio, M., Re, F., Sironi, M., Polentarutti, N., Minty, A., Caput, D., Ferrara, D., Mantovani, A., and Colotta, F., Interleukin-13 induces the production of interleukin-1 receptor antagonist (IL-1ra) and the expression of the mRNA for the intracellular (keratinocyte) form of IL-1ra in human myelomonocytic cells, *Blood*, 83, 1738, 1994.

51. Golde, D. W. and Baldwin, G. C., Myeloid growth factors, in *Inflammation: Basic Principles and Clinical Correlates*, 2nd ed., Gallin, J. I., Goldstein, I. M., and Snyderman, R., Eds., Raven Press, New York, 1992, 291.

52. Cerny, J., Stimulation of bone marrow haemopoietic stem cells by a factor from activated T cells, *Nature*, 249, 63, 1974.

53. Ihle, J. N., Interleukin-3, in *Peptide Growth Factors and Their Receptors I*, Sporn, M. B. and Roberts, A. B., Eds., Springer-Verlag, New York, 1991, 541.

54. Burgess, A. W., Granulocyte-macrophage colony-stimulating factor, in *Peptide Growth Factors and Their Receptors I*, Sporn, M. B. and Roberts, A. B., Eds., Springer-Verlag, New York, 1991, 723.

55. Moore, M. A . S., The clinical use of colony stimulating factors, *Annu. Rev. Immunol.*, 9, 159, 1991.

56. Naccache, P. H., Faucher, N., Borgeat, P., Gasson, J. C., and DiPersio, J. F., Granulocyte-macrophage colony-stimulating factor modulated the excitation-response coupling sequence in human neutrophils, *J. Immunol.*, 140, 3541, 1988.

57. Silberstein, D. D. and David, J. R., The regulation of human eosinophil function by cytokines, *Immunol. Today*, 8, 380, 1987.

58. Nagata, S., Granulocyte colony-stimulating factor, in *Peptide Growth Factors and Their Receptors I*, Sporn, M. B. and Roberts, A. B., Eds., Springer-Verlag, New York, 1991, 699.

59. Warren, M. K. and Ralph, P., Macrophage growth factor CSF-1 stimulates human monocyte production of interferon, turmor necrosis factor, and colony stimulating activity, *J. Immunol.*, 137, 2281, 1986.

60. Sampson-Johannes, A. and Carlino, J. A., Enhancement of human monocyte turmoricidal activity by recombinant M-CSF, *J. Immunol.*, 141, 3680, 1988.

61. Sherr, C. J. and Stanley, E. R., Colony-stimulating factor 1 (macrophage colony stimulating-factor), in *Peptide Growth Factors and Their Receptors I*, Sporn, M.B. and Roberts, A. B., Eds., Springer-Verlag, New York, 1991, 667.

62. Nocka, Buck, J., Levi, E. and Besmer, P., Candidate ligand for the c-kit transmembrane kinase receptor: LL, a fibroblast derived growth factor stimulates mast cells and erythroid progenitors, *EMBO. J.*, 9, 3287,1990.

63. Williams, D. E., Eisenman, J., Baird, A., Rauch, C., VanNess, K., March, C. J., Park, L. S., Martin, U., Mochizuki, D. Y., Boswell, H. S., Burgess, G. S., Cosman, D., and Lyman, S. D., Identification of a ligand for the c-kit proto-oncogene, *Cell*, 63, 167, 1990.

64. Muench, M. O., Firpo, M. T., and Moore, M. A. S., Bone marrow transplantation with interleukin-1 plus *kit*-ligand *ex vivo* expanded bone marrow accelerates hematopoietic reconstitution in mice without the loss of stem cell lineage and proliferative potential, *Blood*, 81, 3463, 1993.

65. Hooks, J. J., Moutsopoulos, H. M., Geis, S., Stahl, N., Decker, J., and Notkins, A. L., Immune interferon in the circulation of patients with autoimmune diseases, *N. Engl. J. Med.*, 301, 5, 1979.

66. Hooks, J. J., Jordan, G. W., Cupps, T., Moutsopoulos, H. M., Fauci, A. S., and Notkins, A. L., Multiple interferons in the circulation of patients with systemic lupus erythematosus and vasculitis, *Arthritis Rheum.*, 25, 396, 1982.

67. Borden, E. C., Interferons: expanding therapeutic roles, *N. Engl. J. Med.*, 326, 1491, 1992.

68. Ezekowitz, R. A. B., Mulliken, J. B., and Folkman, J., Interferon alfa-2a therapy for life-threatening hemangiomas of infancy, *N. Engl. J. Med.*, 326, 1456, 1992.

69. Smalley, R. V., Andersen, J. W., Hawkins, M. J., Bhide, V., O'Connell, M. J., Oken, M. M., and Borden, E. C., Interferon alfa combined with cytotoxic chemotherapy for patients with non-Hodgkins lymphoma, *N. Engl. J. Med.*, 327, 1336, 1992.

70. Spooner, C. E., Markowitz, N. P., and Saravolatz, L. D., The role of tumor necrosis factor in sepsis, *Clin. Imm. Immunopathol.*, 62, S11, 1992.

71. Dinarello, C. A., Role of interleukin-1 and tumor necrosis factor in systemic responses to infection and inflammation, in *Inflammation: Basic Principles and Clinical Correlates*, 2nd ed., Gallin, J. I., Goldstein, I. M., and Snyderman, R., Eds., Raven Press, New York, 1992, 211.

72. Beutler, B., Cachectin/Tumor Necrosis Factor and Lymphotoxin, in *Peptide Growth Factors and Their Receptors I*, Sporn, M. B. and Roberts, A. B., Eds., Springer-Verlag, New York, 1991, 39.

73. Braegger, C. P., Nicholls, S., Murch, S. H., Stephens, S., and MacDonald, T. T., Tumor necrosis factor alpha in stool as a marker of intestinal inflammation, *Lancet*, 339, 89, 1992.

74. Skillings, J., Wierzbicki, R., Eisenhauer, E., Venner, P., Letendre, F., Stewart, D., and Weinerman, B., A phase II study of recombinant tumor necrosis factor in a renal cell carcinoma: a study of the National Cancer Institute of Canada clinical trials group, *J. Immunother.*, 11, 67, 1992.

75. Opal, S. M., Cross, A. S., Kelley, N. M., Sadoff, J. C., Bodmer, M. W., Palardy, J. E., and Victor, G. H., Efficacy of a monoclonal antibody directed against TNF in protecting neutropenic rats from lethal infection with *P. aeruginosa*, *J. Infect. Dis.*, 161, 1148, 1990.

76. Remick, D. G., Colletti, L. M., Scales, W. A., McCurry, K. R., and Campbell, D. A., Jr., Cytokines and extrahepatic sequelae of ischemia-reperfusion injury to the liver, *Ann. N.Y. Acad. Sci.*, 723, 271, 1994.

77. Exley, A. R., Cohern, J., Buurman, W., Owen, R., Lumley, J., Hanson, G., Aulakh, J. M., Bodner, M., Riddell, A., Stephens, S., and Perry, M., Monoclonal antibody to TNF in severe septic shock, *Lancet*, 335, 1275, 1990.

78. Vincent, J. L., Bakker, J., Marecaux, G., Schandene, L., Kahn, R. J., and Dupont, E., Administration of anti-TNF antibody improves left ventricular function in septic shock patients: results of a pilot study, *Chest*, 101, 810, 1992.

79. Cannon, J., Cytokines, in *Manual of Clinical Laboratory Immunology*, 4th ed., Rose, N. R., DeMacario, E. V., Fahey, J. L., Friedman, H., and Penn, G. M., Eds., American Society for Microbiology Publications, Washington, D.C., 1992, 237.

80. Maury, C. P. J. and Teppo, A. M., Serum immunoreactive interleukin 1 in renal transplant recipients, *Transplantation*, 45, 143, 1988.

81. Tewari, A., Buhles, W. C., Jr., and Starnes, H. F., Jr., Preliminary report: Effects of interleukin-1 on platelet counts, *Lancet*, 336, 712, 1990.

82. Smith, J. II, Urba, W., Steis, R., Janik, J., Fenton, B., Sharfman, W., Conlon, K., Sznol, M., Creekmore, S., Wells, N., Elwood, L., Keller, J., Hestdal, K., Ewel, C., Rossio, J., Kopp, W., Shimuzu, M., Oppenheim, J., and Longo, D., Interleukin-1 alpha: results of a phase I toxicity and immunomodulatory trial, *Proc. Am. Soc. Clin. Oncol.*, 9, 717, 1990.

83. Seckinger, P., Lowenthal, J. W., Williamson, K., Dayer, J. M., and MacDonald, H. R., A urine inhibitor of interleukin-1 activity that blocks ligand binding, *J. Immunol.*, 139, 1546, 1987.

84. Cominelli, F., Nast, C. C., Clark, B. D., Schindler, R., Llerena, R., Eysselein, V. E., Thompson, R. C., and Dinarello, C. A., Interleukin-1 (IL-1) gene expression, synthesis, and effect of specific IL-1 receptor blockade in rabbit immune complex colitis, *J. Clin. Invest.*, 86, 972, 1990.

85. Kushner, I., Regulation of the acute phase response by cytokines, in *Clinical Applications of Cytokines: Role in Pathogenesis, Diagnosis and Therapy,* Oppenheim, J. J., Rossio, J. L., and Gearing, A. J. H., Eds., Oxford University Press, New York, 1993, 27.

86. Waage, A. and Espevik, T., Role of cytokines in bacterial infections, in *Clinical Applications of Cytokines: Role in Pathogenesis, Diagnosis and Therapy,* Oppenheim, J. J., Rossio, J. L., and Gearing, A. J. H., Eds., Oxford University Press, New York, 1993, 43.

87. Rossio, J. L. and Gearing, A. J. H., Measurement of Cytokines, in *Clinical Applications of Cytokines: Role in Pathogenesis, Diagnosis and Therapy,* Oppenheim, J. J., Rossio, J. L., and Gearing, A. J. H., Eds., Oxford University Press, New York, 1993, 16.

88. Waldmann, T. A., The IL-2/IL-2 receptor system: a target for rational immune intervention, *Trends Pharm. Sci.*, 14, 159, 1993.

89. Rosenberg, S.A., Lotze, M. T., Muul, L. M., Leitman, S., Chang, A. E., Ettinghausen, S. E., Matory, Y. L., Skibber, J. M., Shiloni, E., Vetto, J. T., Seipp, C. A., Simpson, C., and Reichert, C. M., Observations on the systemic administration of autologous lymphokine-activated killer cells and recombinant interleukin-2 to patients with metastatic cancer, *N. Engl. J. Med.*, 313, 1485, 1985.

90. Rosenberg, S. A., Packard, B. S., Aebersold, P. M., Solomon, D., Topalian, S. L., Toy, S. T., Simon, P., Lotze, M. T., Yang, J. C., Seipp, C. A., Simpson, C., Carter, C., Bock, S., Schwartzentruber, D., Wei, J., P., and White, D. E., Use of tumor-infiltrating lymphocytes and interleukin-2 in the immunotherapy of patients with metastatic melanoma, *N. Engl. J. Med.*, 319, 1676, 1989.

91. Creekmore, S. P., Reynolds, C. W., Hecht, T. T., Urba, W. J., and Longo, D. L., Interleukin-2 therapy for human cancer, in *Clinical Applications of Cytokines: Role in Pathogenesis, Diagnosis and Therapy,* Oppenheim, J. J., Rossio, J. L., and Gearing, A. J. H., Eds., Oxford University Press, New York, 1993, 147.

92. Schreiber, S. L. and Crabtree, G. R., The mechanism of action of cyclosporin A and FK506, *Immunol. Today,* 13, 136, 1992.

93. Kirkman, R. L., Shapiro, M. E., Carpenter, C. B., McKay, D. B., Milford, E. L., Ramos, E. L., Tilney, N. L., Waldmann, T. A., Zimmerman, C. E., and Strom, T. B., A randomized prospective trial of anti-Tac monoclonal antibody in human renal transplantation, *Transplantation,* 51, 107, 1991.

94. Jones, P. T., Dear, P. H., Foote, J., Newberger, M. S., and Winter, G., Replacing the complementarity-determining regions in a human antibody with those from a mouse, *Nature,* 321, 522, 1986.

95. Roildes, E. and Pizzo, P. A., Biologicals and hematopoietic cytokines in prevention or treatment of infections in immunocompromised hosts, *Hemat. Oncol. Clin. N. Am.*, 7, 841, 1993.

96. Ogawa, M., Differentiation and proliferation of hematopoietic stem cells, *Blood,* 81, 2844, 1993.

97. Broxmeyer, H. E., Role of cytokines in hematopoiesis, in *Clinical Applications of Cytokines: Role in Pathogenesis, Diagnosis and Therapy,* Oppenheim, J. J., Rossio, J. L., and Gearing, A. J. H., Eds., Oxford University Press, New York, 1993, 201.

98. Young, N. S. and Dunbar, C. E., Cytokines for treatment of bone marrow failure syndromes, in *Clinical Applications of Cytokines: Role in Pathogenesis, Diagnosis and Therapy,* Oppenheim, J. J., Rossio, J. L., and Gearing, A. J. H., Eds., Oxford University Press, New York, 1993, 207.

99. Gillio, A. and O'Reilly, R. J., Role of cytokines in bone marrow transplantation, in *Clinical Applications of Cytokines: Role in Pathogenesis, Diagnosis and Therapy*, Oppenheim, J. J., Rossio, J. L., and Gearing, A. J. H., Eds., Oxford University Press, New York, 1993, 217.

100. Alving, C. R., Detrick, B., Richards, R. L., Lewis, M. G., Shafferman, A., and Eddy, G. A., Novel adjuvant strategies for experimental malaria and AIDS vaccines, *Am. N.Y. Acad. Sci.*, 690, 265, 1993.

101. Alving, C. R., Glass, M., and Detrick, B., Summary: adjuvants/clinical trials working group, *AIDS Res. Human Retrovir.*, 8, 1427, 1992.

102. Ho., R. J., Burke, R. L., and Marigan, T. C., Liposome-formulated interleukin-2 as an adjuvant of recombinant HSV glycoprotein gD for treatment of recurrent genital HSV-2 in guinea pigs, *Vaccine*, 10, 209, 1992.

103. Playfair, J. H. and DeSouza, J. B., Recombinant gamma interferon is a potent adjuvant for a malaria vaccine in mice, *Clin. Exp. Immunol.*, 67, 5, 1987.

104. Heath, A. W. and Playfair, J.H. I., Cytokines as immunological adjuvants, *Vaccine*, 7, 427, 1993.

105. Hughes, H. P. A. and Babiuk, L. A., The adjuvant potential of cytokines, *Biotechnol. Today*, 3, 101, 1992.

106. Nencioni, L., Villa, L., Tagliohue, A., and Baraschi, D., Adjuvant activity of the 163-171 peptide of human IL-1β administered through different routes, *Lymphokine Res.*, 6, 335, 1987.

107. Taglialive, A. and Baraschi, D., Cytokines as vaccine adjuvants: IL-1 and its synthetic peptide 163-171, *Vaccine*, 11, 594, 1993.

108. Detrick, B. and Hooks, J. J., Autoimmune aspects of ocular disease, in *The Autoimmune Diseases. II*, Rose, N. R. and MacKay, I., Eds., Academic Press, New York, 1992, 345.

109. Phillips, T. M. and Kimmel, P. L., High-perfomance capillary electrophoresis analysis of inflammatory cytokines in human biopsies, *J. Chromatography*, B.656, 259, 1994.

110. Whiteside, T. L., Cytokines and cytokine measurements in a clinical laboratory, *Clin. Diag. Lab. Immunol.*, 1, 257, 1994.

111. Dallman, M. J., Montgomery, R. A., Larsen, C. P., Wanders, A., and Wells, A. F., Cytokine gene expression: analysis using northern blotting, polymerase chain reaction and *in situ* hybridization, *Immunol. Rev.*, 119, 163, 1991.

Chapter **8**

COMPLEMENT

Robert H. McLean and Thomas R. Welch

CONTENTS

0-8493-0134-3/97/$0.00+$.50
© 1997 by CRC Press LLC

I. THE COMPLEMENT SYSTEMS

The complement (C) systems of man[1,2] include the classical complement pathway (CP), the alternative complement pathway (AP), the terminal complement pathway (TP), and control proteins (Figure 1). There are 20 proteins including six serum control proteins in the C pathways (Table 1). The components of the terminal pathway are common to both the CP and AP. In addition, five control proteins of C activation are present within cell membranes (membrane-bound control proteins) (Table 2). The assessment of the concentration and functional

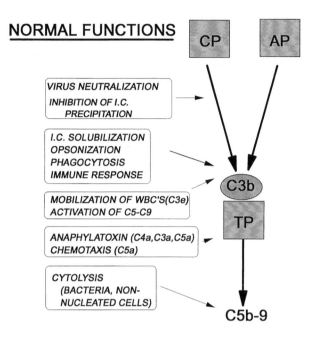

NORMAL FUNCTIONS

VIRUS NEUTRALIZATION
INHIBITION OF I.C.
  PRECIPITATION

I.C. SOLUBILIZATION
OPSONIZATION
PHAGOCYTOSIS
IMMUNE RESPONSE

MOBILIZATION OF WBC'S(C3e)
ACTIVATION OF C5-C9

ANAPHYLATOXIN (C4a,C3a,C5a)
CHEMOTAXIS (C5a)

CYTOLYSIS
  (BACTERIA, NON-
    NUCLEATED CELLS)

CP AP

C3b

TP

C5b-9

Figure 1

The complement pathways and biological functions. C3 is the most abundant C protein in human serum. C3 integrates the alternative C pathway (AP) and classical C pathway (CP) with the terminal C pathway (TP) by serving as the common point of entry into the TP. The TP, also known as the membrane attack complex (MAC), leads to the formation of membrane damage and lysis of target membranes. Susceptible membranes, such as antibody-labeled sheep red cells, provide the basis for the total hemotytic complement assay of the integrity of the entire classical complement pathway (C1–C9). Activation of the alternative complement pathway will not lead to lysis of sheep red cells due to the presence of membrane-bound inhibitor molecules of AP on such red cells. Only certain cells which lack inhibitors of AP, such as rabbit red cells, can be used to measure hemolytic activity of AP. Biologically active fragments of C components, or combinations of C components, mediate important functions (enclosed in boxes).

activity of C proteins are essential in the evaluation of many human diseases. In particular, C assays have diagnostic and therapeutic implications in several common clinical conditions:[3-6]

- In immune complex diseases, such as systemic lupus erythematosus (SLE)[7]

- In many "presumed" immune complex diseases, such as postinfectious glomerulonephritis,[8,9] vasculitis, and idiopathic forms of glomerulonephritis

- In the evaluation of serious and/or recurrent infections[5-7]

- In the diagnosis and monitoring of clinical syndromes due to C control proteins, such as hereditary angioedema (HANE) and paroxysmal nocturnal hemoglobinuria (PNH).

TABLE 1

The Complement Components

	Conc (mg/ml)	Mol wt (kDa)	Primary Function of Active Fragment
Classical pathway			
C1		750	Activates C4
C4	450–750	200	Activates C2
C2	20	102	C2a with C4 forms C3 convertase
C3	1000–1600	190	Opsonin, C5 convertase
Terminal pathway			
C5		191	C5a anaphylatoxin
C6	50–70	104–128	
C7	50–70	92	
C8	55	151	
C9	50–60	71	Cell lysis
Alternative pathway			
Factor B	200	90	AP C3 convertase
Factor D	1	24	AP C3 convertase
Properdin	20	220	Positive regulator of C3bBb
Plasma regulators			
Factor I	35	88	Cleavage of C3b/C34 (with cofactors) — H,C4bp, CR1, MCP
Factor H	480	150	Prevents formation and accelerates decay of C3bBbC3b with factor I
C4-binding protein (C4bp)	250	550	Down-regulates CP C3 convertase
Cl inhibitor	200	110	Inhibits Clr and Cls
Anaphylatoxin inhibitor	35	110	Proteolytic inactivation of anaphylatoxins
S protein	505	83	Binds and inhibits C5b (vitronectin)

Modified from Reference 52. With permission.

A. Evolution of C Pathways

The evolution of the C systems has not been completely defined.[10] C activity is present in modern elasmobranch fishes, whereas invertebrates have no C activity. There is much support for the paradigm that evolution proceeded from the simple to the complex, but Hobart[11] suggested that C6 of the terminal complement pathway may have evolved in the opposite manner.

C3 and components of the alternative pathway are the earliest forms of the C system, antedating the evolution of immune complex mechanism for activation of the CP. The AP persists in primates as a nonantibody-dependent pathway of C3 activation. The terminal complement pathway (C5–C9) first appears in bony fishes.

The evolution of the classical complement pathway may link the protective advantages of the immunoglobulin system with the opsonic

TABLE 2

Membrane-Bound Complement Control Proteins

Component	Mol Wt (kDa)	Ligand	Function
C3/C5 convertase inactivators			
1. Decay-accelerator factor (DAF)(CD55), Cromer blood group	70	C3bBb C4b2a	Dissociates C3/C5 convertases Accelerates decay of C3b, C4b
2. Complement receptor 1 (CR1)(CD35)	190,220	C3bBb	Dissociates C3/C5 convertases With factor I, inactivates C3b
3. Membrane cofactor protein (MCP)(CD46)	48–56 58–68	C3b,(C4b)	With factor I, inactivates C3b
Terminal pathway (MAC) inactivators			
1. P-18, MACIF,HRF-20, MIRL, H19, protectin, (CD59)	18–25	C8,C9	Inhibition of MAC
2. Homologous restriction factor (HRF), C8bp, MIP	65	C8,C9	Inhibition of MAC

Modified from Reference 86. With permission.

TABLE 3

Structural Relationships between Complement and Noncomplement Proteins

Complement Components	Homologous Feature	Examples of Homologous Noncomplement Proteins
C1q	Triple helix	Collagen
Mannan-binding protein		Lung surfactant proteins
C1r, C1s, C2, B, D, I	Protease domain	Serine proteases
C1r, C1s, C2, B, H, C4bp,	60–70 Amino acid unit	Factor XIII
MCP, DAF, CR1, CR2,	(SCR)	β_2-glycoprotein I
C6, C7		IL-2 receptor
		Thyroid peroxidase
		Haptoglobin 2
		Horseshoe crab factor C
		Selectins
C1r, C1s, C6, C7, C8α C8β, C9	Approximately 30-amino acid unit	Epidermal growth factor
C1 Inh	Overall structure	Serpins
C3, C4, C5	Overall structure	α_2-Macrogloblin
		α_1-inhibitor 3
		Pregnancy zone protein
C6, C7, C8α, C8β, C9, P	Approximately 60-amino acid unit	Thrombospondin
C6, C7, C8α, C8β, C9	Membrane-binding domain	Perforin
C6, C7, C8α, C8β, C9, I	30–40 Amino acid unit	LDL receptor
C8γ	Lipocalin structure	α1-Acid glycoprotein
		β-Lactoglobulin
CR3, CR4	α,β Subunits	Integrins
C5α receptor	7 transmembrane helices	G-Protein-linked receptors

Note: SCR: short consensus repeat; MCP: membrane cofactor protein; DAF: decay-accelerating factor; C1INH: C1 inhibitor; B, D, H, and I: complement factors B, D, H, and I, respectively; P: properdin; IL-2: interleukin 2; LDL: low density lipoprotein.
From Farries, T. C. and Atkinson, J. P., *Immunol. Today,* 12, 295, 1991. With permission.

and phagocytic activity of the AP. C1q, a component of the first component of the CP, shares structural similarity to a lectin-like mannan-binding protein, lung surfactant proteins, and conglutinins [12] (Table 3). Each of these molecules shares the capacity to bind to the C1q receptor (C1qR) and may serve to bring Ig and C proteins closer together on the surface of invading microorganisms. The evolution of the other C1 molecules, C1r and C1s esterases, and the appearance of the C3-like protein, C4, may have evolved as links between the immune functions provided by immunoglobulins with the protective functions of C3.

Within the C systems there is sharing of structure and function between C components and with noncomplement proteins (Table 3). One example of this sharing is the existence of three anaphylatoxic fragments C4a, C3a, and C5a (Figure 1). Another instance of shared structure and function includes C3b and C4b which both have opsonic activity and share the complement receptor, CR1. Thus, either the CP or the AP can produce ligands for C3 receptors. Activation of the AP explains, in part, why over one half of patients with congenital absence of C2 suffer no apparent clinical consequences despite the absence of normal CP activity. The complement systems also participate in other amplification systems, such as the coagulation, kinin, and fibrinolytic systems, although the clinical significance of these interactions is presently unclear.

B. The Pathways of Complement Activation

C3 is the most abundant C protein in human serum (Table 1). C3 integrates the alternative C pathway and classical C pathway with the terminal C pathway by serving as the common point of entry into the TP (Figure 1). The TP, also known as the membrane attack complex (MAC), leads to the formation of membrane damage and lysis of target membranes. Susceptible membranes, such as antibody-labeled sheep red cells, provide the basis for an important *in vitro* functional test (the total hemolytic complement assay) of the integrity of the entire classical complement pathway (C1–C9). Activation of the alternative complement pathway will not lead to lysis of sheep red cells due to the presence of membrane-bound inhibitor molecules of AP on such red cells. Only certain cells that lack inhibitors of AP, such as rabbit red cells, can be used to measure hemolytic activity of AP. The clinical importance of the TP in humans is limited to the formation of chemotaxic factor C5a and to protection against certain pathogenic neisserial organisms, although sublytic damage of cells has been suggested to be important in certain diseases.[13]

1. The Classical Complement Pathway (CP)

Activation of the classical pathway commences with the attachment of the **C1q** sub-component of **C1** to C1q receptors on target membranes[1,2] (Figure 2). The binding of C1q produces conformational changes in its substrate, **C1r**, which in turn activates the serine esterase region within **C1s** of the C1 macromolecule. In the presence of calcium, C1r and C1s are each present in C1 in duplication ($C1r_2,C1s_2$) to form a single chain C1 molecule ($C1q,C1r_2,C1s_2$). Human C1q has 18 polypeptide chains at the noncollagenous end. As determined by electron microscopy, these 18 chains form 6 globular heads composed of 3 chains (A,B,C), each attached to one of 6 collagen-like shafts. A group of mammalian lectins bear structural similarities to C1q.[12] Some, such as mannin-binding protein (MBP), can also activate the classical pathway. MBP binds to mannose/N-acetyl D-glucosamine-containing structures of microorganisms. Deficiency of MBP in infants has been associated with increased infections.[12]

C1 inhibitor (C1INH) disassembles C1r,C1s components of C1, leaving the C1q component attached to C1qR. In addition to the activation of subsequent C components, attachment of C1q to its receptor has been reported to promote phagocytosis,[14] antibody-dependent cell-mediated cytotoxicity, cytokine, and immunoglobulin production.

The activated C1 macromolecule cleaves the next component of the CP, **C4,** within the α chain of C4, releasing a 77 residue fragment, **C4a,** and the larger fragment, **C4b.** The resulting conformational changes in C4b expose an internal covalent binding site (a thioester site common to C4,C3, and α-2 macroglobulin), making this binding site accessible to nucleophiles such as water, amino groups (as found on immune complexes), and hydroxyl groups (as found on bacterial cell walls). Several studies have demonstrated relatively greater binding of C4A variants (allotypes) than C4B variants to amino groups,[15] which is consistent with the frequent reports of C4A deficiencies among patients with immune complex disease, such as SLE.[7,16-19]

C2 is the next component in the activation of the CP, and this component is also cleaved by the serine esterase region of $C1r_2,C1s_2$, releasing a small fragment, **C2b,** and a larger fragment, **C2a.** C2 is a single chain molecule which, like factor B of the alternative pathway (see below), is a magnesium-dependent, serine esterase. **C4b,C2a** is known as the **C3 convertase,** since this macromolecule transiently may activate C3 before the convertase is itself inactivated.

Once C2 is activated to form the C3 convertase (C4b2a), C1 is no longer necessary for further CP activation. **C3** is activated by cleavage of the small **C3a** fragment from the α chain of C3. C3a has anaphylatoxin and minor chemotactic activity. A serum inhibitor, **carboxypeptidase B,** is a naturally occurring inhibitor of the C3a,C4a, and C5a anaphylatoxins. Conformational changes of the larger fragment, **C3b,** exposes the thioester region binding site within C3, thereby leading to the formation of the **C5 convertase (C4b,C2a,C3b).** C3b functions as an important opsonin, referring to the ability of C3b to promote phagocytosis (ingestion) of target membranes such as bacteria, yeast, viruses, and immune complexes. C3b participates in stimulating the immune response by a variety of mechanisms and promotes the localization of foreign antigens to lymphoid tissues, stimulates B-cell growth, and participates in stimulating cytokine production.[20] Receptors for degradation products of C3 (C3b, iC3b, C3c, C3d, C3dg) function as mediators of immunological activity (reviewed in Reference 20), participate in the solubilization of immune complexes, primarily through the CP, and mediate the resolubilization of precipitated immune complexes, primarily through activation of the AP.

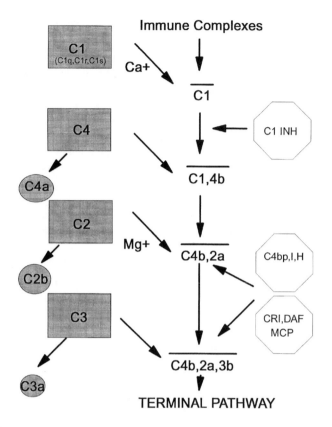

Figure 2

The classical pathway. Activation of the classical pathway components (shaded square symbols) commences with the attachment of the **C1q** subcomponent of **C1** to C1q receptors on target membranes. The binding of C1q produces conformational changes in its substrate, **C1r**, which in turn activates the serine esterase region within **C1s** of the C1 macromolecule.The activated C1 macromolecule cleaves the next component of the CP, **C4**, within the α-chain of C4, releasing a 77-residue fragment, **C4a** (small circles) and the larger fragment, **C4b**. The resulting conformational changes in C4b expose an internal covalent binding site (a thioester site common to C4,C3, and a-2 macroglobulin), making this binding site accessible to nucleophiles. **C2** is the next component in the activation of the CP, and this component is also cleaved by the serine esterase region of $C1r_2,C1s_2$, releasing a small fragment, **C2b**, and a larger fragment, **C2a**. Once C2 is activated to form the **C3 convertase (C4b2a)**, C1 is no longer necessary for further CP activation. **C3** is activated by cleavage of the small **C3a** fragment from the α-chain of C3 and completes the formation of the **C5 convertase (C4b,2a,3b)**. **Factor I** and **factor H** are serum inhibitors (8-sided symbols) of both the classical and alternative pathways. Factor I, in the presence of either factor H or the membrane-bound CR1, removes C3b from the C3 convertase of either the classical or alternative C3 convertase and promotes degradation of C3b. The **C4 binding protein (C4bp)** is a cofactor with factor I in degrading C4b, thereby accelerating the decay of the CP convertase,C4bC2a. **Complement receptor 1 (CR1), decay-accelerator protein (DAF) and membrane co-protein (MCP)** are **membrane-oriented proteins** which function to inhibit the activation and assembly of the C5 convertase (C4b,2a,3b).

2. The Alternative Complement Pathway (AP)

The alternative C pathway was initially recognized with the discovery of properdin by Pillemer et al.[21] and subsequently confirmed by others.[22] In contrast to the CP, the AP is characterized by activation of C3 in the absence of immunoglobulins (Figure 3). Yeast cell walls, particularly zymosan, viruses, and chemicals (inulin) activate C3 through the AP. This activation occurs only in the presence of magnesium, **factor B**, and **factor D** and leads to the cleavage of factor B into **Bb**, the major fragment, and **Ba,** the smaller fragment. Under normal circumstances, hydrolyzed C3 is presumed to exist in plasma in small amounts and causes continuous activation of AP, thereby generating the alternative pathway **C3 convertase, C3bBb**, which then cleaves more C3 by means of a positive feedback mechanism. This amplification of C3 activation produces the macromolecule, **C3bBbC3b**, which functions as the AP **C5 convertase. Properdin** is a normal serum protein of the AP which stabilizes C3bBbC3b by protecting this macromolecule from serum inhibitors. The **C3 nephritic factor (C3nef)** is a circulating antibody which is only found in the serum of patients with certain forms of glomerulonephritis, primarily in membranoproliferative glomerulonephritis[23] and partial lipodystrophy. C3nef, like properdin, protects C3bBbC3b from inhibitors but, unlike properdin, is an autoantibody which is not normally present in serum. Patients with C3nef have low serum concentrations of C3 consequent to abnormally prolonged activity of the AP C3 convertase.

Factor I and **factor H** are serum inhibitors of both the classical and alternative pathways (Figure 3). Factor I, in the presence of either factor H or the membrane-bound CR1, removes C3b from the C3 convertase of either the classical or alternative C3 convertase and promotes degradation of C3b.

The **C4 binding protein (C4bp)** is a cofactor with factor I in degrading C4b, thereby accelerating the decay of the CP convertase,C4bC2a. Both the AP and CP convertases activate the TP, promote phagocytosis, produce cell-mediated cytotoxicity, and stimulate immune functions (Figure 1).

3. The Terminal Complement Pathway (TP)

The **C5 convertases (C4bC2aC3b** and **C3bBbC3b)** cleave C5 into two fragments and initiate activation of the terminal C pathway (Figure 4). Activation of the TP produces hemolytic activity against susceptible cell membranes and produces the most potent chemotactic factor of the C systems, **C5a**. In contrast to the CP and AP, activation of components of the TP (other than C5) are not cleaved, but rather the proteins are altered to form hydrophobic regions. **C6, C7, C8**, and **C9** acquire the ability to assemble within membranes in an orderly fashion

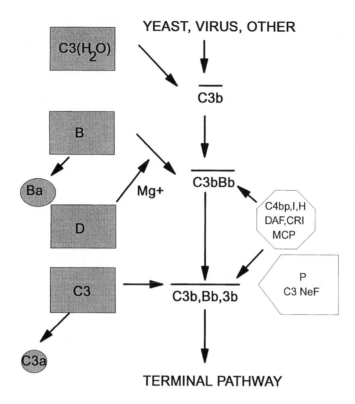

Figure 3
The alternative complement pathway. The AP is characterized by activation of C3 in the absence of immunoglobulins. Yeast cell walls, particularly zymosan, viruses, and chemicals (inulin) activate C3 through the AP. This activation occurs only in the presence of **magnesium, factor B,** and **factor D** and leads to the cleavage of factor B into **Bb,** the major fragment, and **Ba,** the smaller fragment. Under normal circumstances, hydrolyzed C3 is presumed to exist in plasma in small amounts and causes continuous activation of AP, thereby generating **alternative pathway C3 convertase, C3bBb,** which then cleaves more C3 by means of a positive feedback mechanism. This amplification of C3 activation produces the macromolecule, C3bBbC3b, which is the **AP C5 convertase. Properdin** is a normal serum protein of the AP which stabilizes C3bBbC3b by protecting this macromolecule from serum inhibitors. Other **control proteins** (C4bp, factor I, factor H, DAF, CR1, and MCP) function in a similar manner as in the CP (Figure 2).

to form holes within susceptible cell membranes. With the attachment of C9, nonnucleated cells are rapidly lysed by the rapid shift of water to the intracellular space, although some lysis also occurs following the attachment of C8. Nucleated cells are not lysed by C5b–9 because this molecular complex is rapidly internalized, but sublytic damage may occur in certain situations.[13] The components C5b–8 each contribute a single molecule to the macromolecule, whereas C9 is present in the C5b–9 complex as one or more molecules.

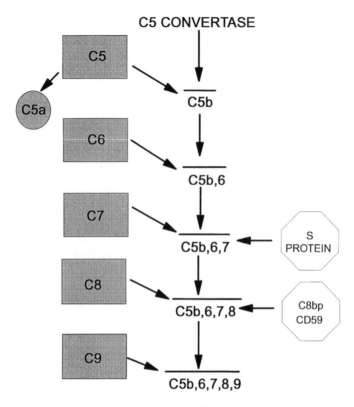

Figure 4
The terminal complement pathway. The **C5 convertases (C4bC2aC3b** and **C3bBbC3b)**
cleave **C5** into two fragments and initiate activation of the terminal C pathway. Activation
of the TP produces **hemolytic activity against susceptible cell membranes** and produces
the most potent **chemotactic factor** of the C systems, **C5a.** In contrast to the CP and AP,
activation of components of the TP (other than C5) are not cleaved, but rather the proteins
are altered to form hydrophobic regions. **C6,C7,C8,** and **C9** acquire the ability to assemble
within membranes in an orderly fashion to form potential holes within susceptible cell
membranes. Control of the TP is mediated by both membrane-oriented factors and by
serum factors. These intrinsic components of the cell membrane include **65 kDa/68 kDa
molecule (C8-binding protein [C8bp],homologous restriction fragment [HRF],MIP)**
and **18 kDa/20 kDa molecule (CD59).** Serum C5b–9 is also inhibited by the abundant
serum protein (**S protein** or **vitronectin**) which binds to C5b–7 complex, preventing
deposition of C5b–9 to target membranes.

Control of the TP is mediated by both membrane-oriented factors
and by serum factors. Two membrane-bound control proteins inhibit
TP activation (Table 2). These intrinsic components of the cell membrane known as **"homologous restriction factors,"** include
**65 kDa/68 kDa molecule (C8 binding protein [C8bp],homologous
restriction fragment [HRF],MIP)** and **18k Da/20 kDa molecule
(CD59).** Serum C5b–9 is also inhibited by the abundant serum protein

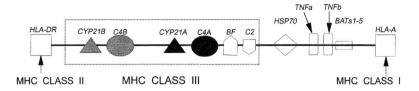

Figure 5
The major histocompatibility complex on chromosome 6. Four genes of the C system, *C4A, C4B, Bf* and *C2*, map to the short arm of chromosome 6 within the major histocompatibility complex. These genes, collectively known as Class III MHC genes, are located downstream of the class II MHC genes (*DR,DQ, DP*) and upstream of the class I MHC genes (*A,B,C*). The class III genes on chromosome 6 span a 120-kb segment approximately 390 kb telomeric to *HLA-DR* and 600 kb centromeric to *HLA-B*. Other genes have been detected between the class III and class I genes.

(**S protein** or **vitronectin**), which binds to C5b–7 complex, preventing deposition of C5b–9 to target membranes (Table 2). Other proteins, including SP40,40/CLI, lipoproteins, proteoglycans, polyanions, and polycations are reported to compete for C5b–7 complex to prevent membrane insertion.

C. Genetics of the Complement Components

1. Structure and Function of Complement Proteins and Genes

Some C components share similar function and structural characteristics (Table 3). C proteins fall into families which may have evolved from common ancestor genes. For example, four genes of the C system, C4A, C4B,Bf, and C2, map to the short arm of chromosome 6 within the major histocompatibility complex (MHC) (reviewed in Reference 26). These genes are collectively known as class III MHC genes (Figure 5).[24] These C genes are located downstream of the class II MHC genes (DR, DQ, DP) and upstream of the class I MHC genes (B and C). C2 and Factor B of the AP share extensive protein sequence homology. Both participate in the formation of macromolecules which activate C3, and both are magnesium-dependent serine esterases. (Figures 2 and 3). Because of the high homology and similar function between the C4A and C4B genes and between the Bf and C2 genes, it is likely that duplication of ancestral genes resulted in these two sets of genes. Two 21-hydroxylase genes, CYP21A (a pseudogene) and CYP21B, are closely linked to the C4 genes and were, presumably, also duplicated along with C4. The MHC genes encode additional proteins involved in the regulation of the immune response but which show no homology in structure to the C genes. Several other genes have been discovered in proximity to the C genes on chromosome 6p. Heat shock protein (HP70), tumor necrosis factors (TNF-α,TNF-β) and several genes of unknown function, the B-associated transcript genes (BATs), have been identified downstream of the class III genes. Preliminary studies have suggested that BATs may be related to immune disease susceptibility (reviewed in Reference 25).

The class III genes on chromosome 6 span a 120-kilobase (kb) segment approximately 390 kb telomeric to HLA-DR and 600 kb centromeric to HLA-B. Specific variants of class III genes have been recognized to segregate more commonly with specific MHC genes.[26] For example, the most common deletion within the C4A gene is invariably found on an HLA haplotype encoding A1,B8,DR3,C4AQ0,B1 allotypes. Such combinations of alleles have been termed "extended haplotypes."[27] The HLA-A1,B8,DR3,C4AQ0,B1 haplotype is significantly associated with several autoimmune diseases such as diabetes, membranoproliferative glomerulonephritis, and systemic lupus erythematosus. The conversion of a C4B gene to a C4A gene (producing an apparent C4B "null" allele) is found commonly on the extended haplotype HLA-B44,DR6 and on the haplotype HLA-B35,DR1,C4A3,2,BQ0.

C2 deficiency is produced by two known genetic mechanisms.[27] One common mechanism which results in a C2 null allele is a 28-base pair (bp) deletion within the C2 gene.[28] C2 deficiency has been estimated to have a prevalence of between 1:10,000 and 1:30,000 and the C2 null allele is strongly linked with the haplotype HLA A25,B18,DR2,BfS,C2Q0,C4A4,B2. This particular 28-bp deletion has been reported to be significantly more common in Caucasian SLE patients (gene frequency of 0.0246) as compared to Caucasian controls (gene frequency 0.0007).[29] In this study, the 28-bp deletion was not detected in 127 African-American SLE patients or in 194 controls.

C1 and C8 are unique among the C components, since the proteins are each encoded by more than one gene. The genes for C1r and C1s are present together on chromosome 12[30] and the serum proteins function as serine proteases as part of the macromolecule, C1. The gene for C1q, which encodes the third molecule that constitutes C1, is located on chromosome 1.[31] C8 has three chains (α, β and γ). The α chain and β chains of C8 are encoded by closely linked genes on chromosome 1,[32] whereas the γ chain is encoded by a gene on chromosome 9 (Table 4).

C5 maps to chromosome 9.[34,35] The C5 protein shares both structure and function with C3 and C4. The genes for C6 and C7, both mapping to chromosome 5,[35] encode proteins that are structurally related and each is activated to participate in the formation of the macromolecule, C5b–9.

On chromosome 1, the group of regulators of complement (RCA) genes encode factor H, C4b-binding protein (C4bp), decay-accelerating factor (DAF), membrane cofactor protein (MCP), and the complement receptors CR1 and CR2 (reviewed in Reference 36). Each of these inhibitors contains varying numbers of the same short consensus repeats

TABLE 4

Polymorphism of Complement Components

	Chromosome Site	No. of Alleles	Alleles
C1q	1p (A and B chains)		
C1r, C1s	12		
C2	6p	9	A-4
			B-4
			C-1
C3	19	31	F,S
			Rare 29
C4	6p	34	C4*A-14
			(Rodgers blood group)
			C4*B-17
			(Chido blood group)
			Others — duplications, hybrids
C5	9	9	
C6	5	21	C6A-1
			C6B-1
			Other-19
C7	5	9	Common-2
			(C7*1,C7*9)
			Rare-7
C8	α and β chains-1		C8A (α-chain)-1
	γ-chain-9q		C8B (β-chain)-1
			Others-5
C9	5		
Factor I	4q25	4	IF*B-I
			IF*A-1
			Rare-2
Factor B	6p	26	BF*F-13
			BF*S-8
			Other-5

From McLean, R. H., *Pediatr. Nephrol.*, 7, 226, 1993. With permission.

(SCR) of 60 to 70 amino acids which indicate the probability of a common ancestor. The SCR are also found on other C components which share the ability of binding to fragments of C3.[36]

2. The Molecular Basis of Complement Polymorphism

Methods have been reported for the determination of C phenotypes. The most common method employs protein electrophoresis combined with specific antibody precipitation or other functionally specific detection systems. Most C proteins have more than one variant (Table 4). Pedigree analysis and techniques of molecular biology have permitted the chromosomal assignment for these C genes.

C4 genes, C4A and C4B (each encoding, respectively, C4A and C4B isotypes or classes), exhibit the most extensive polymorphism of any

C protein.[37] The isotype determinants for C4A and C4B are encoded by 6 base pairs in exon 26 of the C4 genes. Other functional sites within the C4 genes have been determined for the C1 cleavage site,[38,39] the C3b-binding site,[40] the thioester site,[26] and the C5b-binding site.[41-43] At least 14 variants of C4A and 17 variants of C4B have been reported. Rare C4 variants display "mosaic" characteristics in which features of both C4 isotypes can be detected.

The molecular basis of C protein variants, nonfunctional, and "null" variants (undetectable or quantity 0 "Q0" variants) has been described for several variants. Null genes for C4 have been recognized to be surprisingly common.[37,44] Null genes arise from several different mechanisms. The most common cause of a C4 null allele is a large 28-kb deletion on the 5' end of the C4 gene. Another C4A null allele is due to the insertion of thymidine-cytosine.[45] This mutation produces a frameshift and stop codon within this particular allele. A third mechanism producing C4 null alleles is due to the conversion of one isotype to the other, usually C4B to C4A. This mutation results in an "apparently null" allele when phenotyping is assessed by protein electrophoresis. Although two C4 alleles are actually present, they encode only one C4 isotype, leading to the interpretation that the paired C4 isotype gene is absent. Still other C4 null alleles occur from as yet unidentified mutations.

D. Correlations of Complement Abnormalities with Disease

Testing for serum concentrations of C components is an essential step in many clinical situations, but C abnormalities are occasionally discovered incidently in a variety of clinical conditions (Table 5).[5,8,46] In general, abnormally decreased serum concentrations of C components are more useful than elevated levels. Elevated concentrations of C components occur in many conditions, in part, due to the acute phase reaction by C to stress and inflammation. Normal values for C component concentrations at different ages have been reported (Table 6) (summarized in Reference 46).

Hypocomplementemia occurs as a consequence of several pathogenetic mechanisms. Increased consumption of C occurs in immune complex diseases such as SLE and poststreptococcal glomerulonephritis. Hypocomplementemia develops in several conditions due to decreased production or synthesis, as seen in hepatic failure, starvation, or malnutrition, and in conditions of increased loss, as reported in the idiopathic nephrotic syndrome. A rare cause of hypocomplementemia is that due to genetic deficiency or absence of a C component.

TABLE 5

Causes of Hypocomplementemia

Disorders Caused Primarily by Activation and Consumption

Immune complex diseases
Postperfusion, dialysis, and leukapheresis syndromes
Infection
Thermal injury
Adult respiratory distress syndrome
Chronic hypocomplementemic nephritis caused by a C3 nephritic factor
Nephritis with lambda light chain inhibitor of factor H
Acute pancreatitis
Atheroembolic disease
Sickle cell disease
Reaction to radiographic contrast media
C1 inhibitor deficiency with B-cell lymphoproliferative
Disorder of autoantibody to the C1 inhibitor
Hypocomplementemic vasculitis syndrome
Porphyria

Disorders Caused Primarily by Decreased Synthesis

The newborn state
Malnutrition and anorexia nervosa
Liver cirrhosis
Reye's syndrome
Hepatic failure

Disorders Caused Primarily by Increased Catabolism

Increased C1q catabolism associated with hypogammaglobulinemia
Nephrotic syndrome
Disorders caused primarily by deficiency of noncomplement serum or membrane protein
Paroxysmal nocturnal hemoglobinuria
Decreased alternative pathway function associated with hypogammaglobulinemia, beta-thalassemia major, or splenectomy

From Johnston, R. B., *Pediatr. Infect. Dis. J.*, 12, 933, 1993. With permission.

1. Increased Consumption or Activation of Complement

Decreased serum concentrations of C components have been detected in many conditions (Table 5), but in only a relatively small group is hypocomplementemia consistently noted. In these diseases with more consistently detected abnormalities of C component concentrations, the assessment of C concentration constitutes an essential aspect of the clinical management of the patient. Age-related normal values for serum complement levels have been reported [46] (Table 6).

TABLE 6

Normal Serum Concentration of Complement Components by Age

Test	Specimen	Reference Range (mg/dl)	Factor	Reference Range International Units
Classic Pathway Components				
C1q	Serum			
	Cord	1.0–14.9	×10	10–149 mg/l
	1 mo.	2.2–6.2		22–62 mg/l
	6 mo.	1.2–7.6		12–76 mg/l
	Adult	5.1–7.9		51–79 mg/l
C1r	Serum	2.5–3.8	×10	2.5–38 mg/l
C1s (C1 esterase)	Serum	2.5–3.8	×10	25–38 mg/l
C2	Serum			
	Cord	1.6–2.8	×10	16–28 mg/l
	1 mo.	1.9–3.9		19–39 mg/l
	6 mo.	2.4–3.6		24–36 mg/l
	Adult	1.6–4.0		16–40 mg/l
C3				
RID	Serum			
	Cord	65–112	×0.01	0.65–1.12 g/l
	1 mo.	61–130		0.61–1.30 g/l
	Adult	111–171		1.11–1.71 g/l
	Maternal	161–175		1.61–1.75 g/l
Nephelometry	Serum			
	Newborn	58–120	×0.01	0.58–1.20 g/l
C4				
RID	Serum			
	Newborn	16–39	×10	160–390 mg/l
	Adult	15–45		150–450 mg/l
Nephelometry	Serum			
	Newborn	10–26	×10	100–260 mg/l
	Adult	13–37		130–370 mg/l
C5	Serum			
	Cord	3.4–6.2	×10	34–62 mg/l
	1 mo.	2.3–6.3		23–63 mg/l
	6 mo.	2.4–6.4		24–64 mg/l
C6	Serum			
	Cord	1.0–4.2	×10	10–42 mg/l
	1 mo.	2.2–5.2		22–52 mg/l
	6 mo.	3.7–7.1		37–71 mg/l
	Adult	4.0–7.2		40–72 mg/l
C7	Serum	4.9–7.0	×10	49–70 mg/l
C8	Serum	4.3–6.3	×10	43–63 mg/l
C9	Serum	4.7–6.9	×10	47–69 mg/l

TABLE 6 (continued)

Normal Serum Concentration of Complement Components by Age

Test	Specimen	Reference Range (mg/dl)	Factor	Reference Range International Units
Alternative Pathway Components				
C4 binding protein	Serum	18.0–32.0	×10	180–320 mg/l
Factor B				
(C3 proactivator)				
RID	Plasma (EDTA)			
	Cord	7.8–15.8	×10	78–158 mg/l
	1 mo.	6.2–28.6		62–286 mg/l
	6 mo.	16.9–29.3		169–293 mg/l
	Adult	14.7–33.5		147–335 mg/l
Nephelometry	Serum			
	Newborn	14–33	×10	140–330 mg/l
	Adult	20–45		200–450 mg/l
Properdin	Serum			
	Cord	1.3–1.7	×10	13–17 mg/l
	1 mo.	0.6–2.2		6–22 mg/l
	6 mo.	1.3–2.5		13–25 mg/l
	Adult	2.0–3.6		20–38 mg/l
Regulatory Proteins				
β1H-globin	Serum			
(C3b inactivator	Cord	26–42	×10	260–420 mg/l
accelerator)	1 mo.	24–56		240–560 mg/l
	6 mo.	33–61		330–610 mg/l
	Adult	40–72		400–720 mg/l
C1 inhibitor				
(Esterase inhibitor)				
RID	Plasma (EDTA)	17.4–24.0	×10	174–240 mg/l
Complement decay rate (functional)	Serum	<20% decay Deficiency: >50% decay	×0.01	<0.20 (fraction of decay rate) >0.50 (fraction of decay rate)
C3b inactivator (KAF)	Serum			
	Cord	1.8–2.6	×10	18–26 mg/l
	1 mo.	1.5–3.9		15–39 mg/l
	6 mo.	2.3–4.3		23–43 mg/l
	Adult	2.6–5.4		26–54 mg/l
S protein	Serum	41.8–60.0	×10	418–600 mg/l

From Behrman, R. E. and Vaughan, V. C., III, in *Nelson Textbook of Pediatrics,* 13th ed., W. B. Saunders, Philadelphia, 1987, 1540. With permission.

A. Immune Complex Diseases

The abnormally rapid activation of C components which occurs in immune complex (I.C.) diseases results in consumption of classical C components.[14,21,47-50] Normally, immune complexes are eliminated from the blood by the efficient clearing mechanisms by the liver Kupffer cells. Fixation of C3 fragments within immune complex lattices promotes solubilization of immune complexes, thereby serving to direct immune complexes to the C3 receptors in the liver. Effective clearance of immune complexes protects against the phlogistic effects which would occur following local precipitation of immune complexes. Hypocomplementemia occurs as the synthetic capacity of C components is overwhelmed by the consumption of C components. There is also evidence of negative feedback and decreased synthesis of C3 in some patients with immune complex diseases.

In early studies of C in disease, investigators reported depressed serum levels of C3 and decreased titers of total hemolytic complement (CH_{50}) in patients with glomerulonephritis and immune complex disease.[47-50] C assays continue to provide important diagnosis and therapeutic information in these diseases.[49] In the process of studying such selected groups of patients, many heritable deficiencies of C components in humans have been discovered. Some investigators suggested that selection bias may contribute to the increased frequency of immune disorders in C deficient patients. However, there is good evidence for a true predilection to immune disease and/or infections in many congenitally C deficient individuals (see below).

Serum factors which promoted complement activation, in particular the C3 nephritic factor, were first appreciated in patients with membranoproliferative glomerulonephritis (MPGN).[23] Different patterns of C component consumption or "complement profiles" have been reported in hypocomplementemic forms of glomerulonephritis [51] (Table 7).

Patients with MPGN have significantly depressed C3 levels in 77% of cases.[51] West and co-workers have detected characteristic C profiles which are often seen in subgroups of patients with hypocomplementemia (Figure 6).[51] For example, those patients with severely decreased serum C3 levels and type 1 MPGN (subendothelial deposits on renal biopsy) demonstrated activation of the classical C components (low C4) and terminal C pathways (low C6,C7, and C9). Those with intramembranous deposits (dense deposit disease or type II MPGN) had marked depression of only C3. Patients with moderate depression of serum C3 concentration demonstrated less significant activation of components of both the CP or AP. However, it should be noted that the correlation between renal morphology and complement profile is not consistently seen, and C concentrations cannot be used to predict renal morphology.

TABLE 7

Patterns of Complement Abnormalities

	Classical Pathway[a] (C1–C3)	Terminal Pathway[b] (C5–9)
Serum C3 < 30 mg/dl		
1. MPGN I[c]	Low	Low
2. MPGN I, SLE, AGN[c,d] chronic bacteremia	Low	
3. MPGN I, MPGN III[b]		Low
4. MPGN I, MPGN III, AGN		Low C5, P
Serum C3 = 30–86 mg/dl		
1. MPGN I, SLE, chronic bacteremia	Low	
2. MPGN I, MPGN III, AGN		Low C5, P
3. MPGN II		

Note: MPGN I: Type I MPGN refers to the most common form of membranoproliferative glomerulonephritis which demonstrates subendothelial electron deposit on electron microscopy. MPGN II: Type II MPGN is also known as dense deposit disease in which intramembranous deposits are noted on electron microscopy. MPGN III: Type III MPGN refers to the detection of electron dense deposits in the subendothelial areas with disruption of the basement membrane. AGN: acute poststreptococcal glomerulonephritis.

[a] Depression of at least one component.
[b] Depression of C6, C7, and/or C9.
[c] Low early components are uncommon.
[d] Elevated C5b–9 in some patients (Ref. 53).

From Varade, W. S., Forristal, J., and West, C. D., *Am. J. Kidney Dis.,* 16, 196, 1990. With permission.

Decreased serum concentrations of components of the CP and AP are characteristic of patients with SLE and acute poststreptococcal glomerulonephritis (APSGN)[47,52,53] (Table 7, and Figure 6). Activation of the TP in APSGN has also been demonstrated by the detection of decreased C5 and elevated serum levels of the macromolecutar C5b–9.[53] More than 90% of patients with APSGN have decreased serum C3 in the first few weeks of the onset of disease which returns to normal levels within 3 to 4 months. Failure of C3 to normalize is reason to consider diagnostic renal biopsy. For SLE, serum complement is an important reflection of response to therapy. Thus, monitoring the response of serum C3 and C4 is an important adjunct to the diagnosis and management of these conditions [54] (see below).

While less common in the era of ventriculo-peritoneal shunts for hydrocephalus, children with chronic bacteremia and hypocomplementemia, secondary to infected atrial tips of ventriculo-atrial shunts, continue to be encountered.[55] Hypocomplementemia occurs in patients with cryoglobulinemia, hepatitis, and in several clinical conditions which produce C consumption by uncertain mechanisms [8] (Table 5). Presumably, hypocomplementemia in acute pancreatitis is produced by the proteolytic enzymes released by the damage pancreas. In sepsis/ shock syndromes, multifactorial mechanisms of hypocomplementemia

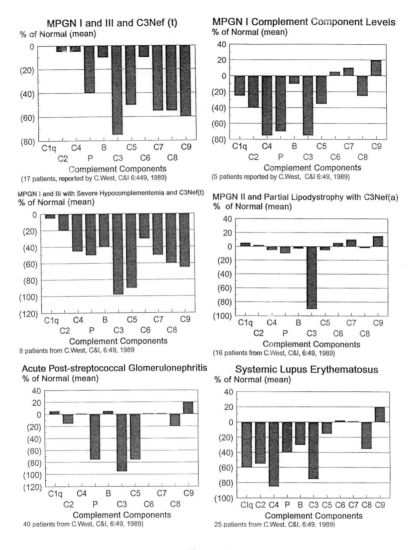

Figure 6

may occur, including both liver damage (the site of synthesis of most C components) and activation of C by the kinin or coagulation systems.

B. Presumed Immune Complex Diseases

Immune complexes are not always identified in patients with consumption of C. Furthermore, the offending antigens within immune complexes, such as DNA in systemic lupus erythematosus, cannot routinely be detected within target organs of the disease process such as the kidney. Despite significantly decreased concentrations of C3, streptococcal antigens are rarely detected within the renal glomeruli of patients with poststreptococcal glomerulonephritis. In the absence of definitive evidence of immune complexes, many immune-mediated diseases in man are best labeled as "presumed immune complex disease." The detection of decreased serum concentrations of C components supports the participation of immune complexes in the disease process, but formal proof is often lacking. Hepatitis B, chronic parasitic infection and *pneumococcal* sepsis have been reported in association with hypocomplementemia.[54]

C. Nonimmune Complex Diseases

Consumption of C occurs in many conditions in which immune complex participation has not been identified (Table 5). The C3 nephritic factor (C3nef) was initially detected in a form of membranoproliferative glomerulonephritis (type 1) characterized by decreased C3. The most active C3nef is associated with type II membranoproliferative glomerulonephritis. The nephritic factor of type II MPGN is commonly seen in association with partial lipodystrophy. This nephritic factor activates the alternative C pathway and has been called the amplification nephritic factor (NF$_a$).[51] Type II MPGN is not considered

---

Figure 6

Patterns of serum complement component concentrations in various glomerulonephritides. Data are shown as percent deviation from the normal. For each diagnosis and each specific component, the heavy vertical bar represents the mean value obtained at diagnosis or with relapses. *Top left*: In membranoproliferative glomerulonephritis type I and type II (MPGN I and II), the presence of the C3 nephritic factor (C3nef) produces activation of the terminal pathway and properdin of the alternative pathway. This complement profile is characteristic of C3nef of the terminal pathway (C3nef$_t$) and is due to a properdin-dependent type of C3nef. *Top right*: Some patients with MPGN I demonstrate predominant abnormalities of the classical pathway and closely resemble the pattern which is seen in SLE (*bottom right*). *Middle left*: eight patients with either MPGN I or III in this series demonstrated more severe hypocomplementemia and had decreased concentrations of components of both the CP and TP. These patients also had C3nef$_t$. *Middle right*: a unique form of nephritic factor, C3nef$_a$, is regularly observed in patients with partial lipodystrophy. Markedly depressed levels of only C3 is seen in these patients, and MPGN type II is seen on renal biopsy. The activation of C3 via the amplification loop stabilizes C3bBb (the alternative pathway C3 convertase), occurs predominantly in the fluid phase, and is properdin-independent, thereby differentiating C3nef$_a$ from C3nef$_t$. *Bottom left*: the hypocomplementemia of acute poststrepococcal glomerulonephritis is characterized by decreased concentrations of C3, C5, and properdin. Activation products of the TP are often noted. Unlike the persistently low levels of C3 noted in patients with MPGN, the hypocomplementemia of acute poststreptococcal glomerulonephritis resolves in several months. *Bottom right*: systemic lupus erythematosus is characterized by evidence of CP activation with decreased concentrations of C1q, C2, C4, and C3. Several studies demonstrate early activation of C4 in relapses of SLE, making this a helpful indication of relapse. A nephritic factor which reacts with C4b has been reported in SLE. (From West, C. D., *Complement Inflammation*, 6, 49, 1989. With permission from S. Karger, AG, Basel.)

to be an immune complex disorder. Decreased serum levels of properdin and C5 and activation of the terminal C pathway have been occasionally noted in type III MPGN [51] (Table 7).

2. Decreased Synthesis of Complement Components

Decreased synthesis is seen in a variety of diseases, particularly in those with severe liver disease and severe malnutrition, and in patients with overwhelming sepsis (Table 5). Hypocomplementemia is a consequence of decreased hepatic synthesis since the liver is the primary site of production of most C components.

3. Increased Loss/Catabolism of Complement Components

Normal or elevated levels for most complement components are present in the nephrotic syndrome.[56] The exceptions include decreased serum concentrations of factor B, C2 (20%) and factor I.[57,58] C1q is decreased in patients with hypogammaglobulinemia for reasons that are uncertain.

Deficiency of control proteins of the C pathway activation reactions result in depletion of specific components. Serum concentration of both C4 and C2 occur in patients with deficiency of C1 inhibitor. Factor H and factor I deficiencies, although uncommon, result in significant hypocomplementemia and clinical disease (see below). The absence of membrane control proteins of C is recognized to be the cause of paroxysmal nocturnal hemoglobinuria. Absence of one or more of these control proteins permits excessive catabolism of C3, lysis of red cells, and hypocomplementemia.

4. Genetic Deficiencies of Complement

Genetically determined deficiencies of each of the nine classical, alternative, and terminal pathway components (C1–C9) have been reported, including deficiencies of each of the three components of C1 (C1q,C1r, and C1s).[59] The onset of diseases associated with C deficiency occurs predominantly during childhood and adolescence. In order for cases to be classified as genetically determined, reported cases need to include the study of family members to rule out an acquired C deficiency. Most cases have had undetectable levels of the affected component. In some, the functional test or protein measurement has shown trace amounts of the serum protein, presumably reflecting the presence of an unstable form of the serum protein which is catabolized more rapidly than normal.

The reported increased incidence of C component deficiencies among patients with immune complex diseases has been explained as due to an ascertainment bias or due to linkage with HLA antigens. However, large population studies in Swiss army recruits did not show any C component deficiency,[60] and in a large group of Japanese blood donors,[61] no classical or alternative C deficiency was detected, arguing against ascertainment as the cause of such an association. In patients with SLE and C deficiency, evidence against a primary role for only HLA antigens, as opposed to the C deficiency itself, include the following observations:

- The occurrence of SLE in C1q and C1INH deficiency; C proteins which are encoded by genes not linked to HLA genes;
- The detection of C4A null allotypes in SLE patients not having the HLA-DR3 antigen, which suggests an important role for the C4A null allotype apart from the HLA antigens;[62]
- The occurrence of quite variable HLA antigens among total C4-deficient cases with SLE, which supports a role for the C4 null allotype alone.[18]

Genetic predisposition to SLE is multifactorial.[63] Deficiency of a C component, the presence of specific HLA antigens, and other genetic characteristics have been demonstrated to be risk factors for the development of SLE.

The most common deficiency of complement is absence of the C1INH and secondary deficiency of C4, consequent to the uninhibited activation of this classical C component, and resulting in the condition known as hereditary angioneurotic edema. Patients with HANE are no longer reported as individual cases, but it is important to recall that angioedema, secondary to C1INH deficiency, is the single most common disorder due to a congenital C component deficiency .

C2 deficiency is the second most common congenital C deficiency, accounting for 24% of 447 cases[3,4] (Figure 7). Deficiencies of the terminal pathway components, C6,C7, and C8, each accounted for 16 to 17% of cases. Congenital absence of factor B has not been reported, and only one case of absent factor D is reported.[4] Deficiency of C3 is one of the least common (4%), emphasizing the importance of this protein in the elaboration of several biologically active products of the C pathways. Patients with congenital C deficiencies fall into recognizable clinical patterns (Figure 8):

- Hereditary angioneurotic edema (HANE)
- Immune complex disease (systemic lupus erythematosus, vasculitis, collagen vascular diseases)
- Susceptibility to infection by pyogenic organisms (*Staphylococcus* or *Streptococcus* organisms)

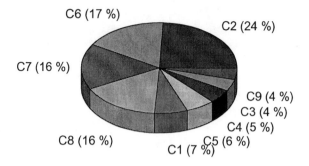

Figure 7
The frequency of complement component deficiencies. The most commonly reported deficiency of complement (other than HANE) is C2 deficiency, accounting for 24% of 447 cases reviewed by Ross and Densen and Gigueroa and Densen.[3,4] Deficiencies of the TP components, C6, C7, and C8 each accounted for 16 to 17% of cases. Deficiency of C3 is the least common (4%).

- Glomerulonephritis (membranoproliferative, anaphylactoid purpura nephritis)
- Infection by *Neisseria* organisms (*N. meningitides*, *N. gonorrheae*).

Some patients, particularly those with C1q and C4 deficiency, have had both infections and immune complex type disease.

A. Deficiencies of Classical Pathway

Patients with deficiencies of the classical components (C1,C2, and C4) have the greatest predilection to be discovered during the investigation of immune complex diseases. Cases with congenital deficiency of C1q present with SLE and related syndromes.[3,4] Pyogenic infections in these individuals have also been common, suggesting the importance for C1q in promoting opsonization and in the enhancement of antibody production.[5] Patients with angioedema secondary to deficiency of C1INH also have a predisposition to the development of SLE and related syndromes. As a consequence of the absence of C1INH, these patients have secondary deficiencies of both C4 and C2, but the primary defect in angioedema is absence of inhibition of the serine proteases C1s and C1r. Individuals with deficiencies of C1 components have had a variety of autoantibodies, including antidouble-stranded DNA and anti-Sm.[5,6] C4- and C2-deficient patients have a lower incidence of autoantibodies than C1 deficient patients, but do have a particular tendency to exhibit anti-Ro(SS-A) antibody.[18]

Congenital deficiency of C2 has frequently been detected during the evaluation of lupus-like disease, vasculitis, or dermatomyositis. Family studies of the proband have demonstrated that as many as 40 to 50% of the C2-deficient individuals are clinically asymptomatic. In

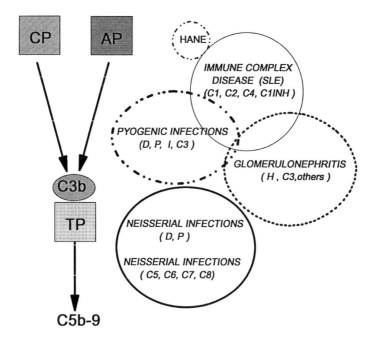

Figure 8

Clinical syndromes associated with congenital complement deficiencies. Patients with congenital C deficiencies fall into four recognizable clinical patterns: (1) immune complex disease such as systemic lupus erythematosus, vasculitis, and other syndromes of collagen vascular diseases (thin solid circle); (2) susceptibility to infection by pyogenic organisms such as *Staphylococcus* or *Streptococcus* organisms (circle of dashes and dots); (3) glomerulonephritis such as membranoproliferative, anaphylactoid purpura, proliferative glomerulonephritis (circle of dots); (4) infection by *Neisseria* organisms including *N. meningitides* and *N. gonorrheae* (thick solid circle); and (5) the most common C deficiency, hereditary angioneurotic edema (HANE).

general, C2-deficient patients with SLE have milder renal involvement than is seen in idiopathic SLE.

C4 deficiency is quite rare. This protein is normally encoded by four genes. The situation in patients with absent C4 has been summarized by Hauptmann.[18] SLE and other immune complex type diseases predominate among the reported individuals. Of all the congenitally C-deficient patients, SLE occurs most commonly among those with C4 deficiency. The remarkably high mortality rate (4/17) demonstrates the importance of C4 in the normal immune defense. The clinical characteristics found in patients with total C4 deficiency (Table 8) and diseases which are associated with partial C4 deficiency (Table 9) have been reported.[18]

Pyogenic infections have been reported commonly in patients with C3 deficiency (Figure 8). These individuals are particularly prone to infections with *N. meningitides*, *S. pneumoniae*, and *Staphylococcus aureus*,

TABLE 8

Clinical and Laboratory Findings in Total C4 Deficiency

General Associations (13/17) Patients

1. Systemic lupus erythematosus (SLE)
2. Discoid lupus erythematosus (DLE)
3. SLE and infections
4. SLE and membranoproliferative glomerulonephritis
5. anaphylactoid purpura (Henöch-Schonlein purpura)

Major Clinical Findings (12 Patients)

1. Digital erythema
2. Facial erythema
3. Photosensitivity
4. Discoid lesions
5. Fever
6. Atrophic scarring
7. Alopecia
8. Raynaud phenomenon
9. Oral ulcers
10. Arthralgias/arthritis
11. CNS involvement

Laboratory Findings

1. Proteinuria
2. Glomerulonephritis
3. Cryoglobulins
4. ANA-positive (7/12)
5. Anti-Ro(SSA) positive (5/12)

Modified from Reference 18.

TABLE 9

Diseases Associated with C4 Null Alleles

1. Systemic lupus erythematosus (SLE) (11.7% vs. 0.9% with C4*Q0)
2. Discoid lupus erythematosus (DLE)
3. Insulin-dependent diabetes (6.9% vs. 2.7% for C4B*Q0)
4. Gougerot-Sjögren disease
5. Systemic sclerosis
6. IgA deficiency
7. Grave's disease
8. Chronic active hepatitis
9. IgA nephropathy
10. Anaphylactoid purpura
11. Recurrent hematuria
12. Subacute sclerosing panencephalitis

Modified from Reference 18. With permission.

which produce meningitis, sepsis, pneumonia, and peritonitis. In view of the importance of C3 fragments in the processing of immune complexes, it is surprising that deficiency of C3 does not predispose more to SLE and related diseases than is reported. Glomerulonephritis (primarily membranoproliferative glomerulonephritis) and partial lipodystrophy have been reported in C3 deficiency, and these conditions are associated with C3(nef).

B. Deficiencies of the Alternative Pathway

Properdin deficiency is the only X-linked deficiency (69 males, 1 female).[3,4] Among the 70 reported cases, three patterns of deficiency have been reported: total absence of properdin, partial deficiency (~10% of normal), and the presence of a dysfunctional properdin protein. As in patients with factor I deficiency, these patients have presented with life-threatening neisserial infections. One pedigree has been reported in which one individual had complete inherited deficiency of factor D. The proband experienced recurrent neisserial infections.

C. Deficiencies of the Terminal Pathway

Deficiency of the terminal C pathways components (C5-C9) are among the most common C deficiencies (Figure 6). TP deficiencies occur in approximately 1 in 10,000 Caucasian and Japanese individuals. No CP or AP component deficiencies were noted in a group of Japanese blood donors,[60] and only one deficient individual was detected among 15,000 individuals screened in England.[59] TP component deficiencies exhibit some ethnic differences, as 99% of reported C9-deficient cases have been among Japanese.

Infection with neisserial organisms constitute the most common clinical association with TP deficiencies (Table 7). Neisseria meningitides has been the most common pathogen in each TP deficiency, although N. gonorrheae has been particularly common among American blacks with C5 deficiency. SLE-like disease and immune complex disease are uncommon among patients with TP component deficiencies.

D. Deficiencies of Control Proteins

Factor I deficiency (14 reported cases)[3,4] mimics the clinical presentation which is seen in C3 deficiency. In these cases, the C3 deficiency is secondary to the uncontrolled and continuous activation of C3 as a consequence of the primary absence of factor I. Factor H deficiency (13 reported cases) is associated primarily with N. meningitides infections and is also reported in association with membranoproliferative glomerulonephritis, SLE, and a hemolytic uremic-like syndrome. C4–binding protein deficiency has only been reported in one pedigree. The proband had angioedema and Bechet's-like syndrome.

The primary defect in patients with paroxysmal nocturnal hemoglobinuria (PNH) is recognized to be failure to produce glycosylphosphatidylinositol anchors for membrane-oriented proteins.[64] Because of this underlying defect, the membrane-oriented C control proteins, CD59 (protectin), DAF (decay-accelerator factor), and HRF (homologous restriction factor) are deficient in PNH. Deficiency of membrane-oriented control proteins in PNH[64] results in clones of red cells that are susceptible to complement-mediated lysis. In the few cases with absence of DAF (Cromer blood group negative), these individuals are completely asymptomatic. In one reported case of CD59 deficiency, the patient had PNH-like clinical findings.

II. METHODS FOR COMPLEMENT ANALYSIS

An array of laboratory options is available when a clinician determines that a patient requires evaluation of the complement system. Some of these analyses are quite straightforward and are available through most clinical laboratories. Complement assays fall into two general categories. Protein measurements determine the expression on tissue or the serum concentration of individual components, their fragments, or their complexes. Functional assays use a biologic effect of complement, such as peptide cleavage or cell lysis, to measure the activity of an individual component or group of components. Before considering the specifics of individual assays, we will provide some general background on these types of measurements.

A. Protein Assays

Both polyclonal and monoclonal antibodies are available for most human complement components. Polyclonal antibodies are employed in assays which require a precipitin reaction with the component being measured.

One of the first such assays employed was rocket immunoelectrophoresis. In this technique, a monospecific polyclonal antibody (usually raised in rabbits or goats) is incorporated into an agarose gel matrix. Wells are cut into the lower edge of the gel, and standard volumes of the serum to be tested are added to the wells. A current is applied to the gel, and an advancing "front" of precipitating antigen–antibody complexes develops in the agarose (the "rocket"). The electrophoresis is stopped and the serum concentration of the component in question is determined by comparing the height of the rocket to that of simultaneously run standards of known concentration.

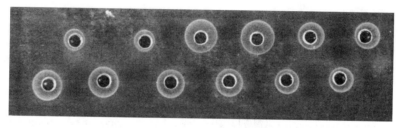

Figure 9
Photograph of a radial immunodiffusion quantitation of human factor H. Paired samples of each specimen were assayed so this gel shows six separate samples. The first (wells 1 and 2) and second (wells 3 and 4) samples have the lowest and highest concentration, respectively.

A labor-intensive procedure, rocket immunoelectrophoresis is hardly ever employed in clinical laboratories today. Its successor, radial immunodiffusion, however, is a mainstay of clinical complement chemistry. As adopted from the work of Mancini et al.,[65] radial immunodiffusion (RID) also involves incorporation of monospecific polyclonal antibody into an agarose gel matrix. Wells are cut in this matrix, and precise volumes of test serum are added to the wells. After an overnight incubation, circular rings surrounding the wells (Figure 9) mark the limit of the diffusion of the component being measured. The protein concentration is proportional to the area of the ring, and is calculated by comparison to the areas of standards placed in the same agarose gel.

The RID method can be used to measure the concentration of any protein for which precipitating polyclonal antibody is available. For several of the commonly measured complement components, kits containing prepoured plates and standards are commercially available. A particular advantage of RID is the capability of adjusting the antibody concentration in the agarose in order to measure particularly high or low serum concentrations of protein with precision. This cannot be done, of course, with commercially prepoured plates.

For components whose concentrations are frequently measured in clinical laboratories, an automated method is available. Rate nephelometry uses the degree of scatter of a light beam, directed through a chamber in which serum is reacted with antibody, to measure protein concentration.[66] Because the technique is automated and can provide a result within minutes, it is used most often in the measurement of complement proteins such as C3, C4, and B, which are frequently monitored in the clinical care of patients with immune-mediated disorders. Nephelometry requires antisera that are free of contaminating particles or turbidity. The technique is most applicable for proteins which are generally present in high concentration; thus the measurement of C2 and the individual terminal components is not well suited to nephelometry. Nephelometry is also limited in the precision with which it can measure very low serum concentrations of proteins and cannot be used to confirm complete deficiency of any component. Nonetheless, the majority of clinical measurements of the complement system today are performed by rate nephelometry.

Neither nephelometry nor RID is suited for the measurement of proteins whose normal serum concentrations are very low. For example, component split products such as $C5a_{des\ Arg}$ cannot be assayed by these methods. For such proteins, enzyme-linked immunosorbant assays (ELISA, EIA) or radioimmunoassays (RIA) are often employed.

There are many variations to the ELISA procedure, which is suited both for the measurement of antigens and antibodies. In a frequently used method, antibody to the peptide being measured is attached to the wells of a microtiter plate. Serum or other fluid containing a component to be measured is then added to the wells. After the protein being measured has had an opportunity to bind to the "capture" antibody, the rest of the serum is washed from the wells. Next, a second antibody, this one linked to an enzyme, is added to the wells. After binding and washing free antibody from the wells, a substrate which undergoes a color change mediated by the enzyme is added. Finally, the color change is quantitated by measuring the absorbance of light at a wavelength specific for the substrate used. Protein concentration is then calculated, based on the absorbance of standards assayed simultaneously.

As is the case for ELISA, there are a number of specific methods employed in RIA. Most methods used in assay of the complement system are variants of a competitive assay, in which the first step is addition of a specific quantity of a radiolabeled protein identical to the one being measured. Next, a precipitating antibody to the components is added and the precipitated radioactivity is determined in a gamma counter. Since the antibody precipitates both native (unlabeled) protein and the added labeled peptide, the amount of radioactivity precipitated is a function of starting protein concentration. Thus, when the component is present in very low concentrations, there will be relatively more precipitated activity than if the component concentration was high. The precipitated radioactivity present with known inputs of unlabeled antigen is used to standardize this assay.

B. Functional Assays

The earliest measurements of complement activity were functional studies based on the lytic effects of the complement on sensitized erythrocytes. Although the availability of specific antisera has greatly lessened the demand for these types of assays, functional tests are employed for screening. For example, the measurement of the entire classical pathway (C1–C9) is accomplished by determining the total hemolytic complement (CH50), and the alternative complement pathway can also be determined by a hemolytic assay (APCH50). Most functional assays rely on the assembly of a membrane attack complex on the surface of an erythrocyte, inducing lysis and releasing hemoglobin into the media. The concentration of hemoglobin released is used as a measure of the number of cells lysed. In screening functional assays (e.g., CH50 and the APCH50), the integrity of a series of components is determined simultaneously, and results are usually expressed as the titer of test serum needed to lyse 50% of target cells.

Functional assays for specific components are variations on the CH50 assay, in which an excess of all components except that of interest is reacted with the sensitized cells. The excess components are added either in the form of purified components or as human serum depleted of the component being measured. Dilutions of test serum then provide the source of the assayed component. Results of functional assays for specific components are reported either as 50% hemolysis units, similar to the CH50 titer, or as "effective molecules" per unit volume. The concept of an "effective molecule" of a complement component is based on the "single hit" concept: that a single MAC is sufficient to produce cell lysis. According to the Poisson distribution, there should be one "effective molecule" per cell at a dilution producing 63% lysis. Since the number of cells and dilution of serum per unit volume is known, effective molecules per ml serum can be easily calculated.[67]

C. Specific Component Assays

1. Specimen Preparation and Handling

More so than for many other clinical tests, the proper preparation and handling of blood samples for complement assays is critical. The coagulation process itself may lead to some complement component activation. Storage at inappropriate temperature or cycles of freezing and thawing may render functional or some immunochemical measurements impossible.

Both serum and plasma are used in complement assays. Although either is acceptable for some tests, there are assays for which one or the other is required. For example, some $C3a_{des\,Arg}$ is generated during coagulation, so EDTA plasma is the appropriate sample for this test. On the other hand, inhibition of complement activation by EDTA renders plasma inappropriate for a CH50. Since laboratories vary in their requirements for specific tests, prior consultation is always advisable.

If serum is to be used, blood is collected into a plain tube without a separator. After clotting at room temperature, the sample is centrifuged, and the serum removed and immediately frozen. Both serum and plasma for complement assays must be stored at –70°C. Overnight shipment to referral labs must be on dry ice.

2. Total Hemolytic Complement (CH50)

The prototype of the functional assays of the complement system is the CH50. This assay measures the dilution of patient serum that will lyse 50% of a target material, sensitized sheep erythrocytes.[67]

To perform the CH50, sheep cells are first coated with a heterologous antiserum to the red cell membrane, hemolysin. Next, serial dilutions of the serum to be tested are added to each of several test tubes. A standardized number of the sensitized sheep cells is then added to each test tube. The tubes are incubated for an hour at 37°C. During this incubation, the complement components of the test serum are sequentially activated by immunoglobulin fixed to the cell surfaces. The activation proceeds until a membrane attack complex is formed through the cell membrane, resulting in lysis. After the 1-hour incubation, the reaction is stopped by the addition of ice cold saline to each tube. The tubes are centrifuged, and the amount of cell lysis that has occurred is determined by spectrophotometrically measuring the absorption of light by the supernatant. The percent lysis in a tube is defined by the light absorption of its supernatant divided by the absorption in a tube with complete cell lysis.

The raw data for this assay consist of the percentage lysis for each of several serum dilutions. These data are either plotted by hand on graph paper or entered into a linear regression program to calculate the dilution at which 50% of the cells lyse. The result of the CH50 is expressed as the reciprocal of the dilution producing 50% lysis. If, for example, this were to occur at a dilution of 1/65, the CH50 would be 65 units.

Since the specific components and conditions of the CH50 will vary from laboratory to laboratory, there is no generally applicable normal value for this test. Centers performing the assay determine their own normal ranges. Most will assay an aliquot of a standard serum with each determination. This permits correction for assay-to-assay variability.

Although the CH50 was once the principal clinical assay of the complement system, it is less readily available today. With the ability to measure precisely the complement components involved in acquired disorders, there is less indication for this test in the management of such disorders. Its major use today is as a screen for inherited disorders. Complete inherited deficiency of any of the classical activation components (C1, C2, C4, C3) or the terminal components C5 through C9 will give a CH50 of 0. In a patient with recurrent *Neisseria* infection, for example, the first test to establish if a deficiency in one of the terminal components is present is a CH50.[3] If this is normal, then no further analysis is probably required. An undetectable CH50 in this situation should then be followed by analysis of terminal component concentrations in order to pinpoint the deficiency.

Although much less commonly employed, a CH50 for the alternative pathway is also available.[68,69] In this test, dilutions of serum are incubated at 37°C with unsensitized rabbit erythrocytes. The reaction is carried out in the presence of the calcium chelator EGTA and added magnesium, in order to minimize any classical pathway activity and maximize conditions for the assembly of the alternative pathway C3 convertase. Complete deficiency of C3, B, or D will result in an APCH50 of zero.

3. C1

Activation of the classical pathway usually begins with binding of C1q to immobilized immunoglobulin. C1 immunochemical and functional levels may be depressed in the face of such activation. A problem in the measurement of C1 is provided by the unique nature of the component as a complex of a single C1q molecule associated with a tetramolecular complex of two C1r's and two C1s's. Antisera are available to each of these molecules, but the usual clinical determination of immunochemical C1 is a C1q concentration by radial immunodiffusion. In the serial follow-up of patients with acquired disorders causing classical pathway activation, there is not usually any advantage to following C1q levels over those of C4. It should also be recognized that C1q levels are usually reduced in any situation in which hypogammaglobulinemia is present.[70]

While antisera to C1r and C1s are also available, immunochemical measurement of these components is much less often performed. Inherited deficiencies of any of the three components of C1 occur, and the detection of such deficiencies constitutes the major indication for such determinations.

The conventional functional measurement of C1 is a hemolytic assay in which excess amounts of C4 and C2 are reacted with sensitized sheep erythrocytes, and dilutions of test serum are used as the C1 source. Addition of an excess of C3 and terminal components then produces cell lysis, the degree of which is a function of the quantity of active C1 input. Hemolytic C1 function would most often be used to confirm a suspected deficiency of one of the components of the C1 complex, and would thus be performed in concert with immunochemical measurements of C1q, C1r, and C1s.[67-69]

4. C2

C2 serum concentrations can be measured by RID or ELISA assays, but are less commonly determined than those of C4 and C3 because antiserum to this component is not widely available. Although C2 concentrations also drop with classical pathway activation, they are rarely helpful in following the course of such activation. C2 is the component for which complete deficiency is most often found.[28] Because of this, low serum concentrations in the presence of otherwise normal component levels are not uncommon and usually reflect heterozygous deficiency.

A hemolytic assay for C2, employing sensitized sheep erythrocytes and purified early components, is also available. Hemolytic C2 activity correlates with serum concentration of the protein, so that test is most often used to confirm a complete deficiency state.[67-69]

5. C3

C3 occupies a central position in the complement cascade since it is the target of both the alternative and classical pathway convertases. Cleavage of C3 produces potent biologic effects itself, as well as initiating activation of terminal components. C3 is the complement component most often measured in clinical laboratories.

Functional determinations of C3 are rarely needed in clinical situations. A hemolytic assay is available based on sensitized sheep cells, purified components, and dilutions of patient serum as a C3 source. Most laboratories capable of undertaking this assay are geared toward research rather than clinical service, however, so prior arrangement and consultation is often necessary.[67-69]

There are several options available for the immunochemical determination of C3. Most of these methods are based on the use of polyclonal antisera raised in rabbits, sheep, or goats. Measurement of C3 in the serum is somewhat complicated by the presence of several antigenic epitopes on the molecule, which may become more or less available as the protein undergoes proteolytic cleavage. Most antisera used in immunochemical measurements of C3 are primarily directed at the C3c and C3d fragments.[20]

Most clinical assays of C3 are performed by rate nephelometry. With the recent availability of C3 standardization by the International Federation of Clinical Chemistry,[71] there should be minimal laboratory-to-laboratory variation in the measurement of this component.

Radial immunodiffusion kits for C3 determination are often employed in laboratories for which test volumes are insufficient to support nephelometric assays. RID with plates incorporating lower antibody concentrations can be used to provide more precise values for C3 concentrations below the measuring range of nephelometry.

6. C3 Breakdown Products

Low serum concentrations of C3 can be found either because of activation with complement consumption or because of diminished synthesis. The latter can either be congenital, as with inherited deficiencies, or acquired. For situations in which it is difficult to distinguish between these possibilities, assay of $C3a_{des\ Arg}$ may be useful. The first step in C3 activation is cleavage of the α chain, releasing a small peptide, C3a, which has anaphylatoxic properties. This molecule is rapidly cleaved by endogenous proteases to $C3a_{des\ Arg}$. Thus, the presence of the latter fragment in the circulation is a measure of C3 activation. $C3a_{des\ Arg}$ levels may be measured by radioimmunoassay. This is a very sensitive determination, capable of measuring nanogram quantities of protein, so very careful specimen handling, including collection into EDTA, is critical to avoid *in vitro* C3 cleavage.[72]

7. C4

Because its serum concentration is as much as tenfold higher than that of the other early C components, C4 levels prove to be much more useful than C1q or C2 in monitoring classical pathway-mediated, acquired diseases.[73] On the other hand, these are some peculiarities specific to C4 which must be considered in interpreting both immunochemical and functional assays of this component. The polyclonal antisera employed in both RID and nephelometric C4 measurements all recognize both C4 isotypes, C4A and C4B. Because of the presence of deletions and duplications of these isotypes, "normal" individuals may express between one and five or more C4 genes. Serum concentrations of the component roughly correlate with the number of expressed genes, although there is considerable overlap.[74] "Normal" C4 concentration ranges are usually based on values derived from large populations, in which most individuals have three or four gene products. Consequently, C4 serum concentrations in some healthy people may fall into the abnormally low range simply because of the presence of two or more null genes.

Awareness of this phenomenon is critical in the serial analysis of complement component concentrations in acquired disorders. In a patient with SLE who has only two expressed C4 genes, for example, it may be impossible ever to obtain a "normal" C4 serum concentration. Thus, in patients with persistently low serum C4 levels, especially if other components are normal, C4 allotyping may be indicated. Such allotyping is generally performed by immunofixation electrophoresis and is most easily interpreted if simultaneous typing of available family members is also performed. Such typing is offered by at least one commercial laboratory, but also can often be arranged through research laboratories with an interest in complement genetics.

C4 functional assays, based on hemolysis of sheep erythrocytes, are also available. In the standard C4 hemolytic assay, sensitized erythrocytes are reacted with an excess of purified C1 and C2. Dilutions of patient serum are added as a source of C4, after which excess C3 and terminal components are added. The degree of lysis in the system is then a function of the amount of C4 input.

C4 hemolytic assays are most often used to confirm complete deficiency of the protein. Like immunochemical measurements, they are also affected by the peculiarities of C4 genetics. C4A isotypes, because of preferential binding to amino-rich surfaces, are less active in erythrocyte hemolysis than are C4B isotypes, which have a greater affinity for carbohydrate-containing surfaces.[15] Therefore, the hemolytic titers per milligram of protein will be highest in individuals whose C4 is all of the B isotype (i.e., those with complete C4A deficiency).[74]

8. C4 Breakdown Products

Similarly to the situation with C3, activation of C4 begins with cleavage of the α chain, releasing a small fragment, C4a, which has anaphylotoxic properties. Endogenous proteases cleave C4a to $C4a_{des\ Arg}$. Elevated $C4a_{des\ Arg}$ levels in the circulation are an indicator of ongoing classical pathway activation. Measurement of this fragment can be performed by radioimmunoassay. Such determinations may be useful in situations in which C4 serum concentrations are persistently low, and it is not clear if such low levels result from actual complement activation (elevated $C4a_{des\ Arg}$) or from inherited deficiencies (normal $C4a_{des\ Arg}$).[75]

9. C5

Serum concentrations of C5 are most often measured by radial immunodiffusion. Reductions in C5 concentration are found in the face of acquired hypocomplementemic states, including several forms of glomerulonephritis.

Since activation and surface binding of C5 is the first step in assembling a membrane attack complex, complete deficiency of C5 results in a total lack of lysis in the CH50 assay. Similarly, complete deficiency is confirmed by a specific C5 hemolytic assay. In this test, sensitized sheep erythrocytes, with all the components of a classical pathway C5 convertase added (C1, C2, C4, C3), are reacted with dilutions of test serum as a source of C5, after which lysis is induced by adding an excess of C6–C9.[67-69]

10. C5 Breakdown Products

As is the case for the analogous molecules C3 and C4, the first step in C5 activation is cleavage of a small fragment (C5a) from the α chain of C5 by either the classical pathway or alternative pathway C5 convertase. This small fragment is proteolytically cleaved immediately to yield $C5a_{des\ Arg}$.[76] $C5a_{des\ Arg}$ levels, thus, provide a valuable marker of C5 activation. This is particularly useful in the interpretation of persistently low serum concentrations, where confusion about the possibility of congenital deficiency or ongoing activation exists.

Given the low molecular weight of this fragment and its very low serum concentration, it is detected by radioimmunoassay. As is also the case for $C4a_{des\ Arg}$ and $C3a_{des\ Arg}$, particular attention needs to be paid to sample collection and handling in this assay, to prevent *in vitro* generations of this fragment.

11. C5b-9 (Terminal Complement Complex [TCC])

Although the membrane attack complex inserts in cell membranes, in situations of ongoing complement activation there is often free MAC in the circulation. Free MAC in the circulation consists of components C5b–9 (also known as the terminal complement complex or TCC) complexed to protein S (vitronectin).

Measurement of TCC in plasma is performed by the measurement of a "neo-antigen." Activation of the components of the MAC expose antigenic determinants which are not present when the proteins are in their native conformations. A monoclonal antibody against such a neoantigen is incorporated into an ELISA. This antibody is used to capture TCCs in the assay wells. The detection antibody is directed at another component of the complex.

Elevation of TCC serum concentration is found in many acquired hypocomplementemic disorders. Glomerulonephritis such as that found in systemic lupus erythematosus or poststreptococcal glomerulonephritis are particularly likely to be associated with free TCC.[53] Nonetheless, there are insufficient data to suggest that serial determination of TCC in such disorders adds anything to management not provided by levels of individual components, such as C3.

12. C6–C9

Most remarks about the measurement and interpretation of serum concentration of terminal pathway components apply to all four of these proteins. These determinations are most often obtained in the investigation of patients with recurrent infection (Figure 8). Occasionally, serial determinations may be of use in patients with acquired hypo-complementemic disorders that involve the terminal components. Membranoproliferative glomerulonephritis type III is the prototype of such disorders.

Terminal component immunochemical concentrations are usually measured by radial immunodiffusion. An undetectable level of a terminal component in the face of a CH50 of zero is good evidence of complete deficiency. C9 deficiency may be an exception, in that some hemolytic activity is present in serum missing this component. This is probably irrelevant however, since no consistent human disturbance occurs with complete C9 deficiency.

Specific functional assays for each component are also available. There are two approaches to these assays. One approach is to use purified components as a source of all proteins except for the one being assayed; dilutions of test serum provide the source of the component being measured. A much simpler procedure involves the use of serum from individuals with complete deficiency of the component being assayed. In this procedure, sensitized sheep erythrocytes are reacted with an excess of depleted serum and dilutions of the serum being tested. Lysis of cells thus depends on the input of the component in the test serum.[67-69]

A particular case is that of C8. This protein is composed of three chains, the gene for one of which (β) is on a separate chromosome from that of the other two (α and γ). C8 deficiency usually results from absence of the α/γ chains, with β chain in the circulation. Most polyclonal antisera to C8 recognize epitopes on all three chains, so individuals with α/γ chain deficiency will have some measurable C8 by RID but will have no hemolytic function.[32]

13. Factor B

Factor B, along with C3, comprises the alternative pathway C3 convertase. Thus, reduction in B level occurs in the face of ongoing alternative pathway-mediated complement activation. B serum concentrations are usually determined using polyclonal antisera. These may be incorporated into agarose for radial immunodiffusion assays or, if of sufficient quality, may be used in rate nephelometric determinations. Since B, after C3 and C4, is the component most frequently measured, many clinical laboratories offer a nephelometric assay of all three as a "panel" measurement of the complement system.

Low serum concentrations of B almost invariably indicate complement activation. Inherited deficiency of B has not been reported. Complement activation producing low B levels may be mediated by immune complexes or may result from impaired regulation. Examples of the latter include H deficiency or an abnormal H binding site on C3.[77]

A functional assay for B is based on the APCH50. Factor B-depleted serum is added to rabbit erythrocytes with dilutions of test serum added as a source of B. The amount of lysis produced in the system is thus a function of B input.[68,69]

14. Factor B Breakdown Products

Proteolytic cleavage of B by D results in two fragments, Ba and Bb. The latter can be measured in plasma with a monoclonal antibody-based ELISA.[78] Elevated levels indicate ongoing alternative pathway activation. Since low levels of B alone are an excellent indicator of activation, there may be little practical reason to assay these fragments.

15. Factor D

D is the complement protein with the lowest molecular weight and lowest serum concentration. One patient with absent factor D has been reported.[79] Because of its low molecular weight, D is lost in the urine in nephrotic syndrome. Although antisera to D are employed in research studies, there is currently no widely available standardized clinical assay for this component.

16. Factor H and Factor I

Serial measurement of the regulatory proteins H and I is probably of little use in the management of acquired abnormalities of the complement system. On the other hand, deficiency or dysfunction of either component can produce secondary complement abnormalities from abnormally regulated C3 consumption.[77] These abnormalities, in turn, have been associated with recurrent infection or glomerulonephritis. Interestingly, a patient with I deficiency was identified and reported as having C3 deficiency before the identity and regulatory function of I was recognized.[80]

Measurement of these proteins should be performed whenever there is evidence of persistent AP-mediated C3 consumption in the absence of C3 nephritic factor or other obvious explanation. Immunochemical determination of both components is generally performed with RID using polyclonal antibodies.

Functional assessment of factors H and I is possible, but not adapted to the clinical laboratory. If functional measurement is indicated to confirm complete deficiency it may be arranged through a complement research laboratory. Such assays are usually performed by size separation of the breakdown products of labeled C3, since the cleavage produced by these regulators results in fragments of specific size.

17. C1 Inhibitor

Genetic deficiency or dysfunction of C1INH produces the syndrome of hereditary angioneurotic edema.[81] Measurement of C1INH serum concentration is most often undertaken in an effort to confirm a diagnosis of HANE. Acquired C1INH deficiency may also occur, both in association with B-cell malignancy of various types and as an isolated disorder. Many of these patients from both groups have an autoantibody to C1INH that interferes with its function.[82] Additionally, ongoing complement activation rarely may deplete C1INH, producing an acquired C1INH deficiency.

The usual immunochemical measurement of C1INH is a RID method employing polyclonal antisera. Deficiency, implying HANE, is usually accompanied by consumption of early classical pathway components, resulting in low serum concentrations of C2 and C4. In acquired C1INH deficiency, the C1q level is also depressed, while C1q is usually normal in HANE. In both situations, C3 serum levels are generally preserved. Complete C1INH deficiency has not been found. Patients with HANE have heterozygous deficiency, with half-normal or lower serum protein concentrations.

In about 15% of patients with HANE, mutations in the C1INH gene result in subtle changes in the molecule which render it functionally abnormal, although immunochemical assays suggest normal or even elevated protein concentrations. This abnormal protein is detected by a functional C1INH measurement.[69] The indications for such a test would be clinical suspicion of HANE, with a normal serum concentration of C1INH and C1q and reduced levels of C2 and C4.

These are a variety of functional assays for C1INH, most of which are primarily available in the research laboratory. Variations of these assays may be offered by some clinical reference laboratories. One popular assay is based on the observation that C1r complexed to C1INH is not detected in an RID employing antibody to C1r. If normal serum is reacted with aggregated immunoglobulin to expose C1r to C1INH, C1r levels by RID fall. This drop in C1r level is attenuated if C1INH is dysfunctional and, thus, does not bind to C1r. Other functional assays include ELISAs, in which C1INH is detected after reacting with a bound target, and reactions which measure the ability of C1INH in test serum to inhibit C1-mediated cleavage of a fluid phase target. Because of the variety of ways in which C1INH function is quantitated, it is important to discuss individual cases with the reference laboratory before submitting specimens. There may be specifics of sample collection, handling, and transport that could be crucial to insuring a reliable result.

18. Properdin

Properdin deficiency is associated with a propensity to overwhelming *Neisseria* infection. Acquired reductions in properdin serum concentration are found in some hypocomplementemic glomerulonephritides.[83] Properdin is usually assayed by RID with polyclonal antisera. There is no clinically available functional assay for properdin. However, absence of this component produces an APCH50 of zero. Thus, absence of protein by RID with normal CH50 hemolysis and absent APCH50 hemolysis would support a diagnosis of properdin deficiency.

19. C4 Binding Protein

Complete C4bp deficiency has not been reported. Serum concentrations of this component may drop with active classical pathway activation.[84] RID with polyclonal antisera or ELISA with monoclonal reagents can be employed to measure this protein.

20. Membrane-Bound Complement Receptors and Inhibitors

Methods are available to assay most of the membrane-bound complement receptors either immunochemically or functionally. There are few situations, however, in which such measurements are of clinical utility. Although active immune complex disease may deplete erythrocyte CR1, serial measurement of receptor expression offers no advantage over more readily available assays of inflammatory activity. Inherited deficiencies of these components are also very unusual. One of the subunits of CR3 and CR4 (CD18) is absent in leukocyte adhesion deficiency and the glycosyl–phosphatidylinositol-anchored regulators MIRL (CD59) and DAF (CD55) are absent from erythrocytes in paroxysmal nocturnal hemoglobinuria.

None of these assays are regularly available in clinical laboratories. Immunochemical measurements generally involve the use of labeled monoclonal antibodies. Cells expressing the component of interest are isolated from peripheral blood and passed through a cell sorter using the specific antibody. Functional measurements of complement receptors frequently employ some variation of a rosetting assay. To detect CR1 on neutrophils, for example, the neutrophils are reacted with sheep erythrocytes bearing C3b. Cells bearing CR1 will bind these erythrocytes, forming rosettes.

21. C3 Nephritic Factor

C3nef is not a complement component. It is an immunoglobulin directed at a C3 convertase, which protects the convertase from decay and, thus, leads to complement consumption.[85] Since C3nef is found in some acquired hypocomplementemic disorders, however, its determination is considered here.

Measurement of C3nef begins with immunochemical assay of the serum C3 level. We have never detected C3nef in serum with a normal concentration of C3. The actual assay for C3nef measures the consumption of C3 in a normal target serum. Equal amounts of target serum and the serum to be assayed are incubated for 20 min at 37°C. The percent consumption of C3 is determined by examining the difference in C3 concentration before and after incubation.

The C3 assay for a C3nef measurement is somewhat complex, limiting the availability of this test to a few reference laboratories. Since the consumption of C3 by C3nef results in the conversion of native C3 to C3b, a method which distinguishes between these must be used. Conventional RID or nephelometry using most polyclonal antisera will not be satisfactory, since these methods recognize both proteins. Since conversion produces a shift in electrophoretic mobility, immunoelectrophoresis is frequently used to assess conversion of native C3 to C3b. A C3 hemolytic assay can also be used in this test, since conversion of C3 to C3b results in a loss of hemolytic activity. Finally, antisera are available with activity against epitopes that are lost when C3 is converted to C3b. These may be incorporated into RID or ELISA assays.

Although a 20-min incubation is typically employed in the C3nef assay, these are situations in which a longer (4 h) incubation is required to produce consumption. C3nef detected after such a prolonged incubation is referred to as "slow" nef or NF_t. The latter term derives from the observation that this C3nef activity is found in patients whose hypocomplementemia includes depression of some terminal components. NF_t is seen often in MPGN type III.[83]

D. Tissue Complement Deposition

In addition to being consumed in the circulation, complement components are frequently deposited at the site of immune injury. Although such deposition has been recognized in a number of areas, it has been best studied in the kidney. Examination of kidney biopsy tissue to establish the pattern of complement deposition is a mainstay in the evaluation of glomerulonephritis. Although labeled monoclonal antibodies are used for these studies in some laboratories, most still rely on fluorescein labeled polyclonal reagents.

Proper tissue handling is critical for successful immunofluorescent examination of biopsy tissue. As soon as a core of kidney tissue is obtained, a segment is cut off and snap-frozen in liquid nitrogen. This sample is stored at –70°C until ready for analysis. The frozen core of tissue is cut in a cryostat and sections are placed on gelatin coated slides. The sections are next reacted with specific antisera conjugated to fluorescein isothiocyanate. Many such conjugated antisera to human complement proteins are commercially available. After incubation with antibody, the slides are washed to remove free antisera, counterstained, and cover-slipped. When conjugated antibody is not available, a "sandwich" procedure is often employed. In such cases, unlabeled antibody is reacted with the section and washed. Following this, a second, labeled antibody directed against the primary antibody is used. For example, if the primary antibody were raised in goats, a labeled rabbit antigoat IgG would be used to detect the primary antibody. The slides are examined with ultraviolet illumination, and the location, distribution, and intensity of positive signal is recorded. Some of the types of pattern seen are illustrated in Figure 10.

III. APPROACH TO COMPLEMENT SYSTEM ANALYSIS

The variety of available tests of the complement system dictates the need for a careful approach to test selection in order to provide meaningful yet cost-effective results. Often, complement analyses are performed sequentially, with one level of testing begun only after the results of a prior level have been reviewed. This approach is particularly important in studying patients with recurrent infection in whom an inherited complement deficiency state is suspected. A systematic approach to such a patient is illustrated in Figure 11, and begins with a CH50 and an APCH50. If both of these are normal, important complement deficiency is virtually excluded. Since the APCH50 is not as widely available as the CH50, another screening approach would be to perform a CH50 along with an immunochemical measurement of B and P. The only deficiency which could exist with a normal value of these three tests is that of D, which probably never occurs.

If the CH50 is zero or very low, then subsequent testing needs to be focused on the classical activation proteins and on the terminal components. If the clinical problem was one of recurrent neisserial infection, then the most direct approach would be to perform an immunochemical determination of C5, C6, C7, and C8. This could be proceeded by a functional assay for C5–C8, if easily available.

If the clinical problem leading to the suspicion of inherited complement component deficiency is angioedema, the initial studies could

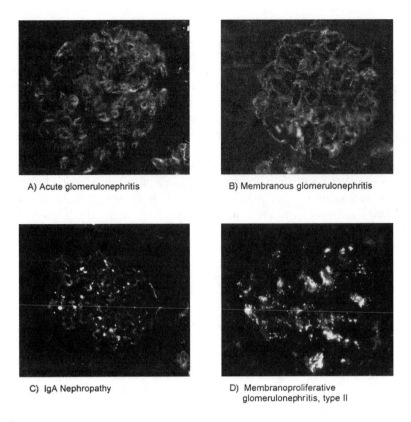

A) Acute glomerulonephritis

B) Membranous glomerulonephritis

C) IgA Nephropathy

D) Membranoproliferative
glomerulonephritis, type II

Figure 10
Patterns of complement (C3) deposition in human glomerulonephritis. (A) Acute glomerulonephritis: fine granular deposits along the capillary basement membrane, a common
pattern in acute glomerulonephritis. Usually associated with similar deposits of IgG,
properdin, and C5. (B) Membranous glomerulonephritis: heavy deposition of granular
deposits outlining capillaries of glomerulus with the epimembranous deposits of membranous glomerulonephritis. Usually associated with a similar deposition limited to IgG.
(C) IgA nephropathy: discrete fine to medium sized granular deposits along the paramesangium in IgA nephropathy. Frequently, the pattern is a more fragmentary and linear
label of the mesangium. There is a constant association in similar pattern with IgA and
fibrinogen and frequently with IgG and IgM as well. The large fluorescing objects represent protein resorption in podocytes. (D) Membranoproliferative glomerulonephritis,
type II: large, discrete, not numerous deposits which are negative for immunoglobulin,
in the paramesangium. The nonspecific linear label of the capillary walls in this example
of early MPGN II is nonspecific and becomes more intense with progression of the
disease. This paramesangial discrete pattern is also seen in one variety of idiopathic
RPGN, but differs by the absence of reactivity for properdin and C5. (Figures kindly
provided by A. James McAdams, Department of Pathology, Children's Hospital Medical
Center, University of Cincinnati, Cincinnati, OH.)

include a C3, C4, C1INH, and possibly a C1q and C2. Normal C3 and
C1q levels, with reduction in C4 and C2, and half-normal serum concentration of C1INH, would confirm type I HANE. A functional C1INH

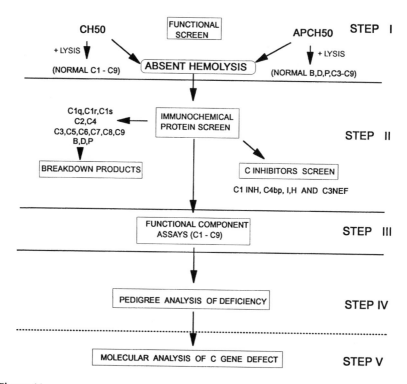

Figure 11
Protocol for the systematic analysis of patients with suspected complement deficiency.

determination could be obtained if immunochemical measurement of this component is normal with characteristic levels of early components.

Acquired disorders of the complement system requiring complement measurement most often involve immune-mediated glomerulonephritis or other autoimmune disorders. The initial approach to such diseases generally involves a nephelometric determination of the C3 and C4 serum concentrations. If these are normal, important acquired hypocomplementemic disturbances are virtually excluded. Subsequent tests if the C3 and/or C4 are abnormal will be dictated by the specific clinical problem. In straightforward acute poststreptococcal glomerulonephritis, for example, serial measurement of C3 will provide evidence of recovery, which will often precede improvement in urinary findings.

In acute glomerulonephritis which is not classical poststreptococcal disease, or in more insidious, chronic glomerulonephritis, further complement analysis may help to establish a precise diagnosis. Characteristic patterns of complement component change have been associated with specific glomerulonephritides. Complete characterization of the individual components (Figure 11) will supplement the data from the renal biopsy. Additionally, determination of C3nef in such settings is appropriate.

Rarely, acquired hypocomplementemic states coexist with isolated inherited component deficiencies. SLE with deficiency of C4 would be an example of this. These situations may result in confusion when it is difficult to distinguish very low or absent component concentrations from consumption or from inherited deficiency. Measurement of component concentration in family members, especially parents, may be helpful. If the component in question has a measurable circulating breakdown product (e.g., $C3_{des\ Arg}$, $C4_{des\ Arg}$, $C5_{des\ Arg}$ for C3, C4, or C5, respectively), the presence of elevated levels of such a product excludes inherited deficiency.

REFERENCES

1. Kinoshita, T., Biology of complement: the overture, *Immunol. Today*, 12, 291, 1991.
2. Müller-Eberhard, H. J., Molecular organization and function of the complement system, *Annu. Rev. Biochem.*, 57, 321, 1988.
3. Ross, S. C. and Denson, P., Complement deficiency states and infection: epidemiology, pathogenesis and consequences of neisserial and other infections in immune deficiency, *Medicine (Baltimore)*, 63, 243, 1984.
4. Figueroa, J. E. and Densen, P., Infectious diseases associated with complement deficiencies, *Clin. Microbiol. Rev.*, 4, 359, 1991.
5. Johnston, R. B., The complement system in host defense and inflamation: the cutting edges of a double edged sword, *Pediatr. Infect. Dis. J.*, 12, 933, 1993.
6. Morgan, B. P. and Walport, M. J., Complement deficiency and disease, *Immunol. Today*, 12, 301, 1991.
7. Howard, P. F., Hochberg, M. C., Bias, W. B., Arnett, F. C., and McLean, R. H., Relationship between C null genes. HLA-D region antigens and genetic susceptibility to systemic lupus erythematosus in Caucasian and Black Americans, *Am. J. Med.*, 81, 187, 1986.
8. Hebert, L. A., Cosio, F. G., and Birmingham, D. J., The role of the complement system in renal injury, *Semin. Nephrol.*, 12, 408, 1992.
9. Davies, K. A., Schifferli, J. A., and Walport, M. J., Complement deficiency and immune complex disease, *Springer Semin. Immunopathol.*, 15, 397, 1994.
10. Farries, T. C. and Atkinson, J. P., Evolution of the complement system, *Immunol. Today*, 12, 295, 1991.
11. Hobart, M. J., Fernie, B., and DiScipio, R. G., Structure of the Human C6 Gene, *Biochemistry*, 32, 6198, 1993.
12. Reid, K. B. M. and Turner, M. W., Mammalian lectins in activation and clearance mechanisms involving the complement system, *Springer Semin. Immunopathol.*, 15, 307, 1994.
13. Torbohm, I., Schonermark, M., Wingen, A.-M, Berger, B., Rother, K., and Hausch, G. M., C5b-8 and C5b-9 modulate the collagen release of human glomerular epithelial cells, *Kidney Int.*, 37, 1098, 1990.
14. Frank, M. M. and Fries, L. F., The role of complement in inflamation and phagocytosis, *Immunol. Today*, 12, 322, 1991.

15. Isenman, D. E. and Young, J. R., The molecular basis for the difference in immune hemolysis activity of the Chido and Rodgers isotype of human complement component C4, *J. Immunol.*, 132, 3019, 1984.
16. Welch, T. R., Beischerl, L., Balakrishnan, K., Quinlan, M., and West, C. D., Major histocompatibility complex extended haplotypes in membrano-proliferative glomerulonephritis, *N. Engl. J. Med.*, 314, 1476, 1986.
17. Fielder, A. H. L., Walport, M. J., Batchelor, J. R., Rynes, R. I., Black, C. M., Dodi, I. A., and Hughes, G. R. D., Family study of the major histocompatibility complex in patients with systemic lupus erythematosus: importance of null alleles of C4A and C4B in determining disease susceptibility, *Br. Med. J.*, 286, 425, 1983.
18. Hauptmann, G., Trappeiner, G., and Schifferli, J. A., Inherited deficiency of the fourth component of human complement, *Immunodefic. Rev.*, 1, 3, 1988.
19. Batchelor, J. R., Fielder, A. H., and Walport, M. J., Family study of the major histocompatibility complex in HLA DR3 negative patients with systemic lupus erythematosus, *Clin. Exp. Immunol.*, 70, 364, 1987.
20. Erdei, A. F., and George, G. J., The role of C3 in the immune response, *Immunol. Today*, 12, 332, 1991.
21. Pillemer, L.L., Blum, I. H., Lepow, O. A., Ross, E. W., Todd, and Wardlaw, A. C., The properdin system and immunity. I. Demonstration and isolation of a new serum protein, *Science*, 120, 279, 1954.
22. Götze, O. and Müller-Eberhard, H. J., The C3-activator system: an alternate pathway of complement activation, *J. Exp. Med.*, 134, 905, 1971.
23. Spitzer, R. E., Vallota, E. H., Forristal, J., Sudopa, E., Stitzel, A., Davis, N. P., and West, C. D., Serum C3 lytic systems in patients with glomerulonephritis, *Science*, 164, 436, 1969.
24. Spies, T., Blanck, G., Bresnahan, M. et al., A new cluster of genes within the human major histocompatibility complex, *Science*, 243, 214, 1989.
25. Moulds, J. M., Krych, M., Holers, V. M., Liszewski, M. K., and Atkinson, J. P., Genetics of the complement system and rheumatic diseases, *Rheumat. Dis. Clin. North Am.*, 18, 893, 1992.
26. Campbell, R. D. and Law, A. SK, Structure, organization, and regulation of the complement genes, *Annu. Rev. Immunol.*, 6, 161, 1988.
27. Awdeh, J. L., Raum, D., Yunis, E. J., and Alper, C. A., Extended HLA/complement allele haplotypes: Evidence for T/t-like complex in man, *Proc. Natl. Acad. Sci. U.S.A.*, 80, 259, 1983.
28. Johnson, C. A., Densen, P., Huford, R. K., Colten, H. R., and Wetzel, A. A., Type I Human complement C2 deficiency, *J. Biol. Chem.*, 267, 9347, 1992.
29. Sullivan, K. E., Petri, M. A., Schmeckpeper, B. J., McLean, R. H., Winkelstein, A., and Jerry, A., Prevalence of a mutation causing C2 deficiency in systemic lupus erythematosus, *J. Rheumatol.*, 21, 1128, 1994.
30. Schreiber, R. D. and Müller-Eberhard, H. J., Fourth component of complement. Description of a three polypeptide chain structure, *J. Exp. Med.*, 140, 1324, 1974.
31. Gigli, I, von Zabern, I. and Porter, R. R., The isolation and structure of C4, the fourth component of complement, *Biochem. J.*, 165, 439, 1977.
32. Kaufman, K. M., Snider, J. V., Spurr, N. K., Schwartz, C. E., and Sodetz, J. M., Chromosomal assignment of genes encoding the alpha, beta and gamma subunits of human complement protein C8. Identification of a close physical linkage between the alpha and beta loci, *Genomics*, 5, 475, 480.
33. Jeremiah, S. J., West, L. F., Davis, M. B., Povey, S., Carritt, B., and Fey, G., Assignment of human complement component C5 to chromosome 9, *Cytogenet. Cell Genet.*, 46, 634, 1987.
34. Lemons, R. S., Le Beau, M. M., Tack, B. F., and Wetsel, R. A., Chromosomal mapping of the gene encoding the fifth component of human complement, *Cytogenet. Cell Genet.*, 46, 647, 1987.

35. Jeremiah, S. J., Abbott, C. M., Murad, Z., Povey, S., Thomas, H. J., Solomon, E., DiScipio, R. G., and Fey, G. H., The assignment of the genes coding for human complement components C6 and C7 to chromonsome 5, *Ann. Hum. Genet.*, 54, 141, 1990.

36. Kalli, K. R., Hsu, P., and Fearon, D. T., Therapeutic uses of recombinant complement protein inhibitors, *Springer Semin. Immunopathol.*, 15, 417, 1994.

37. Mauff, G., Brenden, M., Braun-Stilwell, M., Doxiadia, G., Giles, C. M., Hauptmann, G., Rittner, C., Schneider, P. M., Stradmann-Bellinghausen, B., and Uring-Lambert, B., C4 reference typing reports, *Complement Inflammation*, 7, 193, 1990.

38. Belt, K. T., Carrol, M. C., and Porter, R. R., The structural basis of the multiple forms of human complement C4, *Cell*, 36, 907, 1984.

39. Yu, C. Y., The complete exon-intron structure of a human complement component *C4A* gene. DNA sequences, polymorphism, and linkage to the 21-hydroxylase gene, *J. Immunol.*, 146, 1057, 1991.

40. Kim, Y. U., Carroll, M. C., Isenman, D. E., Nonaka, Masaru, P. P., Takeda, J., Inoue, K., and Kinoshita, T., Covalent binding of C3b to C4b within the classical complement pathway C5 convertase, *J. Biol. Chem.*, 267, 4171, 1992.

41. Anderson, M. J., Milner, C. M., and Cotton, R. G. H., Campbell, R. D., The coding sequence of the hemolytically inactive C4A6 allotype of human complement component C4 reveals that a single arginine to tryptophan substitution at β-chain residue 458 is the likely cause of the defect, *J. Immunol.*, 148, 2795, 1992.

42. Ebanks, R. O., Jaikaran, A. S. I., Carroll, M. C., Anderson, M. J., Campbell, R. D., and Isenman, D. E., A single arginine to tryptophan interchange at β-chain residue 458 of human complement component C4 accounts for the defect in classical pathway C5 convertase activity of allotype C4A6, *J. Immunol.*, 148, 2803, 1992.

43. McLean, R. H., Niblack, G., Julian, B., Wang, T., Wyatt, R., Phillips, J. A. III., Collins, T. S., Winkelstein, J., and Valle, D., Hemolytically inactive C4B complement allotype caused by a proline to leucine mutation in the C5-binding site, *J. Biol. Chem.*, 44, 27727, 1994.

44. Awdeh, A. L., Raum, D., and Alper, C. A., Genetic polymorphism of human complement C4 and detection of heterozygotes, *Nature, (London)*, 282, 205, 1979.

45. Barba, G., Rittner, C. and Schneider, P. M., Genetic Basis of Human Complement C4A Deficiency, *J. Clin. Invest.*, 91, 1681, 1992.

46. Behrman, R. E. and Vaughan, V. C., III, *Nelson Textbook of Pediatrics*, 13th ed., W. B. Saunders, Philadelphia, 1987, 1540.

47. Schur, P. H. and Sandsen, J., Immunologic factors and clinical activity in systemic lupus erythematosus, *N. Engl. J. Med.*, 278, 533, 1968.

48. Kohler, P. F. and ten Bensel, R., Serial complement component alterations in acute glomerulonephritis and systemic lupus erythematosus, *Clin. Exp. Immunol.*, 4, 191, 1969.

49. West, C. D., Northway, J. D., and Davis, N. C., Serum levels of beta-1-C globulin, a complement component, in the nephritides, lipoid nephrosis and other conditions, *J. Clin. Invest.*, 43, 1507, 1964.

50. Gewerz, H., Pickering, R. J., Mergenhagen, S. E., and Good, R. A., The complement profile in acute glomerulonephritis, systemic lupus erythematosus and hypocomplementemic chronic glomerulonephritis, *Int. Arch. Allergy Immunol.*, 34, 556, 1968.

51. Varade, W. S., Forristal, J., and West, C. D., Patterns of complement activation in idiopathic membranoproliferative glomerulonephritis types I, II, and III, *Am. J. Kidney Dis.*, 16, 196, 1990.

52. McLean, R. H., Complement and glomerulonephritis — an update, *Pediatr. Nephrol.*, 7, 226, 1993.

53. Matsell, D. G., Roy, S. III., Tamerius, J. D., Morrow, P. R., Kolb, W. P., and Wyatt, R. J., Plasma terminal complement complexes in acute poststreptococcal glomerulonephritis, *Am. J. Kidney Dis.*, 17, 311, 1991.

54. Hebert, L. E.,Cosio, F. G., and Neff, J. C. Diagnostic significance of hypocomplementemia, *Kidney Int.*, 39, 811, 1991.

55. Strife, C. F., McAdams, A. J., McEnery, P. T., and West, C. D., Hypocomplementemic and normocomplementemic acute nephritis in children: a comparison with respect to etiology, clinical manifestations, and glomerular morphology, *Pediatrics*, 84, 29, 1974.

56. Michael, A. F., McLean, R. H., Roy, L. P., Westberg, N. G., Hoyer, J. R., Fish, A. J., and Vernier, R. L. Immunologic aspects of the nephrotic syndrome, *Kidney Int.*, 3, 105, 1973.

57. McLean, R. H., Forsgren, A., Björkstén, B., Kim, Y., Quie, P. G., and Michael, A. F., Decreased serum factor B concentration associated with decreased opsonization of *Escherichia coli*, in the idiopathic nephrotic syndrome, *Pediatr. Res.*, 11, 910, 1977.

58. Strife, F. S., Jackson, E. C., Forristal, J., and West, C. D., Effect of the nephrotic syndrome on the concentration of serum complement components, *Am. J. Kidney Dis.*, 8, 37, 1986.

59. Reid, K. B., Deficiency of the first component of human complement, *Immunodefic. Rev.*, 1, 247, 1988.

60. Hassig, G. A., Borel, J. F., and Amman, P., Essential hypocomplementemia, *Pathol. Microbiol.*, 27, 542, 1964.

61. Inai, S., Akagaki, Y., Moriyama, T., Fukumori, Y., and Yoshimura, K., Ohnoki, S., Yamaguchi, H., Inherited deficiencies of the late-acting complement components, *Int. Arch. Allergy Immunol.*, 90, 274, 1989.

62. Batchelor, J. R., Fielder, A.H., and Walport M.J., Family study of the major histocompatibility complex in HLA DR3 negative patients with systemic lupus erythematosus, *Clin. Exp. Immunol.*, 70, 364, 1987.

63. Arnett, F. C. and Reveille, J. D., Genetics of systemic lupus erythematosus, *Rheum. Dis. Clin. North Am.*, 18, 865, 1992.

64. Rosse, W., Phosphatidylinositol-linked proteins and paraxysmal nocturnal hemoglobinuria, *Blood*, 75, 1595, 1990.

65. Mancini, G., Carbonara, A. O., and Heremans, J. F. Immunochemical quantitation of antigens by single radial immunodiffusion, *Immunochemistry*, 2, 235, 1965.

66. Alexander, R. L., Comparison of radial immunodiffusion and laser nephelometry for quantitating some serum proteins, *Clin. Chem.*, 26, 314, 1980.

67. Rapp, H. J. and Boros, T., *Molecular Basis of Complement Action*, Meredith Corporation Press, New York, 1970.

68. Whaley, K., Methods in complement for clinical immunologists, in Whaley, K., Ed., Churchill Livingstone, New York, 1985, 77.

69. Harbeck, R. J., Background and general information for complement assays, in Harbeck, R.J. and Giclas P.C., Eds., *Diagnostic Immunology Laboratory Manual*, Raven Press, New York, 1991.

70. Kohler, P. F. and Muller-Eberhard, H. J., Metabolism of human C1q. Studies in hypogammaglobulinemia, myeloma and systemic lupus erythematosus, *J. Clin. Invest.*, 51, 868, 1972.

71. Gochman, N., Beckman, Inc., personal communication, March 11, 1994.

72. Gardinali, M., Padalino, P., Vesconi, S., Calcagno, A., Ciappellano, S., Conciato, L., Chiara, O., Agostoni, A., and Nespoli, A., Complement activation and polymorphonuclear neutrophil leukocyte elastase in sepsis. Correlation with severity of disease, *Arch. Surg.*, 127, 1219, 1992.

73. West, C.D., Relative value of serum C3 and C4 levels in predicting relapse in systemic lupus erythematosus, *Am. J. Kidney Dis.*, 18, 686, 1991.

74. Welch, T. R., Beischel, L., Berry, A., Forristal, J., and West, C. D., The effect of null C4 alleles on complement function, *Clin. Immunol. Immunopathol.*, 34, 316, 1985.

75. Abou-Ragheb, H. H., Williams, A. J., Brown, C. B., and Milford-Ward, A., Plasma levels of the anaphylatoxins C3a and C4a in patients with IgA nephropathy/Henoch-Schonlein nephritis, *Nephron*, 62, 22, 1992.

76. Bergh, K. and Iversen, O. J., Production of monoclonal antibodies against the human anaphylatoxin C5a des Arg and their application in the neoepitope-specific sandwich-ELISA for the quantification of C5a des Arg in plasma, *J. Immunol. Methods*, 152, 79, 1992.

77. West, C.D., Nephritic factors predispose to chronic glomerulonephritis. *Am. J. Kidney Dis.*, 24, 956, 1994.

78. Kolb, W. P., Morrow, P. R., and Tamerius, J. D., Ba and Bb fragments of factor B activation: fragment production, biological activities, neo-epitope expression and quantitation in clinical samples, *Complement Inflammation*, 6, 175, 1989.

79. Hiemstra, P. S., Langeler, E., Compier, B., Keepers, Y., Leijh, J., van den Barselaar, M. Th., Overbosch, D., and Daha, M., Complete and partial deficiencies of complement factor D in a Dutch family, *J. Clin. Invest.*, 84, 1957, 1989.

80. Alper, C. A., Abramson, N., Johnson R. B., Jr., Jandl, J., and Rosen F. S., Increased susceptibility to infection associated with abnormalities of complement mediated functions and of the third component of complement (C3), *N. Engl. J. Med.*, 282, 349, 1970.

81. Davis, A. E., III, Hereditary and acquired deficiencies of C1 inhibitor, *Immunodefic. Rev.*, 1, 207, 1989.

82. Mandle, R., Baron, C., Roux, E., Sundel, R., Gelfand, J., Aulak, K., Davis, A. E., III, Rosen, F. S., and Bing, D. H., Acquired C1 inhibitor deficiency as a result of an autoantibody to the reactive center region of C1 inhibitor, *J. Immunol.*, 152, 4680, 1994.

83. West, C.D., The complement profile in clinical medicine, *Complement Inflammation*, 6, 49, 1989.

84. Welch, T.R., Forristal, J., and Beischel, L., Relationship between the component and regulatory proteins of the classical pathway C3 convertase, *J. Lab. Clin. Med.*, 107, 529, 1986.

85. Daha, M.R., Fearon, D.T., and Austen, K.F., C3 nephritic factor (C3 NeF). Stabilization of fluid phase and cell bound alternative pathway convertase, *J. Immunol.*, 116, 1, 1976.

86. Morgan, B. P. and Meri, S., Membrane proteins that protect against complement lysis, *Springer Semin. Immunopathol.*, 15, 369, 1994.

Chapter **9**

EVALUATION OF PHAGOCYTIC CELL DISORDERS

Naynesh R. Kamani and Steven D. Douglas

CONTENTS

0-8493-0134-3/97/$0.00+$.50

I. INTRODUCTION

The polymorphonuclear leukocyte and the mononuclear phagocyte constitute the major phagocytic cells of the body. They play an
important role in host defense against microbial infections. Neutrophils
are the primary line of defense against bacterial and fungal infections
and are the first cells to arrive at the site of an infection. Phagocytes
arise from the myeloid stem cell, which in turn is derived from the
pluripotent stem cell within the bone marrow. For phagocytic cells to
be able to function properly in their role as antimicrobial effector cells,
they need to get from the blood stream to extracellular sites of infection.
This migration of neutrophils and monocytes occurs via a series of
steps that includes adhesion to endothelial cells, diapedesis through
the endothelial cells into the extravascular space, directed migration
along a chemotactic gradient (chemotaxis), engulfment of the organism,
and subsequent phagocytosis and intracellular killing within the pha-
gosome. These processes require the normal expression and functioning of a myriad of cell surface receptors and ligands, a number of
cytoskeletal proteins, intact degranulation of cytoplasmic granules, and
a normal phagocyte oxidative respiratory burst. Abnormalities of any
of these mechanisms or pathways can result in disorders of phagocytic
cell function. This review will provide a brief overview of tests available
to evaluate these different aspects of phagocytic cell function and a
description of the disorders in which these tests of neutrophil and
monocyte function are abnormal. For a detailed discussion of the
molecular defects, clinical features, and management of these disorders,
the reader is referred to comprehensive reviews of these disorders.[1-3]

II. ASSESSMENT OF PHAGOCYTIC FUNCTION

In the peripheral blood, mature neutrophils and a few band forms (immature neutrophils) and mononuclear phagocytes or monocytes comprise the bulk of the phagocytic cells. The circulating neutrophil pool is in equilibrium with the marrow storage pool so that the number of circulating neutrophils remains relatively constant, except under abnormal circumstances. The marrow storage pool of neutrophils and band forms, consists of 2 to 8×10^9 cells per kilogram of body weight.[4] It takes approximately a week for mature neutrophils to develop from precursor cells in the bone marrow. In an adult, approximately 100 billion neutrophils are produced daily. Of the neutrophils in the blood, there are roughly equal numbers of marginated and circulating cells. The half-life of the neutrophil in the circulation is about 6 h.[5] The absolute neutrophil count in the peripheral blood ranges anywhere from 1500 to 5000 cells per cubic millimeter. The determination of the white blood cell count and the differential count is the most commonly performed laboratory test. Abnormalities in the peripheral blood neutrophil count are quite common. A detailed discussion of the relevance of abnormal findings in the numbers of neutrophils in the circulation is beyond the scope of this chapter, but is thoroughly reviewed in other recent sources.[2,3]

Qualitative defects of neutrophil function are relatively rare. It is thus not surprising that most clinical laboratories do not perform assays of neutrophil function. The evaluation of patients in whom neutrophil dysfunction is suspected thus requires the referral of the patient to institutions with physicians interested in the evaluation of such patients and available clinical immunology laboratories or, alternatively, the sending of blood samples to such institutional laboratories. Unlike lymphocytes, neutrophils do not survive well at room temperatures for long periods of time. It is thus imperative that tests of neutrophil function be performed on fresh samples of blood or on samples that are a few hours old. Samples shipped overnight for evaluation of neutrophil function will not yield interpretable results for most assays of neutrophil function.

Some assays of neutrophil function can be performed on samples of whole blood, whereas others require the isolation of neutrophils. There are a number of techniques currently in use for the isolation of neutrophils. One method utilizes Ficoll-Hypaque sedimentation of anticoagulated blood to remove mononuclear cells followed by dextran sedimentation to remove erythrocytes. Residual erythrocytes can then be eliminated with hypotonic lysis to yield relatively pure populations of neutrophils. A one-step method using a discontinuous Ficoll-Hypaque gradient has also been described wherein the neutrophils are isolated in a discrete band.[6-8]

III. LEUKOCYTE ADHESION

Leukocyte adhesion to endothelial cells constitutes the first step in the migration of leukocytes to extravascular sites of tissue damage or infection. Biochemical messages generated from sites of inflammation result in the activation of both endothelial cells and phagocytic cells, leading to an interaction between their cell surface adhesion molecules (Figure 1).[9] Activation of neutrophils results in an up-regulation of certain cell surface receptors and an increase in oxidative burst activity. In the absence of efficient adhesion to vascular endothelial cells, phagocytic cells are unable to successfully migrate to tissue sites of infection, thus resulting in a susceptibility to recurrent bacterial and fungal infections. Neutrophil adhesion can be evaluated by performing assays designed to detect the presence of adhesion molecules on neutrophil cell surfaces and by measuring neutrophil adherence in *in vitro* assays. Disorders of leukocyte adhesion result in abnormal adhesion of neutrophils to cell surfaces and in abnormalities in neutrophil motility.

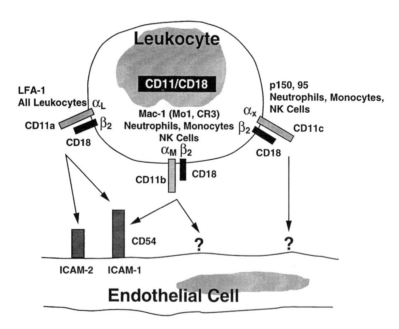

Figure 1
The leukocyte CD11/CD18 complex and its endothelial ligands. LFA-1, lymphocyte function-associated antigen-1; Mac-1, macrophage antigen-1; Mo 1, monocyte antigen 1; CR3, complement receptor type 3; ICAM, intercellular adhesion molecule. (From Harlan, J.M., *Clin. Immunol. Immunopathol.*, 67, S16, 1993. With permission.)

A. Assessment of Adhesion Receptors

Although a number of receptors are involved in mediating adhesion between neutrophils and endothelial cell surfaces, the most important interaction appears to occur between the β2-integrin CD11a/CD18 and CD11b/CD18 molecules on neutrophils and their corresponding ligand, the intercellular adhesion molecule (ICAM-1 and -2) on the endothelial cells. Alternate pathways of neutrophil adherence do exist but are poorly understood.[10] The surface expression of CD11/CD18 molecules on neutrophils can be assessed by using monoclonal antibodies to the α or β chain of the heterodimer. The CD11/CD18 complex exists in three forms characterized by three different α chains a, b, and c. All three β2-integrin molecules have different alpha chains that are noncovalently associated with a common beta chain, CD18.[11-12]

B. Assays of Neutrophil Adhesion

There are a number of assays currently in use for the evaluation of neutrophil adhesion. These *in vitro* assays all involve the assessment of neutrophil adhesion to artificial surfaces such as nylon wool, glass surfaces and plastic surfaces. These assays, however, are *in vitro* models and do not duplicate *in vivo* conditions. Available data suggest that most methods utilized to isolate neutrophils can induce neutrophil activation which may subsequently affect their performance in these assays.[13] McGregor described the first technique for the assay of granulocyte adherence to nylon fibers in 1974. Briefly, venous blood is passed through pipettes packed with nylon fibers prewarmed to 37°C before use. The percentage of granulocyte adherence is then calculated by quantifying the numbers of neutrophils in the effluent compared to the number of neutrophils in the original sample.[14] A number of modifications of this technique have been developed.

Impairment in adherence of neutrophils and monocytes in *in vitro* assays has been seen in two leukocyte adhesion deficiency syndromes, LAD I and LAD II.[15-17] Decreased adherence has also been reported in neutrophils from pre-term neonates and full-term neonates. This may be related to a partial deficiency of CD11b/CD18 on neonatal neutrophils.[18-20] Secondary abnormalities of granulocyte adherence have been reported following ethanol ingestion and corticosteroid therapy.

IV. LEUKOCYTE ADHESION DEFICIENCY SYNDROME

The LAD type I syndrome is characterized clinically by recurrent serious bacterial infections from early infancy, delayed separation of the umbilical cord, and in the laboratory by leukocytosis and defects of neutrophil and monocyte adhesion and chemotaxis. It is an autosomal recessive disorder characterized by mutations in the gene coding for the common β chain. This leads to a defective expression of all three heterodimers (CD11a/18, CD11b/18, and CD11c/18) in affected patients. Absent (<1% expression) heterodimer expression results in a severe phenotype that is fatal in early childhood, and low surface expression (up to 30% expression) leads to a moderate phenotype and the potential for survival into adulthood. Heterozygotes for LAD I are clinically asymptomatic. Since neutrophils are unable to marginate or exit the blood vessels, affected patients often have very high circulating neutrophil counts even in the absence of infection.[15,16]

Several abnormalities of neutrophil and monocyte function result from the absence of CD11/18 adhesion molecules. These include defective adherence to plastic or glass surfaces, defective chemotaxis and aggregation, defective phagocytosis of iC3b-coated particles, and a defective respiratory burst in response to particulate stimuli. The severity of phagocytic cell dysfunction tends to correlate inversely with the degree of adhesion molecule expression. In severely affected patients, the absence of LFA-1 on lymphocytes leads to a number of defects in *in vitro* lymphocyte function, including responses to mitogens, T and natural killer (NK) cell cytotoxicity, and antibody dependent cellular cytotoxicity. These defects may be due to impaired adhesion of T cells to antigen-presenting cells or secondary to defects in monocyte function. These *in vitro* defects of lymphocyte function do not appear to have *in vivo* relevance.

A. Leukocyte Adhesion Deficiency Type II

Etzioni et al. have recently described a syndrome of recurrent infections in two unrelated boys characterized by elevated neutrophil counts and defective neutrophil adhesion and chemotaxis. Their phagocytic cells had normal levels of expression of β-integrins but failed to express Sialyl-Lewis-x (SLeX), a ligand for P-selectin and E-selectin on endothelial cells. Patients with this disorder are believed to have a general defect in fucose metabolism which may involve red blood cells as well. Unlike the β-integrins, SLeX is not expressed on lymphocytes so that lymphocyte functions are preserved in these children.[17,21] Monocyte functions in these patients have not been studied in detail, but migration was reduced *in vivo* in skin-chamber studies.

V. NEUTROPHIL CHEMOTAXIS

Following successful adhesion to endothelial cells and their subsequent diapedesis through the blood vessel wall, neutrophils move to sites of tissue damage and infection along a chemotactic gradient generated by the presence of chemoattractants at those sites. Chemotaxis is the process by which phagocytic cells move in a directed fashion in response to a chemical gradient. Movement in the absence of such a gradient is referred to as random migration or chemokinesis. The primary event in chemotaxis is the sensing of chemical gradients via receptors on neutrophil cell surfaces for chemoattractants such as C5a, platelet activating factor (PAF), and leukotriene B4 (LTB4), etc. The synthetic N-formyl methionyl peptide, f-Met-Leu-Phe (fMLP), serves as a potent chemoattractant for the *in vitro* assessment of chemotaxis. Following interaction of chemoattractants with receptors, there is signal transduction resulting in changes in the neutrophil cytoskeleton. Sequential changes in the actin cytoskeleton lead to lamellar protrusion and a change in the neutrophil shape from spherical to bipolar. These protrusions or lamellipodia contain the necessary molecular machinery including actin microfilaments and other proteins necessary for locomotion.[22,23] Defects in any of the above processes can lead to abnormal neutrophil chemotaxis.

A. Rebuck Skin Window

The Rebuck skin window is the only technique available to assess neutrophil function *in vivo*. Briefly, the cellular exudate at the site of an iatrogenic skin abrasion is analyzed with a glass slide or fluid-filled chamber at specified time intervals. In disorders of neutrophil adherence or chemotaxis, no neutrophils will be seen in the inflammatory cell exudate for longer than 3 h after an abrasion.[7,24] With the development of specific assays for adhesion proteins, neutrophil adherence and chemotaxis, this technique is less frequently utilized. It has the advantage that it is relatively simple to perform and will give abnormal results if either neutrophil adherence or chemotaxis is defective. The technique, however, is poorly standardized and has inconsistent reproducibility. *In vivo* migration of monocytes, which is maximal after 18 to 20 h, can also be studied by this technique.

B. *In Vitro* Assays of Chemotaxis

A number of assays have been developed to measure random neutrophil migration and chemotaxis. The two most commonly used assays employ modifications of the Boyden chamber technique[25] or the "under agarose" method. Both methods require the use of purified populations of neutrophils or monocytes. The Boyden chamber measures the migration of phagocytic cells through cellulose nitrate filters, whereas the under agarose method assesses movement over a plastic surface under an agarose layer.[6,26] Quantitation of chemotaxis can be expressed either as distance values of migration or as numbers of migrating cells both spontaneously and in response to chemoattractants. Both assays fail to distinguish adhesion from true neutrophil locomotion. The polarization assay, which is able to make this distinction, measures the change in the shape of phagocytic cells in suspension in response to the addition of chemoattractants.[22]

VI. DISORDERS OF CHEMOTAXIS

Primary defects of phagocytic cell adhesion (e.g., leukocyte adhesion deficiency) will lead to defects in neutrophil chemotaxis when measured by either *in vivo* or *in vitro* techniques. Transient disorders of neutrophil chemotaxis have been seen in association with a number of viral and other infections and in a variety of other noninfectious conditions. These conditions range from immunologic diseases such as hypogammaglobunemia and complement deficiencies to neoplastic diseases, diabetes, SLE, Schwachman syndrome, Down syndrome, and other diseases.[27,28]

Abnormal neutrophil chemotaxis occurs in most patients with Chediak-Higashi syndrome (CHS). Although the precise underlying defect leading to defective chemotaxis in CHS is unknown, recent evidence suggests that CHS neutrophils fail to polarize in response to chemoattractants. Additional factors contributing to defective chemotactic responses in CHS patients may include the nondeformability of large granule-containing cells and hyperadhesiveness.[22,28] Chemotactic defects can also be demonstrated in some patients with the hyper IgE syndrome. Even in patients in whom chemotactic defects can be documented, the defect appears to be intermittently present. An inhibitor of phagocyte chemotaxis produced by mononuclear cells from patients with the hyper IgE syndrome has been demonstrated in certain patients.[29] It has been partially characterized as being heat stable at 56°C for 30 min and having a molecular weight of 30,000 to 40,000.

Primary neutrophil chemotactic defects have been identified in two patients with distinctly different disorders of host defense. The first was an infant who developed severe recurrent bacterial infections and had omphalitis, marked leukocytosis, and impaired wound healing. LAD could not be documented. Her neutrophils failed to polarize or undergo chemotaxis in response to a number of chemoattractants including PAF, LTB4, and fMLP. Functional responses mediated via chemoattractant receptors including the oxidative burst, degranulation of primary granules, and actin polarization in response to fMLP, were abnormal.[30]

A male infant previously diagnosed as having neutrophil actin dysfunction (NAD) has been confirmed as having an autosomal recessively inherited disorder of neutrophil actin assembly. The infant had a severe defect of neutrophil motility and opsonophagocytosis but normal oxidative burst activity. The inability of the patient's neutrophils to polymerize actin into filaments upon stimulation led to the abnormal neutrophil function and a susceptibility to uncontrollable bacterial infection.[31,32]

A novel inherited syndrome of actin dysfunction has been described in a male infant with severe, recurrent fungal infections. Although both disorders of neutrophil actin dysfunction result in abnormalities in actin polymerization and microfilamentous cytoskeleton, there are distinct clinical, functional, and biochemical features unique to the recently described patient. The exact biochemical defect could not be ascertained but patient neutrophils demonstrated a marked decrease in an 89-kDa protein and an increase in a 47-kDa protein.[33]

VII. DISORDERS OF PHAGOCYTOSIS

After phagocytic cells arrive at the site of infection and prior to intracellular killing, these cells have to be able to engulf and ingest microorganisms. This process of phagocytosis is enhanced by the successful binding of molecules on the microbial cell wall to specific receptors on the phagocyte cell surface. The most important of these are the Fc receptors for IgG1 and IgG3 and receptors for complement components CR1 and CR3. These receptors facilitate the ingestion of opsonized particles and microorganisms by binding opsonized microorganisms. This is followed by the fusion of the phagocytic vacuole and the plasma membrane into the phagolysosome.

The rate of phagocytosis is assessed by measuring the decrease in the number of opsonized extracellular organisms. Several assays have been designed to differentiate between particles that are intracellular, i.e., successfully phagocytosed, and those that are adherent to the surface. Differentiation can be effected by using enzymes (e.g., lysostaphin) that digest extracellularly without penetrating the neutrophil cell wall or by using dyes that stain only uningested organisms. Differential labeling of the cells and the particles being ingested allows accurate assessment of phagocytosis. A number of flow cytometric methods for evaluating phagocytosis have been recently described using fluorescent dyes to stain target microorganisms.[34,35]

There is no known inherited disorder of host defense that is characterized by a primary defect in neutrophil phagocytosis. It is generally believed that such a defect would be incompatible with life since the process of phagocytosis is a very primitive cell function. There are a number of disorders, however, where phagocytosis may be abnormal. In LAD1, an absence or severe deficiency of CR3 (CD11b/CD18) expression on phagocytic cells leads to a secondary defect in particle phagocytosis. Deficiencies of opsonins, i.e., immunoglobulins or complement components, or serum factors may also result in abnormal phagocytosis.

VIII. DEFECTS OF NEUTROPHIL GRANULES

Human polymorphonuclear neutrophils contain three types of cytoplasmic granules. The primary or azurophil granules are the larger and more dense membrane-bound structures which contain a variety of degradative enzymes, including acid hydrolases and myeloperoxidase, and a number of cationic proteins, including the defensins. They have a limiting membrane measuring 70 to 90 Å in width. The secondary or specific granules are smaller but more numerous. They contain lactoferrin and vitamin B12-binding protein. A third type of granule, the tertiary granule, is similar to specific granules but more active in the presence of minimal stimuli that would otherwise not evoke responses from specific granules.[36]

Neutrophil granules play an important role in host defense against a variety of microorganisms. Deficiencies of different granule components result in varying degrees of neutrophil dysfunction ranging from a mild increase in infections to severe recurrent bacterial infections. The demonstration of quantitative defects in the secretion of granule components in the presence of known associated structural defects is diagnostic for the presence of these disorders. Assessment of degranulation is, however, rarely necessary because the abnormalities involving neutrophil granules can be more easily diagnosed by light or electron microscopic techniques. There are at least three disorders of neutrophils in which defects of granules occur. These are (1) myeloperoxidase (MPO) deficiency; (2) specific granule deficiency and (3) Chediak-Higashi syndrome.

A. Myeloperoxidase Deficiency

This is a relatively common autosomal recessive disorder characterized by a partial or complete absence of the iron-containing protein myeloperoxidase in the azurophil granules of neutrophils and monocytes. Myeloperoxidase participates in microbicidal functions by combining with hydrogen peroxide to produce an enzyme–substrate complex that oxidizes halides to form agent(s) toxic to a variety of microorganisms.

TABLE 1

Abnormalities of Neutrophil Function

Disease	Neutrophil Number	Morphology	Adherence	Chemotaxis	Phagocytosis	Granule Products	Oxidative Burst	Microbicidal Actvity
CGD	↔ or ↑	Normal	Normal	Normal	↔	Normal	Absent	Absent
LAD I	↑↑	Normal	Abnormal	Abnormal	Abnormal	Normal	↓a	Normal
LAD II	↑↑	Normal	Abnormal	Abnormal	Abnormal	Normal	Normal	Normal
CHS	↓	Abnormal	Normal	↓	Abnormal	Abnormal	Normal	Delayed
H IgE	↔	Normal	Normal	↔ or ↓	Normal	Normal	Normal	Normal
SGD	↔	Abnormal	Normal	Normal	Normal	↓↓	Normal	Defective
MPO	↔	Normal	Normal	Normal	↓	↓ MPO	Normal	Delayed
NAD	↔	Normal	Normal	↓	Normal	Normal	Normal	Normal
GSD 1b	↔ or ↓	Normal	Normal	↓	Normal	Normal	↓↓	↓

Note: ↔ = Variable; ↑ = Increased; ↓ = Decreased; CGD = Chronic granulomatous disease; LAD = Leukocyte adhesion deficiency; CHS = Chediak-Higashi syndrome; H IgE = Hyper IgE syndrome; SGD = Specific granule deficiency; MPO = Myeloperoxidase deficiency; NAD = Neutrophil actin dysfunction; GSD = Glycogen storage disease.

a Respiratory burst is abnormal in response to particulate stimuli.

Its frequency is estimated at 1:2000 to 1:4000 of the population and has been noted in healthy blood donors. In the absence of MPO, other antimicrobial mechanisms of the phagocyte compensate for the deficiency in MPO such that the majority of affected patients are asymptomatic. Some patients may suffer from recurrent candidal infections.[37,38]

A diagnosis of MPO deficiency can be made by demonstrating the absence of MPO in phagocytic cells by stains that would normally pick up MPO. Alternatively, automated counters that use MPO to characterize neutrophils will give falsely low neutrophil counts on an automated differential count in MPO-deficient patients. Most automated counters currently in use no longer utilize MPO. Evaluation of neutrophil function reveals a slight lag in phagocyte microbicidal activity. All other facets of phagocyte function are normal including a normal oxidative burst.

B. Specific Granule Deficiency

This is an extremely rare disorder of neutrophils and eosinophils characterized by the absence of specific granules. It results in an increased susceptibility to severe, recurrent infections of the skin, lungs and mucous membranes with *Staphylococcus aureus*, pseudomonas, and candida organisms. The defect appears to arise during granulopoiesis, perhaps at the myelocyte-metamyelocyte stage when the synthesis of primary and secondary granule proteins overlaps. Patients show a defect in the transcription of granular proteins.

Neutrophils from patients with specific granule deficiency demonstrate a number of morphologic nuclear abnormalities including bilobed or multilobed nuclei, and nuclear blebs, pockets, or clefts. Specific granules are significantly deficient or absent. Assays designed to measure specific granule constituents show absence of lactoferrin, alkaline phosphatase, vitamin B12-binding protein, and lysozyme. They also have an almost complete deficiency of defensins, a microbicidal/cytotoxic protein constituent of primary granules. Neutrophils from these patients show abnormalities in neutrophil adherence secondary to problems in receptor up-regulation, and abnormalities in chemotaxis and microbicidal activity.[39-41]

IX. CHEDIAK-HIGASHI SYNDROME

Chediak-Higashi syndrome (CHS) is a rare autosomal recessive disorder characterized by partial oculocutaneous albinism, neurologic deficits, recurrent pyogenic infections, and an increased incidence of

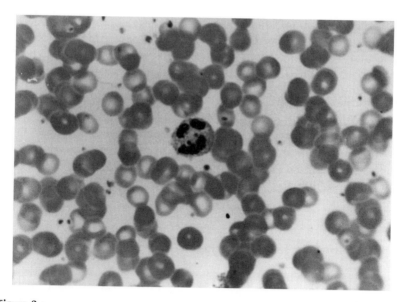

Figure 2
Chediak-Higashi syndrome: polymorphonuclear neutrophil. Note the large cytoplasmic lysosomal granules.

lymphoid malignancies. One of the characteristic findings in affected patients is the presence of giant cytoplasmic membrane-bound granules in phagocytic cells (Figure 2). These giant granules represent fused lysosomal granules. The patients are neutropenic and have demonstrable defects in a number of neutrophil functions. Although they have a normal or enhanced neutrophil oxidative burst, bactericidal assays show delayed or decreased intracellular killing. *In vivo* and *in vitro* neutrophil chemotaxis is also impaired.

Analysis of the neutrophil granules in patients with CHS shows a marked decrease in the amounts of cathepsin G and elastase, both of which are microbicidal/cytotoxic protein constituents of azurophil granules.[41] Although the exact molecular defects contributing to these findings are not known, there appears to be a defect in the regulation of protein synthesis, protein processing, or granule assembly. Investigations of neutrophil granule proteins have shown varying decreases in a number of other proteins, including myeloperoxidase, α-mannosidase, and β-glucuronidase.[42]

X. ASSAYS OF NEUTROPHIL OXIDATIVE METABOLISM

Whenever phagocytic cells are exposed to particulate or soluble stimuli, perturbation of their plasma membranes results in a burst of oxygen consumption. This respiratory oxidative burst is catalyzed by the enzyme NADPH oxidase to produce hydrogen peroxide from molecular oxygen when electrons are transferred from NADPH. This transfer occurs in univalent steps with intermediate production of superoxide anion. The resultant oxidants, superoxide anion (O_2^-), H_2O_2 and $HOCL^-$ are potently microbicidal.[43] The respiratory oxidative burst in neutrophils can be measured by several highly sensitive assays.[44] Although most of these assays are performed in laboratories specializing in neutrophil research, two assays are commonly employed in clinical laboratories. These are the nitroblue tetrazolium (NBT) reduction assay and the flow cytometric assessment of 2',7'-dichlorofluorescin (DCF) oxidation.

A. The Nitroblue Tetrazolium Reduction Assay

This test serves as an excellent screening test for the evaluation of the oxidative burst. It evaluates the ability of neutrophils to reduce NBT dye. In its simplest form, neutrophils in whole blood samples are allowed to adhere to glass slides. They are then incubated in NBT solution in the absence or presence of an agent that activates neutrophils, e.g., opsonized zymosan, lipopolysaccharide, or phorbol myristate acetate (PMA). After a 30-min incubation, the slides are stained and the number of neutrophils with blue formazan (reduced NBT precipitates as blue formazan) are counted.[45] A more quantitative NBT reduction assay can also be performed by using a spectrophotometric assay with neutrophils in suspension.

B. The DCF Oxidation Assay

A flow cytometric assay of DCF oxidation has been used in a number of laboratories for the evaluation of oxidative product formation by neutrophils in response to a stimulus such as PMA. This assay involves the loading of neutrophils with DCF diacetate dye followed by PMA stimulation and subsequent flow cytometric evaluation for fluorescence.[44,46-49] Dihydrorhodamine 123 (DHR) dye can also be used for measuring reactive oxygen species produced during the respiratory burst. DHR 123 is oxidized to a brightly fluorescent compound, rhodamine 123, which localizes to the mitochondria.[50] These assays can be performed in whole blood. They are thus suitable for most clinical laboratories that have flow cytometry capabilities. These flow cytometric assays offer a sensitive and accurate measure of the number of neutrophils that are capable of generating reactive oxygen species.

There are a number of other methods available to quantify the respiratory oxidative burst. These include chemiluminescence assays, iodination, generation of superoxide or hydrogen peroxide, the utilization of glucose via the hexose monophosphate shunt, and microbicidal assays.

C. Microbicidal Assays

Microbicidal assays, which perhaps approximate *in vivo* conditions most closely, are designed to evaluate the ability of patient neutrophils to kill organisms with which the patient is infected. These assays are time consuming and tedious. They measure the reduction in the numbers of viable microorganisms after these have been incubated with patient neutrophils. Since most patients with defects of neutrophil function have recurrent infections with *Staphylococcus aureus*, most *in vitro* bactericidal assays employ these organisms. When phagocytic cells and target bacteria are mixed in the presence of opsonins, intracellular killing of *S. aureus* occurs rapidly, and with normal neutrophil function, more than 90% of the bacteria are killed within 30 min. The number of viable bacteria is quantified by counting the number of colonies growing on agar plates.[6] Flow cytometric assays for measuring phagocytosis and killing of bacteria by polymorphonuclear neutrophils have been developed that allow for the precise evaluation of opsonization and phagocytosis of staphylococcal organisms.[34,35] In this assay, microbial organisms and phagocytes are labeled using different dyes, and phagocytosis is measured by recording dually labeled phagocytes. Using unlabeled phagocytes in parallel, killing of organisms is measured by assessing the decrease in free green fluorescent particles that represent microbial organisms.

XI. CHRONIC GRANULOMATOUS DISEASE

Chronic granulomatous disease is a rare inherited disorder of *ph*agocyte *ox*idative (phox) metabolism characterized by the absence of a respiratory burst in phagocytic cells. Despite this uniform abnormality detectable in all patients with CGD, there is significant heterogeneity in the clinical expression[51] and molecular genetics of this disease.[52] Approximately two thirds of the patients have the x-linked form of the disease with a mutation in the gene for the gp91-phox subunit of the cytochrome b558 component of the NADPH oxidase enzyme. The remaining patients have the autosomal form of the disease with mutations in genes coding for one of the three remaining oxidase components.

TABLE 2

Classification of Chronic Granulomatous Disease (CGD)

Mode of Inheritance	NADPH Component Affected	Gene Locus	Frequency (%)	Defect in Cell-Free System	NBT[a] Score
X linked	gp91-phox	Xp 21.1	60–65	Membrane	0[b]
Autosomal recessive	p22-phox	16p24	7	Membrane	0
Autosomal recessive	p47-phox	7q 11.23	23	Cytosol	0
Autosomal recessive	p67-phox	1q25	6	Cytosol	0

[a] NBT = Nitroblue tetrazolium reduction assay.
[b] A small percentage of these patients have neutrophils that have low levels of oxidase activity; i.e., the cells stain weakly in the NBT test.
Adapted from Cumutte, J.T., *Clin. Immunol. Immunopathol.*, 67, S2, 1993.

These are the p22-phox, p47-phox, or the p67-phox subunits. A classification scheme for CGD based on the component of NADPH oxidase affected is shown in Table 2.[52,53]

The commonest mode of presentation is with recurrent infections of the skin, lungs, gastrointestinal tract and reticuloendothelial organs starting in infancy or early childhood. Since patient phagocytes are unable to kill catalase positive organisms, CGD patients suffer from recurrent bacterial and fungal infections and develop chronic granulomas in the gastrointestinal and genitourinary tracts.

The diagnosis of CGD can be made by demonstrating an absence of a respiratory oxidative burst in phagocytic cells. The NBT slide test or a flow cytometric assay are the best screening tests for this disorder (Figure 3). The diagnosis can be confirmed by additional tests such as abnormal chemiluminescence, absent generation of superoxide, or absence of intracellular killing of catalase positive organisms by neutrophils (Figure 4). In boys in whom an X-linked phenotype of CGD is suspected, carrier states in the mother or female siblings can be documented by the presence of 30 to 70% neutrophils that have a normal oxidative burst upon stimulation in an NBT assay or in a DCF flow cytometric assay. Identification of the genetic defect should be performed to identify new mutations and to confirm the phenotype. These analyses can only be performed in highly specialized research laboratories.

Although fibroblasts obtained at amniocentesis are not suitable for the diagnosis of CGD, prenatal diagnosis can be accomplished by analyzing phagocytes derived from fetal blood sampling. Using either RFLP analysis or cDNA probes, prenatal diagnosis has been performed in early gestation in a number of individuals.[54] Gene therapy of chronic granulomatous disease and other inherited disorders of phagocyte function is now an attainable goal. Peripheral blood-derived hematopoietic progenitors from CGD patients have been used as targets for genetic correction in *in vitro* experiments with some success.[55]

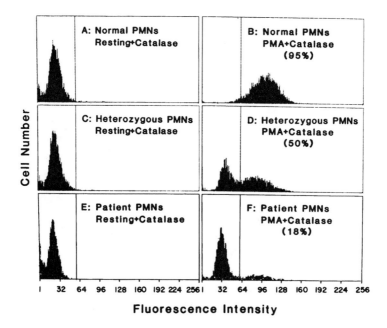

Fluorescence Intensity

Figure 3

Flow cytometric fluorescence histograms of polymorphonuclear neutophils (PMNs) from a normal donor (A and B), from a heterozygous carrier for CGD (C and D), and from her son with CGD who is 58 months after bone marrow transplantation (E and F). PMNs in the absence (A,C,E) or presence (B,D,F) of phorbol myristate acetate (PMA) are illustrated. A total of 3000 cells were analyzed in each assay. Assay allows quantitation of neutrophils with intact oxidative burst. (From Kamani, N. et al., *J. Pediatrics*, 113, 697, 1988. With permission.)

XII. LEUKOCYTE GLUCOSE-6-PHOSPHATE DEHYDROGENASE (G-6PD) DEFICIENCY

Leukocyte G-6-PD catalyzes the first of two reactions that lead to the generation of NADPH, which is the substrate for the respiratory burst oxidase. An absolute or severe (<5% of normal) deficiency of leukocyte G-6-PD thus results in a decrease in respiratory burst activity and a clinical syndrome resembling a milder form of CGD. Even though G-6-PD deficiency is quite common in Mediterranean and African-American individuals, the vast majority of affected patients have levels of leukocyte G-6-PD that do not affect the neutrophil oxidative burst activity. Clinically relevant leukocyte G-6-PD deficiency has been described in only a handful of patients. Deficiencies of other hexose mono-phosphate shunt pathway enzymes such as glutathione reductase can result in abnormalities of respiratory burst activity. These abnormalities,

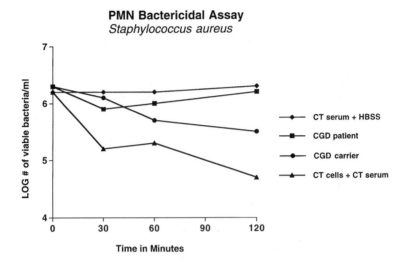

Figure 4

Bactericidal assay using control (CT) or patient (chronic granulomatous disease — CGD) polymorphonuclear neutrophils incubated with *S. aureus* organisms in the presence of control (CT) serum.

however, are probably not clinically relevant, since the rare patients reported with severe glutathione reductase deficiency did not have repeated infections.[56,57]

XIII. GLYCOGEN STORAGE DISEASE TYPE 1B

Glycogen storage disease (GSD), is an inherited disorder in which glucose-6-phosphate cannot be converted to glucose, due to a translocase deficiency. Patients with GSD type 1b variant often have neutropenia and recurrent bacterial infections.[58] Evaluation of phagocyte function in these patients has shown defects in neutrophil chemotaxis, a significant decrease in respiratory burst activity and defective bactericidal activity. Degranulation appears to be normal. Recent studies have shown that these defects in phagocyte function are associated with a decrease in calcium mobilization and calcium stores.[59]

XIV. SECONDARY DEFECTS OF PHAGOCYTE FUNCTION

Varying degrees of impairment of phagocyte chemotaxis and bactericidal activity have been reported in a large number of clinical disorders (Table 3).[28,45,60-65] In many of these conditions, it is unclear if the defect is clinically relevant or whether recurrent infections in these

TABLE 3

Secondary Abnormalities of Neutrophil Function

Disease/Condition	Neutrophil Dysfunction
Neonates	Adherence, degranulation, chemotaxis
Infections	
Viral infections, including HIV	Chemotaxis, killing
Bacterial infections	Chemotaxis
Immunodeficiency	
Wiskott-Aldrich syndrome	Chemotaxis
Hypogammaglobulinemia	Phagocytosis
Complement deficiencies	Phagocytosis
Post bone marrow transplantation	Chemotaxis, killing
Corticosteroid therapy	Adherence, chemotaxis, killing
Malignancies	
Leukemia	Adherence, chemotaxis, phagocytosis, killing
Hodgkin's lymphoma	Chemotaxis
Other malignancies	Chemotaxis
Chromosomal defects	
Down syndrome	Chemotaxis, killing
Monosomy 7	Chemotaxis
Miscellaneous	
Trauma	Chemotaxis
Burns	Chemotaxis, killing
Uremia	Chemotaxis, killing
Diabetes mellitus	Adherence, chemotaxis
Schwachman syndrome	Adherence, chemotaxis, killing
Zinc deficiency	Chemotaxis
Malnutrition	Chemotaxis, phagocytosis, killing
Gaucher disease	Chemotaxis
Alcohol intoxication	Adherence, chemotaxis

conditions are secondary to other associated factors such as malnutrition or unrelated immunologic defects.[66,67] As discussed above, transient defects of neutrophil chemotaxis have been seen in association with a number of viral and bacterial infections. In these situations, reevaluation of phagocyte function after resolution of underlying infection is warranted to document the transient nature of the defect.

XV. SUMMARY

Advances in the understanding of neutrophil and monocyte adhesion, locomotion, phagocytosis, and microbicidal mechanisms have led to a more precise definition of the defects underlying various disorders of phagocytic cell function. It is expected that phagocytic cell dysfunction will be the basis for some heretofore poorly understood disorders of host defense. Defects of phagocyte function present clinically with a propensity to develop recurrent bacterial and fungal infections of the

skin and mucous membranes, lymph nodes, lungs, and reticuloendothelial organs. Heterogeneity in clinical severity is a feature of several
phagocyte dysfunction syndromes and may be secondary to the underlying molecular defect or to the degree of expression of the defective
enzyme or cell surface protein.

Evaluation of phagocyte function should be done in specialized
laboratories with careful interpretation of results of both patient and
control samples. Repeat testing to confirm abnormal results or referral
to research laboratories is highly recommended. Inherited defects of
phagocytic cells usually involve both neutrophils and monocytes,
although it is easier to perform tests on neutrophils because of their
ease of isolation and higher cell numbers. A number of tests of neutrophil function have been developed that allow the assessment of neutrophil function using whole blood samples.

REFERENCES

1. Stiehm, E. R. , *Immunologic Disorders in Infants and Children*, 4th ed., W. B. Saunders,
   Philadelphia, 1995.
2. Williams, W. J., Beutler, E., Erslev, A. J., and Lichtman, M. A., *Hematology*, 4th ed.,
   McGraw-Hill, New York, 1990, 760.
3. Nathan, D. G. and Oski, F. A., *Hematology of Infancy and Childhood*, 4th ed., W. B.
   Saunders, Philadelphia, 1993, 881.
4. Yang, K. D. and Hill, H. R., Neutrophil function disorders: pathophysiology,
   prevention and therapy, *J. Pediatr.*, 119, 343, 1991.
5. Dancey, J., Deubelbeiss, K. A., Harker, L. A., and Finch, C. A., Neutrophil kinetics
   in man, *J. Clin. Invest.*, 58, 705, 1976.
6. Douglas, S. D. and Quie, P. G., *Investigation of Phagocytes in Disease*, Churchill
   Livingstone, New York, 1981.
7. Segal, A. W., Testing neutrophil function, *Clin. Immunol. Allerg.*, 5, 491, 1985.
8. Roos, D. and de Boer, M., Purification and cryopreservation of phagocytes from
   human blood, *Methods Enzymol.*, 132, 225, 1986.
9. Zimmerman, G. A., Prescott, S. M., and Mcintyre, T. M., Endothelial cell interactions with granulocytes: tethering and signaling molecules, *Immunol. Today*, 1992.
10. Furie, M. B., Tancinco, M., and Smith, C. W., Monoclonal antibodies to leukocyte
    integrins CD11a/CD18 and CD11b/CD18 or intercellular adhesion molecule-1
    inhibit chemoattractant-stimulated neutrophil transendothelial migration in vitro,
    Blood, 78, 2089, 1991.
11. Hakkert, B. C., Rentenaar, J. M., van Aken, W. G., Roos, D., and van Mourik, J. A.,
    A three-dimensional model system to study the interactions between human
    leukocytes and endothelial cells, *Eur. J. Immunol.*, 20, 2775, 1990.
12. Etzioni, A., Adhesion molecules in host defense, *Clin. Diagn. Lab. Immunol.*, 1, 1,
    1994.
13. Kuijpers, T. W., Tool, A. T. J., van de Schoot, C. E., Onderwater, J. J. M., Roos, D.,
    and Verhoeven, A. J., Membrane surface antigen expression on neutrophils: a
    reappraisal of the use of surface markers from neutrophil activation, *Blood*, 78,
    1105, 1991.

14. McGregor, R. R., Spagnuolo, P. J., Lentnek, A. L., Inhibition of granulocyte adherence by ethanol, prednisone and aspirin measured with an assay system, *N. Engl. J. Med.*, 291, 642, 1974.

15. Fischer, A., Lisowska-Grospierre, B., Anderson, D. C. et al., Leukocyte adhesion deficiency: molecular basis and functional consequences, *Immunodef. Rev.*, 1, 39, 1988.

16. Harlan, J. M., Leukocyte adhesion deficiency syndrome: insights into the molecular basis of leukocyte emigration, *Clin. Immunol. Immunopathol.*, 67, S16, 1993.

17. Etzioni, A., Frydman, M., Pollack, S. et al., Brief report: recurrent severe infections caused by a novel leukocyte adhesion deficiency, *N. Engl. J. Med.*, 327, 1789, 1992.

18. Hill, H. R., Biochemical, structural and functional abnormalities of polymorphonuclear leukocytes in the neonate, *Pediatr. Res.*, 22, 375, 1987.

19. Anderson, D. C., Neonatal neutrophil dysfunction, *J. Lab. Clin. Med.*, 120, 816, 1992.

20. Bektas, S., Goetze, B., and Speer, C. P., Decreased adherence, chemotaxis and phagocytic activities of neutrophils from preterm neonates, *Acta Paediatr. Scand.*, 79, 1031, 1990.

21. Price, T. H., Ochs, H. D., Gershoni-Baruch, R., Harlan, J. M., and Etzioni A., In vivo neutrophil and lymphocyte function studies in a patient with leukocyte adhesion deficiency type II, *Blood*, 84, 1635, 1994.

22. Wilkinson, P. C., Defects of leukocyte locomotion and chemotaxis: prospects, assays, and lessons from Chediak-Higashi neutrophils, *Eur. J. Clin. Invest.*, 23, 690, 1993.

23. Downey G. P., Mechanisms of leukocyte motility and chemotaxis, *Curr. Opin. Immunol.*, 6, 113, 1994.

24. Shearer, W. T., Paul, M. E., Smith, C. W., and Huston, D. P., Laboratory assessment of immune deficiency disorders, *Immunol. Allerg. Clin. North Am.*, 14, 265, 1994.

25. Boyden, S., The chemotactic effect of mixture of antibody and antigen on polymorphonuclear leukocytes, *J. Exp. Med.*, 115, 543, 1962.

26. Zigmond, S. H. and Hirsch J. G., Leukocyte locomotion and chemotaxis. New method for evaluation and demonstration of cell-derived chemotactic factor, *J. Exp. Med.*, 137, 387, 1973.

27. Boxer, G. J., Curnutte, J. T., and Boxer L. A., Polymorphonuclear leukocyte function, *Hosp. Pract.*, 69, 129, 1985.

28. Brown C. C. and Gallin J., Chemotactic disorders, *Hematol./Oncol. Clin. North Am.*, 2, 61, 1988.

29. Geha, R. S. and Leung, D. Y. M., Hyper immunoglobulin E syndrome, *Immunodef. Rev.*, 1, 155, 1989.

30. Roos, D., Kuijpers, T., Mascart-Lemone, F. et al., A novel syndrome of severe neutrophil dysfunction: unresponsiveness confined to chemotaxin-induced functions, *Blood*, 81, 2735, 1993.

31. Boxer, L. A., Hedley-Whyte, E. T., and Stossel, T. P., Neutrophil actin dysfunction and abnormal neutrophil behavior, *N. Engl. J. Med.*, 291, 1093, 1984.

32. Southwick, F. S., Dabiri, G. A., and Stossel, T. P., Neutrophil actin dysfunction is a genetic disorder associated with partial impairment of neutrophil actin assembly in three family members, *J. Clin. Invest.*, 82, 1525, 1988.

33. Coates, T. D., Torkildson, J. C., Torres, M., Church, J. A., and Howard, T. H., An inherited defect of neutrophil motility and microfilamentous cytoskeleton associated with abnormalities in 47 kD and 89 kD proteins, *Blood*, 78, 1338, 1991.

34. Hampton, M. B., Vissers, M. C. M., and Winterbourn, C. C., A single assay for measuring the rates of phagocytosis and bacterial killing by neutrophils, *J. Leukoc. Biol.*, 55, 147, 1994.

35. Martin, E. and Bhakdi, S., Flow cytometric assay for quantifying opsonophagocytosis and killing of *Staphylococcus aureus* by peripheral blood leukocytes, *J. Clin. Microbiol.*, 30, 2246, 1992.

36. Malech, H. L. and Gallin, J. I., Neutrophils in human diseases, *N. Engl. J. Med.*, 317, 687, 1987.

37. Nauseef, W. M., Myeloperoxidase deficiency, *Hematol./Oncol. Clin. North Am.*, 2, 135, 1988.

38. Parry, M. F., Root, R. K., Metcalf, J. A., Delaney, K. K., Kaplow, L. S., and Richar, W. J., Myeloperoxidase deficiency: prevalence and clinical significance, *Ann. Intern. Med.*, 95, 293, 1981.

39. Gallin, J. I., Neutrophil specific granule deficiency, *Annu. Rev. Med.*, 36, 263, 1985.

40. Rosenberg, H. F. and Gallin, J., Neutrophil-specific granule deficiency includes eosinophils, *Blood* 82, 268, 1993.

41. Ganz, T., Metcalf, J. A., Gallin, J. I., Boxer, L. A., and Lehrer, R. I., Microbicidal/cytotoxic proteins of neutrophils are deficient in two disorders: Chediak-Higashi syndrome and "specific" granule deficiency, *J. Clin. Invest.*, 82, 552, 1988.

42. Holcombe, R. F., Jones, K. L., and Stewart, R. M., Lysosomal enzyme activities in Chediak-Higashi syndrome: evaluation of lymphoblastoid cell lines and review of the literature, *Immunodeficiency*, 5, 131, 1994.

43. Babior, B. M., The respiratory burst of phagocytes, *J. Clin. Invest.*, 73, 599, 1984.

44. Etzioni, A. and Douglas, S. D., Microbial phagocytosis and killing in host defense, *Pediatr. Adolesc. Med.*, 3, 17, 1993.

45. Baehner, R. L. and Nathan, D. G., Quantitative nitroblue tetrazolium test in chronic granulomatous disease, *N. Engl. J. Med.*, 278, 971, 1968.

46. Hassan, N. F., Campbell, D. E., and Douglas, S. D., Clinical evaluation of defects in neutrophil oxidative metabolism, *Clin. Immunol. Newslett.*, 9, 37, 1988.

47. Bass, D. A., Parce, J. W., DeChatelet, L. R., Szedja, P., Seeds, M. C., and Thomas, M., Flow cytometric studies of oxidative product formation by neutrophils: a graded response to membrane stimulation, *J. Immunol.*, 130, 1910, 1983.

48. Hassan, N. F., Campbell, D. E., and Douglas, S. D., Flow cytometric analysis of oxidase activity of neutrophils from chronic granulomatous disease patients, *Adv. Exp. Med. Biol.*, 239, 73, 1988.

49. Hassan, N. F., Campbell, D. E., and Douglas, S. D., Phorbol myristate acetate induced oxidation of 2′, 7′-dichlorofluorescin by neutrophils from patients with chronic granulomatous disease, *J. Leukoc. Biol.*, 43, 317, 1988.

50. Roesler, J., Hecht, M., Freihorst, J. et al., Diagnosis of chronic granulomatous disease and its mode of inheritance by dihydrorhodamine 123 and flow microcytofluorometry, *Eur. J. Pediatr.*, 150, 161, 1991.

51. Kamani, N. R. and Douglas, S. D., Natural history of chronic granulomatous disease, *Diagn. Clin. Immunol.*, 5, 314, 1988.

52. Curnutte, J. T., Chronic granulomatous disease: the solving of a clinical riddle at the molecular level, *Clin. Immunol. Immunopathol.*, 67, S-2, 1993.

53. Curnutte, J. T., Molecular basis of the autosomal recessive forms of chronic granulomatous disease, *Immunodef. Rev.*, 3, 149, 1992.

54. Roos, D., The genetic basis of chronic granulomatous disease, *Immunol. Rev.*, 138, 121, 1994.

55. Thrasher, A., Segal, A., and Casimir, C., Chronic granulomatous disease: towards gene therapy, *Immunodeficiency*, 4, 327, 1993.

56. Mamlok, R. J., Mamlok, V., Mills, G., Daeschner, C. W., Schmalsteig, F. C., and Anderson, D. C., Glucose-6-phosphate dehydrogenase deficiency, neutrophil dysfunction and chromobacterium violaceum sepsis, *J. Pediatr.*, 111, 852, 1987.

57. Beutler, E., Glucose-6-phosphate dehydrogenase: new perspectives, *Blood*, 73, 1397, 1989.

58. Ambruso, D. R., McCabe, E. R. B., Anderson, D. et al., Infectious and bleeding complications in patients with glycogenosis Ib., *Am. J. Dis. Child.*, 139, 691, 1985.

59. Kilpatrick, L., Garty B. A., Lundquist K. F. et al., Impaired metabolic function and signaling defects in phagocytic cells in glycogen storage disease type 1b, *J. Clin. Invest.*, 86, 196, 1990.

60. Krause, P. J., Woronick, C. L., Burke G. et al., Depressed neutrophil chemotaxis in children suffering blunt trauma, *Pediatrics*, 93, 807, 1994.

61. Bell, J. B. and Douglas, S. D., Phagocyte functions and defects: a ten year update, *Pediatr. Ann.*, 16, 379, 1987.

62. Zimran, A., Elstein, D., Abrahamov, A., Dale, G. L., Aker, M., and Matzner, Y., Significance of abnormal neutrophil chemotaxis in Gaucher's disease, *Blood*, 84, 2374, 1994.

63. VanDyke, T. E., Horoszewicz, H. U., and Cianciola, L. J., Neutrophil chemotaxis dysfunction in human periodontitis, *Infect. Immun.*, 27, 124, 1980.

64. Fischer, T. J., Gard, S. E., Rachelefsky, G. S. et al., Monocyte chemotaxis under agarose: defects in atopic disease, aspirin therapy, and mucocutaneous candidiasis, *Pediatr. Res.*, 14, 242, 1980.

65. Liel, Y., Rudich, A., Nagauker-Shriker, O., Yermiyahu, T., and Levy, R., Monocyte dysfunction in patients with Gaucher disease: evidence for interference of glucocerebroside with superoxide generation, *Blood*, 83, 2646, 1994.

66. Brenneis, H., Schmidt, A., Blaas-Mautner, P., Worner, I., Ludwig, R., and Hansch, G. M., Chemotaxis of polymorphonuclear neutrophils (PMN) in patients suffering from recurrent infection, *Eur. J. Clin. Invest.*, 23, 693, 1993.

67. Axtell, R. A., Evaluation of the patient with a possible phagocytic disorder, *Hematol./Oncol. Clin. North. Am.*, 2, 1, 1988.

68. Kamani, N., August, C. S., Campbell, D. E., Hassan, N. F., and Douglas, S. D., Marrow transplantation in chronic granulomatous disease: an update, with six year follow-up, *J. Pediatr.*, 113, 697, 1988.

Chapter 10

CELLULAR IMMUNOLOGY: MONITORING OF IMMUNE THERAPIES

Theresa L. Whiteside

CONTENTS

0-8493-0134-3/97/$0.00+$.50

I. INTRODUCTION

Cellular immunity, as opposed to humoral immunity, encompasses a broad spectrum of immune phenomena mediated by cells of the immune system. The latter comprise various subsets of lymphocytes: T, B, and NK cells, which are derived from a common lymphoid progenitor cell in the fetal liver and bone marrow. Monocytes and granulocytes, hematopoietic cells with lineages distinct from that of lymphocytes, also participate in cellular immune reactions. They have the capability to mediate non-MHC-restricted cytotoxicity and to release a variety of enzymes and cytokines. The cells of the immune system interact with these other hematopoietic cells in the peripheral blood as well as in tissues, and the immune response represents a network of carefully balanced interactions responsible for maintaining homeostasis. A diagram of cells mediating innate or adaptive immunity is given in Figure 1. Any perturbation of the immune network leads to a response —a series of events involving the immune effector cells — which is transient and which culminates in restoration of the baseline level of immune activity.

Cellular immunity includes antigen-driven responses induced by the major histocompatibility complex (MHC)-restricted interactions of the antigen with the specific T-cell receptor (TCR) expressed on a subset of presensitized T lymphocytes (specific immunity) as well as responses which do not require previous sensitization and are largely not restricted by the MHC (nonspecific immunity). While T cells are required for the initiation and are the main mediators of specific cellular

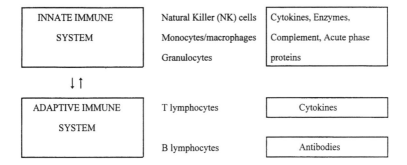

Figure 1
A diagram of components of the innate and adaptive immune systems. The arrows indicate that considerable interactions exist between the two systems. In general, cells of the innate immune system are nonspecific, while those of the adaptive immune system are antigen-specific.

immunity, all cells of the immune system may participate in both types of responses. Soluble products of immune cells, lymphokines, serve as hormones of the immune system, and immune effector cells express receptors for and are responsive to cytokines released by cells in the microenvironment. Immune cells are able to extravasate and migrate in tissues. Consequently, they are found not only in the main lymphoid organs but are distributed throughout the body. Cellular immune responses can be either local or systemic, depending on the route and dose of the antigenic challenge.

Interactions among immune cells and those of immune cells with surrounding tissue cells are highly complex and not yet completely understood. They are necessary for health and, when disturbed, disease may follow. For this reason, a great deal of effort has been invested in studying and monitoring these interactions as well as phenotypic and functional characteristics of immune cells. Today, changes in the number or functions of immune cells can be adequately monitored in health and disease. Furthermore, when immune therapies are administered to patients who have immunologic abnormalities, it is possible to accurately monitor effects of a drug, generally referred to as a biologic response modifier or BRM, on various cellular components of the immune system. In this chapter, I will review the principles and guidelines of immune monitoring during clinical trials with BRMs and consider the usefulness of some of the immunologic assays in such monitoring. The aspects of immune monitoring that are covered appear to be particularly timely today. Increasingly frequently, BRMs are used for immunotherapy, and various diseases are being treated with agents that either stimulate or suppress immune functions. Thus, it has become necessary to assess the impact of these therapeutic interventions on various subsets of immune cells and to define the mechanisms that are involved in clinical responses. In addition, immune effector cells may be used for therapy in conjunction with cytokines, and adoptive transfer of these cells to immunoincompetent patients is dependent on successful *in vitro* generation and activity of the effector cells.

II. CLINICAL TRIALS WITH BRMS

Several categories of BRMs have been available for therapies, as follows: (a) monoclonal antibodies; (b) cytokines ; (c) growth factors; (d) activated cells; (e) cellular products; (f) immunotoxins; and (g) other targeting agents. The basic premise behind the selection of a BRM for therapy is that it can enhance the ability of the innate or adaptive immune system to control a disease process. In general, such a selection is preceded by extensive *in vitro* studies and by *in vivo* experiments in animal models of the disease in order to define the presumed mechanism of action of a BRM.

Following preclinical evaluations, a new BRM is introduced to the clinic as a phase I protocol. The design of a phase I study is based on its mechanism of action tentatively identified in preclinical experiments. The developmental strategy involves determination of the optimal biologic dose (OBD), i.e., the dose of BRM that maximally activates the postulated mechanism of action with tolerable toxicity. A clinical trial designed to determine the OBD is referred to as phase Ib, in contrast to a phase Ia trial, in which only clinical toxicity of the new agent is defined as a maximal tolerated dose (MTD).[1] It is important to remember that biologic agents may exert optimal effects at lower rather than higher doses, resulting in a bell-shaped dose-response curve, and that the OBD may be different from the MTD of the agent. In addition, the same BRM might have quite disparate OBDs for two different immunologic characteristics. A systemically administered cytokine, interleukin-2 (IL-2), for example, which is currently approved for therapy of renal cell carcinoma (RCC), has a much lower OBD for activation of circulating T and natural killer (NK) cells than that for supporting generation of lymphokine-activated killer (LAK) activity.[2]

It appears that in phase Ib trials with BRMs, various or surrogate therapeutic endpoints, such as increased numbers or activity of immune effector cells, are achieved much more easily than clinical responses. In the case of IL-2 therapy in RCC, for example, nearly all patients achieve high levels of endogenous LAK activity during therapy, while only a proportion of these patients will have objective antitumor responses.[2] This reflects the fact that the choice of surrogate endpoints, which is usually based on limited preclinical data, may not reflect the entire spectrum of physiologic mechanisms that are mediated by a BRM, including those responsible for its therapeutic effects.

It could be expected that in phase Ib trials, direct determinations of the dose of a BRM that has the best therapeutic effects, e.g., antitumor effects in a patient with cancer, would be preferable to the use of surrogate measurements. However, the use of surrogate measures remains the only reasonable alternative, since practical and ethical considerations rule out the possibility of directly determining the best therapeutic dose. Antitumor response rates for single agents generally range between 10 and 30% and, therefore, large-scale dose-finding studies would require excessively large number of patients, while exposing many of them to ineffective doses of the agent tested, in an effort to establish the optimal therapeutic dose. In the subsequent clinical trials, it may be possible to expand the earlier clinical observations and begin to ask questions about the biology of the agent or its mechanisms of antitumor response by gradually incorporating additional studies designed to answer more mechanistic questions.

III. SELECTION OF IMMUNE ASSAYS FOR MONITORING

Immunologic monitoring is defined as serial measurements of selected immune parameters over a period of time, generally weeks or months. Such serial measurements are usually taken before, during, and after therapy, as part of a clinical trial. However, they can also be taken during disease, during recovery from disease, or simply to establish immune responses of an individual over time. A baseline measurement (or better, two or three baseline assays) is necessary, because a goal of monitoring is to define changes from the baseline that occur in a designated time period. Biologic fluctuations that are likely to occur in immunologic responses during this period of time, e.g., those associated with hormonal changes, infections, stress, exercise situations, have to be distinguished from changes due to therapeutic interventions. This aspect of monitoring is most difficult, and it requires selection of assays that can reliably measure immunologic changes as well as the ability to accurately correlate physiologic or clinical observations with immunologic results.

A list of assays most frequently used for monitoring is provided in Table 1. Selection of assays for monitoring of immune parameters is best guided by a hypothesis. The hypothesis to be tested in a clinical trial is formulated on the basis of preliminary evidence which is considered by the investigators to be the best indication of mechanisms that lead to therapeutic effects. Obviously, since most BRMs have multiple biologic effects, more than a single hypothesis of action can be postulated, and the choice of the hypothesis to test depends on individual insights of the investigator. Testing of several hypotheses at once is discouraged, however, because it complicates the design of a clinical

TABLE 1

Immunologic Assays Used in Monitoring of Phase I Clinical Trials with BRMs

Categories of Assays	Sample Type
1. Soluble cellular products	
Immunoglobulin levels	Serum, plasma, body fluids
Cytokine levels and pharmacokinetics	Serum, plasma, body fluids
Cytokine receptors and antagonists	Serum, plasma, body fluids
Enzymes (e.g., 2′, 5′-adenylate synthetase, terminal deoxynucleotide transferase)	Serum, plasma, body fluids
Neopterin	Serum, plasma, body fluids
β_2 Microglobulin	Serum, plasma, body fluids
2. Phenotypic assays	
Proportions of cells	Whole blood, tissue biopsy, body fluids
Absolute numbers of cells	Isolated lymphocytes
Cellular subpopulations (e.g., Th1 or Th2 or memory/naive T cells)	Isolated lymphocytes
3. Functional assays	
In vivo DTH skin test	Visual inspection or biopsy
Cytotoxicity: ADCC, LAK, NK, T-cell specific	MNC or subpopulations of MNC
Cytokine production	MNC or subpopulations of MNC
Proliferation	MNC or subpopulations of MNC
Chemotaxis	MNC or subpopulations of MNC
Signal transduction	MNC or subpopulations of MNC
Superoxide generation	MNC or subpopulations of MNC

trial and makes the accompanying monitoring too extensive. There is no way to guarantee that a hypothesis selected for testing in a clinical trial is a correct one and, thus, its selection represents a risk that an investigator is obliged to undertake.

While selection of immunologic assays for monitoring of a clinical trial is primarily guided by the scientific hypothesis that is being tested, a number of other factors might influence the decision to choose a particular assay in preference of another. The frequency of immunologic monitoring is an important component of the trial design. The time points selected for monitoring clearly need to include the baseline (prior to therapy) and final (post therapy) measurements. Beyond that, the schema for monitoring is usually determined by extrapolation from animal models or from previous clinical experience with the same or other BRMs, and it may have to be modified, depending on the frequency and dose of a BRM administered.

A decision to select cellular vs. humoral immunologic assays for monitoring (Table 1) is directly related to the proposed mechanism of action for a BRM. While it may be difficult to prioritize based on the current understanding of such mechanisms, the consideration of practical aspects of monitoring can help in reaching a reasonable decision. Limitations in the frequency or volume of samples obtained from the peripheral blood as well as variability of cell yields restrict the use of cellular assays. Cellular assays are more difficult and more costly to perform than serum assays. Therefore, it is always advisable to consider serum or plasma assays first. A variety of serum assays are available, which can substitute for cellular assays, including those measuring levels of released cytokines, enzymes known to be induced by a particular BRM (e.g., interferon-induced 2′,5′- adenylate synthetase), inhibitors or antagonists of BRMs (e.g., IL-1ra) or products of activated cell subsets (e.g., soluble cytokine receptors, β_2 microglobulin, neopterin). From the practical point of view, it is preferable to use serum or plasma instead of cells for monitoring whenever possible.

In many instances, monitoring of numbers or functions of mononuclear cells (MNC) in the peripheral blood during therapy does not adequately reflect immunologic events that take place at the site of disease. Only about 2% of total lymphocytes are in the peripheral circulation, at any given time point, and monitoring of these cells is not likely to reflect events occurring in tissue. Systemic effects of cytokines and certain other BRMs are often distinct from their local or locoregional effects. Therefore, immunologic monitoring of lesions, tissues, or organs involved in a disease is likely to yield more informative data than will the same assays performed with MNC obtained from the peripheral blood. The obvious difficulties with this strategy are that blood is more readily available than tissues and that only superficial lesions or sites accessible to repeated biopsies can be monitored. Nevertheless, during a clinical trial, it might be feasible to obtain serial biopsies, and this opportunity for *in situ* studies should be taken advantage of as often as possible. An alternative possibility is to obtain body fluids (pleural fluids or ascites), in addition to the peripheral blood to be able to detect changes in the organ-associated immune cells or their products relative to those in peripheral circulation.

Whether immune cells, serum, or plasma are used for immunologic monitoring, the samples have to be recovered from peripheral blood, body fluids, or tissues at time points specified in a protocol schema. For studies of pharmacokinetics, a special effort has to be made to collect the specimens at precisely designated time intervals and to process them in accordance with experimental protocol to avoid degradation, inactivation, or loss of activity. In planning of immunologic monitoring, not only timing of specimen collections, but the nature of anticoagulants used needs to be considered. For example, to measure levels of cytokines in body fluids, plasma rather than serum is preferable, since cytokines tend to be trapped in the clot, with subsequently low levels of cytokines measured in the serum.[3] Separation of

A.

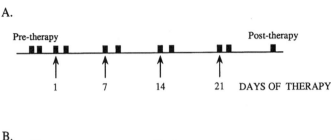

B.

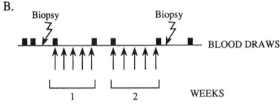

Figure 2

Examples of protocol schemas that might be used for immunologic monitoring. In (A), a BRM is administered systemically at weekly intervals for 3 successive weeks. Blood draws (■) for monitoring are obtained each week just prior to therapy to monitor long-term effects on the immune cells and 24 h after therapy to monitor short-term effects. Three pre-therapy (baseline) and one post-therapy blood draws are obtained. In (B), a BRM is administered locoregionally (e.g., around the tumor) on every working day of the week (5 successive daily treatments) for 2 successive weeks. Tumor biopsy is obtained prior to and after therapy for *in situ* monitoring, in addition to blood samples. Arrows indicate days on which therapy is given.

serum/plasma or MNC from the peripheral blood are routine laboratory procedures, but recovery and fractionation of cells from tissues or body fluids containing tumor or tissue cells is time consuming and requires special expertise and considerable effort.[4] The use of individual separated subsets of tissue infiltrating or blood MNC is not feasible for serial monitoring, mainly due to a need for tissue sampling or large blood volumes, respectively. Also, the lack of uniformly acceptable procedures for cell separations and unpredictable yields of cells that can be recovered from tissues hamper the use of cell separation techniques for monitoring. However, the advantage of studies performed with highly purified subsets of immune cells obtained from the site of disease is obvious, and when it seems feasible to obtain a biopsy, even if it is only prior to and after therapy, investigators are encouraged to incorporate such procedures in their protocol. Two approaches to immunologic monitoring are outlined in Figure 2.

It is often unclear which immunologic assays can be reliably performed with fresh vs. cryopreserved cells. For longitudinal immunologic monitoring, it would be more practical to use serially harvested frozen aliquots of serum/plasma or batched cryopreserved immune cells instead of freshly harvested specimens. The ability to reliably cryopreserve immune effector cells for future use in retrospective studies or for batching of serially collected specimens to eliminate the interassay variability is highly desirable. However, some immunologic measurements are best performed with fresh samples, and investigators may be introducing artifacts in certain functional assays, specifically those measuring cytotoxicity, by utilizing cryopreserved effector cells. Many other functional assays, including proliferation or cytokine production, can be reliably performed with frozen cells, and it may be preferable to select these assays for monitoring rather than those requiring the use of fresh cells. In any case, each monitoring laboratory is obliged to compare fresh vs. frozen cells to ascertain that a test can be reliably performed with either.

In summary, the choice of a strategy for immune monitoring of clinical trials with BRMs is neither simple nor straightforward. No single assay or experimental approach is appropriate for all biologic therapeutic interventions. The choice requires familiarity with principles of immunologic assays, a great deal of judgement, and considerable understanding of biologic, immunologic, and therapeutic effects induced by BRMs.

IV. SERUM AND PLASMA ASSAYS

In Table 1, several serum/plasma assays are listed that have been widely used for immune monitoring. The list is representative rather than inclusive. These assays measure levels of various cellular products in body fluids. Immunoglobulin quantification, for example, has become a routine and highly accurate estimate of quantitative and qualitative changes in B-cell function. More recently, assays for levels of cytokines and enzymes in body fluids have become an important part of immunologic monitoring. Both bioassays and immunoassays are available for assessments of cytokine levels[5] in body fluids, but only the latter (mainly in the form of commercial enzyme-linked immunoassay or ELISA kits) are practical for monitoring of clinical trials. Cytokine bioassays are difficult to perform reliably, are less specific than immunoassays, require neutralization to confirm cytokine identities, and are labor intensive. For these reasons, bioassays are used in special circumstances as confirmatory rather than monitoring assays. In contrast, immunoassays are less sensitive than bioassays but more specific and are easily performed, using commercially available reagents. Figure 3 illustrates the usefulness of these assays in the example of monitoring for plasma levels of sIL2Rα(CD25) in a phase Ib trial, showing rapid and dramatic changes during therapy with IL-2. A number of problems exist with assessments of cytokines in sera, including the ability of cytokines to bind to and form complexes with serum proteins

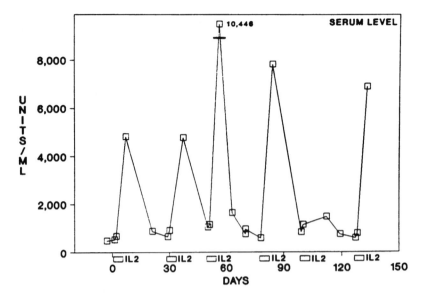

Figure 3

An example of dramatic changes that may occur in plasma levels of sIL2Rα(CD25) during administration of IL-2. In this phase Ib trial, a patient with metastatic melanoma was treated with adoptively transferred autologous A-NK cells and with cycles of IL-2 ($10^6 U/m^2/d \times 5$) administered systemically as continuous infusions. Note that plasma levels of sIL2Rα peaked during the periods of IL-2 therapy and decreased to a near-baseline level when IL-2 therapy was stopped.

or the presence of soluble cytokine receptors or antagonists, natural inhibitors, or anticytokine antibodies.[5] Also, cytokines have a short half-life (minutes) in serum, and their levels are generally low or undetectable by conventional ELISA, even when substantial cytokine production occurs at a disease site. All of these factors may contribute to difficulties in interpretation of cytokine assays, and the knowledge of the cytokine biology is important for accurate assessments and interpretation of cytokine levels in biologic fluids. The latter can be frozen and batched for immunoassays.

V. PHENOTYPIC ASSAYS

In many trials with BRMs, high priorities are given to cell surface phenotype assays, generally performed with fresh whole blood specimens and, less frequently, with MNC separated from the peripheral blood, body fluids, or tissues. As described in Chapter 11, flow cytometry assays are now easily accessible and highly accurate. A broad array of labeled monoclonal antibodies suitable for two-color, three-color, or multiparameter flow analyses are commercially available, allowing for measurements of various cell subsets. Changes in these subsets, as well as the activation level of the cells, can be readily assessed during immunotherapy. Unfortunately, flow cytometry assays are often selected without adequate justification and used in combinations that are not optimally meaningful. For example, the popular use of the CD4/CD8 ratio is often not informative, while determination of the ratio of memory to naive lymphocytes or that of activated to nonactivated cells might be. Large panels of immunologic markers have been used indiscriminately to follow changes induced by biotherapy without considering the hypothesis advanced as part of a clinical trial. Through proper selection of marker panels, it is possible to focus on a single population of effector cells, on several phenotypically distinct subsets, on cells expressing specific activation markers, or on those that express a particular constellation of adhesion molecules. Attempts at correlating phenotypic changes with functional assays may be particularly informative. Various receptors on the cell surface for growth factors and cytokines can further be used to subset the cells and to relate their phenotypes to their functional potential. Thus, phenotypic analysis is a powerful tool for monitoring the effects of therapy on immune cells, given that the selection of markers to be monitored on T, B, NK cells, monocytes, or granulocytes is based on the predicted mechanism of action of the BRM being used.

Two-color flow cytometry is most widely used for monitoring of immune therapies, although three-color flow can provide more specific analysis of cell subsets. The usefulness of three-color or multicolor cytometry is currently limited due to the complexities associated with the analysis of results. From a practical point of view, it is difficult for an average laboratory to analyze a large volume of three-color flow data in a timely fashion. The alternatives are to limit three-color analysis to a single cell type considered the most important or to send the specimens for phenotyping to a specialized laboratory equipped to handle multicolor flow data. This alternative is recommended for monitoring of multicenter or cooperative group trials, as whole blood specimens can be shipped by overnight carriers for flow analysis without compromising their quality.

In addition to surface phenotyping, flow cytometry has been recently used to measure intracytoplasmic markers, using permeabilized cells, as well as to perform certain functional assays. Currently, neither of these technologies have been applied in clinical trials, and they are used in research only. Because of substantial advantages they offer, they may be incorporated in the roster of useful monitoring assays in the future. Intracytoplasmic proteins (including enzymes, cytokines, signal transduction molecules, or transcription factors), measured in phenotypically defined cells by flow cytometry, can provide useful information about the activation state and functional attributes of individual cells or a subset of cells. Proliferation and cytotoxicity can be measured by flow cytometry simply and more efficiently than in the familiar radiolabel assays, providing the identity of effector cells at the population or even single-cell level. Disadvantages of these methods include the requirement for a flow cytometer, relatively complex preparation steps, including cell permeabilization and combination of surface and intracellular staining, and the current paucity of comparative data confirming the validity of these techniques for monitoring.

Interpretation of flow cytometry data in serial monitoring requires stringent controls for interassay variability. Some of the lymphocyte subsets encompass only a small proportion of cells in the gate, and it is necessary to be able to distinguish shifts induced by therapy from daily assay variability. Changes in the phenotype of effector cells should be interpreted in conjunction with changes observed in functional assays. Specifically, it is important to consider whether changes in function induced during therapy correlate with changes in the number of effector cells or are due to the augmentation of effector cell function. It is also possible that therapy alters both the number and function of effector cells, as indicated in Table 2. During therapy, these changes can be dramatic or subtle, and they can occur simultaneously in several subsets of cells. Analysis of these changes and the correlation between their magnitude and frequency requires special statistical approaches, as discussed below. Since entirely different mechanisms may cause alterations in the proportion or absolute number of effector cells vs. functional changes (e.g., increased blood vessel permeability and up-regulation of NK activity during therapy with IL-2, respectively), it should not be expected that phenotypic and functional data will necessarily correlate with each other. Furthermore, it is possible that shifts in one, but not the other parameter, will correlate with clinical response or, more likely, that no significant correlations will be detected, even though profound changes in immune cell numbers or function are registered during therapy. For example, perilesional therapy with escalating doses of IL-2 in 36 patients with advanced head and neck cancer resulted in highly significant increases in the number of CD3$^-$CD56$^+$ cells and NK activity in the peripheral blood of most patients, but no complete clinical responses in a phase I trial at our institution.[6] This reflects the complexity of mechanisms that mediate therapeutic effects of BRMs.

VI. FUNCTIONAL ASSAYS

Functional assays that can be used for monitoring include a variety of technologies, many of which are highly sensitive and adaptable to samples containing a small number of cells or even single cells.

TABLE 2

Changes in the Proportion of NK-Cells Subsets and NK and
LAK Activities in Response to Locoregional Administration
of IL-2 in the Peripheral Blood of Patients with Head and
Neck Cancer[a]

	Pre-Therapy	Post-Therapy	p Value
NK-cell subsets (%)			
CD3⁻ CD56⁺	16 ± 2	22 ± 2	0.003
CD16⁺ CD56⁺	9 ± 2	16 ± 2	0.013
CD16⁺ HLA-DR⁺	1.3 ± 0.2	2.7 ± 0.6	0.003
Cytotoxicity (log LU)[b]			
NK (vs. K562)	2.0 ± 0.07	2.2 ± 0.07	0.005
LAK (vs. Daudi)	2.9 ± 0.08	3.3 ± 0.12	0.006

[a] The data are mean values ± SEM (adapted from Reference 6).
Paired analysis (the signed rank test) was performed for pre- and
post-therapy measurements obtained in 26 patients with inoper-
able head and neck cancer who were treated with perilesional IL-2.

[b] Cytotoxicity data were obtained in 4-h ^{51}Cr-release assays, using
the indicated targets. LAK cells were generated by incubation of
MNC in the presence of 6000 IU of IL-2 for 3 days. The data are
log 10 $LU_{20}/10^7$ effector cells.

Unfortunately, many of these new technologies, such as chemolumi-
nescence, electronchemoluminescence, or molecular/genetic assays,
have not yet been evaluated for performance in serial monitoring. They
will likely be adapted to monitoring in the near future, because of their
advantages of simplicity, substantially lower cost, and elimination of
radioactive labels. In this section, functional assays that are currently
available for monitoring will be briefly described. This overview will
be then followed by more detailed descriptions of monitoring performed for T and NK cells.

A. *In Vivo* DTH Skin Test

The skin test for delayed type hypersensitivity (DTH), is the only
in vivo assay available for measurements of cellular immunity in man.
This test is underutilized in monitoring, largely because of rigorous
requirements for recording of its results. The DTH assay is often mis-
interpreted, because the results are not measured correctly (induration,
not erythema should be measured) or at the proper time (>24 h after
test application). Yet, when performed and read according to the guidelines, the DTH assay remains the best available measure of specific cell-
mediated immunity in patients with immunodeficiencies, particularly
when it is combined with a biopsy to confirm the nature of cells infiltrating the skin.[7] Reagents for diphtheria, tetanus, candida, mycobacteria, and other antigens are commercially available. Other antigens,

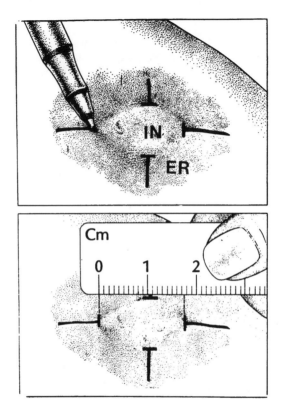

Figure 4
DTH skin test is the only available *in vivo* measure of immunocompetence. The skin test is read 24 to 48 h after intradermal antigen application. Generally, swelling and indura-tion develop, with accompanying redness (erythema). A diagram shows how to correctly read a DTH skin test: the area of induration (IN) has to be measured and recorded as the cross-product or the sum of two greatest perpendicular diameters. In general, indu-ration >5 mm is considered as a positive DTH reaction. ER = erythema.

e.g., tumor-derived purified or synthetic peptides, which are not yet commercially available from vendors, can also be used, provided they have passed safety requirements. A change in the DTH skin test from unreactive to reactive as a result of biotherapy is a significant result.

B. Local vs. Systemic Assays

Since measurements of phenotypic characteristics do not ade-quately convey the functional capabilities of a cell or a population of cells, cellular assays for monitoring of functions of immune effector cells are necessary. These assays are usually performed with peripheral blood MNC and only rarely with effector cells obtained from the site of disease. Thus, functions that are being monitored are not those of the effector cells which may be directly involved in disease but those of substitute cells that are easily accessible for monitoring. This is by far the greatest limitation of monitoring, since systemic effects of BRMs are likely to be different from local or locoregional effects on the immune cells. It should not be expected that the "surrogate" results obtained with peripheral blood lymphocytes will closely reflect biologic activity of the drug on functions of immune cells *in situ*. To overcome this limitation, investigators are attempting to study serial tissue biopsies, utilizing immunostaining and/or *in situ* hybridization (ISH). Another approach utilizes the reverse transcriptase polymerase chain reaction (RT-PCR) for mRNA coding for proteins involved in cytotoxicity (perforin, granzymes, TNF), proliferation (growth factors, cytokines), or signal transduction (the T-cell receptor zeta chain, protein tyrosine kinases). In some cases, it may be possible to recover a limited number of cells from serial biopsies to perform functional studies. Obviously, these studies are very difficult to organize in humans and not applicable when the biopsy cannot be obtained. Nevertheless, they are extremely important, because they allow for a comparison to be made between local and systemic effects of a BRM on immune effector cells and to eventually justify or discredit the common practice of monitoring for alterations in cellular functions in the peripheral blood alone.

C. Cytotoxicity

Among functional assays for lymphocytes, cytotoxicity has occupied a special place, especially in monitoring of immune therapies. There is a good rationale for monitoring cytotoxicity in clinical trials with BRMs, which tend to augment this effector function in many different cell types. In oncology protocols, antitumor cytotoxicity, whether class I MHC-restricted (mediated by the tumor antigen-specific T cells), nonspecific (mediated by NK cells or monocytes), or antibody-mediated (depending on the presence of FcγR on effector cells), has been extensively monitored because of the evidence derived from numerous animal models of tumor metastasis that tumor growth and elimination of metastases are mediated, at least in part, by cytotoxic effector cells. In human studies, it has been reported that autotumor cytotoxicity was the only significant *in vitro* correlate of clinical responses in phase I trials of adoptive therapy with *in vitro*-activated human immune cells and IL-2.[8] More recent data indicate that tumor regression or metastasis elimination are complex tissue events, generally involving cell necrosis, and adequate monitoring of the process of cytotoxicity remains to be established. It is also apparent that a cytotoxicity assay, measuring only the secretory function of effector cells,

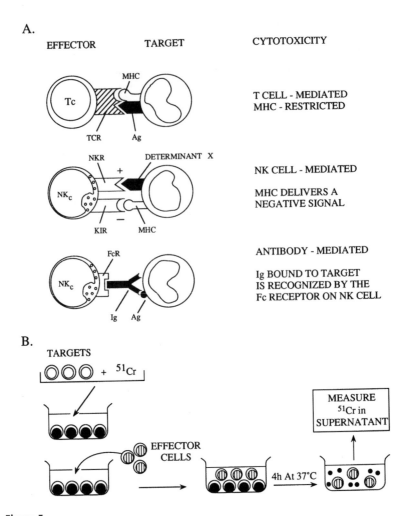

Figure 5

(A) A diagram of interactions between effector cells mediating various types of cytotoxicity and target cells. Cytotoxic T cells (Tc) bind to the target, which presents antigen and class I MHC determinants recognized by the T-cell receptor (TCR). NK cells recognize a triggering determinant X on the susceptible target. Class I MHC molecules on the target are also recognized by the killer cell inhibitory receptors (KIR) on NK cells. Negative signals received by KIRs prevent NK activity, while triggering receptors induce NK-mediated cytotoxicity. Lysis or lack of lysis depend on the balance of negative vs. positive signals received by the NK cell. In the presence of target-specific antibodies, NK cells recognize the Fc portion of IgG bound to antigens on the target cell surface. Cross-linking of FcγRIII on NK cells by target-specific antibodies leads to lysis (ADCC). (B) A diagram of ^{51}Cr-release assay, commonly used to measure cytotoxicity, is shown. Targets are labeled with ^{51}Cr and coincubated with MNC as effector cells. Lysis of targets results in release of ^{51}Cr into the medium. The assay must be performed at a minimum of four different effector (E): target (T) ratios in order to generate a lytic curve, defining the relationship between the percent specific lysis and the number of effector cells used in the assay.

is not able to adequately reflect the many mechanisms involved in the process of cytotoxicity *in vivo*.

The question then arises as to which type of cytotoxicity assays should be selected for monitoring (Figure 5). Once again, the choice depends on the preliminary data available, the hypothesis tested, and practical considerations of investigators' ability to perform the assay reliably during monitoring. Cytotoxicity assays commonly utilized for measurements of T cell or NK cell-mediated lysis are described in a greater detail in subsequent sections.

D. Proliferation Assays

Proliferation of immune cells in response to a BRM or to mitogens/antigens has been a part of the monitoring repertoire for a long time. It is a good measure of immunocompetence and can be performed with banked, cryopreserved cells or as a whole blood assay. In modified versions, it can be nonradioactive. For monitoring, proliferation assays with very few cells can be performed in microtest plates holding only 5 to 20 microliters (Terasaki plates). Two-color flow cytometry can be used for assessment of proliferation to determine the amount of DNA per cell and confirm the phenotype of proliferating cells. Assays measuring proliferation in response to a specific antigen are, perhaps, more useful than mitogen assays, but are more difficult to standardize and perform. Often the stimulating antigens are not available as purified or recombinant reagents, making the interpretation of results difficult. It is important to remember that antigen-presenting cells (APC), which are generally present in the peripheral blood, are necessary for optimal proliferation, and in assays with purified lymphocyte subsets, APC have to be added (Figure 6). Titrations of antigens or mitogens to select the optimal stimulatory concentrations are obligatory. Proliferation assays have to be performed with at least three different doses of the antigen, because lymphocytes obtained from various individuals respond optimally to quite different concentrations of the same stimulatory agent. A stimulation index, calculated as the ratio of experimental to control values, is a measure of the proliferative response. Proliferation assays seem to have been replaced by measurements of cytokines and cytotoxicity in more recent clinical trials, yet they are informative, practical, and easily adjustable to fit the specific trial design or circumstances in a monitoring laboratory.

E. LAK Cell Generation

Assays combining proliferation with cytotoxicity have been often used in monitoring. A good example is the lymphokine-activated killer

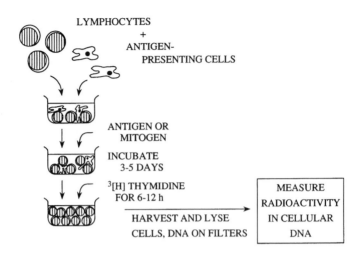

Figure 6

A diagram of a proliferation assay is shown, in which lymphocytes and APC are incubated in the presence of a mitogen or antigen. APC express class II MHC molecules and present antigens to T cells. The initiation of proliferation involves recognition and signaling events. Cytokines, generated as a result of T-cell activation and interaction with APC, are necessary for proliferation. Radioactivity incorporated into DNA of proliferating cells is measured in experimental and control wells.

or LAK cell assay (Figure 7). A population of MNC is activated with IL-2 and cultured for 3 days to generate LAK cells. Subsequently, cytotoxicity of these cells is measured in a 4-h ^{51}Cr-release assay, using a tumor-cell target, such as the NK-resistant cell line, Daudi. The ability to generate LAK activity *in vitro* is a reliable measure of immunocompetence. Lymphocytes obtained from normal donors readily respond to IL-2 by generation of LAK activity, while those obtained from immunoincompetent patients respond partially or not at all.

F.   Cytokine Production

The ability of immune effector cells to produce and release cytokines in response to the drug is a useful monitoring strategy. In contrast to assays of serum levels of cytokines, this strategy calls for incubation of cells alone (spontaneous production) or in the presence of an activating agent (production stimulated) and the subsequent quantitation of cytokines in cellular supernatants.[9] Figure 8 shows the approach for measuring spontaneous and stimulated cytokine production. The assay can be used to measure immune competence of cells by including stimulators, such as PHA or LPS, or the ability to produce cytokines in response to the stimulator of choice. The assay also allows for assessment of *in vivo* activation of cells by measuring spontaneous cytokine

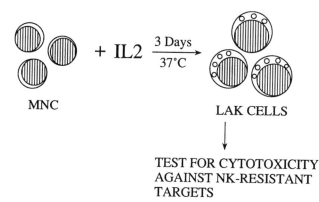

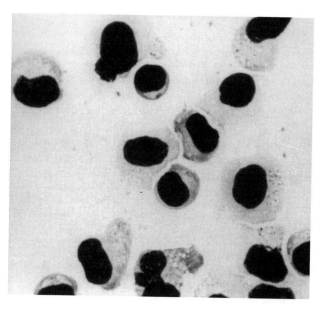

Figure 7

In (A), a diagram of LAK-cell generation is shown. Initially, LAK precursors among MNG, which constitutively express IL2Rβ (a subset of NK cells), respond to IL-2 by up-regulation of high-affinity IL-2R and cytokine secretion. T cells are induced to express IL-2R. Following a period of activation in the presence of IL-2, the cells are tested for cytotoxicity against an NK-resistant target, such as Daudi. LAK cells generated from peripheral blood MNC are mixtures of IL-2-activated NK cells and T lymphocytes. In (B), LAK cells stained with Wright-Gremia are shown after 3-day culture in the presence of IL-2. Note the presence of granules in the cytoplasm of LAK cells. (Magnification × 400.)

release. Unlike cytotoxicity assays, which require fresh and *not* cryo-preserved effector cells, cytokine production assays can be reproduc-ibly performed with either fresh or cryopreserved cells,[9] allowing for batching of cells or of cellular supernatants. Moreover, multiple cytokines

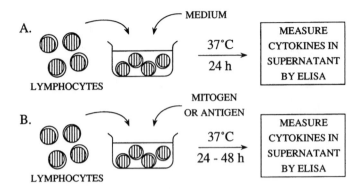

Figure 8

A diagram of spontaneous or stimulated cytokine production *in vitro*. In (A), peripheral blood MNC are incubated in medium alone for 24 to 48 h, and the supernatants are tested by ELISA for the presence of spontaneously produced cytokines. *In vivo*-activated MNC will tend to spontaneously produce cytokines. Alternatively, MNC are incubated in the presence of stimulators (mitogens, antigens) to determine their immunocompetence, i.e., the ability to produce a panel of cytokines in (B).

can be quantified in peripheral blood mononuclear cell (PBMC) supernatants, providing a reasonable assessment of an individual's immunocompetence and allowing for the definition of T-lymphocyte subset (Th0, Th1, or Th2) cytokine profiles.[10,11] Serial monitoring of individuals over a period of several months has demonstrated that stimulated cytokine production is a stable trait.[12] In addition, spontaneous cytokine release by PBMC indicates that they have been activated *in vivo*.[9] While it is recognized that cytokines are produced by a variety of cells, PBMC serve as a convenient vehicle for cytokine assays, primarily because of their accessibility. The ability of PBMC to secrete cytokines *in vitro* has been shown to be modulated by immunotherapies administered *in vivo*.[9] It is possible that this ability may prove to be a more useful correlate of response to therapy than the determination of cytokine levels in plasma. Although the problems associated with testing of plasma, as reviewed above, are largely eliminated in the PBMC system, it requires the use of cells and, as with all indirect procedures, is more time-consuming than serum-based assays. While cytokine measurements in plasma are easily accomplished, those in tissues are more difficult but desirable. Cytokines are local mediators, and their *in vivo* production is probably compartmentalized to achieve optimal physiologic effects. Thus, assays of local cytokine production at the site of inflammation or organ injury and repair are likely more biologically relevant than those in the peripheral blood. At the same time, these assays require tissue biopsy and are technically demanding. Immunocytochemistry for cytokines with cytokine-specific polyclonal or monoclonal antibodies can be used to detect these proteins in tissue samples, with the caveat that it may be difficult to distinguish microscopically cytokines which occupy cellular receptors, having been produced elsewhere in the body, from those that are present in the cytoplasm of the cell.

G. *In Situ* Hybridization

Another approach to evaluation of cytokines in tissue is to measure their gene expression.[7] *In situ* hybridization for cytokine mRNA may be preferable to protein-based assays, although it is by no means simpler or more reliable. Figure 9 illustrates the principle of ISH. Assays for cytokine gene expression are generally difficult to perform and interpret, because mRNAs for cytokines are tightly regulated and rapidly processed. Therefore, very sensitive assays used at the time when the message is likely to be expressed are necessary, e.g., ISH for cytokine mRNA on frozen sections.[13,14] ISH provides information about the number, localization, and distribution of cells expressing cytokine genes in tissue but not about their identity. A combination of ISH with immunocytochemistry is necessary to accomplish the latter. While cryosections have been successfully used for ISH to detect cytokine mRNA in freshly cryopreserved biopsy tissues, the possibility of using archival paraffin-embedded tissues has been explored recently with variable and, so far, not truly convincing results.[15] In our experience, expression of mRNA for cytokines is frequently decreased or absent in archival paraffin-embedded specimens. Like all other RNA determinations, ISH for cytokine mRNA depends on the presence of the undegraded RNA in tissue. To this end, tissues must be snap-frozen immediately after surgery and never allowed to warm up for fear of activating endogenous RNAses. The quality of tissue submitted for ISH or other mRNA studies remains the most critical aspect of this technology. The newest quantitative techniques for cytokine mRNA use the competitive RT-PCR, which combines the exquisite sensitivity of detection with specificity.[16]

H. Molecular Assays for Signaling Molecules

Molecular assays may soon be introduced to monitoring of immune cells. In cancer and certain immunodeficiency diseases, abnormalities in signal transduction have been identified, and they may be responsible for defective functions of immune cells in these diseases.[17] Since it might be possible to reverse these abnormalities and repair immune functions with immunotherapy, monitoring for the presence and extent of signaling defects is indicated at least before and after such therapy. The main concerns about signal transduction studies for monitoring are the large number of cells needed for preparation of cell

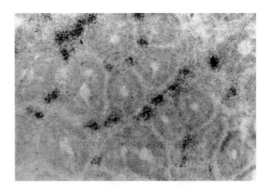

Figure 9
The result of ISH is shown, in which an antisense probe for TNF-α was used for hybridization to show the presence of cells positive for TNF-α mRNA in the intestinal tissue. (Magnification × 120.)

lysates (al least 5 to 10×10^6), the complexity and semiquantitative nature of Western blots, and the possibility of degradation of signaling molecules during the process of lysis. These concerns are being addressed by the development of ELISA assays, which are quantitative and require smaller number of cells (2.5 to 5×10^6) than Western blots, and by using immunostaining *in situ* with antibodies specific for signaling molecules. As an example, decreased expression of absence of the zeta chain, associated with TCR in T cells and FcγRIII in NK cells, has been observed by Western blots in tumor-infiltrating lymphocytes and in the peripheral circulation of patient with advanced cancers.[17] In ELISA assays this decrease can be quantified using cell lysates, and it can be confirmed in tissue biopsies by immunostaining with antibodies recognizing the zeta chain. Both these assays are applicable to monitoring and should contribute to the improved understanding of the mechanism through which BRMs restore immunologic functions.

VII. MONITORING OF T LYMPHOCYTES

T lymphocytes represent 66 to 86% of peripheral blood lymphocytes, with a normal absolute number ranging from 1133 to 2125/mm³ (see Table 3). Changes in the total lymphocyte count generally reflect those in T lymphocytes. However, flow cytometry combined with the differential and WBC counts allows for very precise quantitation of T cells and their subsets in whole blood, other body fluids, or in cells isolated from tissue sites. Monitoring of the percentages of T-cell subsets in the peripheral blood is not adequate, because the total blood lymphocyte number may be altered during therapy with a BRM or in

TABLE 3

Percentages and Absolute Numbers of T Lymphocytes and
T-Cell Subsets in the Peripheral Blood of Normal Individuals[a]

Cell Type	% Positive cells	Positive cells/mm³
T cells		
CD3+	66–86	1,133–2,125
CD4+	38–61	662–1,481
CD8+	21–41	385–897
Activated T cells		
CD3+ HLA-DR+	3–12	48–239
CD4+ HLA-DR+	2–5	39–139
CD8+ HLA-DR+	1–8	26–175
Naive T cells		
CD3+ CD45 RA+	24–48	493–1,237
Memory T cells		
CD3+ CD45 RO+	26–45	495–1,237

[a] The data are mid 80% normal ranges obtained by testing peripheral blood MNC of 100 normal individuals. The percentages of
positive cells were determined by two-color flow cytometry.

the course of disease without a change in proportions of various lymphocyte subsets. By determining only the percentages of T-cell subsets,
changes in their absolute number could be missed, if the WBC or
differential counts fluctuate during therapy. Drug-induced changes in
the T-cell number could be due to altered production, margination,
extravasation, and movement into tissue or destruction, e.g., apoptosis,
of these lymphocytes. It is generally not possible to discern the mechanisms responsible for these changes on the basis of phenotypic analyses, unless more extensive studies are undertaken.

A. Determination of Absolute Numbers and Percentages of T Cells and T-Cell Subsets

Subsets of T lymphocytes associated with distinct functions cannot
be always quantified by phenotypic analysis. This is because many
phenotypic markers do not always discriminate between functional
subpopulations of lymphocytes. For example, two distinct subsets of
human CD4+ T-helper cells, Th1 and Th2, are best defined by mutually
exclusive patterns of cytokine secretion (Figure 10). Th1 but not Th2
cells produce IL-2, IFN-γ, and TNF-β, while Th2, but not Th1, produce
IL-4, IL-5, and IL-10. Different cytokine profiles imply distinct effector
functions. Thus, phagocyte-dependent defense is mediated by Th1
cells, which trigger both cellular responses and production of opsoniz-
ing and complement-fixing antibodies. In contrast, Th2 cells mediate

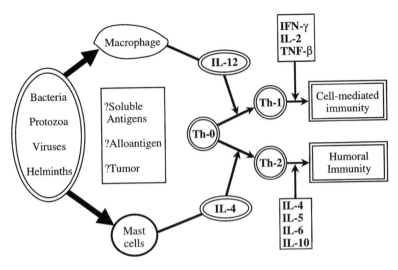

Figure 10
A diagram showing interactions between Th0, Th1 and Th2 subsets of human CD4+ T lymphocytes and distant cytokines produced by these subsets.

phagocyte-independent responses, which include IgE and IgG antibody production, as well as differentiation and activation of mast cells and eosinophils.[18] Many CD4+ T cells exhibit aspects of both Th1 and Th2 subsets, and some of these cells may represent precursors (Th0) of Th1 and Th2 cells. The Th2 subset of CD4+ T cells in humans appears to be associated with expression of a membrane marker, CD30, a member of the TNF/nerve growth factor (NGF) receptor superfamily.[19] Originally described as a surface marker of Hodgkin's and Reed- Steinberg (H-RS) cells, CD30 is strongly and selectively expressed on Th2+ clones of T cells, which are either CD4+ or CD8+. Th2 clones or lines of T cells also release CD30 into their supernatants, and CD30 expression may be a marker of cells predominantly secreting Th2-type cytokines.[19] In combination, phenotypic (e.g., CD30 expression) and functional (e.g., cytokine production) assays can provide an adequate profile of CD4+ T-cell subsets in normal individuals or patients with various disease (reviewed in Reference 20). Subsets of naive or memory T lymphocytes can be distinguished by flow analysis using antibodies specific for isoforms of CD45RA or CD45RO, respectively, which are differentially expressed on the surface of these cells. While a certain degree of overlap may exist between these markers, they are useful in subsetting CD4+ or CD8+ T cells, and they appear to coincide with functional attributes of antigen-primed vs. naive lymphocytes.[21]

To monitor the phenotype or function of tissue-infiltrating T lymphocytes, it is preferable to isolate them from tissue, although *in situ* monitoring can provide a certain amount of useful information about

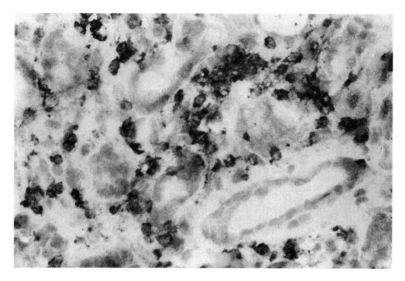

Figure 11
Immunoperoxidase staining for T cells (CD3+) in a cryostat tissue section of kidney. The biopsy was obtained from a renal transplant patient developing rejection. (Magnification × 360.)

their local interactions. *In situ* monitoring is limited by the availability and size of tissue biopsies that can be obtained from patients and by the quality of antibodies or molecular probes available for the definition of phenotypic and functional molecules in tissue. Some of the antibodies, for example, do not work well in paraffin-embedded tissues, and mRNA analyses cannot be performed in tissues which are not fresh or handled in a special way to ensure the integrity of cellular RNA. Despite these limitations, *in situ* monitoring is encouraged in conjunction with T-cell studies in peripheral blood. T lymphocytes (CD3+) as well as CD4+ and CD8+ subsets are readily identifiable in cryosections of tissues (Figure 11), and the creative use of immunostaining with different antibodies specific for, e.g., activation markers, adhesion molecules, or triggering receptors, in combination with ISH can provide crucially important assessments of the ability of effector cells to produce cytokines, enzymes, or signaling molecules at the site of disease.

B. Functional Assays for T Lymphocytes

Functional assays for T lymphocytes that have been used for monitoring include proliferation, cytotoxicity, and cytokine production. The assays for these functions have been described in detail elsewhere.[22] From the monitoring point of view, it is important to distinguish specific, MHC-restricted T-cell responses from those mediated by activated, but not MHC-restricted T lymphocytes. The latter can be easily assessed by a combination of one of the functional assays, e.g., cytotoxicity against a tumor target with flow cytometry to confirm that CD3+ T cells are the effector cells. The former are more difficult to measure, because antigen-specific T cells are rare in the peripheral blood, and their *in vitro* expansion from precursor T cells may be necessary prior to functional assays.

Frequencies of proliferating or cytolytic T-cell precursors can be determined directly in the peripheral blood by limiting dilution and clonal analyses,[23] but this approach does not lend itself easily to serial monitoring, especially that of clinical trials, because it is both labor intensive and expensive. In vaccination trials, where monitoring of cytolytic T-cell precursors (CTL-p) or proliferating T-cell precursors (PTL-p) appears to be necessary, the skillful use of limiting dilution technology and subsequent functional assays with the immunizing antigen or peptide allow for the determination of the frequency of precursor cells.[23] An alternative to the limiting dilution analysis in the fresh peripheral blood is *in vitro* expansion of a population of antigen-specific T cells, followed by specificity testing to confirm the presence of such T cells among lymphocytes that proliferate in cultures routinely supplemented with IL-2 or other cytokines. Such *in vitro* expansion requires repeated sensitization with the immunizing antigen and is both time consuming and highly subjective. The main difficulty with T-cell-specific assays is that the antigen has to be available for *in vitro* sensitization as well as specificity assessments. In bacterial- or viral-specific responses, where the nature of antigenic molecules is known, T-cell-specific responses can, of course, be monitored, but even in these situations, such monitoring is difficult to implement and perform on a large scale. T-cell-specific assays performed with *in vitro* expanded effector cells require a panel of blocking antibodies (anti-TCR, anti-HLA-class I, anti-CD3, etc.) to confirm the specificity of T cells and a panel of targets expressing the relevant antigen or pulsed with the antigen to test the effector cell function. In tumor immunology, the nature of tumor-associated antigens is largely unknown, and T-cell-specific assays are particularly difficult to implement.

If the frequency of precursors in the peripheral blood or in culture of T cells is very low, it may be more practical to measure the number of cells able to secrete cytokines; e.g., TNF-α, in response to the immunizing peptide per 10^5 peripheral blood lymphocytes by the ELISPOT assay,[24] instead of measuring cytotoxicity after limiting dilution. The ELISPOT assay allows for quantitation of single cytokine-producing T cells among the population of T cells obtained from the peripheral blood in response to stimulation with a specific antigen. Another possibility is to perform flow cytometry with antigen-sensitized and permeabilized lymphocytes simultaneously stained for a T-cell surface marker (e.g., CD3) and for a cytokine (e.g., TNF-α) which is detectable in the Golgi of those cells in the population that specifically respond to the antigen. By flow cytometry, it is feasible to rapidly enumerate thousands of cells; thus, even rare TNF-producing T cells in the population can be identified and quantified. However, permeabilization of cells prior to antibody staining requires a careful selection of a permeabilizing agent and of controls to correct for background or nonspecific staining. Since the possibility exists that a cytokine may be released from T cells prior to permeabilization and staining, pretreatments of antigen-sensitized populations with monensin or brefeldin (agents which block the secretory pathway) is recommended.[25]

Among the variety of procedures for determination of cytokine production, single cell assays are particularly useful for defining the cytokine profile of T-cell subsets. As discussed above, either ELISPOT or flow cytometry for quantitation of T cells able to secrete or produce, respectively, a cytokine protein are applicable to clinical monitoring. These methods also allow for the definition of the Th0, Th1, or Th2 subsets of CD4+ T lymphocytes. Changes in these subsets, e.g., from the Th1 to Th2 profile, are known to occur in disease.[20] Alterations induced during therapy may also result in a distinct profile of cytokines produced by the T cells. Changes in the cytokine profile of T-cell subsets are important to monitor, because they might reflect alterations in the functional potential of specific T-cell subsets that accompany the development, progression, or termination of disease or might correlate with responses to therapy. In combination with phenotypic markers, cytokine production assays are particularly applicable to monitoring of abnormalities in T-cell subsets in various body compartments, including those at the site of the disease.

The most common T-cell abnormalities are deficiencies induced by infections and those associated with systemic diseases, including autoimmune disease or cancer. Monitoring of T cell numbers and functions in disease or in response to various therapies has recently become more firmly established in many clinical centers. The possibility of dissecting complex patterns of changes in T-cell subsets and correlating them to clinical responses in patients treated with biologic therapies is an exciting and promising aspect of clinical immunology.

VIII. MONITORING OF NATURAL KILLER (NK) CELLS

NK cells are a subset of effector lymphocytes which, in contrast to T cells, do not require prior sensitization with the antigen and whose lytic functions are regulated by a set of inhibitory receptors recognizing MHC class I determinants on target cells (see Figure 5).[26] NK cells also express triggering receptors responsible for recognition and mediating

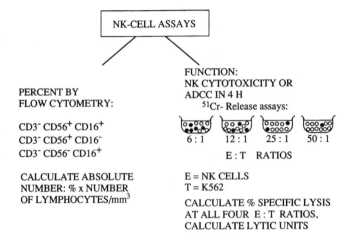

Figure 12

Schematic outline of monitoring for human NK cells and their functions in peripheral blood specimens.

positive signaling, but the nature of these surface structures is presently unknown. Assays for the analysis of NK cells are illustrated in Figure 12.

A. Determination of Absolute Numbers and Proportions of NK Cells and NK Subsets

For the purpose of monitoring, human NK cells are phenotypically identified as CD3- CD56+CD16+ lymphocytes, which represent 5 to 21% of lymphocytes in the peripheral blood (103 to 425 positive cells/mm^3 in normal volunteers (see Table 4). While CD3-CD56+CD16+ cells are the largest subset of peripheral blood NK cells (90%), two smaller subsets, CD56-CD16+ and CD56+CD16-, are also recognized. The CD3-CD56+ NK cells may outnumber CD3-CD16+ cells in the peripheral blood lymphocytes of normal individuals, but the proportions of these subsets fluctuate and much individual variability exists. CD16, which binds IgG complexes with low affinity, has been designated FcγRIII and is responsible for antibody-dependent cellular cytotoxicity (ADCC) mediated by NK cells. CD56 is an isoform of the neural adhesion molecule that serves as a pan NK-cell marker as it is expressed on nearly all NK cells. CD16 expression distinguishes functional subsets of NK cells, since CD16- or CD16^{dim} NK cells produce no IFN-γ, lack the ability to mediate ADCC, respond by proliferation to low concentrations of IL-2, and express abundant CD44 on the cell surface.[27] In contrast, CD16^{bright} NK cells produce IFN-γ, mediate ADCC, proliferate

TABLE 4

Percentages and Absolute Numbers of NK Cells and NK Activity in the Peripheral Blood of Normal Individuals[a]

	% Positive Cells	Positive Cells/mm³
CD3⁻ CD56⁺	6–21	96–425
CD3⁻ CD16⁺	3–20	62–383
DR⁺ CD56⁺	1–4	15–90
NK cell activity		
66–341 $LU_{20}/10^7$ effector cells		

[a] The data are mid 80% normal ranges obtained by testing peripheral blood MNC of 50 normal individuals. The percentages of positive cells were determined by two-color flow cytometry. NK activity was measured in 4-h ^{51}Cr-release assays.

in response to high IL-2 concentrations, and express low levels of CD44 on the cell surface. These two subsets of NK cells are also differently regulated by IL-4.[27]

B. Functional Assays of NK Cells

In addition to eliminating or inhibiting growth of transformed cells, intracellular pathogens and certain immature normal cells, NK cells perform other functions, including a broad range of activities influencing hematopoiesis, immunoregulation, and fetal development. They are also involved in interactions with nonimmune tissue cells.[28] The most commonly used functional assay for NK cells is a 4-h ^{51}Cr-release assay,[29] which can be performed either with isolated MNC or with whole blood.[30] NK cell assays have to be performed at several different effector-to-target-cell ratios in order to be able to construct a lytic curve and calculate lytic units (LU) of activity.[29] The target cell commonly used for monitoring of NK activity is the K562 human leukemia line maintained in culture and passaged frequently to assure that the targets used for the assay are in the log phase of growth (Figure 12). Using this line, it has been possible to measure NK activity in the peripheral blood of healthy individuals and to confirm that it is a stable trait.[29] NK activity is generally higher in males (201 LU/10⁷ effector cells, with n = 49) than females (115LU/10⁷ effector cells, with n = 103). In the author's laboratory, no significant relationship between NK activity and the age of blood donor was detected. In disease, NK activity changes and the NK cell is a sensitive monitor of physiologic alterations occurring during stress, infection, exercise, or other events. NK activity is rapidly up-regulated by cytokines, particularly IL-2 or interferons. In response to IL-2, NK cells acquire LAK activity (Figure 7) and the ability to kill a broad variety of targets. In LAK cultures generated by incubation of peripheral blood MNC in the presence of IL-2, NK cells have been shown to be mainly responsible for cytolytic activity against tumor cell targets.[31] The capability to generate LAK activity *in vivo* may be an important component of innate immunity. In many oncology protocols, LAK activity is monitored by serial assessments of killing of the Daudi cell line (an NK-resistant target) by peripheral blood MNC, because of the expectation that this function of NK cells might correlate with response to therapy. However, it has not been possible so far to demonstrate such correlations in most clinical trials with BRMs. There may be many reasons for this lack of correlation between NK function and clinical response in cancer patients treated with BRMs, but the most likely possibility is that NK cells mediate antitumor effects by more than one mechanism. Thus, 4-h ^{51}Cr-release assays, measuring the perforin/granzyme secretory pathway, may not reflect the true mechanism of antitumor activity used by NK cells *in vivo*.[32] It is highly likely that nonsecretory pathways involving cytokine-mediated DNA fragmentation and apoptosis, which can be measured in ^{3}[H]-thymidine release assays or *in situ* by a terminal deoxynucleotidyl transferase (Tdt)-mediated d-UTP nick-end labeling (TUNEL) assay, may be utilized by NK cells mediating antitumor activities in tissues of patients with cancer.[32] In the future, these assays will probably be included in monitoring of biologic therapies and may prove to be useful in achieving a better understanding of immune NK cell-mediated events associated with clinical response, in cancer and other diseases.

IX. IMMUNOTHERAPY WITH HUMAN T AND NK CELLS

In patients with cellular immunodeficiencies, a good rationale exists for adoptive transfer of *in vitro* activated immune effector cells. When the patients' own immune effector cells are decreased, absent, or nonfunctional, adoptive transfer of competent effector cells, together with cytokines supporting their activities, seems to be indicated. This therapeutic strategy is particularly attractive when other therapies, including attempts at *in vivo* activation of endogenous effector cells, are ineffective. Therapeutic transfer of both T and NK cells, generally in conjunction with high dose IL-2 therapy, have been performed in patients with advanced cancer or AIDS.[33,34] These have largely consisted of the transfer of autologous, *in vitro*-activated and cultured, effector cells. A scheme for the adoptive transfer of immune effector cells is given in Figure 13.

The rationale for adoptive immunotherapy with T cells is to increase the number of specific immunocompetent effector cells and to generate long-term memory T cells. The transfer of antigen-specific

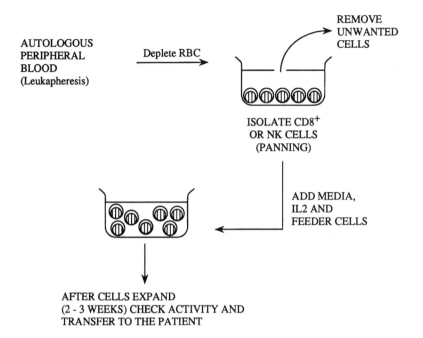

Figure 13

Preparation of human effector cells for adoptive immunotherapy. To enrich autologous MNC in CD8[+] T cells or NK cells, panning on plastic surfaces, which have been coated with monoclonal antibodies for positive selection of effector cells, is first performed. The captured effector cells are then expanded by culturing them in the presence of IL-2 and irradiated feeder cells for 2 to 3 weeks. Prior to reinfusion of effector cells into the patient, phenotypic and functional assays are performed to characterize the cells used for adoptive therapy.

T cells is feasible in only some situations, because of practical difficulties in expanding a sufficiently large number of such T cells in humans. Transfers of human T cells bearing the T-cell receptor α and β chains which recognize specific viral antigens, e.g., CMV proteins, have been performed in recipients of allogeneic bone marrow at high risk of developing CMV disease.[35] Safe and effective restoration of CMV-specific to T-cell responses has been achieved in such patients by the adoptive transfer of *in vitro* expanded, CD8[+] CMV- specific T-cell clones derived from MHC-identical allogeneic bone marrow donors.[36] These clones appear to recognize structural viral proteins. Adoptive immunotherapy with EBV-reactive T cells (unirradiated MNC obtained from the allogeneic EBV seropositive bone marrow donors) has been used in patients who developed a lymphoproliferative syndrome following transplantation with T-cell-depleted allogeneic bone marrow. Clinical trials for the treatment of HIV-1 infections with gag-specific CD8[+] T cell clones are in progress.[37] The goal of these therapies is to provide an antiviral effect by increasing the number of competent virus-reactive T cells present in the host. It is yet unclear whether virus-specific immunologic memory can be induced as a result of adoptive immunotherapy.

In contrast to these successful transfers of virus-specific T cells, adoptive immunotherapy of cancer with tumor-specific T-cell lines has not been so far feasible. Therapy with IL-2-activated tumor-derived T cells (TIL), cannot be considered "specific" because, at best, only a small subset of TIL expanded in culture represent class I MHC-restricted autotumor-reactive T cells. The majority are non-MHC-restricted, IL-2-activated, autotumor-reactive T lymphocytes, whose Vβ TCR repertoire does not correspond to that found *in situ*. In other words, T-cell clones, which are predominant *in situ* and presumably, contain autotumor specific effector cells, tend not to expand *in vitro*,[38] perhaps due to functional suppression in the tumor microenvironment.[39] Nevertheless, therapeutic transfer of activated non-MHC-restricted tumor-reactive T cells has been effective in some patients with melanoma or RCC, resulting in complete and durable responses in about 20% of patients with advanced metastases.[40]

An alternative strategy to therapy with MHC-restricted or non-MHC-restricted T cells is to transfer another type of nonspecific effector cells, such as activated NK (A-NK) cells or subsets of activated NK cells. In oncology, adoptive immunotherapy with a subset of A-NK cells, generated in the presence of high IL-2 concentrations (22 n*M*) from patients' peripheral blood MNC, has been used in phase I trials.[41,42] These effector cells appear to be able to extravasate and actively migrate through tissues. They exert antitumor activities, leading to reduction of established metastases in animal models of metastasis[43] and in some patients who have received this form of adoptive immunotherapy.[41] A-NK cells are IL-2 dependent and are transferred together with IL-2. The mechanisms through which A-NK cells mediate antitumor effects *in vivo* are not understood and are being intensively investigated. The best therapeutic uses of A-NK cells might be in the setting of minimal residual disease, to eliminate residual or occult metastases in patients treated with surgery, or after stem cell or bone marrow transplantation.

X. QUALITY CONTROL AND DATA ANALYSIS

Monitoring of immunologic assays, particularly cellular assays, is difficult and requires that a well designed and rigorously maintained quality control (QC) program be in place in a monitoring laboratory. Such a QC program contains several components: the definition of standard operating procedures (SOP), availability of a SOP manual in the laboratory, training of personnel, implementation of good laboratory practice guidelines, instrument maintenance, review of the quality of performance, and regular proficiency testing. Laboratories monitoring immunologic assays for clinical trials are required to implement their own QC programs to ensure that acceptable results are generated. Currently, no model QC programs exist, but monitoring laboratories are encouraged to follow the good laboratory practice guidelines defined by professional groups such as the College of American Pathologists, or departments of health in some states.

A central and most crucial aspect of immune monitoring is documenting changes from baseline over time. This is only possible when measurements, accumulated over time, are accurate. It is essential to control variability and ensure reproducibility of each assay selected for monitoring. The objective is to assure reproducibility of test results from individual patients tested at different time points, often over a period of weeks, months, or even years. In laboratories involved in preparation of effector cells for immunotherapy, the quality of the therapeutic product must be accurately evaluated. Periodic checks of reagent quality and equipment performance have to be in place. Implementation of a QC program requires considerable effort.

The process of QC begins with sample collection and processing, which have to be organized to meet the protocol schema and occur at specified times of the day and, preferably, before the next cycle of therapy. Bloods for immunologic monitoring need to be routinely harvested in the morning, to avoid diurnal variability. The flow of specimens and recording the collection times and arrival times of samples is a major effort in a monitoring laboratory. Although immunologic monitoring assays should be scheduled in advance, sample collection and arrival times tend to vary. The laboratory must establish strict rules for sample acceptance and handling. Samples are not rejected, unless they are obviously outdated, but rather a precise history of each sample is maintained. Sample processing should be uniform and follow the SOP. The SOP must be available in writing and be reviewed and updated regularly. The decision to cryopreserve cells or use fresh cells should be made prior to the clinical trial and has to be based on preliminary comparative studies, using fresh and cryopreserved lots of the same normal MNC. These comparisons need to be performed and documented for every assay. This is a crucial process, because if assays can be batched (i.e., all samples in the trial testing at the same time), day-to-day variability can be avoided and the cost of monitoring can be decreased considerably.

The importance of the reproducibility of assays used for longitudinal monitoring cannot be overemphasized. Regardless of whether cryopreserved or fresh samples are used, assay standardization has to be performed before a clinical trial begins. The standardization data are obtained by repeatedly performing the assay with cells obtained from normal individuals under the invariant and previously optimized experimental conditions to establish the mean, median, 80% normal range, and coefficient of variation. Intra-assay variability is also determined. When the assay is standardized, a set of appropriate controls has to be selected, and these depend on whether fresh or cryopreserved cells are used. With fresh cells collected at different time points, repeated testing of preserved control samples (e.g., cryopreserved lots of normal MNC with a predetermined range of reactivity) is necessary to control for day-to-day variability. With fresh cells, it may also be advisable to include fresh control cells obtained from a healthy volunteer. A pool of volunteers repeatedly tested over time can be established and used for this purpose. The data obtained from control samples, evaluated in parallel with each patient sample, help ensure the validity of the results for a particular day's assay. With cryopreserved cells or frozen serum/plasma samples, it is best to batch and test all serial samples of a patient in one assay. Even in this case, however, it is necessary to control for day-to-day variability to ensure that the assay performs equally well for all patients on a protocol. If universally accepted standards are available (e.g., the WHO standards for cytokines), these should be regularly included in monitoring assays. Alternatively, internal controls, initially compared to the standards (which are often available only in finite quantities), can replace the latter for routine use. A properly designed QC program will ensure that the values obtained for control samples remain within an acceptable range over time and will specify when patient results are abnormal or altered from baseline values.

Analysis of serial immunologic data should be performed by a qualified biostatistician, working closely with the clinical immunologist. In preparation for final analysis, immunologic data have to be "cleaned," i.e., purged of errors that occur during data entry into computer. All outlier values are checked against the laboratory records, and collection timing of all specimens is verified. The analysis selected depends on the hypothesis tested and the trial design, but it generally seeks to determine if the changes from baseline that occur during various points of therapy or, overall, as a result of therapy, are significant. The monitoring data are generally presented as a series of time plots, which are adjusted by subtraction of the estimated contribution of each patient's baseline level, so that the plots depict the relationship that would exists if baseline values for all patients receiving therapy or a particular dose of therapy were equal to the overall pretreatment average.

XI. SUMMARY

A wide range of immunotherapies for correcting deficiencies or restoring the balance of the immune system altered by disease has become available in recent years. Administration of BRMs to patients with immunologic abnormalities is based on newly obtained insights into functional attributes of immune effector cells. It is now possible to accurately evaluate the number and many functions of effector cells longitudinally in health and in disease as well as during therapy. Cellular products used for immunotherapy can be precisely characterized for phenotypic and functional properties. Newer technologies, utilizing fewer cells and permitting *in situ* studies (i.e., in diseased tissues in addition to peripheral blood), have become available, allowing for more comprehensive monitoring of cellular functions in disease. Molecular technologies in combination with highly specific immunomethods offer a possibility for defining functional defects in unique subsets of immune cells and for documenting a reversal of these defects during therapy. These sophisticated technologies are being gradually introduced to clinical monitoring, and it is reasonable to expect that in the near future, it will be possible to correlate changes in functions of immune effector cells induced by therapy to clinical responses. To achieve this goal, however, monitoring of immune therapies has to be performed under strictly defined and controlled conditions, ensuring that changes that occur in effector cells in response to therapeutic interventions are accurately and precisely measured. The single most important requirement of immunologic monitoring, regardless of the type of assay used, is the day-to-day reproducibility of the assay. For this reason, it is recommended that immunologic monitoring of cellular functions be performed only in clinical immunology laboratories with established QC programs and the capabilities to handle serial specimens and analyze serially acquired results.

REFERENCES

1. Herberman, R. B., Design of clinical trials with biological response modifiers, *Cancer Treat. Rep.*, 69, 1161, 1985.
2. Gambacorti-Passerini, C., Hank, J. A., Albertini, M. R., Borchert, A. A., Moore, K. H., Schiller, J. H., Bechhofer, R., Borden E. C., Storer, B., and Sondel, P. M., A pilot phase II trial of continuous-infusion interleukin-2 followed by lymphokine-activated killer cell therapy and bolus-infusion interleukin-2 in renal cancer, *J. Immunother.*, 13, 43, 1993.
3. Arend, W. P., Inhibiting the effects of cytokines in human diseases, *Adv. Intern. Med.*, 40, 365, 1995.

4. Elder, E. M. and Whiteside, T. L., Processing of tumors for vaccine and/or tumor infiltrating lymphocytes, in *Manual of Clinical Laboratory Immunology*, 4th ed., Friedman, H., Rose, N. R., deMacario, E. C., Fahey, J. L., Friedman, H., and Penn, G. M., Eds., American Society for Microbiology, Washington, D.C., 123, 817, 1992.

5. Whiteside, T. L., Cytokine measurements and interpretation of cytokine assays in human disease, *J. Clin. Immunol.*, 14, 327, 1994.

6. Whiteside, T. L., Letessier, E., Hiraayashi, H., Vitolo, D., Bryant, J., Barnes, L., Snyderman, C., Johnson, J. T., Myers, E., Herberman, R. B., Rubin, J., Kirkwood, J. M., and Vlock, D. R., Evidence for local and systemic activation of immune cells by peritumoral injections of interleukin 2 in patients with advanced squamous cell carcinoma of the head and neck, *Cancer Res.*, 53, 5654, 1993.

7. Smith, D. L. and DeShazo, R. D., Delayed hypersensitivity skin testing, *Manual of Clinical Laboratory Immunology*, 4th ed., Rose, N. R., Conway de Macario E., Fahey, J. L., Friedman, E., Penn, G. M., Eds., American Society for Microbiology, Washington, D.C., 1992, 202.

8. Aebersold, P. M., Hyatt, C., Johnson, S., Hines, K., Korcak, L., Sanders, M., Lotze, M., Topalian, S., Yang, J., and Rosenberg, S. A., Lysis of autologous melanoma cells by tumor-infiltrating lymphocytes: association with clinical response, *J. Natl. Cancer Inst.*, 8, 932, 1991.

9. Friberg, D., Bryant, J., Shannon, W., and Whiteside, T. L., *In vitro* cytokine production by normal human peripheral blood mononuclear cells as a measure of immunocompetence or the state of activation, *Clin. Diag. Lab. Immunol.*, 1, 261, 1994.

10. Maggi, E., Mazetti, M., Ravina, A., Annunziato, F., DeCarli, M., Piccinni, M. P., Manetti, R., Carbonari, M., Pesce, A. M., Del Prete, G., and Romagnani, S., Ability of HIV to promote a Th1 to Th0 shift and to replicate preferentially in Th2 and Th0 cells, *Science*, 265, 244, 1994.

11. Graziosi C., Pantaleo, G., Gantt, K. R., Portin, J. P., Demarst, J. F., Cohen, O. J., Sekaly, R. P., and Fauci, A. S., Lack of evidence for the dichotomy of Th1 and Th2 predominance in HIV-infected individuals, *Science*, 265, 248, 1994.

12. Rossi, M. I., Bonino, P., Whiteside, T. L., Flynn, W. B., and Kuller, L. H., Determination of cytokine production variability in normal individuals over time, *Am. Geriatr. Soc. Suppl.*, 41, SA3, 1993.

13. Vitolo, D., Zerbe, T., Kanbour, A., Dahl, C., Herberman, R. B., and Whiteside, T. L., Expression of mRNA for cytokines in tumor-infiltrating mononuclear cells in ovarian adenocarcinoma and invasive breast cancer, *Int. J. Cancer*, 51, 573, 1992.

14. Vitolo, D., Kanbour, A., Johnson, J. T., Herberman, R. B., and Whiteside, T. L., *In situ* hybridization for cytokine gene transcripts in the solid tumor microenvironment, *Eur. J. Cancer*, 3, 371, 1993.

15. Bromley, L., McCarthy, S., Stickland, J. E., Lewis, C. E., and McGee, J. O'D., Non-isotopic *in situ* detection of mRNA for interleukin 4 in archival human tissue, *J. Immunol. Methods*, 167, 47, 1994.

16. O'Garra, A. and Vieira, P., Polymerase chain reaction for detection of cytokine gene expression, *Curr. Opin. Immunol.*, 4, 211, 1992.

17. Lai, P., Rabinowich, H., Crowley-Nowick, P. A., Bell, M. C., Mantovani, G., and Whiteside, T. L., Alterations in expression and function of signal transduction proteins in tumor associated NK and T lymphocytes from patients with ovarian carcinoma, *Clin. Cancer Res.*, 2, 161, 1996.

18. Romagnani, S., Lymphokine production by human T cells in disease states, *Annu. Rev. Immunol.*, 12, 227, 1994.

19. Romagnani, S., Del Prete, G., Maggi, E., Chilosi, M., Caligaris-Cappio, F., and Pizzolo, G., CD30 and type 2 helper (Th2) responses, *J. Leuk. Biol.*, 57, 726, 1995.

20. Romagnani, S., Biology of human Th1 and Th2 cells, *J. Clin. Immunol.*, 15, 121, 1995.

21. Sanders, M. E., Makgoba, M. W., and Shaw, S., Human naive memory T cells: reinterpretation of helper-inducer and suppressor-inducer subsets, *Immunol. Today*, 9, 195, 1988.

22. *Manual of Clinical Laboratory Immunology*, 4th ed., Rose, N. R., Conway de Macario, E., Fahey, J. L., Friedman, H., and Penn, G. M., Eds., American Society for Microbiology, Washington, D.C., 1992.

23. Moretta, A., Frequency and surface phenotype of human T lymphocytes producing interleukin 2. Analysis by limiting dilution and cell cloning, *Eur. J. Immunol.*, 15, 148, 1985.

24. Czerkinsky, C. C., Nilsson, L. A., Nygren, H., Ouchterlony, O., and Tarkowski, A., A solid-phase enzyme-linked immunospot (ELISPOT) assay for enumeration of specific antibody-secreting cells, *J. Immunol. Methods*, 65, 109, 1983.

25. Jung, T., Schauer, V., Heusser, C., Meumann, C., and Reiger, C., Detection of intracellular cytokines by flow cytometry, *J. Immunol. Methods*, 159, 197, 1993.

26. Karre, K., Express yourself or die: peptides, MHC molecules, and NK cells, *Science*, 267, 978, 1995.

27. Nagler, A., Lewis, L. L., Cwirla, S., and Phillips, J. H., Comparative studies of human FcRIII- positive and negative natural killer cells, *J. Immunol.*, 143, 3183, 1989.

28. Whiteside T. L. and Herberman R. B., Role of human natural killer cells in health and disease, *Clin. Diag. Lab. Immunol.*, 1, 125, 1994.

29. Whiteside T. L., Bryant J., Day R., and Herberman R. B., Natural killer cytotoxicity in the diagnosis of immune dysfunction: criteria for a reproducible assay, *J. Clin. Lab. Anal.*, 4, 102, 1990.

30. Whiteside, T. L. and Herberman, R. B., Measurements of natural killer cell numbers and function in humans, in *Neuroimmunology*, Vol. 24, *Methods in Neuroscience*, M. J. Phillips, and Evans, E. E., Eds., Academic Press, Orlando, 1994, 10.

31. Ortaldo, J. R., Mason, A., and Overton, R., Lymphokine-activated killer cells: analysis of progenitors and effectors, *J. Exp. Med.*, 164, 1193, 1986.

32. Vujanovic, N. L., Nagashima, S., Herberman, R. B., and Whiteside, T. L., The nonsecretory killing pathway of natural killer cells, *Nat. Immun.*, 14, 73, 1995.

33. Whiteside, T. L., Elder, E. M., Moody, D., Armstrong, J., Ho, M., Rinaldo, C., Huang, X., Torpey, D., Gupta, P., McMahon, D., Okarma, T., and Herberman, R. B., Generation and characterization of *ex vivo* propagated autologous CD8+ cells used for adoptive immunotherapy of patients infected with human immunodeficiency virus, *Blood*, 81, 2085, 1993.

34. Rosenberg, S. A., Packard, B. S., Aebersold, P. M. et al., Use of tumor-infiltrating lymphocytes and interleukin 2 in the immunotherapy of patients with metastatic melanoma. A preliminary report, *N. Engl. J. Med.*, 319, 1676, 1988.

35. Riddell, S. R. and Greenberg, P. D., Principles for adoptive T cell therapy of human viral diseases, *Annu. Rev. Immunol.*, 13, 545, 1995.

36. Papadopoulos, E. B., Ladanyi, M., Emanuel, D. et al., Infusions of donor leukocytes to treat Epstein-Barr virus-associated lymphoproliferative disorders after allogeneic bone marrow transplantation, *N. Engl. J. Med.*, 330, 1185, 1994.

37. Riddell, S. R., Greenberg, P. D., Overell, R. W. et al., Phase I study of cellular adoptive immunotherapy using genetically-modified CD8+ HIV-specific T cells for HIV seropositive patients undergoing allogeneic bone marrow transplantation, *Human Gene Ther.*, 3, 319, 1992.

38. Weidmann, E., Elder, E. M., Trucco, M., Lotze, M. T., and Whiteside, T. L., Usage of the T-cell receptor Vβ chain genes in fresh and cultured tumor-infiltrating lymphocytes from human melanoma, *Int. J. Cancer*, 54, 383, 1993.

39. Ioannides, C. G. and Whiteside, T. L., T cell recognition of human tumors: implications for molecular immunotherapy of cancer, *Clin. Immunol. Immunopathol.*, 66, 91, 1993.

40. Rosenberg, S. A., Yannelli, J. R., Yang, J. C., Topalian, S. L., Schwartzentruber, D. J., Weber, J. S., Parkinson, D. R., Seipp, Einhorn, J. H., and White, D. E., Treatment of patients with metastatic melanoma with autologous tumor-infiltrating lymphocytes and interleukin 2, *J. Natl. Cancer Inst.*, 86, 1159, 1994.
41. Lister, J., Rybka, W. B., Donnenberg, A. D., deMagalhaes-Silverman, M., Pincus, S. M., Bloom, E. J., Elder, E. M., Ball E. D., and Whiteside T. L., Autologous peripheral blood stem cell transplantation and adoptive immunotherapy with A-NK cells in the immediate post-transplant period, *Clin. Cancer Res.*, 1, 607, 1995.
42. Kirkwood, J. M., Ernstoff, M. S., Vlock, D. R., Herberman, R. B., and Whiteside, T. L., New approaches to the use of IL2 in melanoma: adoptive cellular therapy utilizing purified populations of A-LAK effectors, in Hersey, P., Ed., Biological Agents in the Treatment of Cancer: Proc. Conf., held in Newcastle, September 4 to 7, 1990, Government Printing, Newcastle, NSW, 1990.
43. Yasumura, S., Lin, W.-c., Hirabayashi, H., Vujanovic, N. L., Herberman, R. B., and Whiteside, T. L., Immunotherapy of liver metastases of human gastric carcinoma with interleukin 2-activated natural killer cells, *Cancer Res.*, 54, 3808, 1994.

Chapter **11**

CLINICAL APPLICATIONS OF FLOW CYTOMETRY

Alan Winkelstein (deceased) and Albert D. Donnenberg

CONTENTS

0-8493-0134-3/97/$0.00+$.50
© 1997 by CRC Press LLC

I. INTRODUCTION

One of the major advances in laboratory medicine has been the ability to immunologically identify specific subsets of leukocytes. This process, termed **immunophenotyping**, employs antibodies reactive against cell-associated determinants to distinguish specific subsets. Quantification of a subset of interest can be readily accomplished by use of a **flow cytometer**, an instrument which electronically detects the presence of the marker antibody.

In clinical laboratories, immunophenotyping by flow cytometry has been invaluable for defining the cell of origin of specific neoplasms, particularly in patients with acute leukemia or non-Hodgkin's lymphoma. A second major application is to provide information critical for the staging and management of HIV-1-infected patients; the data derived from analysis of T-cell subsets play an important role in guiding therapeutic decisions. A third and growing use of these procedures is for the quantification of hematopoietic stem cells, particularly those needed for marrow reconstitution after myeloablative therapy.

In addition to clinical considerations, these cell analytic techniques provide essential information concerning the structure and functions of the cells comprising normal hematopoietic and lymphoid systems. This review will focus on the use of immunophenotyping as a means of studying both normal and abnormal hematopoietic cell populations.

Flow cytometry is a relatively new technique: it was introduced as a clinical tool less than 20 years ago. However, the early clinical instruments were of limited usefulness. They were difficult to operate and did not have extensive analytical capabilities. Most were restricted to the measurement of a single fluorescent parameter; this compromised their ability to analyze complex clinical samples. Advances in hardware, software, and reagents have resulted in the development of instruments and procedures that are readily adaptable to most clinical laboratories. These instruments are comparatively simple to use and do not require extensive operator training. In addition, they possess markedly increased analytic capabilities; most can measure two different physical and three to four fluorescent characteristics on each incident cell. Several publications extensively detail the principles and techniques for operating a flow cytometer in detail.[1-7] These are summarized below.

Another technologic development that has greatly enhanced immunophenotyping is the production of a wide variety of monoclonal antibodies, particularly those capable of identifying specific features of human hematopoietic cells. By definition, a monoclonal antibody is a single homogenous immunoglobulin that specifically recognizes and binds to a single antigenic determinant. Clinically, most of the monoclonal antibodies used to identify hematopoietic cells are of murine origin. The antibodies are generated to membrane-bound determinants, including complex proteins, glycoproteins, glycolipids, and carbohydrates. Most of the targeted antigens have important biological functions. These include serving as membrane receptors or ligands for soluble and contact-dependent signaling, acting as enzymes, or acting as cell adhesion molecules. The latter are responsible for cell-to-cell or cell-to-tissue interactions.

Antibodies recognize and react against small peptide sequences of complex antigenic molecules. Thus, each antigenic protein contains numerous small peptide fragments, termed epitopes, which can elicit specific antibody responses. Antibodies to any epitope of the parent molecule can be used to identify the entire molecule. Initially, this led to a "hodgepodge" of nomenclatures; each laboratory and commercial source had unique designations for its monoclonal antibodies. In order to facilitate communication, International Workshops[8,9] established a consensus nomenclature. Cell surface antigens were assigned a **cluster of differentiation** (CD) number based on their recognition by monoclonal antibodies. All antibodies to the same antigen, regardless of their epitope specificity, were grouped together. Thus, two or more antibodies, each reactive with a different epitope on the same antigen are considered as directed against the same CD. In general, the antigens themselves are identified by CD number (e.g., CD3 on T cells, see below) and the monoclonal antibodies recognizing them are grouped as **anti-CD number** (e.g., anti-CD3).

At the International Workshop held in Vienna in 1989, 78 CD groups were designated. [9] At the most recent workshop, held in Boston in 1993, 130 CD clusters were defined.[10] Table I presents a current listing of all CD antigens. It is important to recognize that virtually none of the CD antigens are truly restricted to a single cellular lineage. With rare exceptions, lineage assignments cannot be made on the basis of a single CD antigen. Rather, they are determined by the presence (and absence) of a combination of markers.

To detect the presence of a cell-bound monoclonal antibody, the antibody must be coupled either directly or indirectly to a dye (fluorochrome). These are dyes that, when excited by a light beam of a specific wavelength, emit light at a different wavelength. In most clinical flow cytometers, light is supplied by an argon laser that emits a major band at a wavelength of 488 nm. The three most commonly used fluorochromes are fluorescein isothiocyanate (FITC), phycoerythrin (PE), and peridinin chlorophyll protein (PerCP). When excited by an argon laser, FITC emits a green color that has a maximum wavelength intensity of 520 nm, phycoerythrin is an orange-red emitting dye that is most intense at 578 nm, and PerCP is a red emitting dye with a relatively sharp peak at 680 nm. These differences enable the individual fluorochromes to be clearly distinguished by photodetectors that measure the intensity of emitted light after passage through a series of wavelength-specific optical filters.

For the direct staining procedure, a cell suspension is initially incubated with a dye-coupled monoclonal antibody directed against the

CD determinant of interest. The indirect assay uses a second antibody labeled with a fluorochrome to detect the presence of an unlabeled cell-bound antibody. In both the direct and indirect procedures, the labeled cell suspension is pumped "single file" into the flow cell, where they are illuminated by one or more lasers. Figure 1 schematically depicts the operation of a flow cytometer. Both physical characteristics of the individual cells and the amount of bound antibody can be assessed by detecting scatter of the incident light and light emitted by the fluoro-chromes, respectively. The physical characteristics are measured both by the angle of the light reflected from the cell's surface and the amount of the incident light that is absorbed or scattered by the cell's internal structures. Flow cytometers measure light scatter at a small angle (for-ward scatter) as a surrogate for cell size, and at 90° (side scatter) as an indicator of granularity or internal complexity. In peripheral blood, small cellular debris, lymphocytes, granulocytes, and monocytes can be distinguished on the basis of their intrinsic light-scattering proper-ties alone. The quantity of labeled antibody attached to the cell surface is measured by photomultiplier tubes (PMTs) which, with the aid of a series of filters, register the intensity of the color emitted by a particular fluorochrome (e.g., with FITC, the amount of green light emitted). The analog output from the photomultiplier tubes is amplified, digitized, and captured by a computer which stores the measurements made on each cell in a data file called a **list mode** file. In a typical file, several discrete parameters (forward light scatter, side light scatter, green, orange/red, and red fluorescence intensity) are measured on 10,000 or more events. In the parlance of flow cytometrists, events are signals which may, or may not, represent cells. The process of data collection, in which cells are run through the cytometer and parameters describing individual events are stored in data files, is known as **acquisition**. Depending on the complexity of the data, they can either be analyzed in real time during sample acquisition, or after the fact by recalling the stored list mode data files.

Assays can be performed using anticoagulated blood (heparin, EDTA, or ACD), bone marrow aspirates, or isolated cell suspensions. After lysing residual erythrocytes and excluding platelets and other small particles from the analytic gate (on the basis of their low light scatter), a predetermined number of events are collected. As mentioned, normal leukocytes can be segregated into three distinct groups, corre-sponding to lymphocytes, monocytes, and granulocytes, on the basis of light scatter. Lymphocytes comprise the leukocyte population with the smallest cell diameter and the least internal complexity. Monocytes are larger cells and have greater internal complexity; neutrophils are cells of approximately the same size as monocytes but with still greater internal complexity. A typical three-part differential is shown in Figure 2.

TABLE 1

CD Designations from the Fifth International Workshop on Human Leukocyte Differentiation Antigens, Boston 1993[10]

CD	Reactivities	Other Name(s)	Characteristics
CD1a, b, c	Thy, LHC, DC, B sub	T6	Glycoprotein noncovalently associated with β2M; MHC relatedness
CD2	T, NK	T11, Tp50, sheep RBC receptor	Cytoadhesion molecule binding to CD58 molecule (LFA-3); Abs can activate T cells or inhibit T-cell activation, depending upon the experimental conditions and antibodies used
CD3	T	CD3 complex, T3	Abs recognize the ε chain of CD3 complex
CD4	T sub	T4	Cytoadhesion structure binding to MHC class II molecules. Abs can block or mediate T-cell activation
CD5	T, B sub	Tp67	Type I transmembrane glycoprotein
CD6	T, B sub	T12	Abs can induce accessory cell dependent proliferation
CD7	T sub		Mature T cells and prethymic bone marrow T cells
CD8, CD8β	T sub, NK sub	T8	Adhesion structure to MHC class I; Ab inhibits cytotoxic T cells
CD9	Pre B, M, Plt, Eo	p24	Tetraspans family; Abs activate plts, induce B-cell homotypic adhesion
CD10	Lymphoid progenitors, cALL, GC B cells	CALLA	Neural endopeptidase
CD11a, b, c	Leukocytes	α chains of LFA-1, CR3, and CR4, respectively	Type I integral membrane glycoprotein; member of LCAM family
CDw12	M, G, Plt		Abs induce oxidative burst in M
CD13	M, G	Aminopeptidase N, gp150	GPI-linked glycoprotein; Abs induce oxidative burst in M
CD14	M, G	LPS receptor	Present on a variety of proteins and lipids
CD15, CD15s	G, M	My1, sLe-x	Abs activate NK cells and granulocytes
CD16, CD16b	NK, G, M	Fcγ-receptor type IIIa	Recognize membrane lipid moiety lactosyl ceramide
CDw17	G, M, Plt	Lactosyl ceramide	Type I transmembrane glycoproteins noncovalently linked to CD11a, CD11b, or CD11c molecules
CD18	Leukocytes	Integrin β2 chain	
CD19	B	Bgp95	Part of B-cell antigen receptor complex

CD	Alternative names	Cellular distribution	Function
CD20	B1, Bgp35	B	Phosphoprotein expressed on B cells
CD21	CR2	B sub	Part of the B-cell antigen receptor complex; functions as CR2 and as receptor for EBV
CD22	Bgp135	Cytoplasm: pan B; surface: B sub	Member of the sialoadhesion family; augments anti-Ig-mediated B cell activation
CD23	FcɛRII	B sub	Soluble CD23 has an autocrine-like B-cell growth factor activity; identical to IgE binding factor
CD24	Heat-stable antigen homolog	B, G	Induces oxidative burst in granulocytes, costimulates B cells in proliferation, inhibits PWM induced B-cell differentiation
CD25	Il-2 receptor α chain, Tac antigen	T act, B act, M act	Low-affinity IL-2 binding capacity
CD26	Ta1, gp120	T act, B act, M	Abs trigger lymphokine secretion, proliferation, and cytotoxicity of preactivated T cell
CD27	T14	T sub	Member of TNF/NGF receptor family
CD28	Tp44	T sub	Cosignaling molecule in T cell activation: counter-receptor for CD80, CD86, and B7-3
CD29	Integrin β1 chain, 4B4	Broad	Major β chain of VLA protein family (CD49 molecule family)
CD30	Ki-1 antigen	B act, T act	Member of TNF/NGF receptor family
CD31	PECAM-1	Plt, M, G, B, T sub	Oxidative burst and cytokine production in monocytes; inhibition of cell adhesion and migration, activation of β1 and β2 integrins
CD32	FcγRII	M, G, B, Eo	Activates monocytes and granulocytes; low-affinity receptor for IgG
CD33	My9	M, normal and malignant myeloid Prog	Type I transmembrane glycoprotein; member of the Ig supergene family
CD34	My10	Prog, EC	Stem-cell marker
CD35	CR1, C3b/C4b receptor	G, M, B, some T/NK	Member of the RCA gene family; mediates erythrocyte clearance of immune complexes
CD36	Platelet GPIV	M, Plt	Involved in platelet–platelet, platelet–monocyte, platelet–tumor cell interactions
CD37	gp40-45	B	Member of the tetraspans family
CD38	T10	PC, Thy, T act	ADP cyclase

TABLE 1 (continued)

CD Designations from the Fifth International Workshop on Human Leukocyte Differentiation Antigens, Boston 1993[10]

CD	Reactivities	Other Name(s)	Characteristics
CD39	B sub	gp80	Homotypic adhesion of B cells
CD40	B		Member of TNG/NGF family
CD40L	T act	TRAP-1, CD40 ligand	Type II integral membrane protein belonging to TNF family
CD41	Plt	GPIIb/IIIa, α IIb Integrin	Activation-dependent receptor for fibrinogen, fibronectin, and von Willebrandt factor
CD42a, b, c, d	Plt	Platelet glycoprotein GPIX, GPIb-α, GPIb-β, GPV	Glycoprotein, subunit of CD42 complex
CD43	T, G, M, NK, Plt	gp115	Member of cell surface mucin family
CD44, CD44R	T, B, G, M	Hermes antigen	Member of cartilage link protein family; receptor for hyaluronate and proteoglycin serglycin; lymphocyte homing
CD45	Leukocytes	LCA	CD45 has intrinsic cytoplasmic protein tyrosine phosphatase activity; specific signal transduction pathways via protein tyrosine dephosphorylation
CD45RO	T sub, G, M	gp180, UCHL1	180-kDa isoform of the CD45 molecule family; does not contain exon A, B or C
CD45RA	T sub, B, G sub, M	gp220, 2H4	220 kDa isoform of the CD45-sharing exon A
CD45RB	T sub, B, G, M	T200	Isoform of the CD45-sharing exon B
CD46	Leukocytes	MCP	Member of the RCA gene family; receptor for measles virus and the M protein of A streptococcus
CD47	Extremely broad	Integrin-associated protein	Abs inhibit binding to vitronectin and induce oxidative bursts in neutrophils
CD48	Leukocytes	BLAST-1	GPI-linked glycoprotein; member of the Ig superfamily
CD49a, b, c, d, e, f	Plt, cultured T, M, B, Thy, memory T	VLA-1, 2, 3, 4, 5, 6 α- chain	Noncovalently associates with CD29
CD50	Broad, not on EC	ICAM-3	Counter-receptor for LFA-1

CD	Expression	Other names	Description
CD51	EC, fibroblasts	Vitronectin receptor, α chain	Glycoprotein cleaved into 2 disulfide-linked subunits that noncovalently associate with $\beta1$, $\beta3$, $\beta5$, $\beta6$, or $\beta8$ integrins
CD52	Leukocytes	Campath-1	Extremely glycosylated protein; target for complement-mediated cell lysis
CD53	Exclusively leukocytes		Member of tetraspans family
CD54	Broad	ICAM-1	Adhesion ligand of LFA-1, CR3, CD43
CD55	Broad	Decay-accelerating factor	Member of the RCA gene family; receptor for echoviruses
CD56	NK, lymphocytes act	NKH1, N-CAM	Homotypic adhesion molecule
CD57	NK, T, B sub, brain	HNK1	Carbohydrate structure
CD58	Leukocytes, epithelial	LFA-3	Binds to T-lymphocyte CD2 molecule with high affinity
CD59	Broad	HRF-20	Mediates inhibition of the complement membrane attack complex
CDw60	T sub		Acetylated form of ganglioside GD3
CD61	Plt	Platelet glycoprotein GPIIIa	Forms a calcium-dependent complex with platelet glycoprotein GPIIb
CD62E	EC act	E-selectin, EC act	Related to selectin family
CD62L	Broad	L-selectin; LAM-1	Structural organization similar to CD62E
CD62P	Plt act, EC act	P-selective	Similar to CD62E; recognizes carbohydrate ligands
CD63	Plt act, M	LIMP	Heavily glycosylated lysosomal protein; from tetraspans family; translocated to the surface upon activation of the platelets
CD64	M, G act	FcγRI, high affinity Fc-IgG	Associates with γ chain of Fcε receptor type I
CDw65	G	VIM2 antigen	Strongly stains monocytes and AML blasts
CD66 family	G, colon carcinoma	BGP, CGM6, p100, NCA, CGM1, CEA	Carcinoembrionic antigen gene family within the Ig superfamily
CD67			Now CD66b
CD68	M, M	Macrosialin	Best macrophage marker in immunohistochemistry; mucin-like molecule
CD69	T and B early act, M act	AIM, MLR, Leu23	Member of the Ca^{2+}-dependent lectin superfamily of type II transmembrane receptors
CD70	T and B act, Sternberg-Reed cells	Ki-24	Member of TNF family; counter-receptor for CD27

TABLE 1 (continued)

CD Designations from the Fifth International Workshop on Human Leukocyte Differentiation Antigens, Boston 1993[10]

CD	Reactivities	Other Name(s)	Characteristics
CD71	T and B act, M, proliferating cells	Transferrin receptor, T9 antigen	Mediates cellular iron uptake and regulation of cell growth
CD72	B	Lyb-2	Member of Ca^{2+}-dependent lectin superfamily of type II transmembrane receptors; counter-receptor for the CD5 molecule
CD73	B sub, T sub	ecto-5′-NT	GPI linked membrane glycoprotein
CD74	B, M	MHC-class II-associated invariant chain	Involved in intracellular transport and surface expression of MHC class II proteins
CDw75	Mature B		Strongly expressed by GCB, weakly by mantle zone B cells
CDw76	B, T sub, EC	previously CD76	Strongly expressed by mature B cells and mantle-zone B cells, weakly expressed by GCB cells
CD77	B sub	Burkitt's lymphoma-associated antigen	Interacts with CD19 molecules on B cells
CDw78	B	Ba	Not yet fully characterized
CD79a, b	B	B29, Igβ	Molecules function as a coupling molecule for signal transduction of B-cell antigen receptor
CD80	B, B act, M, DC, T act	B7-1, BB1	Counter-receptor of the T-cell accessory molecules CD28 and CTLA-4
CD81	Broad	TAPA-1	Member of the tetraspans family
CD82	M, B, B act, T act, LGL	4F9	Member of the tetraspans family
CD83	LHC, DC, reticulum cells	HB15	Expressed predominantly by dendritic cells
CDw84	B, M, Plt	p75	Function unknown
CD85	B, M, PC	VMP-55	Function unknown
CD86	B act, M	B7-2, B70	Related to the CD80 molecule; counter-receptor for the T-cell accessory molecules CD28 and CTLA-4
CD87	M, G, EC	Urokinase plasminogen activator-receptor	Involved in cell migration

CD88	G, M, smooth muscle cells	C5a receptor	Member of rhodopsin superfamily; couples to GTP-binding proteins
CD89	G, M, B sub, T sub	Fcα-receptor	Binds serum and secretory IgA1 or IgA2
CDw90	Prog sub	Thy-1	Abs inhibit proliferation of Thy-1+/CD34+ cord blood cells
CD91	M	α2-Macroglobulin receptor	Glycoprotein cleaved into β transmembrane chain and α extracellular chain
CDw92	G, M	p70	Function unknown
CD93	M, EC	p 120	Function unknown
CD94	NK, T sub	KP43	Member of the Ca^{2+}-dependent lectin superfamily of type II transmembrane receptors
CD95	T act, M act	APO-1, FAS	Member of TNF/NGF receptor family; Abs induce cytolytic process known as apoptosis
CD96	T, T act	Tactile	Type I integral membrane protein
CD97	G, M, T act, B act	p74/80/89	7-Span transmembrane protein belonging to the secretin receptor superfamily
CD98	T, B, Plt	4F2	Abs inhibit lectin-induced T-cell proliferation but not MLR, ADCC, T-cell mediated cytotoxicity
CD99	Broad	E2, MIC2	MIC2 gene locus is in the pairing region of the human X and Y chromosomes; first pseudoautosomal gene to be described in man
CD99R	T sub	CD99 Mab restricted	CD99 epitopes whose expression is restricted to T-cell subpopulations
CD100	Broad	p150	Abs inhibit or augment CD2- or CD3-induced T-cell proliferation
CDw101	G, M, T sub	p140	Possible T-cell signaling function
CD102	Broad, EC	ICAM-2	Counter-receptor for the CD11a/CD18 (LFA-1) complex
CD103	Intestinal IEL, hairy cells	α Chain of HML1, integrin αE	Involved in adhesion of intraepithelial T lymphocytes to epithelial cells
CD104	Epithelia, Schwann cells	Integrin β4-chain	Type I transmembrane glycoprotein
CD105	EC, M act	Endoglin	Type II transmembrane glycoprotein
CD106	EC act	VCAM-1	Binds to VLA-4 and CD49d/integrin β7 complexes
CD107a, b	Plt act	LAMP1, LAMP2	Lysosome associated membrane protein
CDw108	ALL, T act (spleen)	GPI-gp80	Bears the JMH blood group antigen

TABLE 1 (continued)

CD Designations from the Fifth International Workshop on Human Leukocyte Differentiation Antigens, Boston 1993[10]

CD	Reactivities	Other Name(s)	Characteristics
CDw109	EC, T act, Plt	Platelet activation factor, 8A3 7D1 GR56	GPI-anchored cell-membrane glycoprotein
CD115	M, M	CSF-1 receptor; macrophage-CSF receptor	Belonging to the Ig and receptor tyrosine kinase family; Interaction with its ligand M-CSF induces dimerization
CDw116	M, G	GM-CSF receptor α-chain	Belonging to the cytokine receptor (hematopoietin) superfamily; binds GM-CSF with low affinity; upon association with the β-chain it forms the high-affinity GM- CSF receptor
CD117	Mast cells, myeloid Prog	Stem cell factor receptor, steel factor receptor, c-kit	Belongs to the Ig and receptor tyrosine kinase family
CDw119	M, G	Interferon-γ receptor	Type I transmembrane protein
CD120a, b	M, G	55-kDa TNF receptor, 75-kDa TNF receptor	Member of TNF/NGF receptor family; binds both TNF α and β with high affinity
CDw121a, b	G	IL-1 receptor type I, IL-1 receptor type II	Binds both IL-1α and IL-1β with high affinity
CDw122	T act, NK	IL-2 receptor β chain	Cytokine receptor superfamily; binds IL-2 with low affinity; noncovalently associates with the CD25 molecule and the "interleukin-2-receptor-γ-chain" to form the high-affinity IL-2–receptor complex
CDw124	B, T, Prog	IL-4 receptor	Member of cytokine receptor superfamily; noncovalently associates with the "interleukin-2-receptor-γ-chain"
CD126	B act, PC	IL-6 receptor	Member of cytokine receptor superfamily; binds IL-6 with low affinity; noncovalently associates with the CDw130 molecule to form the functional high-affinity IL-6 receptor
CDw127	T	IL-7 receptor	Cytokine receptor superfamily; noncovalently associates with the "interleukin-2-receptor-γ-chain", resulting in augmentation of binding affinity and internalization of IL-7

| CDw128 | G | IL-8 receptor | Rhodopsin superfamily; couple to GTP binding proteins |
| CDw130 | B act, PC, L, EC | gp130 | Cytokine receptor superfamily; binds oncostatin M with low affinity; noncovalently associates with the CD126 molecule to form the high-affinity IL-6 receptor |

Note: Table I key:

act = activated	M = monocyte/macrophage
ADCC = antibody-dependent cellular cytotoxicity	MLR = mixed lymphocyte reaction
ALL = acute lymphocytic leukemia	NGF = nerve growth factor
B = B cell	NK = natural killer cell
CR = complement receptor	PC = plasma cell
DC = dendritic cell	Plt = platelet
EBV = Epstein-Barr virus	Prog = progenitor
EC = endothelial cell	PWM = pokeweed mitogen
Eo = eosinophil	RCA = regulator of complement activation
G = granulocyte	sub = subset
GCB = germinal center B cell	T = T cell
GM-CSF = granulocyte-monocyte colony-stimulating factor	Thy = thymus
IEL = intraepithelial lymphocyte	TNF = tumor necrosis factor
LGL = large granular lymphocyte	VLA = very late activation antigen
LHC = Langerhans cell	

Adapted from Schlossman, S., Bowmsell, L., Gilks, W. et al., Eds., *Leukocyte Typing V*, Oxford University Press, Oxford, 1995.

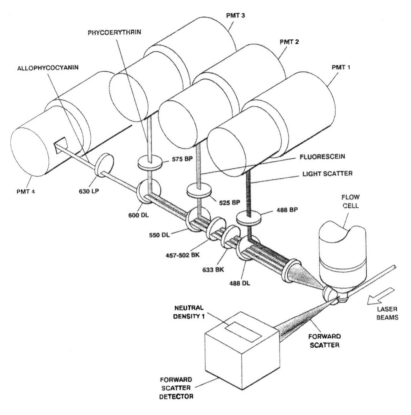

Figure 1

Since the scatter and fluorescence characteristics of each event are recorded in the list mode file, analysis of collected data can be performed on all events or can be restricted to gated events (i.e., cells which meet predetermined scatter and fluorescence criteria).

The measurement of the percentage of peripheral blood T lymphocytes illustrates the principals of flow cytometry. A unique characteristic of mature T cells is the presence of the CD3 membrane determinant, a polypeptide that is part of the T-cell antigen receptor complex.[11,12] To quantify T cells, the cell suspension is incubated with a FITC-labeled monoclonal antibody specific for an epitope present on CD3. The characteristics of each cell in the suspension are then analyzed and recorded; this includes the two inherent physical characteristics, size and internal complexity, and the intensity of the green fluorescent signal emitted by each cell.

Based on the physical characteristics (i.e., light scatter), a **gate** is established to delineate the lymphocyte population. The subsequent analysis of fluorescence is then limited to events with scatter parameters falling within this "lymphocyte" gate. In this example, only T cells that have bound the labeled antibody will fluoresce green. A frequency distribution histogram, which records the number of events at each fluorescent intensity, is then generated. Figure 3 shows a histogram of a CD3 analysis; the initial peak (on the left) represents cells that are negative for green fluorescence and thus lack CD3 (non-T cells). The peak on the right constitutes the positive events indicating the presence of bound anti-CD3 antibody (T cells). This is overlaid by an isotype control, a FITC-labeled mouse IgG without specific reactivity to human leukocytes and of the same isotype as the anti-CD3 antibody. The upper limit of staining with the isotype control can be used to set a fluorescence cutoff; higher fluorescence is considered to indicate specific antibody binding, and therefore presence of the target antigen. Although such interpretations are subject to several pitfalls, the use of isotype controls is routine in most laboratories (e.g., control antibodies should be matched with respect to concentration and fluorescence as well as

---

Figure 1
Schematic operation of a 3-color dual laser flow cytometer. The fluorochrome-labeled cells are pumped through the flow cell, where they enter the collinear light paths of argon and helium–neon lasers. A photodiode aligned with the laser path captures light scatted between 1.5° and 19° (forward scatter). Before encountering this forward scatter detector, the scattered laser light is attenuated by a neutral density filter; the laser beam itself is blocked by an obscuration bar. A collection lens is positioned 90° from the incident laser light. This light (which consists of both laser light scattered by the cell, and light emitted by the fluorochomes on the cell surface) passes through a series of filters and dichroic mirrors which are able to distinguish between the light sources on the basis of their wavelengths. In the instrument depicted here, a Coulter Elite cytometer, light from the argon laser (488 nm) is deflected to photomultiplier tube 1 (PMT 1) by a 488 dichroic long pass (DL) mirror. Before reaching PMT 1, this light passes through a 488 nm band pass (BP) filter, which blocks all other wavelengths. The use of these filters ensures that PMT 1 measures only light emitted by the argon laser and scattered at 90° by the cell (side scatter). The light transmitted through the 488 DL mirror then passes through two blocking (BK) filters which attenuate any remaining scattered laser light (including that from the helium–neon laser), leaving only the light emitted by the cell-bound fluorochromes. This emitted light is then deflected to PMT 2 using 550 nm DL and 525 BP filters. Thus PMT 2 captures a narrow bandwidth of light centering on 525 nm (green fluorescence emitted by the dye fluorescein isothiocyanate, FITC). In the three-color instrument shown here, this process is repeated two more times, with PMTs 3 and 4 capturing orange-red (575 nm) and red (630 nm) light emitted by the fluorochromes phycoerythrin (PE) and allophycocyanin (APC), respectively. FITC and PE are excited by the argon laser, APC by the helium–neon laser. By using different combinations of fluorochromes (e.g., FITC, PE, and PerCP) single laser instruments can be used to detect three fluorochromes. Four-color cytometry is becoming more widely available with the advent of several "tandem dyes" in which two fluorochromes are conjugated to a single antibody (e.g., PE-Cy5). The first dye is excited by the laser light and emits light at a higher wavelength. The emitted light excites the second dye, which in turn, emits at an even higher wavelength. Commercially available cytometers with multiple lasers and photodetectors have been used to measure as many as seven fluorochromes simultaneously. (Diagram reproduced with permission of Coulter Corporation, Miami, FL.)

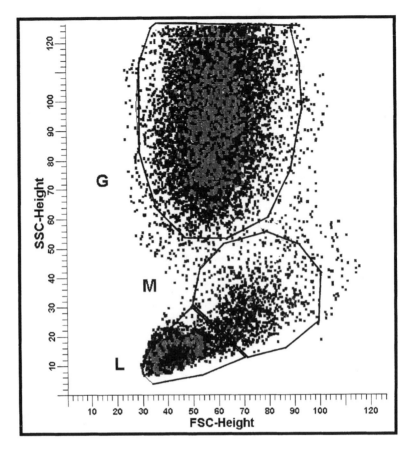

Figure 2
A three-part white cell differential can be obtained by analyzing forward scatter (FSC-Height), a measure of cell size and side scatter (SSC-Height), a measure of internal complexity. Lymphocyte (L), monocyte (M), and granulocyte (G) populations are resolved. The lymphocyte region is particularly important since it is frequently used as a **gate** for analysis of lymphocyte subpopulations. The border between lymphocytes and monocytes is sometimes difficult to resolve. The purity (percent of events within the lymphocyte scatter gate that are true lymphocytes) and recovery (percent of true lymphocytes that fall within the lymphocyte scatter gate) can be independently assessed using antibodies to CD45 and CD14 (see Table 3).

isotype; specific binding can compete with nonspecific binding, such that the negative peak in the control antibody is brighter than the negative peak in the test sample; positive and negative populations are not always discretely bimodal, but may fuse to form a single skewed distribution which overlaps with the negative control, to name a few of the problems commonly encountered). Once a cutpoint between fluorescence positive and negative has been established, the proportion

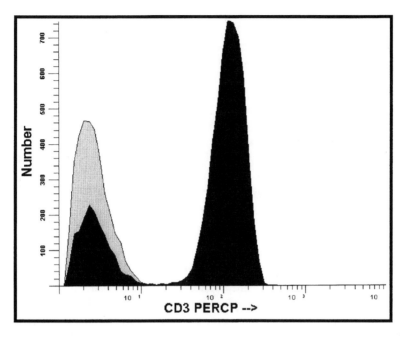

Figure 3
Single-color histogram showing CD3+ (right peak) and CD3negative lymphocytes (dark-shaded left peak). Only events falling within the lymphocyte scatter gate (see Figure 2) were analyzed. Anti-CD3 was directly conjugated with PerCP. Overlaid on the CD3− peak are the results obtained when an independent sample of the same leukocytes were stained with a PerCP-conjugated irrelevant murine monoclonal antibody of the same isotype (IgG1) as the anti-CD3 antibody (isotype control, light-shaded left peak).

of CD3+ lymphocytes can be determined. The circulating T-cell count can be calculated by multiplying the percentage of reactive cells in the lymphocyte scatter gate by the total concentration of circulating lymphocytes (cells/μl). This latter value can determined independently with a hematology instrument, or directly by comparison to reference beads added to the sample at a known concentration.

A major advantage of the current generation of flow cytometers is their capacity to analyze several different properties simultaneously. This can be illustrated by measuring subsets of T lymphocytes, an important determination used in following HIV-infected individuals.[13] Mature, peripheral blood T lymphocytes can be subdivided into two mutually exclusive populations: the T-helper/inducer cells and T-suppressor/cytotoxic cells.[14] These two populations each possess unique and largely mutually exclusive cell membrane determinants. T-helper/inducer and T-suppressor/cytotoxic cells are characterized by the presence of membrane-bound glycoproteins, termed CD4 and CD8, respectively. An example of three color flow cytometric analysis for the simultaneous quantification of these subsets on CD3+ cells (T cells) falling within the "lymphocyte gate" is shown in Figure 4.

In this example, T-helper/inducer cells are labeled with FITC-conjugated anti-CD4; T-suppressor/cytotoxic cells are identified by anti-CD8 coupled to PE; and the T-cell gate is defined by PerCP-conjugated anti-CD3. CD4 staining is divided into positive and negative populations, whereas CD8 resolves negative dim and bright populations. T cells staining **double positive** for CD4 and CD8 are rare in the peripheral circulation, but can usually be resolved if enough events are acquired. Four- to seven-color analyses can be performed on the latest instrumentation. Often this requires the use of novel fluorochromes, multiple lasers, and special electronics that can track individual cells as they pass sequentially through the laser paths.

II. NORMAL BLOOD LYMPHOCYTES

A major clinical use of flow cytometry is to enumerate subsets of normal peripheral blood lymphocytes. These cells can be broadly subdivided into three functional groups: T (thymic dependent) cells, B (bone marrow-derived) cells, and non-T non-B cells. Most non-T non-B cells are natural killer (NK) cells. The percentages and total number of each cell type are summarized in Table 2.

A. T Lymphocytes

T cells are defined as lymphocytes that have productively rearranged and transcribed the T-cell antigen receptor (TCR) genes.[15] Each T cell and its clonal descendants expresses a receptor with a unique specificity. The T-cell receptor (TCR) is a heterodimer consisting of two polypeptide chains.[16-18] Each of the chains consists of a constant and a variable region; the variable regions of the two polypeptide chains determine the antigen specificity of the receptor. Two different types of T-cell receptors have been identified; the vast majority of cells in the peripheral blood and organized lymphoid tissues (~95%) bear a receptor consisting of an alpha and a beta chain. These cells are responsible for the specific recognition of foreign peptides presented in association with self major histocompatability complex (MHC) class I and II antigens.[17] A minor population of T cells have receptors composed of alternate polypeptide chains, termed gamma and delta.[11,12] To date, the functions of these gamma–delta T cells have not been defined with certainty.

Studies have indicated that for both the alpha–beta and gamma–delta receptors, the intracytoplasmic portion of the T-cell receptor is

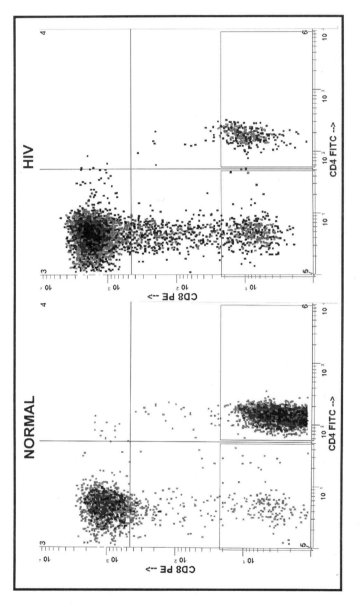

Figure 4

Bivariate scatter plots of peripheral blood leukocytes from healthy control (left panel) and HIV-1-infected (right panel) subjects. Cells were stained with antibodies to CD4 (FITC conjugated), CD8 (PE conjugated), and CD3 (PerCP conjugated). Events were gated on $CD3^+$ and lymphocyte scatter (not shown). This gating strategy confines the analysis to T lymphocytes. For analysis, the scatter plot was divided into six nonoverlapping regions corresponding to two categories for CD4 (negative and positive) and three categories for CD8 (negative, dim, and bright). T cells from the control subject were predominantly $CD4^+$ (68%). $CD8^{dim}$ cells and double negative cells comprised minor populations (3.6% and 3.4%, respectively). In the HIV-1-infected subject, $CD4^+$ cells accounted for only 6.7% of the total T cells. $CD8^{dim}$ cells and double negative cells were more prominent (10%, and 8.9%, respectively).

TABLE 2

Lymphocyte Immunophenotypic Panel

Cell Surface Markers	%[a]	Number[b]
T cells		
CD3	72.9 ± 9.0	1484 ± 499
CD2	80.6 ± 6.7	1683 ± 520
CD5	72.0 ± 8.7	1464 ± 512
T-cell subsets		
CD4	45.2 ± 8.7	909 ± 266
CD8	29.1 ± 7.3	606 ± 270
CD4/CD8 ratio	0.92–4.11	
CD4/CD29	23.6 ± 6.6	476 ± 178
CD4/CD45RA	24.8 ± 8.5	484 ± 169
CD8/CD57	7.3 ± 5.9	147 ± 132
T-cell activation		
CD3/HLA-DR	7.1 ± 4.7	153 ± 138
CD3/CD25 (IL-2R)	4.8 ± 2.9	102 ± 87
B cells		
CD20	11.7 ± 4.8	245 ± 153
CD1 9	11.8 ± 4.6	248 ± 151
NK cells		
CD16	12.3 ± 8.3	263 ± 204
CD56	18.3 ± 8.7	376 ± 213
CD57	11.3 ± 8.2	239 ± 195

[a] Percent of lymphocytes as determined by light scatter (mean ± SD).
[b] Absolute peripheral cell count expressed as cells/μL (mean ± SD).

insufficient to transduce signals required for T-cell activation.[11,18] Rather, it appears antigen binding to the receptor initiates a complex process by which the activation signal is transmitted via interaction with the noncovalently bound proteins comprising the T-cell receptor complex. TCR-mediated signal transduction is the first step in the process which transforms a resting T cell into an activated effector cell. The relationship between the T-cell receptor and the associated CD3 polypeptide is shown in Figure 5.

Most laboratories quantify the number of post-thymic T lymphocytes on the basis of surface CD3 antigen expression. All immunologically competent T cells are CD3⁺; very early immature thymocytes do not express this antigen on their membranes. However, the CD3 molecule can be identified intracytoplasmically. It appears the presence of CD3, either membrane-bound or intracytoplasmically, is the single most specific marker of T cells.[19,20] However, intracytoplasmic CD3 has also been observed in some natural killer (NK) cells[21] and in rare cases of acute myeloid leukemia.[20]

Several other **T-cell antibodies** have been described, most of which react with both immature and mature cells. These include antibodies

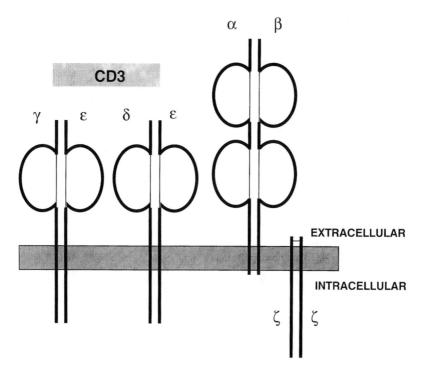

Figure 5

The T-cell receptor (TCR) complex. The antigen receptor itself consists of two polypeptide chains, each consisting of variable and constant regions. The variable regions determine the antigenic specificity of the receptor. The accessory molecules, including those of the CD3 cluster, transduce signals when the antigen receptor is engaged. Less commonly, γ and δ antigen receptor chains (not to be confused with the γ and δ chains that are part of CD3) replace α and β in the antigen-binding structure. These T cells comprise a small proportion of total T cells. Monoclonal antibodies directed against CD3 recognize both αβ and γδ T-cell subsets. Membrane-bound CD3 is only expressed on T lymphocytes.

to the CD7, CD5, and CD2 antigens. However, none have absolute T-cell lineage specificity. For example, CD2 is also expressed on a high percentage of NK cells; CD7 is found on platelets and NK cells; and CD5 is present on a subset of B cells. T cells were first identified and quantified by their surprising ability to form rosettes (complexes consisting of a T cell surrounded by red cells) with sheep erythrocytes. The CD2 antigen identifies the receptor for sheep erythrocytes, which, physiologically, functions in T-cell activation; it specifically binds to a cellular ligand, CD58 (LFA-3), an antigen expressed on many tissues. Engagement of CD2 can be mitogenic or comitogenic to T cells. The functions of the CD5 and CD7 antigens have not been definitively established. CD3$^+$ T cells are the most numerous type of circulating lymphocyte; typically they comprise 60 to 80% of peripheral blood lymphocytes.

1. T Helper/Inducer and T Suppressor/Cytotoxic Cells

The two mutually exclusive subsets of peripheral T lymphocytes, the T helper/inducer (CD4⁺) and the T suppressor/cytotoxic (CD8⁺), appear to function in an analogous manner. T cells require a minimum of two distinct signals for activation. The first consists of TCR-mediated binding of a peptide antigen, presented in the context of an MHC molecule (class I or class II) on the membrane of an antigen-presenting cell (APC). CD4 or CD8 glycoproteins also stabilize and transduce signals during this interaction: CD4 specifically interacts with the MHC class II determinants, CD8 with class I. In addition to TCR engagement, T-cell activation requires a second signal to proceed. Physiologically, the interaction of CD28 on the T cell with CD80 on the APC, provides a strong "second signal."

The structures of both the CD4 and CD8 complexes are similar. Both are heterodimers, composed of two polypeptide chains. The two polypeptides of the CD4 molecule, termed alpha and beta chains, both contain constant and variable regions. The variable regions of the two peptides determine its MHC class II specificity. The CD8 complex consists of only one polypeptide chain that has MHC class I specificity; the other polypeptide is an invariant chain identified as beta-2 microglobulin.

In addition to the T-cell receptor, CD4, and CD8 molecules, several other membrane determinants are important in the interactions between T cells and APC. T cells also express integrin family adhesion molecules, the lymphocyte-function-associated antigens (LFA). These heterodimers consists of a 95-kDa beta subunit (CD18), noncovalently associated with one of three different α chains (CD11a, CD11b, and CD11c). These CD11/CD18 complexes bind specifically to membrane counter-receptors designated intracellular adhesion molecules (ICAM). Three ICAM, ICAM-1 (CD54), ICAM-2, and ICAM-3 have been defined; these are widely distributed on many tissues, including APC. Stimulation of the T-cell receptor results in transient activation of LFA-1 receptors, thereby enhancing the binding of the T cell to ICAM-1.[22] The interactions between T cells and APC are depicted in Figure 6.

As noted above, CD2 binds to another receptor, LFA-3 (CD58), and a second antigen, CD59. Similarly the B7 antigen (CD80), which is present on activated B cells, monocytes, and dendritic cells, specifically interacts with another T-cell–associated antigen, CD28. Other interactions between antigen-stimulated T cells and AP include CD5 and CD43 on T cells with CD72 and ICAM-1 on APC, respectively.[22]

In normal individuals, CD4⁺ cells comprise approximately two thirds of the circulating T cells. The normal concentration range for CD4 cells is 800 to 1200/μl and for CD8, 250 to 500/μl. Clinically, the distribution may be expressed as a CD4/CD8 ratio; the normal range for this ratio is 1.2 to 3.0.

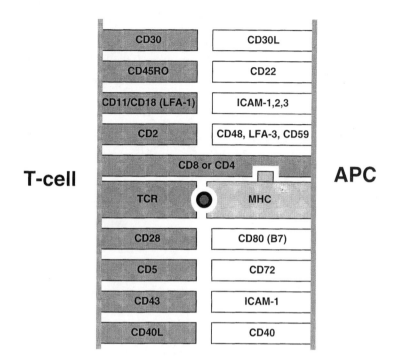

Figure 6
Interactions between surface determinants present on T cells and antigen-presenting cells (APC). These molecules function in a coordinate fashion to regulate adhesion, T cell and APC activation, and subsequent lymphoproliferation and expression of effector functions. Some, like CD40L, are expressed only transiently after activation. (Modified from Lanier, L., *Ann. N.Y. Acad. Sci.*, 673, 86, 1993. With permission.)

2. T-Cell Activation

T-cell activation is a complex process marked by a series of morphological, biochemical, and immunological changes. Prior to antigen stimulation, immunologically competent T lymphocytes are present as small resting cells. Stimulation results from the presentation of an antigenic peptide on APC to the appropriate T-cell receptor–CD3 complex. The early biochemical events leading to activation include the release of intercellular Ca^{2+} have been described in detail.[23] Morphologically, activation results in the transformation of small resting T lymphocytes into a larger, less differentiated appearing cells. These activated cells synthesize both RNA and DNA and undergo repetitive mitotic division. In mitogen-stimulated cultures, the initial division occurs between 24 and 48 h. Following proliferative expansion, which is accompanied by apoptotic death, a proportion of the daughter cells revert to small lymphocyte morphology. Immune response effector mechanisms result from either induction of a cytolytic injury to target cells or the release

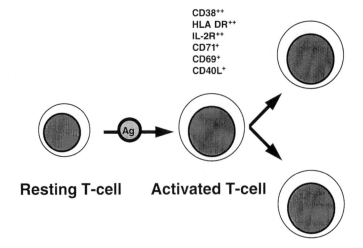

CD38++
HLA DR++
IL-2R++
CD71+
CD69+
CD40L+

Resting T-cell   Activated T-cell

Proliferative Expansion

Figure 7
Acquisition of T-cell **activation markers** following encounter with antigen and APCs.
Many of these determinants are also expressed during *de novo* lymphopoiesis.

of soluble mediators (lymphokines) which activate other cells, such as
those belonging to the monocyte/macrophage series.

The process of activation and division can be traced by immunophenotypic changes (Figure 7).[23-28] Resting T cells do not express (or
express at low levels) membrane-associated receptors for growth factors or MHC class II determinants. However, within a few hours after
in vitro mitogenic or antigenic activation, responsive T lymphocytes
display early activation markers such as CD69, and shortly thereafter,
up-regulate membrane receptors for the lymphocyte growth factor IL-2.
The interaction between the growth factor receptor and IL-2 constitutes
a necessary prerequisite for the subsequent proliferative expansion of
stimulated cells.

Recent studies have demonstrated there are at least three different
types of IL-2 receptors.[28] Biochemically, the receptor with the highest
affinity is a heterotrimer consisting of three different polypeptide
chains termed alpha, beta, and gamma. The 55-kDa α chain (CD25) has
low affinity for IL-2. Furthermore, it is incapable of transmitting signals
intracellularly because of its short cytoplasmic tail. However, it can
rapidly bind IL-2 to the cell membrane. By contrast, the 75-kDa beta
and 64-kDa gamma chains form a complex that is effectively able to
mediate signal transduction. In addition, the beta–gamma chain complex binds IL-2 with high affinity, serving to slow the rate of dissociation.

Thus, the heterotrimeric receptor combines the rapid association rate of the α chain with the slow dissociation rate and signal transducing capacities of the beta–gamma chains to form an active receptor. Binding of IL-2 to this receptor induces T-cell proliferation.

In addition to this heterotrimeric complex, two α chains can associate with each other to form a low affinity receptor. As expected, these are ineffective in signal transduction. Despite a lack of activity, the number of receptors consisting of two α chains greatly exceeds that of the alpha–beta–gamma receptors on activated T cells. The low affinity α chain receptors are not specific for activated T cells; they are present on other cells, including activated B lymphocytes and the B cells of chronic lymphocytic leukemia.

The third type of IL-2 receptor, one with intermediate affinity for IL-2, is found on approximately 90% of natural killer cells. They differ from the other two types of receptors in that they lack the alpha polypeptide chain. In clinical practice, a monoclonal antibody to the α chain (CD25) is commonly used to detect activated T cells.

Shortly after the appearance of IL-2 receptors, stimulated T cells express a second activation antigen, the receptor for the iron-binding protein transferrin (CD71).[29] Both CD25 and the CD71 antigens appear prior to the onset of DNA synthesis; thus, they are referred to as early activation antigens. These antigens persist through the mitotic cycle but cease to be expressed after completion of the proliferative expansion phase.

The next phase, which occurs after 24 to 48 h, is marked by MHC class II expression on stimulated T cells. These antigens appear concurrently with the DNA synthetic phase of the mitotic cycle. In contrast to CD25 and CD71, MHC class II expression persists for indeterminate periods after the cells have completed their proliferative expansion. Clinically, the coexpression of HLA-DR on CD3+ lymphocytes is considered an indicator of T-cell activation, although hyporesponsive T cells produced during lymphopoietic stress also share this phenotype. Up-regulation of another activation antigen, CD38, tends to parallel that of HLA-DR.

Another group of antibodies that are useful in studying T-cell activation are those directed against isoforms of the CD45 antigen. This antigen, termed the common leukocyte antigen, is expressed on all hematopoietic cells except erythrocytes and platelets. By contrast, it is absent from nonhematopoietic cells.[30]

CD45 antigens belong to a family of membrane-associated glycoproteins; there are at least four discrete isoforms that differ in their carbohydrate and protein structure.[31] Expression of these isoforms is regulated at the level of RNA splicing. Among the isoforms, CD45RA and CD45RO antigens are differentially expressed on T lymphocytes. These two antigens appear to identify *"naive"* and *"memory"* T cells, respectively,[32] although naive cells *masquerading* as memory cells, and vice versa have been reported. *In vitro* studies have shown that CD45RO+, but not CD45RA+ T cells, proliferate in response to recall antigens and can provide help to B lymphocytes in their response to antigens. Similarly, the majority of T cells in inflammatory lesions are CD45RO+. It should be noted, however, that the earliest thymic T cells are CD45RO+ (whereas thymic émigrés and cord blood T cells are CD45RA+), as are virtually all of the T cells in the peripheral circulation of bone marrow transplant recipients (autologous as well as allogeneic) studied early after engraftment. These cells have been hypothesized to comprise a maturational stage prior to the CD45RA+ resting naive T cell, induced under conditions that favor extrathymic lymphopoiesis.[33]

CD4+ T cells have been subdivided as Th0, Th1, or Th2 on the basis of cytokine production patterns. Th1 is equated with the production of IL-2 and IFN-γ (limited B cell help, delayed-type hypersensitivity, macrophage activation, cytotoxicity) whereas Th2 produce IL-4, IL-5, IL-9, and IL-10 (B cell help). Th0 cells, which in some schemes are thought to represent a common precursor of Th1 and Th2, produce IL-2, IL-4, IL-5, GM-CSF, and IFN-γ. In mouse and in man, characterization of Th subsets has been accomplished by the analysis of cytokines secreted by long-term T-cell lines and clones (usually by ELISA of culture supernatants). In short-term bulk-activated cells, these characteristic cytokine secretion patterns are easily obscured by the heterogeneity of responsive cells and the presence of cells of transitional phenotypes. The recent finding that the sensitivity of cytokine detection by flow cytometry could be greatly increased by inhibiting cytokine secretion has facilitated the detection of multiple intracellular cytokines produced in single cells. Cells are incubated in short-term culture with agents such as brefeldin A or monensin (which inhibit Golgi function). They are next stained for surface determinants, then fixed and permiabilized and stained for intracellular cytokines. Studies in normal and helminth-infected subjects indicate that CD27 can be used to resolve populations of CD4+ T cells which produce IL-4 plus IFN-γ, vs. IL-4 or IL-5 or IFN-γ alone (15).[34]

CD8+ T cells have been subdivided based on the expression of CD11. The CD8+CD11+ subset has been shown to suppress mitogen-induced T-cell proliferation and differentiation of B lymphocytes, whereas the CD8+CD11− subset contains both precursors and effectors for cytotoxic reactions.[35]

The CD8+ subset has also been divided on the basis of their expression of the CD57 antigen. In normal individuals, CD8+CD57+ cells comprise 10 to 40% of the circulating CD8+ cells. Greater than 90% are also CD3+, indicating a T-cell lineage. Yamashita et al. found that almost all CD8+CD57+ cells express the CD45RA antigen, a marker associated with *"naive"* T cells.[36] Even after *in vitro* stimulation, they did not become CD45RO⁺, the isoform associated with memory T cells.

The numbers of CD8⁺CD57⁺ subset have been found to be increased in several clinical disorders including cytomegalovirus and HIV-1 infections, inflammatory bowel disease, and following bone marrow and solid organ transplantation.[36] The functions of these CD8⁺CD57⁺ cells are not known. Phillips and Lanier[37] showed they can exert lectin- and anti-CD3-induced cytolytic activity; the significance of this *in vitro* phenomenon is not known. By contrast, they do not appear to be capable of effecting antigen-specific cytotoxicity against allogenic cells, suggesting they are not either precursors or cytolytic effectors. It has been suggested they may function as immunoregulatory cells.[36]

B. B Lymphocytes

B lymphocytes are defined as cells that rearrange and productively transcribe immunoglobulin heavy and light chain genes.[38-41] Their function is primarily to mediate humoral immune responses, although they can also serve as antigen-presenting cells. Humoral responses are effected by the terminal differentiation of B cells into plasma cells capable of synthesizing and secreting large quantities of specific antibodies. B lymphocytes constitute a minority of the peripheral blood lymphoid population, typically between 5 to 15%.

One of the principal methods for B-cell identification relies upon detecting the presence of membrane-associated immunoglobulins. Each B cell is programmed to synthesize antibodies with a single antigenic specificity. These immunoglobulins are incorporated into the cell membrane, where they serve as antigen receptors. Triggering these receptors, in conjunction with other contact-dependent and -independent signals, induces B-cell activation.

B cells may express any of the immunoglobulin isotypes (IgG, IgA, or IgM), but the majority of circulating cells display either IgM alone or IgM plus IgD. In the process of maturation, B lymphocytes initially express IgM; subsequently they coexpress both IgM and IgD. These two immunoglobulin isotypes, which differ with respect to their heavy chain sequences, have the same antigenic specificity and display the same light chain isotype.[42] Only a small fraction of circulating lymphocytes switch isotype expression to either IgG or IgA.

In addition to the membrane-associated immunoglobulins, B lymphocytes express a series of lineage- and differentiation-specific antigens. To date, over 20 different antigens have been identified on B lymphocytes.[43] Clinically, CD19 and CD20 are the most widely used markers for B lymphocytes, as they provide a much stronger signal than membrane immunoglobulin. Both antigens are initially expressed during the pre-B cell stage of development, a maturation phase extending from the commitment of stem cells to the B-cell lineage until the expression of membrane lg. These antigens persist until the cell differentiates into a plasma cell. The CD19 molecule is a glycosylated 90- to 95-kDa glycoprotein that functions as a component of a multimolecular complex with the complement component C3 receptor (CD21) and possibly other antigens. It is believed to act as an accessory molecule for signal transduction.[44,45] The CD20 molecule is a 35- to 37-kDa phosphoprotein primarily expressed on B lymphocytes; it appears to be involved in regulation of Ca^{2+} influx, a process required for cell activation.[45]

The most specific antigen for B cell lineage appears to be CD22. Like CD3 on T cells, CD22 can be identified as a cytoplasmic component during early stages of B-cell ontogeny. With subsequent maturation, this antigen is translocated to the cell membrane, normally in conjunction with IgD. CD22 has tyrosine kinase activity, is thought to participate in adhesion and signal transduction, and can enhance B-cell proliferation.[46]

B cells constitutively express MHC class II; this is in accord with recent findings indicating that these cells can function as APCs.[44] MCH class II (HLA-DR) antigens are expressed during all stages of B-cell development; they initially appear on the most immature pre-B cells and persist until they differentiate into antibody producing plasma cells. Other B-cell antigens include CD24, a marker that also appears early in the pre-B cell stage, and CD21, the complement receptor type 2 (CR2 receptor) which binds C3d and Epstein-Barr virus (EBV).[44]

CD23, the low affinity receptor for IgE, may be identified at the stage in which B cells express both IgM and IgD.[47,44] However, its expression markedly increases during B-cell stimulation; as such, it is generally considered to be an activation antigen. Like other B-cell antigens, CD23 is lost at the plasma cell stage. In murine and human studies, this antigen has been shown to focus antigen presentation to T cells after internalization of IgE-antigen complexes[48,49] and to be spatially[50] and functionally[51] associated with MHC class II molecules. It can be secreted and may serve as an autocrine growth factor.

C. Natural Killer Cells

Natural killer (NK) cells are lymphoid-like cells capable of mediating non-MHC–restricted cytotoxicity against certain malignant and virus-infected cells.[52] They have also been shown to produce cytokines upon stimulation. NK cells do not productively rearrange either the T-cell receptor or immunoglobulin genes. Further, NK cells differ from conventional cytotoxic T cells, which require that the target express autologous MHC antigens. Cytologically, most NK cells are identified as large granular lymphocytes (LGL).

At present, no single antibody selectively identifies the entire NK cell population. Clinically, these killer cells are usually recognized by the presence of either the CD56 or the CD16 antigens and the lack of the CD3 antigen. The CD56 antigen is a glycoprotein which is functionally characterized as a neural cell adhesion molecule; its role in mediating cytolytic reactions is unknown. In addition to true NK cells, CD56 is also present on a minor subset of T-cytotoxic lymphocytes; these cells can effect non-MHC–restricted cytotoxicity. This T-cell subset is CD3$^+$ and typically weakly coexpresses CD8.

The CD16 antigen is a receptor for the Fc region of IgG. It is expressed at much higher levels on NK cells than CD56. However, about 10% of NK cells lack CD16 (CD3$^-$CD16$^-$CD56$^+$). CD16$^+$ cells are also able to mediate antibody dependent cellular cytotoxicity (ADCC), a cytolytic mechanism by which killer cells lyse target cells coated with IgG antibodies.

Other antigens present on a proportion of NK cells include CD2, CD8, CD11b, and CD57. CD2 is expressed on approximately 50% of the NK cells; CD8 is weakly expressed on 30 to 40%. CD11b is an adhesion molecule that may be important in target cell attachment. A monoclonal antibody to the CD57 antigen was the first reagent used to identify NK cells. Subsequently, the antigen, which is a carbohydrate of unknown function, was shown to identify only approximately 50% of the NK cells. It is also found on a subset of T lymphocytes, typically those coexpressing CD8.[36]

Because of the multiplicity of antigens on NK cells, investigators have attempted to assess the functional activities of different subsets. Lanier et al.,[53] using antibodies to CD16 and CD57, identified four distinct cell populations. The most potent killer cells were phenotypically characterized as CD16$^+$CD57$^-$. Substantial cytolytic activities were also present in the CD16$^+$CD57$^+$ subset. By contrast, CD16$^-$CD57$^+$ cells were poor effectors, and no target cell killing was associated with the CD16$^-$CD57$^-$ population.

About 15% of normal blood lymphocytes express the CD56 antigen. These cells can be segregated into three subsets, CD56$^+$CD16$^-$CD3$^-$, CD56$^+$CD16$^+$CD3$^-$ and CD56$^+$CD16$^-$CD3$^+$. Most CD56$^+$CD16$^-$CD3$^+$ cells also express CD8. Both the CD56$^+$CD16$^+$CD3$^-$ and CD56$^+$CD16$^-$CD3$^+$ subsets mediate non-MHC–restricted cytotoxicity against K562 cells, the classic target for NK cell assays.[53] Morphologically, both populations are identified as large granular lymphocytes.

Approximately two thirds of the CD56$^+$ cells are CD16$^+$CD3$^-$; comparatively, these are the most potent cytolytic effectors. The CD56$^+$CD16$^-$CD3$^+$, identified as non-MHC–restricted cytotoxic T cells, comprise slightly less than one third of the CD56+ cells. They are less potent effectors than the CD56+CD16+CD3- subset.

CD56+CD16-CD3- cells represent a rare subset (<2% of the blood lymphocytes); morphologically, these cells are identified as either large agranular or large granular lymphocytes. Like the other subsets, these cells can effect non-MHC-restricted cytotoxicity. The relationships between the CD56+CD16-CD3- cells and cytolytic cells expressing either the CD3+ or the CD16+ antigens are unknown. It has been shown that CD56+CD16-CD3- cells predominate in a proportion of patients recovering from bone marrow transplants.[54] Srour et al.,[55] examined six phenotypically different subsets of peripheral blood lymphocytes to determine their relative NK cell activities. Effectors were selected by reactivity with a "two antibody cocktail" consisting of CD16 and CD56. The cells most active in mediating cytolysis lacked the CD3 antigen. The single most effective killers had the following phenotype: CD3-(CD16+CD56)+CD8+. Substantial cytolytic activity was also present in the CD3+(CD56+CD16+) subpopulations. The levels of CD57 and CD8 expression were substantially higher on CD3+ than on CD3- populations.

D. Lymphocyte Changes with Age

Sansoni et al.[56] recently defined the major age-related changes in lymphocyte subset analysis in healthy elderly people and centenarians. They reported that: (1) there was an age-related decrease in the absolute number of CD3 lymphocytes. This affected both the CD4+ and CD8+ subsets; thus there was no apparent significant change in the CD4/CD8 ratio. However, there was a marked increase in the number of apparently activated T cells (CD3+); (2) there was a pronounced reduction in the number of B lymphocytes (CD19+); (3) they also found a progressive increase in the number of NK cells (CD16, CD56, and CD57) and T lymphocytes capable of mediating non-MHC-restricted cytotoxicity (CD3+/CD56+). The proportion of CD45RO+ T cells has also been reported to increase with age.

III. HEMATOPOIETIC CELL MATURATION

A. Stem Cells

Several studies have shown that hematopoietic cell recovery following myeloablation is mediated by a minor population of cells characterized as CD34+. Isolated CD34+ cells alone can reconstitute bone marrow hematopoiesis following myeloablation.[57] Moreover, cells bearing this antigen contain virtually all hematopoietic cells capable of *in vitro* colony formation.[58-61] In peripheral stem cell products, there is an excellent correlation between the proportion of circulating CD34+ cells in the product and its hematopoietic colony-forming activity.[62]

In hematopoietic tissues, CD34+ cells comprise 1 to 3% of the cells in normal bone marrows and <0.1% of peripheral blood mononuclear cells.[58,60,63,64]

The CD34 antigen is a transmembrane 115-kDa glycoprotein. Its expression is restricted to immature hematopoietic precursors, endothelial cells, and some skin cells. The precise function of this glycoprotein is not known, but it may function as an adhesion molecule regulating the attachment of hematopoietic stem cells to marrow stromal elements.[65-67] A recent report showed that the CD34 glycoprotein on endothelial cells is a ligand for the adhesion molecule L-selectin.[68]

CD34+ cells are heterogeneous; they include both pluripotential stem cells and progenitors committed to specific cell lineages. Furthermore, there appears to be an orderly maturation process characterized by the concomitant appearance of new antigens and the progressive diminution in CD34 expression. The most primitive hematopoietic stem cells are characterized by their bright expression of the CD34 antigen. These cells lack lineage-specific antigens as well as the differentiation/activation markers which are present on more mature hematopoietic progenitors.[69,70] The vast majority of these early CD34+ cells are in the G0/G1 phase of their cell cycle.[71]

The CD34+CD38-HLA-DR- (lineage negative) cells are extremely rare; they comprise approximately 1% of the marrow CD34+ cells. Morphologically, these cells consist of a homogenous population whose members are slightly larger than small lymphocytes. Nuclear structure is characterized as an irregular shape, with evenly dispersed chromatin and prominent nucleoli. They contain only scanty cytoplasm.[69]

The initial phases of CD34+ maturation consist of the acquisition of both CD38 and HLA-DR.[69,70] This may reflect their transition into an active phase of their proliferative cycle.[71] CD34+CD38+HLA-DR+ cells are not lineage committed.

During the subsequent stages of maturation, CD34+CD38+HLA-DR+ cells acquire antigens consistent with specific cell lineages, e.g., CD33 on myeloid precursors,[69] high density CD71 on erythroid precursors,[69,72] CD19 and CD10 on cells destined to become B lymphocytes[69,73] and CD7, CD5, and CD2 on pre-T cells. *In vitro* studies have shown that the CD34+ cells can give rise to T lymphocytes,[74] megakaryocytic cells,[75] mast cells and basophils,[76] and natural killer cells.[77]

Additional antigens have also been used to distinguish immature CD34+ cells from more committed progenitors. Expression of the adhesion molecule LFA on CD34+ cells appears to distinguish between committed and uncommitted CD34+ cells; the uncommitted stem cells are LFA 1-.[78,79] Similarly, changes in the expression of CD45 isoforms

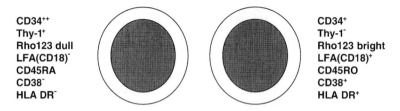

CD34++
Thy-1+
Rho123 dull
LFA(CD18)⁻
CD45RA
CD38⁻
HLA DR⁻

CD34+
Thy-1⁻
Rho123 bright
LFA(CD18)+
CD45RO
CD38+
HLA DR+

Primitive CD34+ cell
Multipotential

Committed CD34+ cell
Unipotential

Figure 8

Characteristics of primitive and lineage-committed CD34+ stem cells. Early stem cells exclude the dye rhodamine 123, which cannot be actively pumped from more mature cells. HLA-DR, CD38 (see Figure 10) and the RO isoform of CD45 are expressed on more differentiated CD34+ cells.

can be used to follow stem cell maturation. Early CD34 precursors predominately express CD45RA; maturation is associated with its conversion to CD45RO.[80,81]

The Thy-1 antigen is also useful in defining primitive CD34+ cells. This is a nonclustered 25- to 35-kDa antigen that is present on 14% of fetal liver cells, cord blood cells, and about 25% of CD34+ cells. It is also present on mature CD3+CD4+ lymphocytes. CD34+Thy-1+ cells have the functional characteristics of immature stem cells.[82] During further development, this antigen is lost. Baum et al.[83] showed a rare subset (0.05 to 0.1%) of CD34+Thy-1+ lineage negative fetal bone marrow cells were capable of long-term multilineage cultures, a functional measure of early hematopoietic progenitors.

CD34+ stem cell maturation can also be assessed by the uptake of the dye rhodamine.[84] The earliest CD34+ cells exclude this dye. As maturation proceeds, the intensity of the staining increases.

Approximately one third of cells identified as CD34+HLA-DR⁻ expressed receptors for the c-kit (stem cell factor) ligand. However, 50% of the more differentiated CD34+HLA-DR+ cells also are c-kit ligand positive.[85] The properties of primitive vs. more committed CD34+ stem cells are diagrammed in Figure 8.

Terstappen et al.[69] used a combination of physical and flow cytometric characteristics to follow CD34 cell maturation. Using two-color fluorescence (CD34 and CD38), size and complexity criteria (Figure 9), the smallest stem cell population (termed PI) brightly expresses CD34; these cells were CD38⁻. These C34+CD38⁻ cells are extremely rare, comprising a small proportion of CD34+ cells. The next maturation phase (P II) is characterized by the dim expression of CD38 on the CD34bright cells. This subset represents approximately 10 to 15% of the CD34+ cells.

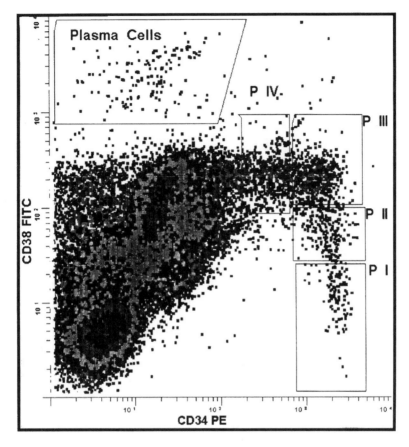

Figure 9

Maturation of bone marrow progenitor cells. The most primitive cells (P I) are CD34[bright] and CD38[-]. With maturation, CD38 expression increases and the intensity of CD34 staining decreases. Terstappen et al. [69] postulated a maturational hierarchy (P I through P IV) based on these parameters. These populations differ with respect to light scatter properties (not shown here), plating efficiency in culture, and coexpression of lineage specific markers. Analysis of rare events, such as CD34 subsets, requires acquisition of a large number of events. In this example 136,000 events were acquired; only 1500 (1.1%) were CD34[+] and only 110 (7% of CD34[+] cells) were in the P I region. Plasma cells, a very rare population in normal bone marrow (0.11% in this example), are easily visualized as intensely CD38[+] and CD34[-].

Morphologically, P II cells are indistinguishable from the CD34[+]CD38[-] P I subset.

In the next maturation phase, termed P III, cells are larger, less intensely CD34[+,] and strongly express CD38. The P IV cells are also large cells that were CD34[dim] and CD38[bright]. Both P III and P IV cells morphologically contained blast cells of erythroid, myeloid, and lymphoid origin. Three-color fluorescence studies showed that these cells are committed to myeloid, erythroid, or B lymphoid differentiation, identified by coexpression of the CD33, CD71, and CD10 antigens, respectively.

Culture of isolated CD34[+] cells has provided useful information concerning the relationship between maturation and the expression of membrane-associated antigens. Purified CD34[+]CD38[-] cells, stimulated with hematopoietic growth factors, acquire CD38 between days 2 and 5. CD34 is lost between days 5 and 11; this loss is accompanied by the acquisition of a new antigen, CD15. Myeloid differentiation is initially demonstrated by the appearance of CD33 and CD71. Further maturation along neutrophilic pathways results in the acquisition of CD11b, followed by CD16, whereas monocytic development is characterized by the appearance of the CD11b and CD14 antigens.[86]

In another study, Bernstein et al.[87] showed CD33[-]CD34[+] human bone marrow cells are capable of giving rise to colony-forming cells in long-term marrow cultures (LTMC), but are largely depleted of progenitors that directly form colonies in semi-solid media. In addition, blast colony-forming cells, a population capable of self renewal is present in the CD33[-]CD34[+] but not in the CD33[+]CD34[+] fractions. By contrast, CD33[+]CD34[+] cells contain most of the colony-forming cells but not the precursors of these cells as detected in LTMC assays.

A recent report indicated that in adult bone marrow, CD34[+] maturation can be traced by the sequential acquisition of CD13 followed by CD33. Raymakers et al.[88] found that approximately 50% of marrow CD34[+] cells expressed CD13. The CD34[+]CD13[+]CD33[-] population was enriched for progenitors of CFU-GEMM colonies, a multipotential type of colony. By contrast, the CD34[+]CD13[+]CD33[+] cells contained most of the precursors for CFU-GM colonies. They also reported the CD34[+]CD13[-] population could be subdivided into those expressing CD19 (pre-B cells), CD7 (pre-T cells) and CD36 (precursors of erythroid colonies).

In fetal bone marrows, Huang and Terstoppen[70] made the interesting observation that the CD34[+]HLA[-] DR[-]CD38[-] population was not only capable of giving rise to hematopoietic colonies but also to stromal cells able to support the differentiation of hematopoietic cells. By contrast, CD34[+]HLA[-] DR[+]CD38[-] cells were restricted to forming hematopoietic colonies only.

Although CD34 cells can be identified as a rare population in the peripheral blood, there are distinct differences between the blood and marrow in the relative proportions of committed and uncommitted stem cells. One study found that 83% of the CD34[+] cells in unstimulated peripheral blood coexpressed the myeloid committed antigen CD33. By contrast, only 44% of marrow CD34[+] cells were positive for this lineage-associated antigen.[64] Different distributions of CD34[+] subsets, isolated by immunoaffinity columns, were found in unstimulated peripheral blood, bone marrow aspirates, and cells collected after G-CSF and chemotherapy priming. The percentages of CD34+CD38-HLA-DR- cells in the three isolates were 6.5%, 1.3%, and 0.1%, respectively.[89]

As mentioned above, CD34 is also expressed on lymphocyte precursors. Cells destined to become T cells can be identified in the marrow; these CD34+ progenitors coexpress the T-cell antigens CD7, CD5, and CD2. In fetal marrows, this fraction represents approximately 2% of the marrow CD34+ cells.[90] These data suggest that T lineage features are initially acquired within the bone marrow. During early development through childhood, these committed cells then migrate, via the blood, to the thymus, where they mature and undergo selection. Later, after thymic involution, extrathymic maturation of bone marrow-derived pre-T cells may become more important. Likewise, pre-B cells which express both CD34 and the B cell antigens, CD19 and CD10, are found in hematopoietic tissues.[73,91] CD34+ cells coexpressing CD7+ and CD19+ have been identified in fetal marrows. It is unclear whether these CD7+CD19+ cells are committed to the B-cell lineage or represent a pluripotential lymphoid stem cell capable of either T- or B-cell maturation.[92,93]

Clinically, enumeration of CD34+ cells is assuming increasing importance, particularly in determining the numbers of cells needed for marrow repopulation after myeloablative therapy. Because of the relative rarity of these cells in both marrow harvests and peripheral blood stem cell harvests, a number of techniques for enumeration have been proposed.[59,60,64,94-98] Probably the most widely accepted method for quantifying CD34+ cells measures them by plotting side scatter vs. CD34 fluorescence intensity (Figure 10).[62,70,80,94,99,100] Others employ two-color procedures using "antibody cocktails" to eliminate mature cells coexpressing lineage-specific antigens.[64,98] Despite these advances, flow cytometric progenitor quantification suffers from two drawbacks: (1) we are as yet uncertain of the phenotypic characteristics of the most desirable progenitor cells (especially with respect to long- and short-term repopulating activity); (2) the clinical goal is to determine the absolute number of progenitor cells in the graft preparation. It is difficult to relate the proportion of CD34+ cells measured by cytometry to the cell count determined using a hematology instrument such as a Coulter counter. Nucleated red blood cells (RBC) and debris are seen differently by these instruments, and sample preparation requires RBC lysis for flow determinations and stomalysis (isolation of nuclei) for cell counts. The use of *no wash* RBC lysing and staining techniques in conjunction with calibration beads added at a known concentration allows absolute cell counts to be obtained directly from the flow cytometer, and has been proposed as a solution to the latter problem.

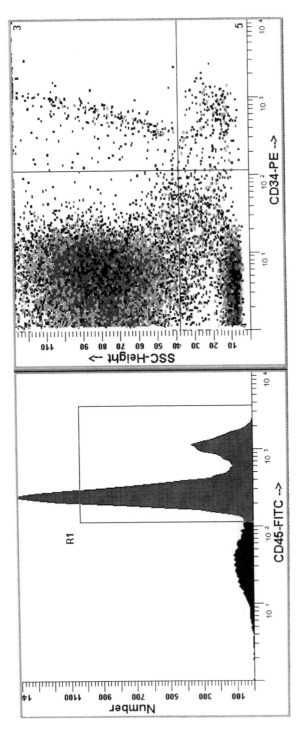

Figure 10

Detection of CD34⁺ cells in human bone marrow. The fluorescence signal from these cells, which comprise 1 to 2% of nucleated cells in the marrow, can be obscured by the autofluorescence and nonspecific antibody binding of more mature myeloid cells. Recently, the International Society of Hematotherapy and Graft Engineering (ISHAGE) has recommended that CD45 be used as a gating antibody to eliminate interference caused by CD45⁻ and dim events. In the present example, bone marrow cells were stained with antibodies to CD45 (FITC conjugated) and CD34 (PE conjugated). A gate was first created which includes only CD45 intermediate and bright events (left panel, R1). This gate was then applied to a bivariate plot of CD34 vs. side scatter (right panel). Since CD34⁺ cells have relatively low side scatter, and autofluorescent myeloid cells typically have high side scatter, this strategy, in conjunction with CD45 gating, helps to identify the CD34⁺ population (right panel, lower right quadrant) that would otherwise be contaminated by false positive events (upper right quadrant). In this example, CD34⁺ events accounted for 1.2% of CD45 gated events, and 1.4% of total events.

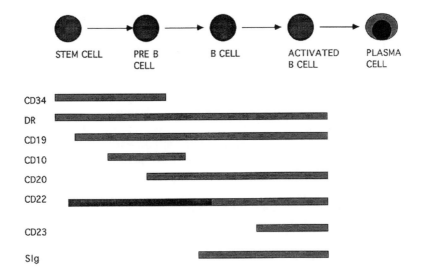

Figure 11
Maturation of B lymphocytes. As they mature, B cells lose CD34 and CD10 and gain
lineage-specific markers (CD19, CD20) and surface immunoglobulin (SIg).

B. B Cells

Although B-cell maturation is a continuous process, the ontogeny
of these cells can be operationally divided into discrete stages. These
have been designated pre-B cell, resting B cell, activated/proliferating
B cells, and terminally differentiated plasma cells (Figure 11). These
different stages can be defined by the presence of specific membrane-
associated and cytoplasmic antigens. In parallel to the other cells of the
lymphohematopoietic system, the earliest pre-B cells coexpress the
CD34 antigen and have been identified as CD34+CD19+CD10+HLA-DR+
cells.[73,91] The B-cell lineage can established by the presence of cytoplasmic CD22. The sequence of antigen acquisition is believed to be: CD19,
cytoplasmic CD22,[20,101,102] followed by CD10. Other studies have shown
rearrangement of the heavy chain gene, and expression of CD24, a
B-cell marker, occurs at a stage between expression of CD19 and CD10.

Further maturation of early pre-B cells result in both a disappearance of CD34 and the acquisition of CD20. The final phase of pre-B cell
maturation is the appearance of intracytoplasmic μ immunoglobulin
heavy chains. These are not associated with light chains. Pre-B cells do
not express membrane-associated immunoglobulins.

The transition from a pre-B cell to an immunologically competent
B lymphocyte is initially characterized by the appearance of membrane-
associated IgM. Concomitantly, there is a loss of the CD10 antigen.
Based on studies in patients with acute leukemia, there appears to be

an intermediate state between the pre-B cell and the IgM-bearing B cell. These intermediate cells express both cytoplasmic and membrane-associated μ heavy chains but lack an associated immunoglobulin light chain.[103]

The IgM-bearing B lymphocyte undergoes further maturation into a cell coexpressing both IgM and IgD. As described previously, these two immunoglobulin isotypes share the same immunologic specificity. At this stage, CD22 is translocated from the cytoplasm to the cell membrane. Several other physiologically important receptors are also expressed on these immunologically competent B cells; these include the receptor for the Fc portion of IgG (CD16).

Resting B-cell activation is initiated by engagement of membrane Ig by the cognate antigen in the context of cytokine and contact-mediated signals provided by T cells and APCs. This results in a series of cytological, biochemical, and phenotypic changes. Morphologically, responsive B lymphocytes are transformed into large cells with basophilic-staining cytoplasm and a less differentiated nuclear structure. A prominent nucleolus may be apparent. Accompanying these cytologic changes, the cells enter an active phase of the mitotic cycle; *in vitro* studies indicate that DNA synthesis commences approximately 24 h after stimulation and reaches a maximum at 72 h.

Activation and subsequent differentiation can be followed by a series of phenotypic changes. Within the first 24 h, stimulated B cells show decreased expression of membrane-bound IgD, CD21 and CD22; these membrane-associated features are lost after 72 to 96 h. Concomitantly, new antigens are expressed, including CD71 (the transferrin receptor), CD54 (the ligand for LFA-1), CD80 (the ligand for the T cell antigen, CD28), CD23, and CD25 (IL-2 receptor). Antibody synthesis increases and complete immunoglobulin molecules can be demonstrated both in the cytoplasm and on the membrane.

Following their proliferative expansion, activated B cells terminally differentiate into plasma cells. These specialized cells are capable of synthesizing and secreting large quantities of antigen-specific antibodies. The transition between a B lymphocyte and a plasma cell is phenotypically characterized by a diminution, or loss, of B-cell–associated antigens, including CD19 and CD20. Plasma cells do not express membrane associated immunoglobulins but contain large amounts of Ig in their cytoplasm. No plasma cell specific antigens have been identified. However, they express certain nonlineage-specific determinants including PCA-1, PC-1 and CD38.

Because of the rarity of plasma cells in hematopoietic tissues, most of the phenotypic studies have been performed on the malignant plasma cells present in patients with multiple myeloma. Harada et al.[104] recently reported a difference between normal and malignant plasma cells; the former express the CD19 antigen.

C. T Cells

The maturation of thymocytes into immunologically competent T cells has been well studied in children and in small animal models. It should be noted that this is an ontogenic paradigm, based largely on events which begin late in fetal development and continue through childhood. In young adulthood, the thymus involutes and ceases to be a major site of lymphopoiesis. Extrathymic maturation of T cells, through probably of great significance in the adult, is at present only poorly characterized. T-cell maturation in the thymus follows a sequence of events that parallels B-cell development (Figure 12). As mentioned above, T-cell precursors have been identified in the bone marrow. These pre-thymocytes are CD34+CD7+ cells; a proportion of these cells may express CD5 and CD2. Barcena et al.[105] analyzed CD7 subsets among primitive human fetal hematopoietic cells. Based on fluorescent intensity of the CD7 staining, they subdivided these cells into three groups. The CD7bright cells coexpressed CD56 and were thought to be the precursors of natural killer cells. These cells were CD34−. The CD7dim and CD7 populations were capable of differentiating into phenotypically mature T cells. The acquisition of other early T-cell markers, such as CD2, CD28, and CD5, is thought to occur primarily within the thymus.

After migration to the thymus, CD34+CD7+ stem cells undergo an orderly maturation which can be followed by the appearance and disappearance of thymic-related antigens. The most immature thymocytes are located in the outer cortex. Using multiparameter flow cytometry, Terstappen et al.[90] showed that these early thymocytes were CD34+CD7+CD2+CD5+. These cells were also CD38+ and CD71+ and expressed the nuclear enzyme, terminal deoxynucleotide transferase (TdT). Cytoplasmic, but not membrane-associated, CD3 could be demonstrated. Morphologically, these immature thymocytes were identified as atypical blasts. In fetal and pediatric thymi, this population comprises less than 2% of the total thymic cells.

The second stage of maturation is marked by the acquisition of the common thymocyte antigen CD1 and the simultaneous expression of CD4 and CD8. Galy et al.[106] used a fetal thymic organ culture system to show that CD34+ thymocytes first acquire CD1 and subsequently express both CD4 and CD8 (double positives). CD4 appears slightly before CD8. During the second phase of maturation, there is a progressive decrease in the intensity of CD34 staining. Other phenotypic characteristics of these stage II thymocytes include the persistence of the T-cell antigens, CD7, CD5, and CD2, along with continued expression of membrane-associated CD38 and nuclear TdT. Numerically, stage II thymocytes represent the predominant cell in the thymus; they comprise >70% of total cells.

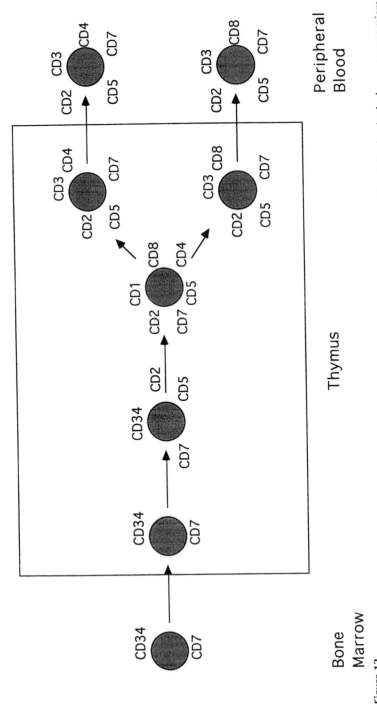

Figure 12

Maturation of T lymphocytes. From late fetal development through late childhood, lymphoid progenitor cells originating in the bone marrow migrate to the thymus, where they differentiate into T lymphocytes. During this sequence, early T cells simultaneously express both CD4 and CD8. Concomitant with the appearance of the CD3–TCR complex, the developing T lymphocytes segregate into two populations, expressing either CD4 or CD8.

Late in the second stage of maturation, the CD3 antigen, but not the T-cell receptor complex, is expressed on the cell membrane. At this time, the beta chain of this receptor can be identified intracytoplasmically. Concomitantly, the cell no longer expresses the nuclear antigen TdT.

It is generally believed that only a small proportion of the cells coexpressing CD4 and CD8 escaped apoptosis or programmed cell death.[107] The process is the major mechanism by which potentially autoreactive T cells are eliminated. The selection process is regulated by T-cell receptor/MHC and appropriate CD4–CD8/MHC interactions.

The final stage of intrathymic maturation (stage III) is characterized by the disappearance of the CD1 antigen. Following this maturation process, immunologically competent cells, which express either CD4 or CD8 (but not both) are exported from the thymus to the peripheral lymphoid tissues.

D. Natural Killer Cells

The maturation of NK cells is, at present, poorly understood. It is generally believed that the development of these cells is independent of the thymic microenviroment.[108] However, NK cells share lytic activities and express many membrane antigens in common with T cells, including CD2, CD7, CD8, and CD56.[109] Recently, it has been shown that they can also express cytoplasmic CD3.[21] Barcena et al.[105] reported that CD7[bright] cells from human fetal livers express CD56; this suggests that NK cells can arise from primitive hematopoietic tissues. In another study, it was shown that NK cells can be generated from cultured bone marrow-derived CD34+ cells.[110] Sanchez et al.[108] found a CD56+CD5- population present in the thymus that represent a population of lineage-committed NK cells. Based on the functional studies using subsets of thymocytes, they postulated a CD34+ cell which is a common T and NK precursor.

E. Myeloid Cells

Until recently, myeloid maturation was primarily determined by the ability of progenitors to form colonies in semisolid media. The introduction of antibodies directed against different myeloid-associated antigens has greatly expanded the study of myelopoiesis. Specific precursor stages can now be phenotypically recognized.

The most primitive myeloid progenitors, cells bearing only the CD34 antigen, are capable of long-term growth in liquid media. Further maturation of these cells give rise to cells capable of forming CFU-GEMM; these colonies are believed to represent the progeny of multipotential cells capable of differentiating into granulocytes, monocyte/macrophages,

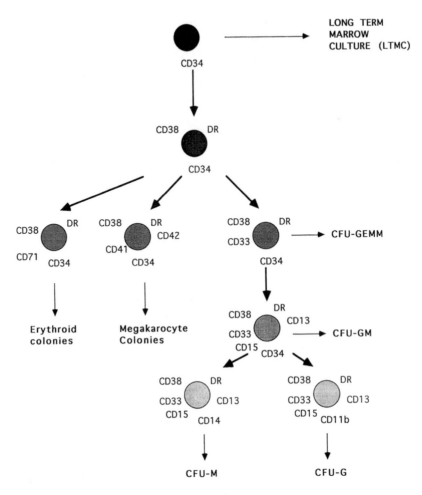

Figure 13

Phenotypic maturation of myeloid elements and presumed relationships between phenotypic stages and *in vitro* colony formation.

erythrocytes, and megakaryocytes. Phenotypically cells capable of CFU-GEMM formation are characterized as CD34$^+$, HLA-DR$^+$, CD38$^+$, and CD33$^+$. They also weakly express the CD15 antigen. The maturation sequence is depicted in Figure 13.

Further differentiation of progenitors results in stem cells committed to more specific cell lineages. One type is capable of maturing into granulocytes and monocyte/macrophages; these precursor cells can be functionally identified by their ability to give rise to CFU-GM (colony-forming unit–granulocyte/macrophage) colonies in semisolid media. A second subset, destined to develop into erythrocytes, are designated BFU-E (burst-forming unit — erythroid) colonies. A third, BFU-MK

(burst-forming unit — megakaryocyte) can give rise to megakaryocytes. The CFU and BFU nomenclature results from the cautious atti-
tude of early experimental hematologists who recognized that a **colony
forming unit** may not always be a single cell, depending on the experimental conditions. The *burst* in BFU refers to the fact that erythroid
colonies have a starburst appearance resulting from the formation of
satellite clusters. The phenotype of cells capable of CFU-GM has been
determined to be $CD34^+CD33^+CD13^+CD15^+CD11b^-$. BFU-E- and BFU-
MK-forming cells have similar phenotypes and express neither the
CD13 nor CD15 antigens. The BFU-E precursors can be recognized by
the expression of high concentrations of CD71.

Subsequent maturation of all cell lines is accompanied by a disappearance of CD34. Cells destined to become neutrophils express the
CD11b antigen. Monocytic precursors are $CD14^+$. Recent studies have
shown that CD14 defines a 55-kDa glycoprotein which functions as a
receptor for lipopolysaccharide.[111] Erythroid precursors can be recognized by the expression of glycophorin and early megakaryocytic cells
by the appearance of platelet-specific antigens including CD41 and
CD42.

IV. LYMPHOCYTE CHANGES IN PATIENTS INFECTED WITH HIV

Among the major factors leading to the widespread clinical acceptance of flow cytometry are its utility for monitoring and managing
HIV-1 infected patients. This virus, the etiologic agent of the acquired
immunodeficiency syndrome (AIDS), has the ability to infect and
destroy $CD4^+$ T cells. This eventually results in a profound depletion
of these cells and a severe immunodeficiency. The consequence of this
deficiency is susceptibility to opportunistic infections and certain
malignancies, including Kaposi's sarcoma and non-Hodgkin's lymphoma. Managing HIV-1–infected patients depends upon following
the $CD4^+$ T-cell number (cells/µl) and therapeutically intervening
when these counts have fallen to specified values. The importance of
the $CD4^+$ count is illustrated by the Centers for Disease Control's (CDC)
recent decision to broaden the definition of AIDS to include HIV-
infected individuals with $CD4^+$ counts less than 200/µl or 20% of the
total T cells.[112]

A brief discussion of the HIV life cycle is useful in understanding
the pathogenesis of this infection (Figure 14). An envelope glycoprotein
of this retrovirus, gp120, specifically binds to cell membrane-expressed
CD4. Following this interaction, the viral RNA core is internalized into
the cell's cytoplasm. Through the activity of the enzyme reverse transcriptase, viral RNA is transcribed into a complementary strand of

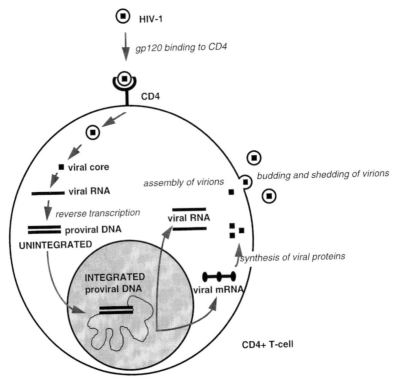

Figure 14
Life cycle of HIV. CD4 on T cells (and also monocytes) serves as a receptor for the viral envelope glycoprotein gp120. Following binding, the viral core is internalized and its RNA is transcribed into a corresponding strand of DNA by the retroviral enzyme reverse transcriptase. Proviral DNA is subsequently integrated into the cell's own DNA and serves as the template for transcription of viral RNA.

DNA and integrated into the cell's own nuclear DNA. Subsequently, the virus-derived DNA is transcribed into new RNA and ultimately translated into viral proteins. One of the consequences of this viral replication cycle is the destruction of CD4+ T cells.

In an HIV-1 infected individual, the interval between initial infection and the development of symptomatic manifestations is highly variable. However, the majority of patients experience a long asymptomatic or latent period, approximately 10 years on average.[113] During this period there is a progressive decline in the number of CD4+ cells; however, the rate of CD4 decline varies at different stages of the infection.

In a large prospective study of the natural history of HIV-1 disease, the Multicenter AIDS Cohort Study (MACS),[114,13] four stages of CD4+ cell loss were discerned. In the first stage, which occurs during the initial 12 to 18 months after seroconversion, the mean absolute CD4+ lymphocyte count rapidly declines from about 1000/μl to about 600/μl.

The CD8 count increases in a compensatory fashion, such that the absolute number of CD3[+] lymphocytes remains virtually constant. In the second stage, the CD4 count declines at a slower rate. As in the first stage, CD8 number increases, and total T-cell number remains essentially unchanged. This phase of the illness, which corresponds to the latent phase, can persist for several years. The third stage is characterized by a rapid decline in the remaining CD4[+] T cells, accompanied by a decline in CD8[+] T cells. The decline of both CD4[+] and CD8[+] populations signals the failure of T-cell homeostasis and precedes the onset of symptomatic disease by 12 to 18 months.[114] During the last stage, the interval between the development of symptomatic disease and death, there is a further reduction in CD4 cell numbers.

The causes of the CD4 lymphopenia are not fully known. In asymptomatic individuals, infectious virus can be recovered from about one in a thousand peripheral blood CD4 lymphocytes. However, recent flow cytometric studies, using a new technique to detect PCR amplification products,[115] indicate that the proportion of peripheral CD4[+] cells expressing viral message may be closer to one in one hundred, and the proportion with proviral DNA as high as one in ten. Further, virus isolation studies indicate that a higher proportion of CD4[+] cells may be infected in the lymph nodes than in the periphery. This leads to speculation that the organized lymphoid tissues may be major sites of cell destruction.[113] Lymphocyte death by apoptosis can readily be demonstrated in the lymph nodes of infected individuals.[116] Similarly, a large proportion of peripheral blood T cells (both CD4[+] and CD8[+]) from late stage patients apoptose in short-term unstimulated culture. Although HIV-1 infection can directly cause apoptosis of CD4[+] T cells, apoptosis of CD8[+] T cells has been attributed to the increase in lymphopoiesis that accompanies CD4[+] T-cell destruction. According to this interpretation, newly generated replacement T cells (CD4[+] and CD8[+]) are far more susceptible to apoptosis than stable resting naive or memory T cells.[117]

The CD4 count is used as a benchmark to follow disease progression in infected patients. For the past several years, it has been recommended that asymptomatic HIV-1 infected subjects be treated prophylactically with zidovudine (AZT) when their CD4[+] T-cell count falls below 500 cells/μl.[118] However, the Concorde trial, a European cooperative study, provided data indicating early treatment does not prolong the asymptomatic phase of the illness.[119] Based on these findings, it is now recommended that decisions regarding treatment for asymptomatic patients with CD4[+] counts <500/μl should be made on an individual basis. All available data, however, demonstrate that treatment with antiretroviral agents can prolong survival in symptomatic HIV-1 infected patients.[120,121] Recent advances in administration of multidrug regimens, including nucleoside combinations and protease inhibitors, promise further improvement in survival. The U.S. Public Health Service has recommended that the CD4 count should be monitored in HIV-1–infected individuals at 3- to 6-month intervals.[122]

Treatment of HIV-1 infection with the available antiretroviral drugs results in only a transient and modest increase in CD4 counts. The major effects of these agents are to interfere with viral replication. In general, when therapy is instituted, the CD4+ count can be expected to increase by approximately 50 cells/µl; this increase lasts for a period of 4 to 12 weeks.

The second benchmark in the management of an HIV-1–infected patient is a CD4+ count of 200/µl. At this time point, prophylactic treatments, including those designed to prevent *pneumocystis carinii* pneumonia (PCP), are instituted.[123] Once the count has declined to less than 200/µl, there is little clinical value in following this parameter.

Early in infection, the reduction in CD4 cells does not appear to preferentially affect a specific subset of CD4+ cells. Both CD4+CD45RA+ and CD4+CD45RO+ cells appear to decline at similar rates.[124] Late in HIV-1 disease, CD45RO+ cells comprise the majority of remaining CD4+ T cells. Although the CD45RO+ phenotype is usually associated with memory T cells, there is evidence that the earliest naive T cells may bear phenotypic markers similar to those displayed by activated memory cells.[125]

In AIDS patients, there is an apparent increase in the number of activated CD4+ cells, as judged by the coexpression of either CD38 or HLA-DR antigens.[13] As mentioned above, it is not certain whether these are truly activated memory cells, responding to HIV-1 or other infectious agents, or alternatively, hypofunctional replacement T cells destined for apoptosis. It is conceivable that they could be either, depending on the extent of disease progression. In keeping with the later interpretation, CD25 expression (IL-2 receptor α chain), another indicator of T-cell activation, is not increased coordinately with CD38 or HLA-DR. Residual CD4+ cells have impaired *in vitro* ability to express IL-2 receptor after stimulation.[126,127]

As detailed above, CD4 loss is offset by an increase in CD8+ T cells throughout the asymptomatic phase of HIV-1 infection, such that the total number of lymphocytes remains relatively stable. This change is accompanied by an increase in the frequency of HIV-1–specific cytotoxic T cells, which may play a vital role in maintaining the asymptomatic phase.[128-130] Consistent with this observation, an elevated proportion of CD8+ T cells express CD38 [125,131-133] and HLA-DR.[13,134] This increase in "activated" CD8 cells is not unique to HIV-1 infection. It is a characteristic of systemic viral infections, including those due to EBV and CMV. This phenotype is also seen during the early phases of immune reconstitution after bone marrow transplantation,[125] where it identifies a population of hypofunctional replacement T cells, rather than activated memory cells. This may explain the finding that persistently elevated numbers of either CD8+CD38+ or CD8+-HLA-DR+ T cells are poor prognostic signs in HIV-infected subjects.[134,133]

The percentage of natural killer cells, as measured by expression of CD16, has been reported to be essentially unchanged in the three groups of HIV-infected homosexuals: seropositive asymptomatic men, symptomatic patients, and individuals with AIDS. By contrast, the number of NK cells, determined by cells coexpressing both CD16 and CD56, is reduced. The decrease in CD16+CD56+ cells tends to parallel the decline in CD4 counts. As CD16+CD56+ cells are potent mediators of non-MHC–restricted cytolytic activities, it is not surprising that there is a concomitant diminution in functional killing activity. It has been reported that this killing defect can be corrected *in vitro* by addition of either interleukin-2 or interferons.

Another abnormality, which at present is unexplained, is a prominent increase in the number of cells reacting with the CD57 antibody.[134-138] This increase appears to be due primarily to a selected elevation of CD57+ on CD8+ T cells; CD16+CD57+ cells are not increased. However, in AIDS patients, the absolute number of CD57+ cells is actually reduced, due to lymphopenia.[114] Some studies report that the percentage of CD57+ cells is increased in seronegative homosexuals; however, the total numbers of these cells is within the normal range.[114] Stites et al. provided evidence suggesting that increased CD8+CD57+ cells were an independent predictor of progression to AIDS.[134]

The CDC recently published revised recommendations for phenotyping lymphocyte subsets in patients with HIV-1 infection.[122] They suggested employing a monoclonal antibody panel using two-color fluorescence (Table 3). One of the major recommendations was to quantify both CD4 and CD8 cells on CD3+ cells, rather than using either a single-color analysis or dual staining with CD4 and CD8 alone. Triple staining is also readily available which permits simultaneous measurement of CD3, CD4, and CD8. These modifications eliminate the inclusion of non-T cells expressing either the CD4 or CD8 antigen. Low concentrations of the CD4 antigen are present on monocytes, and CD8 is weakly expressed on a subset of natural killer cells. The CDC also suggests that the panel includes measurements of both B lymphocytes and NK cells, and provides guidelines for standardizing lymphocyte scatter gates.

A. Idiopathic CD4+ T Lymphopenia

At the Ninth International AIDS Conference, a syndrome was reported consisting of markedly depressed CD4+ T cell counts in the absence of evidence for HIV-1 infection or other recognizable causes of immunosuppression. This led to speculation that another, as yet

TABLE 3

Guidelines for Lymphocyte Testing in HIV-Infected Patients

FITC Mab/PE MoAb	Purpose
CD45/CD14	To set lymphocyte gate[a]
Isotype/isotype	To set negative thresholds
CD3/CD19	To enumerate total T and B cells
CD3/CD4	To specifically identify CD4[+] T cells; excludes monocytes which weakly express CD4.
CD3/CD8	To specifically identify CD8[+] T cells; excludes NK cells which may be CD8[dim]
CD3/CD16 and/or CD56	To quantify NK cells

[a] The CDC has established guidelines for determining the adequacy of a lymphocyte gate created using forward and side scatter. Purity (the exclusion of nonlymphocytes) and recovery (the inclusion of lymphocytes) are evaluated. Lymphocytes (T cells, B cells, and NK cells) form a discrete CD45[bright], CD14[negative] population. Monocytes (the major culprit to contaminate the lymphocyte scatter gate) are CD45[bright], but also CD14[bright], and therefore easily distinguished from lymphocytes. Debris is CD45[dim] or negative. Lymphocyte and monocyte populations are identified on the basis of fluorescence, and their respective scatter profiles are determined. Optimally, the lymphocyte scatter gate is adjusted to include at least 95% of the lymphocytes (recovery) with a maximum of 10% nonlymphocytes (90% purity).[122]

unknown, virus causes an AIDS-like syndrome. The syndrome, termed idiopathic CD4[+] lymphopenia, appears to be rare. To date, only a small number of cases have been identified. The clinical features and demographic characteristics of this syndrome are extremely heterogeneous. Less than half of the identified patients have risk factors for HIV-1 infection and there is wide geographic and age distribution of the cases.

Several aspects of this syndrome have been defined.[139-144] Major differences between this syndrome and the CD4[+] lymphopenia occurring as part of HIV-1 infection have been observed. In many patients with idiopathic CD4[+] lymphopenia, the CD4 count remained low but stable for prolonged periods or spontaneously increased. CD8 counts tended to vary widely. There is no epidemiological or microbiological evidence to suggest that this syndrome is caused by a transmissible agent.

The provisional case definition for idiopathic CD4[+] T-lymphocytopenia used for national surveillance includes the following: a documented absolute CD4[+] lymphocyte count of <300 cells/μl or of less than 20% of total T cells on more than one occasion, no evidence of infection on HIV testing, and the absence of any defined immunodeficiency or therapy associated with decreased levels of CD4[+] T cells.[141]

V. ACUTE LEUKEMIA

Acute leukemia is defined by the clonal expansion of neoplastic hematopoietic cells which often appear to be arrested at an early stage

TABLE 4

FAB Classification of Acute Leukemia

1. Acute Lymphoblastic Leukemia

L1	Small cell, high nucleus to cytoplasm ratio, regular or clefted nucleus, small inconspicuous nucleolus
L2	Larger blasts with irregular nuclear membranes, one or more prominent nucleoli, relative abundance of cytoplasm
L3	Large cells with round or oval nuclei, prominent nucleoli, intense basophilic cytoplasm; may have prominent vacuoles

2. Acute Myeloid (Nonlymphocytic) Leukemia

M0	Acute myeloblastic leukemia with no maturation
M1	Acute myeloblastic leukemia with minimal maturation (myeloblasts, with or without scant granules)
M2	Acute myeloblastic leukemia with maturation (myeloblasts with granules, promyelocytes, and few myelocytes)
M3	Acute promyelocytic leukemia
M4	Acute monomyelocytic leukemia
M5a	Acute monoblastic leukemia without differentiation
M5b	Acute monoblastic leukemia with differentiation
M6	Acute erythroleukemia
M7	Acute megakaryocytic leukemia.

of maturation. However, the discordant expression of maturation and differentiation markers often serves as a hallmark of leukemic transformation. Neoplastic transformation can occur in either lymphoid or myeloid precursors. Depending upon the lineage of the precursor, the resultant leukemia is classified as either an **acute lymphoblastic leukemia** (ALL) or an **acute myeloid leukemia** (AML). The latter has also been designated as **acute non-lymphoblastic leukemia**.

Traditionally, acute leukemias have been classified on the basis of morphological and cytochemical features, using the system originally proposed by the French-American-British (FAB) cooperative group in 1976[145] and subsequently modified several times.[146-149] (Table 4). Clinically, the most important distinction is between leukemias of myeloid and lymphoid origins; these two forms differ in their demographic and clinical features, their responses to therapy and their ultimate prognoses. The acute lymphoblastic leukemias have been subdivided into three subgroups, and the acute myeloid leukemias into eight subgroups.

Despite the widespread usage of the FAB classification system, it is now well recognized that it has numerous limitations.[149,150] Most important, morphological features, by themselves, are often unable to fully discriminate between the different types of leukemia.

Flow cytometric analysis of leukemic cells has been an valuable adjunct to the management of affected patients.[149,151,152] It is of use both in the recognition and in the classification of these malignancies. The principal uses of immunophenotyping include: (1) defining cell lineages, including differentiation of the lymphoid from myeloid forms and recognizing lymphoblastic leukemia of the B- and T-cell lineages; (2) identifying characteristic features of certain forms of acute myeloid leukemia; (3) determining the lineage of morphologically unclassifiable cells; (4) recognizing unusual or rare forms of leukemia, such as acute erythroleukemia and acute megakaryocytic leukemia; (5) detecting leukemias that show mixed lineage or biphenotypic characteristics, such as acute myeloid leukemias that coexpress one or more lymphoid-associated antigens, or acute lymphoblastic leukemias expressing myeloid determinants (the prognostic significance of these mixed lineage leukemias is, at present, controversial[6]); (6) distinguishing acute leukemias from other hematological and non-hematological malignancies.[149]

In addition, leukemia phenotyping may provide prognostic information and be of value in recognizing the presence of minimal residual disease in a patient who has achieved a complete clinical remission after chemotherapy or bone marrow transplantation.

Historically, the lack of leukemia-specific antigens imposed a major limitation on the use of flow cytometry for leukemia detection, diagnosis, and classification. Antibodies used to classify these malignancies are directed against antigens which are also expressed on normal hematopoietic cells. Thus, the presence of a single specific antigen cannot distinguish normal hematopoietic precursors from leukemic cells. This problem was especially evident when cells were analyzed using single-color fluorescence procedures. Through multiparameter flow cytometry, it is now possible to find a unique signature for each leukemia (i.e., a constellation of "normal" determinants expressed in abnormal combination or intensity). This poses a new classification problem, since at some level of detail, these signatures become unique to a particular patient. New studies comparing clinical outcome with the results of multiparameter flow cytometry and traditional histopathology are needed before the potential of flow cytometry can be fully realized.

To phenotype an acute leukemia, most laboratories employ a panel of monoclonal antibodies, subdivided into those with specificity for myeloid cells and those that react with B- or T-lymphoid cells. In the vast majority of cases, these panels can accurately define the leukemic cell's lineage. A leukemic panel proposed for the diagnosis and classification of acute myeloid leukemia is presented in Table 5.

A. Acute Lymphoblastic Leukemia

The neoplastic transformation of lymphoid precursors is the predominant form of leukemia in children. However, these malignancies

TABLE 5

Three-Color Antibody Panel for Phenotyping Acute Myelocytic Leukemia (AML)

FITC	PE	PerCP	Comment
CD7	CD13	CD2	FAB M0
CD38	CD34	HLA-DR	FAB M0
CD15	CD34	CD56	FAB M1
CD33	CD13	HLA-DR	FAB M1
CD16	CD32	CD64	FAB M2
CD11b	CD13	CD33	FAB M5
CD45	CD14	HLA-DR	Differential

Note: The creation of panel sets for the diagnosis and classification of leukemia is a continuous process which evolves as flow data, morphology, traditional classification data, and clinical outcomes are compared. This particular set was created by Carleton Stewart, Ph.D., Roswell Park Cancer Institute, and can be used to recognize AML populations which are well correlated with some of the FAB categories (see Table 4). The use of CD45 and side scatter to *gate* the leukemic population (in conjunction with other lineage markers) is also proving increasingly useful.

can occur at any age. Based on the cell of origin, ALL is typically subdivided into three groups: the malignant transformation of T lymphocytes (T-ALL), those which are the neoplastic counterparts of surface immunoglobulin-positive B lymphocytes (B-ALL), and a third and numerically predominant group, non-T- non-B-cell leukemia. The vast majority of these non-T- non-B-cell diseases are due to the malignant transformation of pre-B cells. T-cell leukemia comprises between 15 to 25% of the cases of lymphoblastic leukemias; B-cell leukemia, 2 to 5%, and the non-T- non-B-cell (pre-B cell) forms, 70 to 75%.[151,153,154]

B. Pre-B Cell Acute Lymphoblastic Leukemia

Pre-B-ALL can be considered to represent the neoplastic transformation of cells arrested at any stage in the normal B lymphocyte maturation sequence from its initial commitment to the appearance of membrane-associated immunoglobulins (Figure 15). Nadler et al.[155] subdivided pre-B–cell leukemias into discrete stages which appear to recapitulate normal B-cell maturation (Figure 17). The first stage represents the transformation of the earliest cell committed to the B-cell lineage; these cells express HLA-DR antigens but lack specific B-cell determinants. The neoplastic cells often coexpress CD34. Their B cell origin can be established by detecting the presence of cytoplasmic CD22, a lineage-specific determinant.[20]

The second stage is defined by leukemic cells which coexpress HLA-DR and the B-cell antigen CD19. Other B-cell lineage-specific membrane-associated antigens are not demonstrable. Cells at this stage

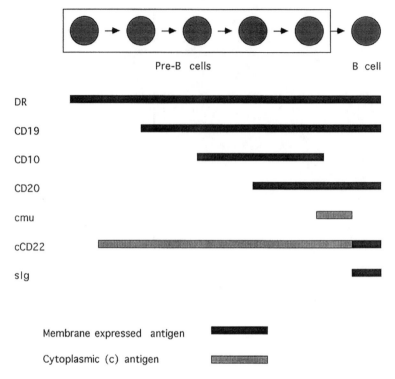

Figure 15
Maturation of pre-B cells. Appearance of cytoplasmic CD22 (cCD22) is an early landmark
in B-cell differentiation. Expression of cytoplasmic μ chain is the final event; expression
of surface immunoglobulin (SIg) marks the transition from pre-B to B lymphocyte.

of maturation may have undergone heavy chain gene rearrangement,
but the light chain genes are still in the germ line configuration. In early
infancy (<1 year of age), stage I and stage II tend to be the predominant
forms of ALL.

In the third stage, the leukemic cells acquire CD10. This antigen
was initially designated the **common acute lymphoblastic leukemia
antigen** or CALLA and was thought to be leukemia specific. However,
CD10 is present on pre-B cells, a subset of normal B cells, and early
thymocytes. Numerically, HLA-DR+CD19+CD10+ pre-B ALL is the most
prevalent type. In stage IV, leukemic cells bear the three previously
described antigens plus the CD20 antigen. The final stage of pre-B-cell
leukemia is characterized by the acquisition of cytoplasmic μ heavy
chains. These immunoglobulin heavy chains are not associated with
light chains.

CD34 is commonly expressed on leukemic pre-B cells. Pui et al.[156]
found that this antigen was expressed in more than 75% of children
with newly diagnosed pre-B-ALL. In addition, the presence of CD34

was significantly associated with favorable presenting features, including young age (1 to 10), Caucasian race, absence of central nervous system (CNS) disease, low LDH, CD10 positivity, and leukemic cell hyperdiploidy (>50 chromosomes). Event-free survival was clearly superior for patients with CD34+ leukemia.

C. B-Cell Acute Leukemia

The surface immunoglobulin-positive B-cell acute lymphoblastic leukemias (B-ALL) constitute the neoplastic equivalent of cells arrested at the next stage of B cell maturation. In addition to the presence of membrane-associated surface immunoglobulins, the leukemic cells express B-cell markers, including CD19 and CD20. Most are also CD22+. B-ALL, which represents only a small minority of the acute lymphoblastic leukemias, has been associated with the poorest prognosis. Patients with this form of ALL are usually characterized by FAB L3 morphology, male sex, Caucasian race, older age at diagnosis, and extramedullary disease.

D. T-Cell Acute Leukemia

T-cell acute leukemia is less common than the pre-B-cell variant.[20] Clinically, this form is rare in infancy. It usually occurs in older age children and in adults. In one large series, T-ALL accounted for 26% of the cases of adult ALL.[153] The leukemia is often complicated by such features as the presence of mediastinal mass, CNS involvement, and an extremely high white cell count.

T-ALL can be subdivided using a model similar to the B-cell leukemias (Figure 16).[151,157-159] T-ALL are clonal diseases in which the neoplastic cells are arrested at a stage that closely corresponds to a phase of normal thymocyte maturation. Stage I is phenotypically characterized by cells expressing the T-cell antigens, CD7, CD5, and CD2, and cytoplasmic but not membrane-associated CD3. Stage II is marked by the appearance of the common thymocyte antigen CD1 and the coexpression of both CD4 and CD8. Stage III cells express the CD3–T-cell receptor complex and either CD4+ or CD8+.

Immunophenotypic studies in patients with T-ALL indicate that almost all react with antibodies to the CD7 antigen.[102,160] However, this antigen is not specific for cells of the T lineage; it may be expressed on some myeloid leukemias. CD5 is also commonly present on T-ALL cells, and the combination of CD5 and CD7 is regarded as highly specific for this form of leukemia.[151,160]

Leukemic cells with the stage I phenotype (CD7+, CD5+, CD2+, CD3+, CD1-,CD4-,CD8-) account for 30 to 40% of all cases of T-cell ALL.

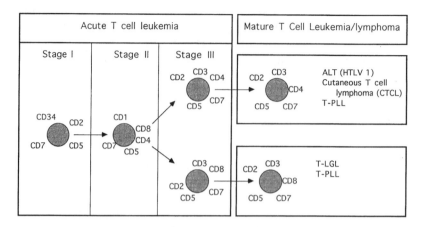

Figure 16
Acute T-cell leukemias and lymphomas express surface markers which correspond to
normal stages of T-cell maturation.

These neoplastic cells commonly coexpress CD34 and HLA-DR antigens and may express other myeloid-related antigens.[161] Another 30 to
50% of patients with T-ALL have phenotypes corresponding to the
intermediate stages of normal thymocyte development (CD1+, CD4+,
and CD8+). Leukemias corresponding to the terminal stage of maturation (CD3+, CD4+, CD8−, or CD3+, CD4−, CD8+) are the least common
(10 to 25%).

In contrast to pre-B ALL, CD34+ expression on T-ALL cells is correlated with poor prognostic features including initial CNS disease and
CD10 negativity.[156] It has not been determined whether expression of
CD34 itself has independent prognostic significance. CD34 is present
on 46% of T-ALL cases and is not confined to leukemias corresponding
to the early stages of T-cell maturation; in children, 52% of CD3+ T-
ALL are CD34+.

E.   Acute Myeloid Leukemias

Leukemias arising from myeloid precursors are more heterogeneous than ALL. Immunophenotyping has added considerably to the
recognition of certain myeloid leukemias as such and to the subclassi-
fication of these malignancies. Traditionally, myeloid leukemias are
subdivided into eight FAB groups. Although these correlate only
weakly with published immunophenotypic descriptions,[162] the application of multiparameter flow cytometry, where several markers and
physical characteristics are used simultaneously to identify and characterize myeloid leukemia cells (Table 5), will likely meet or exceed the
traditional capabilities to predict prognosis and response to therapy. A

TABLE 6

Frequency of Antigens Expressed on AML Cells

Antigen	Drexler[a]	Vaickus et al.[b]
CD11	66%	56%
CD13	84%	57%
CD14	40%	71%
CD15	60%	91%
CD33	81%	71%
HLA-DR	81%	—
CD34	—	45%

[a] Review of multiple studies.[162]
[b] CALGB study.[151]

relatively new area lies in the marriage between analytic flow cytometry and traditional histology. High speed cell sorters are now being used to identify and sort putative leukemia cells onto microscope slides so that they can be examined by more traditional techniques (personal communication, Carleton Stewart, Roswell Park Cancer Institute, Buffalo, NY). This may prove especially useful for the definitive detection of residual disease after therapy and will greatly clarify the relationships between immunophenotype and morphology.

The antibodies most useful in identifying AML include those directed against the CD34, CD33, CD13, CD14, CD15, HLA-DR, and CD11b.[151,162] CD15, CD33, and CD13 are the determinants most commonly expressed on the myeloblastic leukemic cells.[149] Table 6 shows the reported immunophenotyping of AML cells from two large series, one a review of published data[162] and the other, the results of the CALGB series.[151] In order to define a leukemic population as positive for a specific antigen, most investigators use the criterion that the determinant must be expressed on >20% of the neoplastic cells.

The frequency of antigen expression varies in different series, and none are present on the malignant cells of all AML patients. CD34 can be identified on AML cells in approximately one third of the patients. Its presence has been reported to portend a poorer prognosis.[163] CD34 expression correlates with the more undifferentiated forms of AML, FAB class M0, M1, or M2. It is generally believed that expression of the CD34 antigen indicates an arrest at a very early stage of myeloid development. CD13 and CD14 expression have been correlated with a low complete remission rate.[149]

CD14 and CD11b are present on a proportion of the monocytic forms of acute myeloid leukemias (M4 and M5).[149,162] A subgroup of M4, termed M4EO and cytogenetically characterized by the inversion of chromosome 16, has been found to commonly express the CD2 antigen.[164] Acute promyelocytic leukemia (M3) is almost uniformly negative for HLA-DR. Two of the less common forms of AML, acute erythroleukemia (M6) and acute megakaryocytic leukemia (M7), can generally be recognized by the expression of either glycophorin on the former, or platelet-associated antigens such as CD41, on the latter.[152]

M0 is a newly recognized variant of AML in which there is minimal cell differentiation and cytochemistry for myeloid features is negative. This form is recognized by the expression of myeloid antigens and negative lymphoid markers. These cells are typically positive for both CD33 and CD13.[148]

F.   Mixed Leukemias

One of the more perplexing problems related to the immunophenotyping of acute leukemic cells is the simultaneous presence of antigens of different cell lineages. In both morphologically and cytochemically typical AML, it is not infrequent to find that the malignant cells express one or more lymphoid-associated antigens. Similarly, in otherwise typical ALL, expression of myeloid-associated antigens is a relatively common event. Not only do these aberrations contribute ambiguity with respect to the classification of the neoplastic elements, but they raise important biological questions as to the origin of the leukemic cells and their relation to normal hematopoietic progenitors.

The problem of categorizing these mixed lineage leukemias is further complicated by findings that in some patients, there may be two distinct populations of leukemic cells, one that appears to contain only myeloid antigens and a second with only lymphoid associated antigens. These are designated as **bilineal leukemias**. The more common finding is that of a single population of leukemic cells which react with antibodies of both lineages, **biphenotypic leukemias**. Within this latter group, some antigens are expressed on only a proportion of the leukemic cells (heterogeneous expression), whereas others are equally expressed on all neoplastic cells (homogeneous expression). It has been postulated that antigens expressed in a heterogeneous manner may imply that the leukemic cells possess a capacity for maturation.

There are at least two interpretations concerning the biological significance of mixed lineage marker coexpression. One suggests that mixed expression is due to abnormal gene regulation, and therefore represents an example of **lineage infidelity**.[165] The other postulates that mixed lineage markers are expressed at discrete stages of normal progenitor cell development; in the leukemic process the malignant clone with mixed markers is arrested at one such stage. This has been termed **lineage promiscuity**.[166]

Numerous reports document the occurrence of aberrant marker expression. Because of differences in study designs (study populations, number of antibodies used, definition of mixed lineage, staining, and analytic techniques), the true incidence of these mixed leukemias is difficult to determine from the available literature. For example, many investigators have used the arbitrary criterion that an antigen must be expressed on a minimum of 20% of the leukemic cells to be considered positive. However, in reported studies on mixed leukemias, the minimum criteria have ranged from expression on 5 to 30% of the malignant cells.

Myeloid-associated antigens are frequently observed on acute lymphoblastic leukemic cells (My⁺ALL). The incidence varies widely; in a recent review of 14 separate studies including a total of 3817 patients, Drexler et al.[167] reported the frequency of My⁺ALL ranged from 5 to 46% with an average of 12%. There was a significant difference in the incidence of myeloid antigen expression between childhood and adult forms of ALL. The incidence in children averaged 7%, whereas 18% of adult cases coexpressed myeloid antigens. In children, coexpression of myeloid antigens was not of prognostic significance; however, in adults, My⁺ALL patients did not fare as well as those lacking these myeloid antigens.[168]

The most common myeloid antigens detected on ALL cells were CD13, CD33, CD14, CDw65, and CD15. In a small number of studies, the presence of a myeloid-associated antigen correlated with expression of CD34. This suggests the leukemia may have resulted from the transformation of a pluripotential stem cell which has undergone limited differentiation after transformation. However, in CD34⁺ ALL, there is no predominance of any single myeloid antigen. Aberrant expression was more common in patients with B-cell lineage neoplasms than in those with the T cell variants.

In patients with AML, as judged by FAB criteria, the incidence of leukemic cells coexpressing lymphoid antigens also varied considerably between independent studies. Drexler et al.[169] published a comprehensive review of this topic and concluded the incidence of AML-bearing lymphoid differentiation markers (Ly⁺AML) was relatively low. However, in the series reviewed by these authors, the incidence ranged from 13 to 60%. The most commonly expressed lymphoid-associated antigens were CD1, CD2, CD3, CD5, CD8, CD10, CD19, CD20, CD21, and CD22. However, none of these antigens occurred in more than 10% of the AML cases.

CD4 and CD7 were detected in 24% and 15% of Ly⁺AML, respectively.[170] However, these two antigens are not lineage specific. CD4 and CD7 may be a component of immature myeloid precursors, and CD4 is expressed on monocytes. The presence of CD4 correlated with FAB M4 and M5 morphology; CD7 was seen more commonly in the less differentiated forms, especially FAB Ml, and was often associated with expression of CD34.[171] With the exception of CD7, lymphoid markers on AML cells did not appear to portend prognosis. However, the presence of CD7 without other T cell antigens suggests a poor prognosis.[172]

By immunophenotypic criteria, it is often difficult to distinguish between poorly differentiated myeloid leukemias expressing CD7 and T-cell ALL expressing CD34 or other myeloid antigens. Additional studies to determine the presence of cytoplasmic CD3 or myeloperoxidase staining may be required to appropriately classify these leukemias.

The expression of the B-lymphocytic marker CD19 on AML cells shows extreme heterogeneity; the reported incidence ranges from 0 to 61%. Likewise, expression of the CD2 antigen, a marker for T cells and NK cells, varies from 9 to 57%. Ball et al. reported 21% AML cases were positive for the T-cell antigen CD2 and 14% for CD19. Patients expressing these antigens appeared to have a more favorable prognosis.[173]

G. Minimal Residual Disease

One of the most promising new areas in which flow cytometry is being used to assist the management of patients with acute leukemia is in the detection of residual neoplastic cells after therapy. The classical criterion by which remission is determined is the presence of <5% blasts in bone marrow aspirates. However, small numbers of persistent blasts could be either recovering normal myeloid precursors or residual leukemic cells. Morphologically, these two cannot be distinguished.

Several techniques, including cytogenetics, *in situ* hybridization, PCR-based gene rearrangement studies, and immunophenotyping, have been proposed as methods useful in defining residual or recurrent disease. The identification of residual leukemia cells by flow cytometry depends upon the finding that, given the ability to simultaneously detect enough lineage and differentiation markers, every leukemia will have its unique signature that distinguishes it from its normal counterparts. This signature might include the presence of lymphoid antigens on myeloid cells, myeloid antigens on lymphoid cells, discordant expression of early and late differentiation markers, or a phenotypic pattern that differs from normal with respect the intensity of staining or light scatter properties. Definitive quantification of these cells after therapy is greatly assisted by their identification prior to therapy. At this time, the leukemic cells predominate and thus can be easily characterized. Once the patient has responded to potentially curative therapy, the marrow aspirate is then screened for cells expressing known leukemic phenotype. For example, if at presentation a leukemia is $CD34^+CD33^+CD19^+$, cells coexpressing these markers could be measured after an apparent clinical remission is achieved. Great sensitivity and specificity are obtained using three-color staining (and light scatter properties) because the *signature* of the leukemic clone (which can be thought of as a cluster in multiparameter space) lies well outside the space occupied by normal hematopoietic cells, nonspecifically stained cells, autofluorescent cells, or random noise. It should be cautioned that the leukemic *signature*, or in some cases *signatures*, are not always stable in time, and that a great deal of selection occurs when a florid leukemia is reduced by therapy to minimal residual disease. Practically, a *panel* of multiantibody combinations is run in order to detect such changes, if they occur. Several early studies have shown promising results,[174-176] but this field is evolving rapidly.

H. Chronic Myelogenous Leukemia (CML)

CML is a clonal myeloproliferative disease characterized by a unique chromosomal abnormality, the Philadelphia chromosome, a reciprocal 9:22 translocation.[151,177] This results in the approximation of the *c-abl* oncogene on chromosome 9 to the breakpoint region (*bcr*) of chromosome 22.[178] The new gene, *bcr-abl*, codes for a high molecular weight tyrosine kinase.[179]

The typical clinical course of CML consists of a chronic phase characterized by leukocytosis and the presence of immature myeloid elements. This phase can persist for years, but ultimately terminates in a blast crisis: the emergence of an acute leukemia. Approximately 70% of these acute leukemias are myeloblastic in origin; most of the others are of B lymphoid lineage. T-cell ALL are extremely rare.[180]

Immunophenotyping is particularly useful for distinguishing the lineage of the acute leukemic cells when the patient enters blast crisis. The myeloid forms express typical myeloid antigens, including CD33, CD13, CD15, and CD14.[181] By contrast, the lymphoid forms display antigens typically seen in pre-B-cell ALL (CD19, CD20, CD10).[182-187] Rare cases express T-cell antigens and are presumed to be of T-cell origin.[188-190] Many of the acute lymphoid and myeloid leukemias are CD34+.

VI. LYMPHOCYTE PHENOTYPES FOLLOWING BONE MARROW TRANSPLANTATION

Patients undergoing autologous or allogenic bone marrow transplant comprise a unique group for studying lymphocyte regeneration. As a result of myeloablative and immunoablative therapy, reconstitution of the lymphoid system results from the proliferation and maturation of transplanted cells. These include both prelymphoid stem cells and mature lymphocytes, a proportion of which retain their self-replicative capacity. The graft origin of repopulating lymphocytes can be

TABLE 7

Changes in Lymphocyte Phenotypes after Bone Marrow Transplantation

1. Reduction in the numbers of CD4+ cells
2. Inversion of the CD4/CD8 ratio
3. Increased numbers of T cells with *activation markers* HLA-DR and CD38
4. Decreased numbers of T cells with *activation marker* CD25
5. Increased numbers of CD8+CD57+ cells
6. Unusual expression of antigens on NK cells; approximately one third of transplanted patients have a high proportion of CD56bright CD16- NK cells
7. Increased proportion of CD5+ B cells
8. Increased proportion of apoptotic T cells (CD4 and CD8)
9. Increased proportion of CD45RO+, CD29bright, S6F1+ T cells

substantiated in allogeneic BMT by the detection of donor specific markers.[191]

In a successful transplant, T and B lymphocytes repopulate the blood to near normal levels within 3 months. However, the recovery of T-cell subsets, and the return of functional immunity occurs at different rates. One of the consequences is an inversion of the normal CD4/CD8 ratio. This is due to both a proportional increase in the number of CD8+ cells and a decrease in the absolute numbers of CD4+ cells.[191-193] There is also a persistent increase in the number of T cells expressing markers normally associated with activation, such as CD38 and HLA-DR. As discussed in Section IV on HIV, the functional capacity of these cells cannot be determined from the presence of these phenotypic markers alone. Another difference between the phenotypes of normal individuals and those who have undergone marrow transplantation is an increased number of CD8+CD57+ cells in the latter.[194,195] These changes are summarized in Table 7. These phenotypic abnormalities reflect functional deficits, most prominently an inability of the CD4+ population to provide normal helper functions.

Natural killer cells, as measured by the numbers of CD16+ cells, appear to increase by 2 weeks after transplant and reach a maximum at 3 weeks.[196] In a study that examined the recovery of NK cells after transplant, it was noted that approximately one third of the transplanted patients had two phenotypically distinct NK cell subsets, a CD56dimCD16+ and CD56brightCD16-. Cells with the latter phenotype comprise only a minor population in normal blood. In the transplant group, CD56bright CD16- cells persist for a mean of approximately 4 months. Furthermore, these unique cells can comprise as much as 70% of all NK cells and 40% of peripheral blood lymphocytes.[54]

The absolute number of peripheral B lymphocytes usually normalizes within 2 months of transplantation. However, a high proportion of these cells also express CD5, a marker present on virtually all T cells, and on 15 to 25% of normal peripheral B cells. As discussed below, the significance of CD5 on B lymphocytes is ambiguous and may identify early B cells or activated mature B cells, depending upon the context.

In allogeneic bone marrow transplant (BMT) recipients who do not develop graft-vs.-host disease (GVHD), the CD4/CD8 ratio normalizes within the first year. However, patients with chronic GVHD continue to show elevated numbers of CD8[+] cells.

These observations have been further extended by examining CD8[+] subsets. *In vitro*, functionally distinct CD8[+] T cells can be resolved based on the expression of CD11. CD8[+]CD11[+] T cells suppress mitogen-induced T-cell proliferation and differentiation of B lymphocytes. By contrast, CD8[+]CD11[-] lymphocytes contain both precursors and effectors for cytotoxic reactions.[35,197] A second method of subdividing normal CD8[+] cells is based on the coexpression of CD57 antigen. Patients with long-term chronic GVHD have increased numbers of three CD8[+] lymphoid subsets: both CD8[+]CD11[+] and CD8[+]CD11[-] cells and CD8[+] cells coexpressing CD57[+]. The numbers of each of these subsets tend to correlate with disease activity. By contrast, the presence of increased numbers of CD8[+]HLA-DR[+] T cells does not appear to be related to GVHD activity.[198] In fact, these cells are prominent early after both autologous and allogeneic BMT.

BMT is also accompanied by alterations in the distribution of CD4 subsets. In healthy subjects, CD45RA expression and CD29[bright] expression on CD4[+] T cells are largely mutually exclusive. Thus, in healthy subjects the monoclonal antibodies 2H4 (CD45RA) and 4B4 (CD29) can be used to define distinct CD4[+] populations. Early after BMT, virtually all CD4[+] T cells are CD29[bright]. In patients with chronic GVHD, the CD4[+]CD45RA[+] cells show delayed recovery. In contrast, there is no difference in the rate of reconstitution of CD4[+]CD29[bright] cells in transplanted patients with or without chronic GVHD.

Immunophenotyping may also provide useful information for determining the cause of graft failure after allogenic transplantation. In diseases where autologous transplantation is not possible, matched unrelated, or partially matched familial donors serve as alternative graft sources. In order to prevent GVHD, which is prevalent and severe in such alternative donor settings, bone marrow allografts are often depleted of mature T lymphocytes. T-cell depletion is effective for preventing or reducing the severity of acute graft vs. host disease, but often at the cost of an increased incidence of graft rejection, which is relatively rare among leukemia patients receiving unmodified allogeneic grafts. In such cases it is important to distinguish between active graft rejection, mediated by residual host cells that have survived the marrow ablative regimen, and other causes of failure to engraft (e.g., insufficient stem cell dose). The rejection of T-cell–depleted marrow grafts has been associated with the emergence of host-derived T lymphocytes, predominantly of the CD8[+]CD57[+] phenotype.[119,200] A high

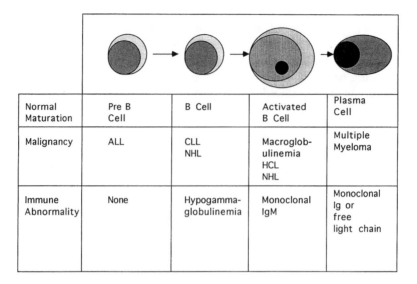

Normal Maturation	Pre B Cell	B Cell	Activated B Cell	Plasma Cell
Malignancy	ALL	CLL NHL	Macroglob-ulinemia HCL NHL	Multiple Myeloma
Immune Abnormality	None	Hypogamma-globulinemia	Monoclonal IgM	Monoclonal Ig or free light chain

Figure 17

Nearest normal counterparts of pre-B cell and B-cell malignancies. Many of these neo-plastic diseases are complicated by profound humoral immune abnormalities.

proportion of these cells also express HLA-DR suggesting *in vivo* activation.[199,201] CD3+CD8+CD57+ cells have been shown to inhibit normal hematopoiesis *in vitro*.[202]

In graft rejection, another immunophenotypic change is an increase in the proportion of CD8+CD11b- cells. These are believed to be the CD8 cells with cytotoxic potential;[196] this is in accord with other findings indicating peripheral blood lymphocytes from patients undergoing graft rejection are capable of killing donor cells.[199]

VII. NON-HODGKIN'S LYMPHOMA AND CHRONIC LYMPHOID LEUKEMIAS

Tumors of mature B and T lymphocytes constitute a heterogeneous group of malignancies which, by definition, are clonal in origin. These malignant clones often closely resemble normal cells at a particular stage of differentiation (Figure 17).

One of the earliest clinical insights stemming directly from flow cytometry was the recognition that lymphoid neoplasms can arise from either B or T cells. In actuality, the vast majority (>80%) are of B-cell origin. For discussion purposes, it is useful to segregate B-cell lymphoid malignancies into two general categories, those in which there is prominent blood involvement (the lymphocytic leukemias) and those in which the disease is primarily restricted to lymphoid tissues (non-Hodgkin's lymphomas). This is an arbitrary distinction; differences between the two are often obscure. For example, although the major feature of B-cell chronic lymphocytic leukemia (B-CLL) is a persistent excess in the number of circulating blood lymphocytes, these patients may present with lymphadenopathy. The pathologic and immunophenotypic findings of involved nodal tissue do not differ from those observed in patients with diffuse forms of small cell lymphomas. Likewise, individuals with classical lymphoma, primarily limited to lymphoid tissues, often show varying numbers of circulating neoplastic cells.

The *sine qua non* of a B-cell malignancy is the clonal expansion of cells which, because they underwent malignant transformation subsequent to immunoglobulin gene rearrangement, display identical surface immunoglobulins. Flow cytometry has been an invaluable aid in identifying B-cell clonality. Although clonality is rigorously demonstrated by determining that each cell produces identical (monoclonal) antibody, in clinical practice clonality can usually be inferred from the ratio of *kappa* and *lambda* light chain-positive cells. This is typically performed by two- or three-color fluorescence. Antibodies to the kappa light chain are labeled with one fluorochrome and those to lambda chains with a second. In a normal subject, approximately 50% of the B cells will react with each antibody. Thus, the ratio of kappa- to lambda-bearing cells is about 1 (normal range 0.5 to 3.0). Marked variations from this range strongly suggest a clonal B cell expansion (Figure 18).

The sensitivity for detecting monoclonal B lymphocytes by light chain expression can be significantly enhanced by *gating out* non-B cells which nonspecifically bind immunoglobulins (e.g., monocytes). This can be accomplished by positively identifying B lymphocytes based on their reactivity with CD19 or CD20. In the two color method, the presence of kappa- and lambda-bearing cells is determined in separate samples, using antibodies to each light chain in combination with an antibody to a B cell marker (e.g., CD19) (Figure 18). Alternatively, three-color cytometry is used to simultaneously stain for kappa, lambda, and CD19. These modifications increase the ability to detect relatively small numbers of tumor cells among normal B cells. Recently, the Kolmogorov-Smirnov test (a nonparametric statistical test based on the maximum difference between two cumulative distribution functions) has been employed to even further increase the ability to detect circulating lymphoma cells.[203]

The B cell clonal neoplasms can be considered as a spectrum of diseases that correspond in phenotypic and functional characteristics to resting and antigen-activated normal B cells (Figure 17). The malignant

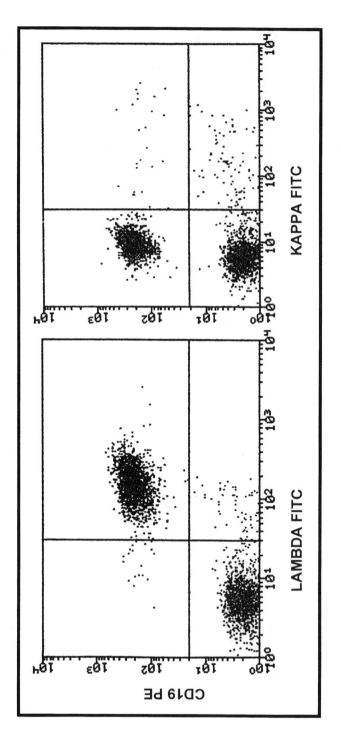

Figure 18
Expression of *kappa* and *lambda* light chains on CD19+ B cells in a patient with a lymphoid malignancy. The marked excess of B cells expressing *lambda* light chains (left panel) and paucity of B cells expressing *kappa* light chains (right panel) are indicative of a clonal expansion.

counterparts of the normal small, resting B lymphocytes are chronic lymphocytic leukemia and the low grade small cell non-Hodgkin's lymphomas. Following antigen binding to surface Ig accompanied by appropriate signals from T cells and APCs, a normal small B cell is transformed into an activated B cell. The malignant equivalents include prolymphocytic leukemia (PLL), hairy cell leukemia (HCL), and the intermediate and high grade lymphomas. During this stage, activated B cells begin to assume the morphologic characteristics of plasma cells. The neoplastic counterpart of cells in this transition phase is Waldenstrom's macroglobulinemia. Finally, the terminal stage of B-cell maturation is the formation of plasma cells; the corresponding malignancy is the disease multiple myeloma.

A. Chronic Lymphocyte Leukemia (CLL)

CLL is the most common leukemia occurring in adults in the U.S.[204] Most cases are due to the neoplastic transformation of B lymphocytes; T-cell CLL comprises less than 5% of all cases. In fact, it has been suggested that the designation CLL should be reserved only for chronic lymphoid leukemias showing a B-cell phenotype.[205,206]

The hallmark of B-CLL is a persistent elevation of the blood lymphocyte count. In general, the lymphocyte count exceeds 10,000/µl (normal lymphocyte counts range from 1500 to 4000/µl, with B-lymphocyte counts averaging 250/µl). Using flow cytometry to demonstrate clonality, a diagnosis can often be made with a count as low as 5000/µl. In most established cases of CLL, the lymphocyte counts range from 30,000 to 50,000/µl, and it is not unusual for it to exceed 100,000/µl.

In association with peripheral lymphocytosis, there is an increase in the number of marrow lymphocytes. By definition, in stage 0 B-CLL (the earliest stage recognized by the Rai classification), lymphocytes must exceed 30% of the total marrow cellularity. As the disease progresses, affected patients develop generalized lymphadenopathy and hepatosplenomegaly. In advanced stages anemia and/or thrombocytopenia result from bone marrow compromise or associated autoimmune disorders.

Morphologically, the neoplastic lymphocytes found in patients with B-CLL closely resemble normal mantle zone B lymphocytes. The cells are relatively homogeneous: usually small cells with scant cytoplasm, a nucleus with clumped chromatin, and no discernible nucleolus. A proportion of the cells may be larger, with a single prominent nucleolus (prolymphocytes); these generally comprise less than 10% of the total lymphocytes and consist of activated T as well as B lymphocytes.

The continued presence of an unphysiologically large mass of B cells, which are competent to present antigen to T cells and can produce a variety of cytokines, has interesting consequences for T- and B-cell–mediated immunity. In affected patients, there is a high incidence of humoral immune abnormalities. The most prominent is an inability to mount appropriate antibody responses to exogenous antigens. This often culminates in hypogammaglobulinemia.[204] Between 60 to 90% of patients with CLL will have a deficiency in at least one immunoglobulin isotype and up to 50% are panhypogammaglobulinemic.[207] This humoral immune deficiency correlates with a increased susceptibility to infections with encapsulated pyogenic bacteria.[208]

In addition to this immune deficiency, these patients often develop various autoimmune phenomena.[204,209] The best studied is the occurrence of autoantibodies to red blood cells (positive direct antiglobulin or Coombs tests); these can be found in up to 20% of affected patients at some time during the course of their illness.[210] Approximately one quarter of these patients will have an overt autoimmune hemolytic anemia. Other autoantibodies include those directed at platelets and granulocytes. These autoantibodies are not synthesized by the malignant cells. Rather, they are produced by residual normal B cells. This is suggested by the isotype of the autoantibodies which are typically polyclonal and belong to the IgG class. By contrast, the malignant cells in CLL are programmed to produce either monoclonal IgM or IgM plus IgD.

B-CLL shares functional and phenotypic markers with normal mantle zone B cells.[211,212] These small clonal B-lymphocytes usually express low levels of membrane immunoglobulin (IgM, IgD, or both) and CD5, a glycoprotein present on follicular B cells, a subset of peripheral B cells, and almost all normal T lymphocytes (Figure 19). In addition, most B-CLL cells express HLA-DR, CD19, CD20, CD21, CD24, and CD37, which are also present on normal mature B cells. Most B-CLL also express CD23, which has received notice as a potential B cell autocrine growth factor. Most do not express CD10 (common acute lymphocytic leukemia antigen) or other early markers found in other B cell neoplasms. B-CLL are also commonly CD27$^+$, CD39$^+$, NuB1$^+$, KiB3$^\pm$, 7F7$^\pm$, and CD25$^\pm$ which, taken together with the markers described above, correspond to cellular subsets in the mantle zone.[213] In addition, expression of bcl-2 is high in B-CLL cells and in normal tonsillar follicular mantle zone B cells, but not in germinal center B cells or normal peripheral CD5$^+$ B cells.[214] Thus, for the majority of early B-CLL cases, which do not express lineage- or differentiation-discordant markers and may not have detectable chromosomal abnormalities, this normal phenotype contrasts strikingly with the remarkable tumor mass regularly attained by the B-CLL clone.

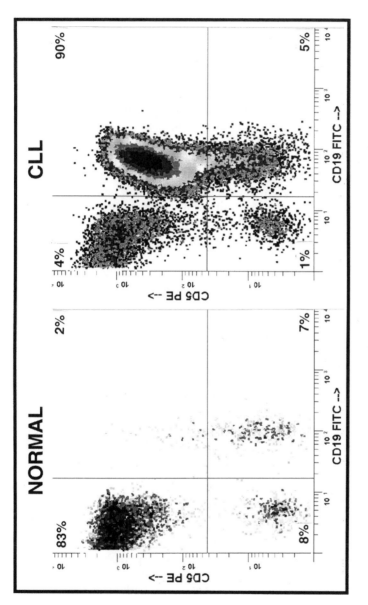

Figure 19

Comparison of CD5 vs. CD19 in a healthy subject and a patient with B-CLL. Events were gated on lymphoid scatter (see Figure 2). For each antibody, positive and negative cells are resolved into quadrants. The percent of lymphocytes within each quadrant is shown. In the healthy subject, CD5+CD19- T lymphocytes predominate. CD19+ cells (B cells) are mostly CD5-, although CD5dim B cells are also demonstrable (17.4% of B cells). In the patient sample, normal T cells (CD5+CD19-) and B cells represent minor populations. The predominant phenotype is CD5+CD19+, which represents 99.1% of B cells and 90% of lymphocytes.

The significance of CD5+ expression in B-CLL is controversial. CD5 is a monomeric glycoprotein expressed on virtually all T cells and on a subset of B cells. Although the function of CD5 is unknown, antibodies directed against CD5 can be costimulatory in culture. The relative scarcity of CD5+ peripheral B cells in healthy adults (<30% of normal peripheral B cells are CD5+), their abundance in cord blood and lymph node follicles, as well as their association with autoimmune diseases and B-cell malignancies have led to conflicting interpretations concerning the significance of CD5 expression on CLL B cells. CD5+ B cells have been proposed to comprise a separate B-cell lineage,[215] or alternatively a stage of maturation[216] or a subpopulation with suppressor activity.[217] CD5+ B cells have been characterized as being particularly responsive to IL-5; their repertoire of VH and VL usage has been reported to be restricted and prone to expression of autoantibodies primarily restricted to the IgM isotype. The functional significance of CD5 expression in CLL is particularly important, since the great majority of B CLL clones are CD5+. However, the results of a recent report indicate that functional assumptions based on the expression of the CD5+ phenotype must be viewed with caution.[218] In contrast to CD5+ cells in the lymph node, which are membrane IgM+, CD5+ B cells isolated from the peripheral blood of healthy subjects express levels of IgG and IgA comparable to their CD5− counterparts. Further, CD5− cells rapidly and transiently became CD5+ upon exposure to PMA and anti-CD3 activated T cells. In cell separation experiments, the CD5− B cells, which became CD5+ in culture, produced the greatest amounts of immunoglobulin. CD5-positive and -negative peripheral B cells produced comparable levels of autoantibody. Taken together with the reports cited above, it is clear that CD5 can be expressed on normal B cells displaying a broad spectrum of activities and ranging widely in maturational status. According to this interpretation, CD5 expression on B cells may be analogous to the expression of certain T-cell-activation markers. For example, CD38 is constitutively expressed on late thymocytes, is expressed at low levels on resting naive T cells, but is induced to high levels on mature memory T cells during activation. In B-CLL cells, as on their normal mantle zone counterparts, the expression of CD5 on predominantly small resting cells may reflect a recent history of activation and proliferation. Thus CD5 may reveal more about the recent experience of a B cell than it does about its pedigree or maturational state. Accordingly, it is not surprising that a variety of pathologic processes involving B-cell activation have been associated with CD5 expression.

This interpretation may also help explain the finding that increased numbers of circulating CD5+ B cells have been identified in two other situations in which there is reduced capacity for immunoglobulin synthesis: in neonates[219,220] and in bone marrow transplant recipients.[221] In both conditions, the eventual decline in the number of CD5[+] B cells reflects the acquisition of immunocompetency.

A second distinguishing feature of CLL cells relates to the density of membrane-bound immunoglobulins. B-CLL cells express much lower concentrations of membrane-associated immunoglobulins than normal peripheral B cells.[204] Because of this low density, surface immunoglobulins cannot be detected by routine flow cytometric analysis in 15 to 20% of the cases. It has been postulated that B-CLL cells may not differ from normal B cells in their total content of immunoglobulins. Rather, in normal cells, there is a high density of immunoglobulins on the membrane and very low concentrations in the cytoplasm. With B-CLL cells, the amount of membrane immunoglobulins is decreased, but there is a larger pool in the cytoplasm. In most cases the membrane-bound immunoglobulins are of the IgM or IgM plus IgD isotypes; those that bear the two isotypes appear to have the same idiotypic specificity.[222]

As mentioned above, increased numbers of nonmalignant CD5[+] B cells are seen in both experimental models of autoimmunity and in certain connective tissue diseases. The latter include Sjogren's syndrome, a disorder often characterized by polyclonal hypergammaglobulinemia and rheumatoid arthritis.[223,224]

In patients with B-CLL, the absolute number of circulating T lymphocytes is often increased several fold, although this increase is masked by a far greater expansion of B cells.[204] Recent data indicate that stable clonal expansions of T cells (as determined by TCR Vβ expression[225]) and activated large atypical CD4[+] T cells[226] are common findings. The possible roles of these T cells include: (1) mediators of immune surveillance, suppressing growth of the B-CLL clone; (2) promiscuously activated cells recruited because of the B-CLL cell's ability to act as both antigen presenter[227] and cytokine source[228]; or (3) helper/inducer cells which promote B-CLL growth through contact-dependent and cytokine mediated signals. The notion that T cells are polyclonally activated by B-CLL cells could explain antibody-mediated autoimmune processes, such as anemia and thrombocytopenia, which frequently develop in B-CLL. As mentioned above, these are otherwise difficult to explain, since the specificities of the autoantibodies are different from that of the B-CLL. Indiscriminate T-cell activation could have the unfortunate consequence of inducing antibody expression in previously silent autoreactive B-cell clones. Finally, the third possibility opens the possibility that CLL B cells, like their normal counterparts, require the collaboration of helper T cells for their expansion. It should be noted that these roles may not be mutually exclusive. Clonal or pauci-clonal T cell expansions account for only a small proportion of

TABLE 8

Phenotypes of B-Cell Malignancies

	CD19, CD20	CD 5	FMC-7	Surface Ig	CD11 c	CD25	CD10
CLL	+	+	−	Faint	±	+	−
PLL (*de novo*)	+	−	+	Strong	−	−	−
(2% to CLL)	+	+	+	Strong	−	−	−
HCL	+	−	−	Strong	+	+	−
Variant HCL	+	−	−	Strong	+	−	−
SLVL	+	−	+	Strong	−	−	−
Follicular lymphoma	+	−	+	Strong	−	−	+
Mantle zone lymphoma	+	+	+	?	−	−	±

the expanded T cells seen in CLL. Thus, T cell expansion and activation in B-CLL appears to be quite heterogeneous.

Flow cytometry may also be useful to distinguish B-CLL from other B-cell malignancies. Whereas 40 to 50% of normal peripheral blood B cells express CD1c, only a small proportion of B-CLL cells react with antibodies to this antigen.[229] This distinction may be clinically useful because a high proportion of patients with B-cell prolymphocytic leukemia (PLL), hairy cell leukemia (HCL), and B-cell non-Hodgkin's lymphomas have neoplastic cells which are CD1c+. Another difference is in the expression of the antigen FMC-7; CLL cells are negative, whereas this antigen regularly occurs in PLL and HCL.

In a study by Newman et al.,[230] the myeloid-associated antigen, CD11b, was demonstrated on leukemic cells from 18% of the patients. The presence of CD11c and CD11b correlated with less aggressive forms of this disease. Other adhesion molecules show variable expression. CLL cells generally lack LFA-1 (CD11a/CD18) and its ligand, ICAM-1 (CD54). By contrast, most express the lymphocyte homing receptor antigen CD44 and L-selectin; the latter serves to bind lymphocytes to high endothelial venules.

Although immunophenotyping is useful in recognizing B-CLL, its value for patient management or as a prognostic aid has not been determined. In most patients, the disease is compatible with a prolonged survival. Death usually results from either infection or refractory disease. In a small percentage of patients, the malignancy transforms into a more aggressive type of leukemia, PLL, or to a high-grade lymphoma (Richter's syndrome). Table 8 shows a comparison of the phenotypic findings in CLL, PLL, and other B cell lymphomatous disorders.

VIII. OTHER TYPES OF B-CELL LEUKEMIA

A. Prolymphocytic Leukemia

This malignancy occurs in two forms, one that arises *de novo* and a second resulting from the transformation of classic B-CLL. In both, there is a predominance of a homogeneous population of **prolympho-cytes**. These large lymphocytes are characterized by nuclei containing a single prominent nucleolus. By definition, in PLL, prolymphocytes must comprise >55% of the circulating lymphocytes. The *de novo* form is usually characterized by a extremely high lymphocyte count, often in excess of 100,000/µl. Typically, patients with this disease show massive splenomegaly with little or no lymphadenopathy. The mean survival of patients with PLL is relatively short.

Phenotypically, *de novo* PLL can be readily distinguished from typical B-CLL. As would be expected, both malignancies express the B-cell markers CD19 and CD20. However, PLL cells are generally characterized by the expression of high density surface immunoglobulins, and react with a specific B-cell antigen, FMC-7. CD5, which is characteristically expressed on most B-CLL leukemias is not present in *de novo* PLL. In those B-CLL leukemias which do transform into PLL, the malignant clone usually maintains the CD5 antigen. It should be noted that prolymphocytic leukemias almost always arise from the B-CLL clone, whereas about half of the large B-cell lymphomas, acute lymphoblastic leukemias, and multiple myelomas developing after B-CLL arise from a distinct clone as determined by immunoglobulin idiotype.[232]

B. Hairy Cell Leukemia

This neoplasm has activated B cells as its closest normal counterpart. Cytologically, the malignant cells are larger than those found in B-CLL; often they have an enlarged nucleus with a discernible cleft. The cells are characterized by the presence of the fine cytoplasmic projections which gives the disease its name. HCL cells also possess a unique cytoplasmic acid phosphatase enzyme which is resistant to tartrate degradation (tartrate-resistant acid phosphatase, or TRAP). The clinical features of the disease include splenomegaly, often massive, and pancytopenia.[231] Affected patients may manifest a profound monocytopenia, a defect that may be pathogenically related to their increased susceptibility to opportunistic infections. Bone marrow biopsies show both a malignant cell infiltration and fibrosis. Hairy cell leukemia is compatible with a long survival; major clinical problems primarily result from the pancytopenia due to decreased marrow production and splenic sequestration.

Phenotypically, the HCL cells react with a variety of B-cell markers (CD19, CD20, CD21, CD22, and sometimes CD23 and CD24)[233,234] and show membrane associated monoclonal immunoglobulins with a single light chain isotype. The characteristic feature is the presence of CD11c, an antigen usually expressed on cells of the myeloid/monocytic series.[235] Other determinants often present include the PCA-1 antigen, a plasma cell-associated determinant[236] and CD25, the α chain of the IL-2 receptor.[237] These characteristics are consistent with the concepts that the malignant hairy cell represents the neoplastic counterpart of an activated B lymphocyte.

Robbins et al.[238] used two-color flow cytometry to determine the phenotypic patterns seen in 161 cases of HCL. In cases in which there were more than 10 to 15% leukemic cells, the abnormal population was readily identifiable on the forward vs. side scatter plot as a distinct population of large cells overlapping with the normal monocyte region. All cases expressed B cell lineage markers CD19, CD20, and CD22 and monoclonal surface immunoglobulins were identified on virtually all of the cases. CD11c was present on the leukemic cells in all patients and CD25 on 99%. CD10 (CALLA) was present in on HCL cells in 26% of the cases.

These investigators[238] also compared the phenotypic expression in HCL with B-CLL. They found that, in 50 CLL cases, 74% were positive for CD11c and 68% for CD25. However, they noted a distinct difference in the staining patterns. In HCL, CD19+ cells showed intense uniform staining with CD11c. By contrast, CLL cells showed only weak to moderate staining. Likewise, CD25 reactivity was consistently intense on HCL cells whereas in CLL, there was a broad range of fluorescence intensity.

Several other differences were noted between HCL and CLL. HCL cells reacted strongly with antibodies to CD22. With rare exceptions, they were consistently negative for CD5+. Immunoglobulin staining differed from CLL in that it was of moderate intensity. Using the B-Ly7 antibody, which does not react with a defined CD antigen, all cases of HCL were positive whereas reactivity was consistently absent in patients with CLL. An interesting finding was that antibodies to CD20 consistently caused aggregation of hairy cells. Because aggregates were not scored as CD20+, the apparent proportion of CD20+ cells was lower than that of CD19+ lymphocytes.

1. Variant Hairy Cell Leukemia

This is a disorder which is morphologically intermediate between typical hairy cell leukemia and prolymphocytic leukemia.[231] It occurs most frequently in elderly individuals. Typically, affected patients present with splenomegaly but not lymphadenopathy. High lymphocyte counts, often in excess of 100,000/μl, are common. The malignant cells have the cytological features of typical hairy cell leukemia. In addition, they show a large nucleus with a prominent nucleolus, a finding generally associated with PLL. As in classic HCL, monocytopenia is a common feature. Despite the high lymphocyte count, the course of this disease is typically benign. Immunophenotyping reveals a pattern similar to that seen in typical HCL except that the neoplastic cells are generally negative for CD25.

C. Splenic Lymphoma with Circulating Villous Lymphocytes (SLVL)

This disorder is an indolent lymphoid neoplasm characterized by dominant splenomegaly with minimal or absent lymphadenopathy.[231] In approximately two thirds of affected patients, the presence of a small monoclonal immunoglobulin **spike** can be identified in the serum. The white count ranges from 5000 to 40,000/μl. Circulating lymphocytes are typically larger than those seen in B-CLL and have short villi, often localized to one pole of the cell. Anemia and thrombocytopenia, due to hypersplenism, are common. Unlike HCL, the marrow is easily aspirable and usually shows a lymphocytic infiltrate. By contrast, marrow fibrosis, which is common in HCL, is not present. Another difference between SLVL and HCL is the pattern of splenic infiltration; the former predominantly involves the white pulp whereas HCL primarily affects the red pulp.

The antigen profile of SLVL is similar to PLL; the cells are moderate to strongly positive for membrane-associated immunoglobulins and express the typical B-cell markers including CD22 and FMC-7, but usually lack CD5, CD11c, CD25, and CD38.

D. Leukemic Phase of Non-Hodgkin's Lymphoma

1. Follicular Lymphoma

Although follicular lymphomas are primarily neoplasms affecting lymphoid tissues and the bone marrow, they may be prominent in the peripheral blood as well. In these instances, the clinical features closely resemble those seen in B-CLL. Morphologically, the circulating follicular lymphoma cells are often pleomorphic with small prominent nucleoli, nuclear clefting, a finer chromatin pattern than that seen in B-CLL, and a high nuclear/cytoplasmic ratio. Chromosomal abnormalities, especially t(14:18) with rearrangements of the *bcl-2* oncogene are frequent.

Phenotypically, these malignant cells usually show intense staining for membrane-associated immunoglobulins. They react with the B cell lineage markers and are typically positive for both the CD10 and the FMC-7 antigens. Most follicular lymphomas are CD5⁻.

2. Leukemic Phases of Mantle Zone Lymphoma

The leukemic phase of mantle zone lymphomas is an aggressive disease with a median survival of less than 2 years. Morphologically, the neoplastic cells are pleomorphic, medium-sized lymphoid cells.[231] They contain a moderate amount of cytoplasm and show irregular, often clefted, nuclei, frequently with nucleoli. Immunophenotyping indicates strong expression of membrane-associated immunoglobulins, the presence of B-cell markers including CD22, as well as the coexpression of CD5 and FMC-7. CD10 is present on the lymphoma cells in approximately 50% of the cases.

3. Large Cell Lymphoma

The leukemic phases of these malignancies are quite rare. They are difficult to recognize in the absence of immunophenotypic studies. Approximately two thirds are due to the malignant transformation of B lymphocytes.[231] Typically, both the T- and B-cell forms are characterized by large undifferentiated cells which are difficult to distinguish from other hematopoietic malignancies, including acute myeloid leukemias.

E. Variant CLL

In 1990, Wormsley et al.[239] described a form of apparent B-CLL in which the leukemic cells coexpressed both the CD5 and CD11c antigens. This suggested a disorder that had characteristics of both CLL and HCL. The clinical features were more consistent with the former: none of the patients had pancytopenia, splenomegaly, or by cytological examination, cells with cytoplasmic villi. All were TRAP negative. The cells were slightly larger than those seen in typical CLL and had a lower nuclear/cytoplasmic ratio. Although there were cytological features suggestive of PLL, the malignant cells did not react with the FMC-7 antibody. The intensity of immunoglobulin staining varied from weak, as seen in typical CLL, to the more intense staining characteristic of other lymphoid neoplasms. Leukemic cells from all cases were CD10⁻. Further studies in normal subjects, using three-color fluorescence, suggested the existence of a minor population of CD20⁺CD5⁺CD11c⁺ B lymphocytes.

F. Waldenstrom's Macroglobulinemia

Although not a leukemia, macroglobulinemia belongs in the spectrum of B-cell neoplasms. In most affected patients, this disorder clinically manifests itself as a low grade lymphoma-like neoplasm with the additional feature of a marked overproduction of monoclonal IgM. The concentration of the paraprotein is often sufficiently high in the serum as to produce the hyperviscosity syndrome.

The neoplastic cells are pleomorphic with features ranging from those of a small lymphocytes to plasma cells; typically, a proportion are intermediate cells with characteristics of lymphocytes and plasma cells (plasmacytoid lymphocytes). They are predominantly localized in lymphatic tissues and the bone marrow. Rarely, peripheral blood involvement can be demonstrated. Phenotypically, they express B cell markers and also react with the PCA-1 antibody. As mentioned above, the malignant cells in Waldenstrom's macroglobulin are capable of substantial immunoglobulin synthesis and thus, by immunophenotypic criteria, show both surface and cytoplasmic IgM.[151]

G. Multiple Myeloma and Other Plasma Cell Dyscrasias

The terminal stage of normal B-cell maturation is the formation of antibody-producing plasma cells. The principal malignant equivalent of this terminal stage of differentiation is the disorder multiple myeloma. Major features of this neoplasm include a plasma cell infiltration of the bone marrow and the presence of a monoclonal immunoglobulin in the serum or monoclonal light chains in the urine. A third diagnostic criterion is the occurrence of characteristic "punched out" bone lesions on X-ray. Associated features include bone marrow failure, primarily due to the infiltration by the malignant cells, renal failure, increased susceptibility to infection (in part due to a failure of normal polyclonal immunoglobulin synthesis), hypercalcemia, amyloidosis, and pathologic bone fractures.

The malignant plasma cells do not express CD19 or CD20. Similarly, immunoglobulins are not expressed on the cell membrane. However, these neoplastic cells show large intracytoplasmic pools of immunoglobulin.[212] They usually express certain nonlineage antigens, PCA-1, PC-1, and CD38.[151,240,241] Most myeloma cells have been reported to be CD56+.[242,243] In a proportion of myeloma patients, the malignant cells are CD10+; the presence of this antigen has been correlated with a poorer prognosis.

Harada et al.[104] suggested that there are phenotypic differences between normal plasma cells and myeloma cells. In a series of 20 patients, myeloma plasma cells in bone marrow aspirates were identified

TABLE 9

Phenotypes of T-Cell Malignancies

	CD3	CD4	CD8	CD57	CD56 CD16	CD7	CD25
T–LGL	+	−	+	+	−	+	−
NK–LGL	−	−	−	−	+	?	−
T–PLL	+	±	±	−	−	+	−
CTCL	+	+	−	−	−	−	+
ATL	+	+	−	−	−	−	+

by the presence of intense staining with CD38. Two-color analysis indicated that, in 13 patients, the neoplastic plasma cells were CD19⁻CD56⁺. Five others were CD19⁻CD56⁻ and two were CD56⁺CD19⁺. By contrast, normal plasma cells from various tissues proved to be CD38^bright, CD19⁺CD56⁻; none of the myeloma cells had this phenotype.

Other plasma cell dyscrasias include cryoglobulinemia, primary amyloidosis, idiopathic cold agglutinin hemolytic anemia, and a heterogeneous entity termed monoclonal gammopathy of undetermined significance (MGUS). The last is characterized by the presence of a monoclonal gammopathy without other evidence of either multiple myeloma or other plasma cell dyscrasia. Long-term follow-up of these individuals indicates that only a small proportion ultimately progresses to myeloma. None of these diseases can be specifically identified by immunophenotyping. In Harada's series,[104] CD19⁺CD56⁻ and CD19⁻CD56⁺ cells were found in patients with MGUS, suggesting the presence of phenotypically normal plasma cells and a clonally derived population. Sonneveld et al.[243] showed CD56 was not expressed on the plasma cells from 23 patients with MGUS.

IX. T-CELL LEUKEMIAS

T-cell lymphoproliferative malignancies constitute a spectrum of diseases that result from the clonal expansion of neoplastic T lymphocytes. These diseases appear to arise from T cells which have already undergone thymic maturation; thus they are referred to as post-thymic diseases.[206] Included in this group of neoplasms are: (1) large granular cell leukemia (LGL), also called T-CLL or T-gamma disease; (2) T-cell prolymphocytic leukemia (T-PLL); (3) cutaneous T-cell lymphomas, a collective term that includes mycosis fungoides (MF) and Sezary syndrome (SS); and (4) adult T-cell leukemia. A comparison of the immunophenotypic profiles of these diseases is shown in Table 9.

A. Large Granular Cell Leukemia

Cells morphologically classified as large granular lymphocytes comprise 10 to 15% of the normal peripheral blood mononuclear cells. This population, however, is not homogenous. Based on expression of the CD3 antigen, two distinct subtypes can be distinguished. The CD3⁻ subset contains the true natural killer cells; the CD3⁺ cells may be non-MHC–restricted cytotoxic T cells. As expected, the CD3⁻ cells do not express membrane-bound T-cell receptors, and the T-cell receptor genes are in a germ cell configuration. By contrast, the CD3⁺ population shows rearranged T-cell receptor genes. Both the CD3⁺ and the CD3⁻ subsets of LGL can undergo neoplastic transformation.[244]

Because the clonal origin of LGL may be either CD3⁺, indicating a T-cell origin, or CD3⁻, which is consistent with a NK cell origin. Loughran[245] suggested this entity be subdivided into two groups, T-LGL and NK-LGL. He presented evidence indicating that there are distinct differences in the clinical features of these two disorders.

T-LGL is a chronic leukemia, primarily affecting middle aged or elderly individuals.[206] Clinically, it is characterized by a modest lymphocytosis; the median lymphocyte count is 7800/µl (range 10,000 to 49,000). The characteristic finding on peripheral blood smears is the presence of an increased number of LGL. These cells are larger than normal lymphocytes and have abundant, pale cytoplasm and prominent azurophilic granules. However, morphological variations are quite common, including the presence of large, agranular cells and, in a minority of patients, cells that resemble small lymphocytes.

On physical examination, splenomegaly is a common finding; by contrast, lymphadenopathy and skin infiltration are rare. The latter is in distinct contrast to other T-cell lymphoproliferative diseases which are frequently complicated by cutaneous involvement.

Other hematological findings include a high incidence of neutropenia, which is often severe.[244] Thrombocytopenia, by contrast, is rare. Almost half of the patients with T-LGL have neutrophil counts less than 500/µl. The causes of the neutropenia have not been fully defined; only a minority of patients have antineutrophil antibodies. Furthermore, although marrow infiltration by LGL occurs in more than 85% of affected patients, it is usually does not replace normal hematopoietic elements. There is evidence suggesting that cells with the same phenotypes as T-LGL are capable of suppressing *in vitro* hematopoiesis.[202]

Another complication of T-LGL is the development of a severe aregenerative anemia.[244,246] In some affected patients, the bone marrow shows almost a complete absence of erythroid precursors, an entity designated as pure red cell aplasia (PRCA). In a recent study of 21 patients with T-LGL,[246] 12 were severely anemic. Four of these patients had PRCA. Other investigators have shown neoplastic cells from patients with PRCA associated with T-LGL can directly suppress erythroid colony formation *in vitro*.[247,248]

T-LGL may be discovered incidentally. In symptomatic patients, the most frequent clinical manifestation is recurrent bacterial infections resulting from the neutropenia. There is a close association between T-LGL and rheumatoid arthritis;[244] of affected patients, 25 to 30% have this connective tissue disease. In addition, over half of the affected patients have positive tests for rheumatoid factor. Multiple other serological abnormalities have been found in patients with T-LGL: these include the presence of antinuclear antibodies (ANA), unexplained polyclonal gammopathies, and, in up to 20% of affected patients, hypogammaglobulinemia.[244] It is noteworthy that skin and CNS involvement, common manifestations of other T-cell neoplasms, are very rare in T-LGL.

By definition, the leukemic cells in T-LGL are CD3$^+$. Greater than 95% express the CD8 antigen and are negative for CD4. Another common finding is the coexpression of CD57$^+$. By contrast, there is variable expression of the other NK-associated antigens, CD56 and CD16. There may be an increased number of apparently activated cells (CD3$^+$/HLA-DR$^+$). Rare cases of CD3$^+$CD4$^+$CD8$^-$ T-LGL have been described.

It appears that some patients with "Felty's syndrome" (rheumatoid arthritis, splenomegaly, and neutropenia) may have an occult form of T-LGL. Although these patients do not have an elevated lymphocyte count, a subset of patients with otherwise typical Felty's syndrome show a clonal rearrangement of T cells and immunophenotypic findings similar to patients with classic T-LGL.[249-255]

NK-LGL is also a clonal disease of large granular lymphocytes. However, this leukemia differs from T-LGL, both in its clinical manifestations and its immunophenotypic features. NK-LGL generally occurs in a younger population (median age 39). Patients often have unexplained fevers, weight loss, and night sweats. Unlike T-LGL, NK-LGL tends to follow an acute clinical course. Coexisting rheumatoid arthritis has not been observed. The hematological findings also differ; severe neutropenia is unusual, whereas pronounced thrombocytopenia occurs in approximately 75% of affected patients. Lymphocytosis is generally present and often increases at a rapid rate. Massive hepatosplenomegaly associated with evidence of hepatic failure is common.

Cytologically, NK-LGL cells are indistinguishable from those of T-LGL. The typical phenotype of NK-LGL is CD3$^-$, CD4-, CD8$^-$, CD16$^+$, CD56$^+$, and CD57$^-$. As expected, T-cell receptor genes are not rearranged.

B. T-Prolymphocytic Leukemia

Like the B-cell variant, T-cell PLL is characterized by a high white cell count, splenomegaly, and, in approximately half of affected patients, hepatomegaly. Skin lesions and serous effusions occur more commonly than in B-PLL. T-PLL has a poor prognosis; the median survival is 7 months. Morphologically, T-PLL is characterized by the presence of monomorphic cells which are large lymphocytes with moderate amounts of agranular, basophilic cytoplasm. The nucleus can have either a regular or on irregular shape with condensed chromatin. A prominent nucleolus is normally apparent. Rare small cell variants of this neoplasm have also been described. Phenotypically T-PLL cells react with the anti-T-cell antibodies including CD2, CD3, and CD5. T-PLL cells are strongly CD7+; by contrast, other postthymic T-cell leukemias do not express this antigen. T-PLL cells can express either CD4 or CD8; rarely they coexpress both antigens.

C. Adult T-Cell Leukemia/Lymphoma (ATL)

This malignancy is believed to be caused by the retrovirus, HTLV–1.[206] The virus is endemic in discrete geographical areas including southwestern Japan, the Caribbean Basin, Melanesia, and in parts of Africa. In the U.S., clusters have been reported in the southeast and in immigrants from HTLV-1–endemic areas living in Brooklyn.[256] The major clinical features are lymphadenopathy, hepatosplenomegaly, skin infiltration, and hypercalcemia with or without osteolytic bone lesions.

The leukemic cells generally are pleomorphic, varying in size and degree of nuclear chromatin condensation. The nucleus is generally irregular and polylobed. ATL cells have the phenotype of mature T-helper cells (CD4+).[257,258] They display typical T-cell markers, except for CD7. One noteworthy feature of these leukemic cells is their intense expression of the CD25 antigen, (IL-2 receptor α chain).[257] Antibodies to CD25 have been successfully used to treat selected patients in experimental protocols. Despite expression of the helper/inducer phenotype, functionally these cells act as potent *in vitro* suppressors of B cell differentiation.[257,258]

D. Cutaneous T-Cell Lymphoma (CTCL)

This term refers to a T-cell lymphoma, caused by T-helper/inducer cells, in which the primary site of involvement is the skin.[151] CTCL includes two clinically defined entities, mycosis fungoides and Sezary syndrome, and a series of neoplasms with overlapping features. Mycosis fungoides is usually considered to be a neoplasm in which the predominant feature is skin infiltration leading to plaque and tumor formation. Extensive blood stream involvement in classic MF is rare. By contrast, SS is characterized by a diffuse skin reddening and the presence of numerous circulating Sezary cells. These are large lymphoid cells with a distinct irregular nucleus with deep and narrow indentations. Because of their resemblance to the anatomical structure of the brain, these lymphoid cells have been described as **cerebriform**. In most patients with CTCL, careful examination reveals overlapping features of MF and SS, including the presence of a variable number of circulating Sezary cells.

Clinically, the dominating feature of CTCL is a chronic indolent skin rash. The initial rashes are often nonspecific and the actual diagnosis may not be made for several years. Phenotypically, the malignant cells resemble mature T-helper/inducer cells, bearing T-cell lineage markers and expressing CD3, CD4, and CD5, but not CD8.[259-261] In most cases, the circulating Sezary cells are CD7-. By contrast, this antigen is present on mycosis fungoides cells in the skin.[184]

X. NON-HODGKIN'S LYMPHOMA AND HODGKIN'S DISEASE

A. Non-Hodgkin's Lymphoma

These malignancies show marked diversity in their clinical manifestations, their prognoses, and their responses to therapy. An understanding of these diseases is further complicated by the existence of multiple classification systems. Although each has its proponents, none have yet proven to be clearly superior. In addition, none are based on immunophenotypic criteria, information that has significant prognostic value. Immunophenotyping also provides information applicable to both the classification and management of these disorders. Except in the leukemic phases, immunophenotyping of non-Hodgkin's lymphoma is typically performed on histological or frozen sections. Flow cytometric analysis requires a cell suspension be prepared from freshly biopsied tissue. Thus, it is used primarily as an adjunct diagnostic procedure. Clinically, the two most important reasons to perform immunophenotyping are to distinguish between a reactive and neoplastic process and to determine the cell lineage in a lymphoid malignancy.

Most lymphoid tumors are of B-cell origin and characteristically exhibit a monoclonal surface immunoglobulin. Clinically, this can be recognized by showing a excess of B cells displaying a single light chain determinant.[262] In a recent series, light chain monoclonality was identified in over 90% of NHL. This study proposed the normal range to be a kappa/lambda ratio between 0.5 to 3.0.[263] Among the lymphomas, the low grade tumors have a higher incidence of membrane lg positivity; high grade tumors were often membrane lg negative.[264]

Reactive lymphoid tissue generally presents with a polyclonal distribution of both T and B cells. Using flow cytometry, de Martini[264] analyzed 94 cases of reactive lymphoid hyperplasia. These investigators reported a mean of 37% (range 9 to 71%) of the cells was membrane lg⁺. CD3⁺ cells comprised an average of 54% of the cellularity (range 22 to 81%); the CD4/CD8 ratio was 2.6 (range 0.7 to 83). In this study, there was a normal distribution of *kappa/lambda* stained cells (normal range defined as 0.7 to 5.5).

In addition, specific determinants appear to have prognostic implications. For example, CD11a is generally strongly expressed on cells from low or intermediate grade lymphomas, whereas most of the high grade lymphomas are CD11a⁻. Lack of expression of HLA-DR and LFA-1 and high level expression of Ki-67 (reflecting a high proliferative activity) are all associated with a poor prognosis in diffuse large cell lymphomas.[265] Approximately 25% of follicular lymphomas are CD10⁺, whereas the diffuse forms are almost always negative.[264]

B. Hodgkin's Disease

In many respects, this disease has been an enigma. The pathological hallmark of Hodgkin's disease is the presence of the Reed Sternberg cell, a binucleated or multinucleated giant cell, or its mononuclear variants. Collectively, these cells have been designated as Hodgkin's cells (HC). These cells are considered to be the neoplastic elements in this disease. Despite extensive investigations, the origin of HCs is a subject of much debate. In fact, there is evidence suggesting they arise from B lymphocytes,[266] T lymphocytes,[267,268] undifferentiated lymphoid cells, macrophages or reticulum (dendritic) cells.[269] These conflicting data suggest Hodgkin's disease may not be a single entity. Rather, current opinions suggest the different histologic forms may be due to the malignant transformation of several different precursors. This is supported by evidence suggesting HC in the lymphocyte predominant form is of B cell origin, whereas the mixed cellularity type may result from the neoplastic transformation of T cells.

In part, the difficulty in determining the origins of HCs result from the pathological findings that HC comprise only a small minority of the cells in involved tissue. The vast majority of cells are reactive elements. It appears the greater the number of T cells, the better the prognosis.[270] In nodular sclerosing and mixed cellularity forms of Hodgkin's disease, most cells are found to be activated CD4 T cells.

Immunophenotypic studies have shown that HC generally express several activation antigens including CD30, CD25, HLA-DR, and CD71.[271] In fact, the expression of CD30 (Ki-1 antigen) has been widely used to confirm a pathological diagnosis; the only major disease that also expresses this antigen is the large anaplastic cell non-Hodgkin's lymphomas (Ki-1+ lymphoma).[272] CD30 is a member of the TNF receptor family; its expression is normally confined to activated T cells. Its expression of HC cells may play a role in the pathologic process.

Other studies indicate HC frequently express several myeloid/macrophage antigens, including CD11a, CD11b, and CD15. A recent study found the B7/BB1 antigen (CD80), a molecule expressed on antigen-presenting cells and the natural ligand for CD28 and CTLA-4 on T cells, was strongly expressed on Reed Sternberg cells in all 47 patients with Hodgkin's disease. Of note, these were frequently surrounded by CD28+ T cells. These data suggest an accessory cell function for HC cells.[273]

Nodular lymphocyte predominant Hodgkin's disease (NLPHD) may represent a distinct form of this malignancy.[274] By immunophenotypic criteria, the malignant cell, strongly expresses B-cell–associated markers and lacks CD15.

Recent studies on the cellular origins of Hodgkin's disease have been facilitated by the development of HC cell lines. Ellis et al.[275] described the expression of several adhesion molecules in HC, including CD11a and CD11c in high density. CD44 (Hermes antigen), the lymphocyte homing receptor, is also strongly expressed. In addition, CD54 (ICAM-1), CD58 (LFA-3), ICAM-2, PECAM, and, rarely, CD2 (LFA-1), may be found on HC lines. These findings suggested that cultured HC have a phenotypic profile similar to dendritic cells.

REFERENCES

1. Andreeff, M., *Clinical Cytometry*, The New York Academy of Sciences, New York, 1986.
2. Shapiro, H., *Practical Flow Cytometry*, 3rd ed., Alan R. Liss, New York, 1995.
3. Melamed, M., Lindmo, T., and Mendelsohn, M., Eds., *Flow Cytometry and Sorting*, 2nd ed., Wiley-Liss, New York, 1990.
4. Coligan, J., Kruisbeck, A., Margulies, D., Shevach, E., and Strober, W., Eds., Immunofluorescence and cell sorting, in *Current Protocols in Immunology*, Wiley-interscience, New York, 1991, 5.0.
5. Kipps, T., Meisenholder G., and Robbins, B., New developments in flow cytometric analyses of lymphocyte markers, *Clin. Lab. Med.*, 12, 237, 1992.
6. Givan, A., *Flow Cytometry. First Principles*, Wiley-Liss, New York, 1993.

7. Robinson, J., *Handbook of Flow Cytometry Methods,* Wiley-Liss, New York, 1993.
8. IUIS-WHO Nomenclature Subcommittee, Nomenclature for clusters of differentiation (CD) of antigens defined on human leukocyte populations, *Bull. WHO,* 62, 809, 1984.
9. Clark, E. and Lanier, L., Report from Vienna: in search of all surface molecules expressed on human leukocytes, *J. Clin. Immunol.,* 9, 265, 1989.
10. Schlossman, S., Boumsell, L., Gilks, W., et al., Eds., *Leukocyte Typing V,* Oxford University Press, Oxford, 1995.
11. Fowlkes, B. and Pardoll D., Molecular and cellular events of T cell development, *Adv. Immunol.,* 44, 207, 1989.
12. Rothenberg, E., The development of functionally responsive T cells, *Adv. Immunol.,* 51, 85, 1992.
13. Landay, A., Ohisson-Wilhelm, B., and Giorgi, J., Application of flow cytometry to the study of HIV infection, *AIDS,* 1990, 4, 479, 1990.
14. Parnes, J., Molecular biology and function of CD4 and CD8, *Adv. Immunol.,* 44, 265, 1989.
15. Kronenberg, M., Siu, G., Hood, L., and Shastri, N., The molecular genetics of the T-cell antigen receptor and T-cell antigen recognition, *Annu. Rev. Immunol.,* 4, 529, 1986.
16. Marrack, P. and Kappler, J., The T-cell receptor, *Science,* 238, 1073, 1987.
17. Miceli, M.C. and Parnes, J.R., The roles of CD4 and CD8 in T-cell activation, *Semin. Immunol.,* 3, 133, 1991.
18. Altman, A., Coggeshall, K., and Mustelin, T., Molecular events mediating T-cell activation, *Adv. Immunol.,* 48, 227, 1990.
19. Campana, D., Janossy, G., Coustan-Smith, E., et al., The expression of T-cell receptor associated proteins during T-cell ontogeny in man, *J. Immunol.,* 142, 57, 1989.
20. Pui, C.-H., Behm, F., and Crist, W., Clinical and biologic relevance of immunologic marker studies in childhood acute lymphoblastic leukemia, *Blood,* 82, 343, 1993.
21. Lanier, L., Spits, H., and Phillips, J., Expression of cytoplasmic CD3 epsilon proteins in activated human adult natural killer (NK) cells and CD3 gamma, delta, epsilon complexes in fetal NK cells, *J. Immunol.,* 149, 1876, 1992.
22. Lanier, L., Distribution and function of lymphocyte surface antigens, *Ann. N.Y. Acad. Sci.,* 677, 86, 1993.
23. Weiss, A. and Imboden, J., Cell surface molecules and early events involved in human T lymphocyte activation, *Adv. Immunol.,* 41, 138, 1987.
24. Ko, H.-S., Fu, S., Winchester, R., Yu, D., and Kunkel, H., Ia determinants on stimulated human T lymphocytes, *J. Exp. Med.,* 150, 246, 1979.
25. Reinherz, E., Kung, P., Pesando, J., Ritz, J., Goldstein, G., and Schlossman, S., Ia determinants on human T-cell subsets defined by monoclonal antibody, *J. Exp. Med.,* 150, 1472, 1979.
26. Cotner, T., Williams, J., Christenson, L., Shapiro, H., Strom, T., and Strominger, J., Simultaneous flow cytometric analysis of human T-cell activation antigen expression and DNA content, *J. Exp. Med.,* 157, 461, 1983.
27. Holter, W., Majdic, O., Liszka, K., Stockinger, H., and Knapp, W., Kinetics of activation antigen expression by *in vitro*-stimulated human T lymphocytes, *Cell. Immunol.,* 90, 322, 1985.
28. Smith, K., Lowest dose interleukin-2 immunotherapy, *Blood,* 81, 1414, 1993.
29. Neckers, L. and Cossman, J., Transferrin receptor induction in mitogen-stimulated human T lymphocytes is required for DNA synthesis and cell division and is regulated by interieukin 2, *Proc. Natl. Acad. Sci. U.S.A.,* 80, 3494, 1983.
30. Thomas, M., The leukocyte common antigen family, *Annu. Rev. Immunol.,* 7, 339, 1989.

31. Hall, L., Streuli, M., Schlossman, S., and Saito, H., Complete exon-intron organization of the human leukocyte common antigen (CD45) gene, *J. Immunol.*, 141, 2781, 1988.

32. Clement, L., Isoforms of the CD45 common leukocyte antigen family: markers for human T-cell differentiation, *J. Clin. Immunol.*, 12, 1, 1992.

33. Donnenberg, A.D., Margolick, J.B., and Donnenberg, V.S., Lymphopoiesis, apoptosis and immune amnesia. *Ann. N.Y. Acad. Sci.*, 770, 213, 1996.

34. Elson, L.H., Nutman, T.B., Metcalfe. D.D., and Prussin, C., Flow cytometric analysis for cytokine production identifies T helper 1, T helper 2, and T helper 0 cells within the human CD4+CD27-lymphocyte subpopulation, *J. Immunol.*, 154(9), 4294, 1995.

35. Clement, L., Dagg, M., and Landay, A., Characterization of human lymphocyte subpopulations: alloreactive cytotoxic T-lymphocyte precursor and effector cells are phenotypically distinct from Leu²⁺ suppressor cells, *J. Clin. Immunol.*, 4, 395, 1984.

36. Yamashita, N., Nguyen, L., Fahey, J., and Clement, L., Phenotypic properties and cytotoxic functions of human CD8+ cells expressing the CD57 antigen, *Nat. Immunol.*, 12, 79, 1993.

37. Phillips, J. and Lanier, L., Lectin-dependent and anti-CD3 induced cytotoxicity are preferentially mediated by peripheral blood cytotoxic T lymphocytes expressing leu-7 antigen, *J. Immunol.*, 136, 1579, 1986.

38. Korsmeyer, S., Hieter, P., Ravetch, J., Poplack, D., Waldmann, T., and Leder, P., Developmental hierarchy of immunoglobulin gene rearrangements in human leukemic pre-B cells, *Proc. Natl. Acad. Sci. U.S.A.*, 78, 7096, 1981.

39. Korsmeyer, S., Antigen receptor genes as molecular markers of lymphoid neoplasms, *J. Clin. Invest.*, 79, 1291, 1987.

40. Waldmann, T., The arrangement of immunoglobulin and T-cell receptor genes in human lymphoproliferative disorders, *Adv. Immunol.*, 40, 247, 1987.

41. Cooper, M., B lymphocytes. Normal development and function, *N. Engl. J. Med.*, 317, 1452, 1987.

42. Fu, S., Winchester, R., and Kunkel, H., Similar idiotypic specificity for the membrane IgD and IgM of human B lymphocytes, *J. Immunol.*, 114, 250, 1975.

43. Uckun, F.M., Regulation of human B-cell ontogeny, *Blood*, 76, 1908, 1990.

44. Banchereau, J., Rousset, F., Human B lymphocytes: phenotype, proliferation, and differentiation, *Adv. Immunol.*, 52, 125, 1992.

45. Kipps, T., Meisenholder, G., and Robbins, B., New developments in flow cytometric analyses of lymphocyte markers, *Clin. Lab. Med.*, 12, 237, 1992.

46. Clark, E., CD22, a B cell-specific receptor, mediates adhesion and signal transduction, *J. Immunol.*, 150, 4715, 1993.

47. Kikutani, H., Suemura, M., Owaki, H., et al., Fc epsilon receptor, a specific differentiation marker transiently expressed on mature B cells before isotype switching, *J. Exp. Med.*, 164, 1455, 1986.

48. Kehry, M. and Yamashita, L., Low-affinity IgE receptor (CD23) function on mouse B cells: role of Independent antigen focusing, *Proc. Natl. Acad. Sci., U.S.A.*, 86, 7556, 1989.

49. Pirron, U., Schlunck, T., and Prinz, J., Riedber E. IgE-dependent antigen focusing by human B lymphocytes is mediated by the low-affinity receptor for IgE, *Eur. J. Immunol.*, 20, 1547, 1990.

50. Bonnefoy, J., Guillot, O., Spits H, Blanchard D, Ishizaka K, and Banchereau J. The low affinity receptor for IgE (CD23) on B lymphocytes is spatially associated with HLA-DR antigens, *J. Exp. Med.*, 167, 57, 1988.

51. Flores-Romo, L., Johnson, G., Ghaderi, A., Stanworth, D., and Gordon, J., Functional implication for the topographical relationship between MHC class II and the low-affinity IgE receptor: occupancy of the CD23 prevents B lymphocytes from stimulating allogeneic mixed lymhocyte responses, *Eur. J. Immunol.*, 20, 2465, 1990.

52. Moretta, L., Ciccone, E., Pende, D., Tripodi, G., Bottino, C., and Moretta, A., Human natural killer cells: clonally distributed specific functions and triggering surface molecules, *Lab. Invest.*, 66, 138, 1992.

53. Lanier, L., Le, A., Civin, C., Loken, M., and Phillips, J., The relationship of CD16 (leu-11) and leu-19 (NHK-1) antigen expression on human peripheral blood NK cells and cytotoxic T lymphocytes, *J. Immunol.*, 136, 4480, 1986.

54. Jacobs, R., Stoll, M., Stratman, G., Leo, R., Link, H., and Schmidt, E., CD16-CD56⁺ natural killer cells after bone marrow transplantation, *Blood*, 79, 3239, 1992.

55. Srour, E., Leemhuis, T., Jenski, L., Redmond, R., and Jansen, J., Cytoloytic activity of human natural killer cell subpopulations isolated by four-color immunofluorscence flow cytometric cell sorting, *Cytometry*, 11, 442, 1990.

56. Sansoni, P., Cossarizza, A., Briznti, V., et al., Lymphocyte subsets and natural killer cell activity in healthy old people and centenarians, *Blood*, 82, 2767, 1993.

57. Berenson, R., Andrews, R., Bensinger, W., et al. Antigen CD34⁺ marrow cells engraft irradiated baboons, *J. Clin. Invest.*, 81, 951, 1988.

58. Strauss, L., Rowley, S., La Russa, V., Sharkis, S., Stuart, R., and Civin, C., Antigenic analysis of hematopoiesis. V. Characterization of My-10 antigen expression by normal lymphohematopoietic progenitor cells, *Exp. Hematol.*, 14, 878, 1986.

59. Civin, C., Trischman, T., Fackler, M., et al., Report on the CD34 cluster workshop, in *Leukocyte Typing IV, White Cell Differentiation Antigens*, Knapp, W., Dorken, B., Gilks, W., Eds., Oxford University Press, New York, 1989, 818.

60. Andrews, R., Singer, J., and Bernstein, I., Monoclonal antibody 12-8 recognizes a 115-kd molecule present on both unipotent and multipotent hematopoietic colony-forming cells and their precursors, *Blood*, 67, 842, 1986.

61. Civin, C., Trishman, T., and Fackler, M., et al., Report on CD34 cluster workshop. in *Leukocyte Typing IV. White Cell Differentiation Antigens*, Knapp, W., Dorken, B., Gilks, W., Eds., Oxford University Press, New York, 1989, 818.

62. Serke, S., Sauberlich, S., and Huhn, D., Multiparameter flowcytometrical quantitation of circulating CD34⁺-cells: correlation to the quantitation of circulating haemopoietic progenitor cells by *in vitro* colony-assay, *Br. J. Haematol.*, 77, 453, 1991.

63. Civin, C., Strauss, L., Brovall, C., Fackler, M., Schwartz, J., and Shaper, J., Antigenic analysis of hematopoiesis. Ill. A hematopoietic progenitor cell surface antigen defined by a monoclonal antibody raised against KG-la cells, *J. Immunol.*, 133, 157, 1984.

64. Bender, J., Unverzagt, K., Walker, D., et al., Identification and comparison of CD34-positive cells and their subpopulations from normal peripheral blood and bone marrow using multicolor flow cytometry, *Blood*, 77, 2591, 1991.

65. Simmons, D., Satterthwaite, A., Tenen, D., and Seed, B., Molecular cloning of a CDNA encoding CD34, a sialomucin of human hematopoietic stem cells, *J. Immunol.*, 148, 267, 1992.

66. Silvestri, F., Banavali, S., Baccarani, M., and Preisler, H., The CD34 hemopoietic progenitor cell associated antigen: biology and clinical applications, *Haematologica*, 77, 265, 1992.

67. Greaves, M., Brown, J., Molgaard, H., et al., Molecular features of CD34: A hemopoietic progenitor cell-associated molecule, *Leukemia*, 6 (Suppl. 1), 31, 1992.

68. Baumhueter, S., Singer, M., Henzel, W., et al., Binding of L-selectin to the vascular sialomucin CD34, *Science*, 262, 436, 1993.

69. Terstappen, L., Huang, S., Safford, M., Lansdorp, P., and Loken, M., Sequential generations of hematopoietic colonies derived from single nonlineage-committed CD34⁺CD38- progenitor cells, *Blood*, 77, 1218, 1991.

70. Huang, S. and Terstappen, L., Formation of haematopoietic microenvironment and haematopoietic stem cells from single human bone marrow stem cells, *Nature*, 360, 745, 1992.

71. Srour, E., Brandt, J., Leemhuis, T., Ballas, C., and Hoffman, R., Relationship between cytokine-dependent cell cycle progression and MHC class 11 antigen expression by human CD34+ HLA-DR- bone marrow cells, *J. Immunol.*, 148, 815, 1992.

72. Loken, M., Shah, V., Dattilo, K., and Civin, C., Flow cytometric analysis of human bone marrow: I. Normal erythroid development, *Blood*, 69, 255, 1987.

73. Loken, M., Shah, V., Dattilio, K., and Civin, C., Flow cytometric analysis of human bone marrow. II. Normal B lymphocyte development, *Blood*, 70, 1316, 1987.

74. Tjonnfjord, G., Veiby, O., Steen, R., and Egeland, T., T lymphocyte differentiation *in vitro* from adult human prethymic CD34+ bone marrow cells, *J. Exp. Med.*, 177, 1531, 1993.

75. Debili, N., Issaad, C., Masse, J.-M., et al., Expression of CD34 and platelet glycoproteins during human megakaryocytic differentiation, *Blood*, 80, 3022, 1992.

76. Kirshenbaum, A., Kessler, S., Goff, J., and Metcalfe, D., Demonstration of the origin of human mast cells from CD34+ bone marrow progenitor cells, *J. Immunol.*, 146, 1410, 1991.

77. Miller, J., Verfaillie, C., and McGlave, P., The generation of human natural killer cells from CD34+/DR- primitive progenitors in longterm bone marrow culture, *Blood*, 80, 2182, 1992.

78. Kansas, G., Muirhead, M., and Dailey, M., Expression of the CD11/CD18, leukocyte adhesion molecule 1, and CD44 adhesion molecules during normal myeloid and erythroid differentiation in humans, *Blood*, 76, 2483, 1990.

79. Gunji, Y., Nakamura, M., Hagiwara, K., et al. Expression and function of adhesion molecules on human hematopoietic stem cells: CD34+LFA1- cells are more primitive than CD34+LFA-l+ cells, *Blood*, 80, 429, 1992.

80. Lansdorp, P., Sutherland, H., and Eaves, C., Selective expression of CD45 isoforms on functional subpopulations of CD34+ hematopoietic cells from human bone marrow, *J. Exp. Med.*, 172, 363, 1990.

81. Fritsch, G., Buchinger, D., Fink, F., et al., Rapid discrimination of early CD34+ myeloid progenitors using CD45-RA analysis, *Blood*, 81, 2301, 1993.

82. Craig, W., Kay, R., Cutler, R., and Lansdorp, P., Expression of Thy-1 on human hematopoietic progenitor cells, *J. Exp. Med.*, 177, 1331, 1993.

83. Baum, C., Weissman, I., Tsukamoto, A., Buckle, A.-M., and Peault, B., Isolation of a candidate human hematopoietic stem-cell population, *Proc. Natl. Acad. Sci. U.S.A.*, 89, 2804, 1992.

84. Udomsakdi, C., Eaves, C., Sutherland, H., and Lansdorp, P., Separation of functionally distinct subpopulations of primitive human hematopoietic cells using rhodamine-123, *Exp. Hematol.*, 19, 338, 1991.

85. Briddell, R., Broudy, V., Bruno, E., Brandt, J., Srour, E., and Hoffman, R., Further phenotypic characterization and isolation of human hematopoietic progenitor cells using a monoclonal antibody to the ckit receptor, *Blood*, 79, 3159, 1992.

86. Terstappen, L., Buescher, S., Nguyen, M., and Reading, C., Differentiation and maturation of growth factor expanded human hematopoietic progenitors assessed by multidimensional flow cytometry, *Leukemia*, 6, 1001, 1992.

87. Bernstein, I., Andrews, R., and Zsebo, K., Recombinant human stem cell factor enhances the formation of colonies by CD34+ and CD34+lin-cells, and the generation of colony-forming cell progeny from CD34+lin- cells cultured with interleukin-3, granulocyte colony stimulating factor, or granulocyte-macrophage colony-stimulating factor, *Blood*, 77, 2316, 1991.

88. Raymaker, R., Viewinden, G., Pennings, A., Dolstra, H., and DeWitte, T., Phenotypic make-up of myeloid, erythroid and mixed progenitor cells. Analysis by single cell sorting and cloning from CD34+ bone marrow cells, *Blood*, 82 (Suppl. 1), 12a, 1993.

89. Pincus, S., Nimgaonkar, M., Roscoe, R., Patel, A., Ball, E., and Winkelstein, A., A comparative study of blood and marrow derived CD34+ cells: subset analysis reveals differences in the frequencies of primitive hematopoietic stem cells, *Blood*, 82 (Suppl. 1), 12a, 1993.

90. Terstappen, L., Huang, S., and Picker, L., Flow cytometric assessment of human T-cell differentiation in thymus and bone marrow, *Blood*, 79, 666, 1992.

91. Schmitt, C., Eaves, C., and Lansdorp, P., Expression of CD34 on human B cell precursors, *Clin. Exp. Immunol.*, 85, 168, 1991.

92. Grumayer, E., Griesinger, F., Hummel, D., Brunning, R., and Kersey, J., Identification of novel B-lineage cells in human fetal bone marrow that coexpress CD7, *Blood*, 77, 64, 1991.

93. Panzer-Grumayer, E., Panzer, S., Wolf, M., Majdic, O., Haas, O., and Kersey, J., Characterization of CD7+CD19+ lymphoid cells after Epstein-Barr virus transformation, *J. Immunol.*, 151, 92, 1993.

94. Serke, S., Sauberlich, S., Abe, Y., and Huhn, D., Analysis of CD34-positive hemopoietic progenitor cells from normal human adult peripheral blood: flow-cytometrical studies and *in vitro* colony (CFU-GM, BFU-E) assays, *Ann. Hematol.*, 62, 45, 1991.

95. Siena, S., Bregni, M., and Brando, B., et al., Flow cytometry for clinical estimation of circulating hematopoietic progenitors for autologous transplantation in cancer patients, *Blood*, 77, 400, 1991.

96. lkematsu, W., Teshima, T., Kondo, S., et al., Circulating CD34+ hematopoietic progenitors in the harvesting peripheral blood stem cells; enhancement by recombinant human granulocyte colonystimulating factor, *Biotherapy*, 5, 131, 1992.

97. Wunder, E., Sovalat, H., Fritsch, G., Silvestri, F., Henon, P., and Serke, S., Report on the European workshop on peripheral blood stem cell determination and standardization — Mulhouse, France, February 6–9 and 14–15, 1992, *J. Hematother.*, 1, 131, 1992.

98. Roscoe, R., Rybka, W., Winkelstein, A., Houston, A., and Kiss, J., Enumeration of CD34+ hematopoietic stem cells for reconstitution following myeloablative therapy, *Cytometry*, 16, 74, 1994.

99. Egeland, T., Steen, R., Quarsten, H., Gaudernack, G., Yang, Y.-C., and Thorsby, E., Myeloid differentiation of purified CD34+ cells after stimulation with recombinant human granulocyte-monocyte colony stimulating factor (CSF), granulocyte-CSF, monocyte-CSF, and interleukin-3, *Blood*, 78, 3192, 1991.

100. Smeland, A., Funderud, S., Kvalheim, G., et al., Isolation and characterization of human hematopoietic progenitor cells: an effective method for positive selection of CD34+ cells. *Leukemia*, 6, 845, 1992.

101. Campana, D., Janossy, G., Bofill, M., et al., Human B cell development. I. Phenotypic differences of B lymphocytes in the bone marrow and peripheral lymphoid tissue, *J. Immunol.*, 134, 1524, 1985.

102. Janossy, G., Coustan-Smith, E., and Campana, D., The reliability of cytoplasmic CD3 and CD22 antigen expression in the immunodiagnosis of acute leukemia: a study of 500 cases, *Leukemia*, 3, 170, 1989.

103. Koehler, M., Behm, F., Hancock, M., and Pui, C.-H., Expression of activation antigens CD38 and CD71 is not clinically important in childhood acute lymphoblastic leukemia, *Leukemia*, 7, 41, 1993.

104. Harada, H., Kawano, M., and Huang, N., et al. Phenotypic difference of normal plasma cells from mature myeloma cells, *Blood*, 81, 2658, 1993.

105. Barcena, A., Muench, M., Galy, A., et al. Phenotypic and functional analysis of T-cell precursors in the human fetal liver and thymus: CD7 expression in the early stages of T- and myeloid-cell development, *Blood*, 82, 3401, 1993.

106. Galy, A., Verma, S., Barcena, A., and Spits, H., Precursors of CD3+CD4+CD8+ cells in the human thymus are defined by expression of CD34. Delineation of early events in human thymic development, *J. Exp. Med.*, 178, 391, 1993.

107. Cohen, J., Programmed cell death in the immune system, *Adv. Immunol.*, 50, 55, 1991.

108. Sanchez, M., Spits, H., Lanier, L., and Phillips, J., Human natural killer cell committed thymocytes and their relation to the T cell lineage, *J. Exp. Med.*, 178, 1857, 1993.

109. Lanier, L., Spits, H., and Phillips, J., The developmental relationship between NK and T cells, *Immunol. Today*, 13, 392, 1992.

110. Miller, J., Verfaille, C., and Philip, M., The generation of human natural killer cells from CD34+/DR- primitive progenitors in long-term marrow culture, *Blood*, 80, 2182, 199.

111. Ziegler-Heitbrock, H., and Ulevitch, R., CD14: Cell surface receptor and differentiation marker, *Immunol. Today*, 14, 121, 1993.

112. CDC, 1993 Revised classification system for HIV infection and expanded surveillance case definition among adolescents and adults, *Morbid. Mortal. Weekly Rep.*, 41 RR-17, 1, 1993.

113. Pantaleo, G., Graziosi, C., and Fauci, A., The immunopathogenesis of human immunodeficiency virus infection, *N. Engl. J. Med.*, 328, 327, 1993.

114. Margolick, J.B., Muñoz, A., Donnenberg, A.D., Park, L.P., Galai, N., Giorgi, J.V., O'Gorman, M., and Ferbas, J., for the multicenter AIDS cohort study. Failure of T-cell homeostasis preceding AIDS in HIV-1 infection, *Nature Medicine*, 7, 674, 1995.

115. Patterson, B.K., Goolsby, C., Hodara, V., Lohman, K.L., and Wolinsky, S.M., Detection of CD4+ T cells harboring human immunodeficiency virus type 1 DNA by flow cytometry using simultaneous immunophenotyping and PCR-driven in situ hybridization: evidence of epitope masking of the CD4 cell surface molecule in vivo, *J. Virol.*, 69(7), 4316, 1995.

116. Muro-Cacho, C.A., Pantaleo, G., and Fauci, A.S., Analysis of apoptosis in lymph nodes of HIV- infected persons. Intensity of apoptosis correlates with the general state of activation of the lymphoid tissue and not with stage of disease or viral burden, *J. Immunol.*, 154(10), 5555, 1995.

117. Donnenberg, A.D., Margolick, J.B., Beltz, L.A., Donnenberg, V.S. and Rinaldo, C.R., Apoptosis and lymphopoiesis in bone marrow transplantation (BMT) and HIV disease, *Res. Immunol.*, 146, 11, 1995.

118. Volberding, P., Lagakos, S., Koch, M., et al., Zidovudine in asymptomatic human Immunodeficiency virus infection: a controlled trial in persons with fewer than 500 CD4-positive cells per cubic millimeter, *N. Engl. J. Med.*, 322, 941, 1990.

119. Aboulker, J.-P. and Swart, A., Preliminary analysis of the Concorde trial, *Lancet*, 341, 889, 1993.

120. Fischl, M., Richman, D., Grieco, M., et al., The efficacy of azidothymidine (AZT) in the treatment of patients with AIDS and AIDS-related complex: a double-blind, placebo-controlled trial, *N. Engl. J. Med.*, 317, 185, 1987.

121. Bartlett, J., Zidovudine now or later?, *N. Engl. J. Med.*, 329, 351, 1993.

122. CDC, 1994 Revised guidelines for the performance of CD4+ T-cell determinations in persons with human immunodeficiency, M.M.W.R., 44 RR-3, 1, 1994.

123. Masur, H., Prevention and treatment of pneumocystis pneumonia, *N. Engl. J. Med.*, 327, 1853, 1992.

124. Giorgi, J., Nishanian, P., Schmid, I., Hultin, L., Cheng, H., and Detels, R., Selective alterations in immunoregulatory lymphocyte subsets in early HIV (human T-lymphotropic virus type II/lymphadenopathyassociated virus) infection, *J. Clin. Immunol.*, 7, 140, 1987.

125. Donnenberg, A.D., Margolick, J.B. and Donnenberg, V.S., Lymphopoiesis, apoptosis and immune amnesia, *Ann. N.Y. Acad. Sci.*, 770, 213, 1996.

126. Winkelstein, A., Kingsley, L., Klein, R., et al., Defective T-cell colony formation and IL-2 receptor expression at all stages of HIV infection, *Clin. Exp. Immunol.*, 71, 417, 1988.

127. Winkelstein, A., Kingsley, L., Weaver, L., and Machen, L., Defective T cell colony formation and IL-2 receptor expression in HIV-infected homosexuals: relationship between functional abnormalities and CD4 cell numbers, *J. Acq. Immune Def. Synd.*, 2, 353, 1989.

128. Walker, C., Moody, D., Stites, D., and Levy, J., CD8+ lymphocytes can control HIV infection *in vitro* by suppressing virus replication, *Science*, 234, 1563, 1986.

129. Walker, C., Moody, D., Stites, D., and Levy, J., CD8+ T-lymphocyte control of HIV replication in cultured CD4+ cells varies among infected individuals, *Cell. Immunol.*, 119, 470, 1989.

130. Walker, B. and Plata, F., Cytotoxic T lymphocytes against HIV, *AIDS*, 4, 177, 1990.

131. Gupta, S., Abnormality of Leu 2+7+ cells in acquired immune deficiency syndrome (AIDS), AIDS-related complex, and asymptomatic homosexuals, *J. Clin. Immunol.*, 6, 502, 1986.

132. Ziegler-Heitbrock, H., Stachel, D., Schlunk, T., et al., Class II (DR) antigen expression on CD8+ lymphocyte subsets in acquired immune deficiency syndrome (AIDS), *J. Clin. Immunol.*, 8, 473, 1988.

133. Giorgi, J., Liu, Z., Hultin, L., Cumberland, W., Hennessey, K., and Detels, R., Elevated levels of CD38+ CD8+ T cells in HIV infection add to the prognostic value of low CD4+ T cell levels: results of 6 years of follow-up, *J. Acq. Immune Def. Synd.*, 6, 904, 1993.

134. Stites, D., Moss, A., Bacchetti, P., et al., Lymphocyte subset analysis to predict progression to AIDS in a cohort of homosexual men in San Francisco, *Clin. Immunol. Immunopathol.*, 52, 96, 1989.

135. Giorgi, J., Fahey, J., and Smith, D., Early effects of HIV on CD4 lymphocytes *in vivo*, *J. Immunol.*, 138, 3725, 1987.

136. Prince, H., Kreiss, J., and Kasper, C., Distinctive lymphocyte subpopulation abnormalities in patients with congenital coagulation disorders who exhibit lymph node enlargement, *Blood*, 66, 64, 1985.

137. Ziegler-Heitbrock, H., Schramm, W., and Stachel, D., Expansion of a minor subpopulation of peripheral blood lymphocytes CD8+/Leu7+ in patients with hemophilia, *Clin. Exp. Immunol.*, 61, 633, 1985.

138. Lewis, D., Puck, J., Babcock, G., and Rich, R., Disproportionate expansion of a minor T cell subset in patients with lymphadenopathy syndrome and acquired immunodeficiency syndrome, *J. Infect. Dis.*, 151, 555, 1985.

139. CDC. Unexplained CD4+ T-lymphocyte depletion in persons without evident HIV infection — United States, *M.M.W.R.* 41, 541, 1992.

140. Fauci, A., CD4+ T-lymphocytopenia without HIV infection — no lights, no camera, just facts, *N. Engl. J. Med.*, 328, 429, 1993.

141. Smith, D., Neal, J., and Homberg, S., Centers for Disease Control Idiopathic CD4+ T-lymphopenia Task Force, Unexplained opportunistic infections and CD4+ T-lymphocytopenia without HIV infection — An investigation of cases in the United States. *N. Engl. J. Med.*, 328, 373, 1993.

142. Ho, D., Cao, Y., Zhu, T., et al., Idiopathic CD4+ T-lymphocytopenia Immunodeficiency without evidence of HIV infection, *N. Engl. J. Med.*, 328, 380, 1993.

143. Spira, T., Jones, B., Nicholson, J., et al., Idiopathic CD4+ T lymphocytopenia — an analysis of five patients with unexplained opportunistic infections, *N. Engl. J. Med.*, 328, 386, 1993.

144. Duncan, R., von Reyn, F., Alliegro, G., Toossi, Z., Sugar, A., and Levitz, S., Idiopathic CD4+ T- lymphocytopenia — four patients with opportunistic infections and no evidence of HIV infection, *N. Engl. J. Med.*, 328, 393, 1993.

145. Bennett, J., Catovsky, D., Daniel, M., et al., Proposals for the classification of the acute leukemias, *Br. J. Haematol.*, 33, 451, 1976.
146. Bennett, J., Catovsky, D., Daniel, M., et al., Proposed revised criteria for the classification of acute myeloid leukemia, *Ann. Intern. Med.*, 103, 626, 1985.
147. Bennett, J., Catovsky, D., Daniel, M.-T., et al., Criteria for the diagnosis of acute leukemia of megakaryocytic lineage (M7), *Ann. Intern. Med.*, 103, 460, 1985.
148. Bennett, J., Catovsky, D., Daniel, M.-T., et al., Proposal for the recognition of minimally differentiated acute myeloid leukaemia (AML-MO), *Br. J. Haematol.*, 78, 325, 1991.
149. Hirsch-Ginsberg, C., Huh. Y., Kagan. J., Liang. J., and Stass, S., Advances in the diagnosis of acute leukemia, *Hematol./Oncol. Clinics N.A.*, 7, 146, 1993.
150. Browman, G., Neame, P., and Soamboonsrup, P., The contribution of cytochemistry and immunophenotyping to the reproducibility of the FAB classification in acute leukemia, *Blood*, 68, 900, 1986.
151. Vaickus, L., Ball, E., and Foon, K., Immune markers in hematologic malignancies, *Crit. Rev. Oncol./Hematol.*, 11, 267, 1991.
152. Catovsky, D. and Matutes, E., The classification of acute leukemia, *Leukemia*, 6(Suppl 2), 1, 1992.
153. Thiel, E., Kranz, B., and Raghavachar, A., et al., Prethymic phenotype and genotype of pre-T (CD7+/ER-)-cell leukemia and its clinical significance within adult lymphoblastic leukemia, *Blood*, 73, 1247, 1989.
154. Pui, C.-H., Rivera, G., Hancock, M., et al., Clinical significance of CD10 expression in childhood acute lymphoblastic leukemia, *Leukemia*, 7, 35, 1993.
155. Nadler, L., Korsmeyer, S., Anderson, K., et al., B cell origin of non-T cell acute lymphoblastic leukemia. A model for discrete stages of neoplastic and normal pre-B cell differentiation, *J. Clin. Invest.*, 74, 332, 1984.
156. Pui, C.-H., Hancock, M., Head, D., et al., Clinical significance of CD34 expression in childhood acute lymphoblastic leukemia, *Blood*, 82, 889, 1993.
157. Reinherz, E. and Schlossman, S., The differentiation and function of human T lymphocytes, *Cell*, 19, 821, 1980.
158. Reinherz, E., Kung, P., Goldstein, G., Levey, R., and Schlossman, S., Discrete stages of human intrathymic differentiation: Analysis of normal thymocytes and leukemic lymphoblasts of T cell lineage, *Proc. Natl. Acad. Sci. U.S.A.*, 77, 1588, 1980.
159. Crist, W., Shuster, J., Falletta, J., et al., Clinical features and outcome in childhood T-cell leukemia-lymphoma according to stage of thymocyte differentiation: a pediatric oncology group study, *Blood*, 72, 1891, 1988.
160. Freedman, A. and Nadler, L., Cell surface markers in hematologic malignancies, *Semin. Oncol.*, 14, 193, 1987.
161. Garand, R., Voisin, S., Papin, S., et al., Characteristics of pro-T ALL subgroups: comparison with late T-ALL, *Leukemia*, 7, 161, 1992.
162. Drexler, H., Classification of acute myeloid leukemias — a comparison of FAB and immunophenotyping, *Leukemia*, 1, 697, 1987.
163. Geller, R., Zahurak, M., Hurwitz, C., et al., Prognostic importance of immunophenotyping in adults with acute myelocytic leukaemia: the significance of the stem-cell glycoprotein CD34 (My10), *Br. J. Haematol.*, 76, 340, 1990.
164. Adriaansen, H., de Boekhorst, P., van der Schoot, C., Ruud Delwel, H., and van Dongen, J., Acute myeloid leukemia M4 with bone marrow eosinophilia (M4Eo) and Inv(16)(p13q22) exhibits a specific immunophenotype with CD2 expression, *Blood*, 81, 3043, 1993.
165. McCulloch, E., Stem cells in normal and leukemic hemopoiesis (Henry Stratton Lecture, 1982), *Blood*, 62, 1, 1983.
166. Greaves, M., Chan, L., Furley, A., Watt, S., and Molgaard, H., Lineage promiscuity in hemopoietic differentiation and leukemia, *Blood*, 67, 1, 1986.

167. Drexler, H., Thiel, E., and Ludwig, W.-D., Review of the incidence and clinical relevance of myeloid antigen-positive acute lymphoblastic leukemia, *Leukemia*, 5, 637, 1991.

168. Sobol, R., Mick, R., Royston, I., et al., Clinical importance of myeloid antigen expression in adult acute lymphoblastic leukemia, *N. Engl. J. Med.*, 316, 1111, 1987.

169. Drexler, H., Thiel, E., and Ludwig, W.-D., Acute myeloid leukemias expressing lymphoid-associated antigens: diagnostic incidence and prognostic significance, *Leukemia*, 7, 489, 1993.

170. Terstappen, L., Safford, M., Konemann, S., et al., Flow cytometric characterization of acute myeloid leukemia. II. Phenotypic heterogeneity at diagnosis, *Leukemia*, 6, 70, 1992.

171. Kondo. S., Okamura, S., Harada, N., et al., CD7-positive acute myeloid leukemia: further evidence of cellular immaturity, *J. Cancer Res. Clin. Oncol.*, 118, 386, 1992.

172. Jensen, A., Hokland, M., Jorgensen, H., Justesen, J., Ellegaard, J., and Hokland, P., Solitary expression of CD7 among T-cell antigens in acute myeloid leukemia: identification of a group of patients with similar T-cell receptor beta and delta rearrangements and course of disease suggestive of poor prognosis, *Blood*, 78, 1292, 1991.

173. Ball, E., Davis, R., and Griffin, J., et al., Prognostic value of lymphocyte surface markers in acute myeloid leukemia, *Blood*, 77, 2242, 1991.

174. van Dongen, J., Breit, T., Adriaansen, H., Beishuizen, A., and Hooijkaas, H., Detection of minimal residual disease in acute leukemia by immunological marker analysis and polymerase chain reaction, *Leukemia*, 6(Suppl 1), 47, 1992.

175. Drach, J., Drach, D., Glassi, H., Gattringer, C., and Huber, H., Flow cytometric determination of atypical antigen expression in acute leukemia, *Cytometry*, 13, 893, 1992.

176. Gerhartz, H. and Schmetzer, H., Detection of minimal residual disease in acute myeloid leukemia, *Leukemia*, 4, 508, 1990.

177. Nowell, P. and Hungerford, D., Chromosome studies on normal and leukemia human leukocytes, *J. Natl. Cancer Inst.*, 25, 85, 1960.

178. Rowley, J., Identification of the constant chromosome regions involved in human hematologic malignant disease, *Science*, 216, 749, 1982.

179. Konopka, J. and Witte, O., Activation of the abi oncogene in murine and human leukemias, *Biochim. Biophys. Acta*, 823, 1, 1985.

180. Smith, M., Mohamed, A., and Karanes, C., CD7+ TdT+ chronic myelogenous leukemia blast crisis with null genotype, *Leukemia*, 7, 177, 1993.

181. Bettelheim, P., Lutz, D., Majdic, O., et al., Cell lineage heterogeneity in blast crisis of chronic myeloid leukemia, *Br. J. Haematol.*, 59, 395, 1985.

182. Martin, P., Najfield, V., Hansen, J., Penfold, G., Jacobson, R., and Fialkow, P., Involvement of the B- lymphoid system in chronic myelogenous leukemia, *Nature*, 287, 49, 1980.

183. Fauser, A., Kanz, L., Bross, K., and Lohr, W., T-cells and probably B-cells arise from the malignant clone in chronic myelogenous leukemia, *J. Clin. Invest.*, 73, 1080, 1985.

184. Janossy, G., Greaves, M., Revesz, T., et al., Blast crisis of chronic myeloid leukemia (CML). II Cell surface marker analysis of "lymphoid' and myeloid cases, *Br. J. Haematol.*, 34, 179, 1976.

185. LeBien, T., Hozier, J., Minowada, J., and Kersey, J., Origin of chronic myelocytic leukemia in a precursor of pre-B-lymphocytes, *N. Engl. J. Med.*, 301, 144, 1979.

186. Greaves, M., Verbi, W., Reeves, B., et al., "Pre-B" Phenotypes in blast crisis on Phl positive CML. Evidence for a pluripotent stem cell "target," *Leuk. Res.*, 3, 181, 1979.

187. Bakshi, A., Minowada, J., Arnold, A., et al., Lymphoid blast crisis of chronic myelogenous leukemia represent stages in the development of B-cell precursors, *N. Engl. J. Med.*, 309, 826, 1983.

188. Soda, H., Kuriyama, K., Tomonaga, M., et al., Lymphoid crisis with T cell pheno-type in a patient with Philadelphia chromosome negative chronic myeloid leuke-mia, *Br. J. Haematol.*, 59, 671, 1985

189. Griffin, J., Tantravahi, R., Canellos, G., et al., T-cell surface antigen in a patient with blast crisis of chronic myeloid leukemia, *Blood*, 61, 640, 1983;.

190. Hernandez, P., Carnot, J., and Cruz, C., Chronic myeloid leukaemia blast crisis with T-cell features, *Br. J. Haematol.*, 51, 175, 1982.

191. Lum, L., The kinetics of immune reconstitution after human marrow transplan-tation, *Blood*, 69, 369, 1987.

192. Witherspoon, R., Lum, L., and Storb, R., Immunologic reconstitution after human marrow grafting, *Sem. Hematol.*, 21, 2, 1984.

193. Fox, R., McMillan, R., Spruce, W., Tani, P., and Mason, D., Analysis of T lympho-cytes after bone marrow transplantation using monoclonal antibodies, *Blood*, 60, 578, 1982.

194. Leroy, E., Calvo, C., Divine, M., et al., Persistence of T8+/HNK-l+ suppressor lymphocytes in the blood of long-term surviving patients after allogeneic bone marrow transplantation, *J. Immunol.*, 137, 2180, 1986.

195. lzquierdo, M., Balboa, M., Fernandez-Ranada, J., et al., Relation between the in-crease of circulating CD3+CD57+ lymphocytes and T cell dysfunction in recipients of bone marrow transplantation, *J. Immunol.*, 82, 145, 1990.

196. Aotsuka, N., Asai, T., Oh, H., Yoshida, S., Itoh, K., and Sato, T., Lymphocyte subset reconstitution following human allogeneic bone marrow transplantation: differ-ences between engrafted patients and graft failure patients, *Bone Marrow Trans-plant*, 8, 345, 1991.

197. Clement, L., Grossi, C., and Gartland, G., Morphologic and phenotypic features of the subpopulation of Leu-2+ that suppresses B cell differentiation, *J. Immunol.*, 133, 2461 1984.

198. Yabe, H., Yabe, M., Kato, S., Kimura, M., and Iwaka, K., Increased numbers of CD8+CD11+,CD8+CD11-, and CD8+Leu7+ cells in patients with chronic graft-ver-sus-host disease after allogeneic bone marrow transplantation, *Bone Marrow Trans-plant.*, 5, 295, 1990.

199. Bosserman, L., Murray, C., Takvorian, T., et al., Mechanism of graft failure in HLA-matched and HLA-mismatched bone marrow transplant recipients, *Bone Marrow Transplant.*, 4, 239, 1989.

200. Bordignon, L., Keever, C., Small, T., et al., Graft failure after T-cell depleted human leukocyte antigen identical marrow transplants for leukemia: II. *In vitro* analyses of host effector mechanisms, *Blood*, 74, 2237, 1989.

201. Voltarelli, J., Przepiorka, D., Shankar, P., Kopecky, K., Martin, P., and Torok-Storb, B., CD8+/DR+/CD25- T-lymphocytes associated with graft failure, *Bone Marrow Transplant.*, 4, 647, 1989.

202. Vinci, G., Vernant, J., Nakazawa, M., et al., *In vitro* inhibition of normal human hematopoiesis by marrow CD3+, CD8+, HLA-DR+, HNK1+ lymphocytes, *Blood*, 72, 1616, 1988.

203. Nakano, M., Kuge, S., Kuwabara, S., et al., The basic study on *kappalambda* imaging delta-curve for the detection of monoclonal B-cell population in the peripheral blood, *Blood*, 72, 1461, 1988.

204. Foon, K. and Piro, L., Lymphocytic leukemias: new insights into biology and therapy, *Leukemia*, 6(Suppl. 4), 26, 1992.

205. Foon, K. and Gale, R., Is there a T-cell form of chronic lymphocytic leukemia?, *Leukemia*, 6, 867, 1992.

206. Matutes, E., Brito-Babapulle, V., Worner, I., Sainati, L., Foroni, L., and Catovsky, D., T-cell chronic lymphocytic leukaemia: the spectrum of mature T-cell disorders, *Nouv. Rev. Fr. Hematol.*, 30, 347, 1988.

207. Winkelstein, A. and Jordan, P., Immune deficiencies in chronic lymphocytic leukemia and multiple myeloma. in *IVIG Therapy Today,* Ballow M, Ed., Humana Press, Totowa, NJ, 1992, 39.

208. Chapel, H. and Bunch, C., Mechanisms of infection in chronic lymphocytic leukemia, *Semin. Hematol.,* 24, 291, 1987.

209. Kipps, T. and Carson, D., Autoantibodies in chronic lymphocytic leukemia and related systemic autoimmune diseases, *Blood,* 81, 2475, 1993.

210. Hamblin, T., Oscier, D., and Young, B., Autoimmunity in chronic lymphocytic leukemia, *J. Clin. Pathol.,* 39, 713, 1986.

211. Baldini, L., Cro, L., Calori, R., Nobili, L., Silvestris, I., and Maiolo, A.T., Differential expression of very late activation antigen-3 (VLA-3)/VLA-4 in B-cell non-Hodgkin lymphoma and B-cell chronic lymphocytic leukemia, *Blood,* 79(10), 2688, 1992.

212. Dighiero, G., Travade, P., Chevret, S., Fenaux, P., Chastang, C., and Binet, J.L., B-cell chronic lymphocytic leukemia: present status and future directions. French Cooperative Group on CLL, *Blood,* 78(8), 1901, 1991.

213. Baldini, L., Cro, L., Cortelezzi, A., Calori, R., Nobili, L., Maiolo, A.T., and Polli, E.E., Immunophenotypes in "classical" B-cell chronic lymphocytic leukemia. Correlation with normal cellular counterpart and clinical findings, *Cancer,* 66(8), 1738, 1990.

214. Schena, M., Larsson, L.G., Gottardi, D., Gaidano, G., Carlsson, M., Nilsson, K., and Caligaris-Cappio, F., Growth- and differentiation-associated expression of bcl-2 in B-chronic Lymphocytic leukemia cells, *Blood,* 79(11), 2981, 1992.

215. Stall, A.M., Adams, S., Herzenberg, L.A., and Kantor, A.B., Characteristics and development of the murine B-1b Ly-1 B sister cell population, *Ann. N.Y. Acad. Sci.,* 651, 33, 1992.

216. Shirai, T., Okada, T., and Hirose, S., Genetic regulation of CD5$^+$ B cells in autoimmune disease and in chronic lymphocytic leukemia, *Ann. N.Y. Acad. Sci.,* 651, 509, 1992.

217. Fernandez, L.A., MacSween, J.M., and Robson, D.A., Feedback suppression of normal and leukemic B cell colony growth by CD5$^+$ B cells, *Ann. N.Y. Acad. Sci.,* 628, 379, 1991.

218. Vernino, L.A., Pisetsky, D.S., and Lipsky, P.E., Analysis of the expression of CD5 by human B cells and correlation with functional activity, *Cell. Immunol.,* 139(1), 185, 1992.

219. Bofill, M., Janossy, G., Janossa, M., et al., Human B cell development. II. Subpopulations in the human fetus, *J. Immunol.,* 134, 1531, 1985.

220. Antin, J., Emerson, S.G., Martin, P., Gadol, N., and Ault, K., Leu-1$^+$ (CD5$^+$) B cells. A major lymphoid subpopulation in human fetal spleen: phenotypic and functional studies, *J. Immunol.,* 136, 505, 1986.

221. Ault, K., Antin, J., Ginsburg, D., et al., Phenotype of recovering lymphoid cell populations after marrow transplantation, *J. Exp. Med.,* 161, 1483, 1985.

222. Saisano, F., Froland, S., Natvig, J., and Michaelsen, T., Same idiotype of B lymphocyte membrane IgD and IgM. Formal evidence for monoclonality of chronic lymphocytic leukemic cells, *Scand. J. Immunol.,* 3, 841, 1974.

223. Plater-Zyberk, C., Maini, R., Lam, K., Kennedy, T., and Janossy, G., A rheumatoid arthritis B cell subset expresses a phenotype similar to that in chronic lymphocytic leukaemia, *Arthritis Rheum.,* 86, 971, 1985.

224. Hardy, R. and Hayakawa, K., Development and physiology of ly-1 B and its human homologue, leu-1 B, *Immunol. Rev.,* 93, 81, 1986.

225. Farace, F., Orlanducci, F., Dietrich, P.Y., Gaudin, C., Angevin, E., Courtier, M.H., Bayle, C., Hercend, T., and Triebel, F., T cell repertoire in patients with B chronic lymphocytic leukemia. Evidence for multiple *in vivo* T cell clonal expansions, *J. Immunol.,* 153(9), 4281, 1994.

226. Donnenberg, A.D., Donnenberg, V.S., and Meisler, A.I., Activated CD4+ T-cells in RAI stage 0 chronic B-cell lymphocytic leukemia, *Blood*, 84(10), 456a (abstr.), 1994.

227. Decker, T., Flohr, T., Trautmann, P., Aman, M.J., Holter, W., Majdic, O., Huber, C., and Peschel, C., Role of accessory cells in cytokine production by T-Cells in chronic B-cell lymphocytic-leukemia, *Blood*, 86(3), 1115, 1995.

228. Lahat, N., Aghai, E., Maroun, B., Kinarty, A., Quitt, M., and Froom, P., Increased spontaneous secretion of IL-6 from B cells of patients with B chronic lymphatic leukaemia (B-CLL) and autoimmunity, *Clin. Exp. Immunol.*, 85(2), 302, 1991.

229. Orazi, A., Cattoretti, G., Polli, N., Delia, D., and Rilke, F., Distinct morphophenotypic features of chronic B-cell leukaemias identified with CD1c and CD23 antibodies, *Eur. J. Haematol.*, 47, 28, 1991.

230. Newman, R., Peterson, B., Davey, F., et al., Phenotypic markers and BCL-1 gene rearrangement in B-cell chronic lymphocytic leukemia: a cancer and leukemia group B study, *Blood*, 82, 1239, 1993.

231. Mulligan, S. and Catovsky, D., The chronic B-cell leukaemias, *Aust. N.Z. J. Med.*, 23, 42, 1993.

232. Foon, K.A., Thiruvengadam, R., Saven, A., Bernstein, Z.P., and Gale, R.P., Genetic relatedness of lymphoid malignancies. Transformation of chronic lymphocytic leukemia as a model, *Ann. Intern. Med.*, 119(1), 63, 1993.

233. Worman, C., Brooks, D., Hogg, N., Zola, H., Beverley, P., and Cawley, J., The nature of hairy cells — a study with a panel of monoclonal antibodies, *Scand. J. Haematol.*, 30, 223, 1983.

234. Divine, M., Farcet, J., Gourdin, M., et al., Phenotype -study of fresh and cultured hairy cells with the use of immunologic markers and electron microscopy, *Blood*, 64, 547, 1984.

235. Schwarting, R., Stein, H., and Wang, C., The monoclonal antibodies alpha S-HCL1 (alpha Leu-M5) allow the diagnosis of hairy cell leukemia, *Blood*, 65, 974, 1985.

236. Anderson, K., Boyd, A., Fisher, D., et al., Hairy cell leukemia: a tumor of pre-plasma cells, *Blood*, 65, 620, 1985.

237. Korsmeyer, S., Greene, W., Cossman, J., et al., Rearrangement and expression of immunoglobulin genes and expression of Tac antigen in hairy cell leukemia, *Proc. Natl. Acad. Sci. U.S.A.*, 80, 4522, 1983.

238. Robbins, B., Ellison, D., Spinosa, J., et al., Diagnostic application of two-color flow cytometry in 161 cases of hairy cell leukemia, *Blood*, 82, 1277, 1993.

239. Wormsley, S., Baird, S., Gadol, N., Rai, K., and Sobol, R., Characteristics of CD11c+CD5+ chronic B-cell leukemias and the identification of novel peripheral blood B-cell subsets with chronic lymphoid leukemia immunophenotypes, *Blood*, 76, 123, 1990.

240. Anderson, K., Bates, M., Slaughenhoupt, B., Schlossman, S., and Nadler, L., A monoclonal antibody with reactivity restricted to normal and neoplastic plasma cells, *J. Immunol.*, 132, 3172, 1984.

241. Hamilton, M., Ball, J., Bromidge, E., Franklin, I., Surface antigen expression of human neoplastic plasma cells includes molecules associated with lymphocyte recirculation and adhesion, *Br. J. Hematol.*, 78, 60, 1991.

242. Van Camp, B., Durie, B., Spier, C., et al., Plasma cells in multiple myeloma express a natural killer cell-associated antigen: CD56 (NKH1;Leu 19), *Blood*, 76, 377, 1990.

243. Sonneveld, P., Durie, B., Lokhorst, H., Frutiger, Y., Schoester, M., and Vela, E., Analysis of multidrug-resistance (MDR-1) glycoprotein and CD56 expression to separate monoclonal gammopathy from multiple myeloma, *Br. J. Haematol.*, 83, 63, 1993.

244. Reynolds, C. and Foon, K., T gamma-lymphoproliferative disease and related disorders in human and experimental animals: a review of the clinical, cellular, and functional characteristics, *Blood*, 64, 1146, 1984.

245. Loughran, T., Jr., Clonal diseases of large granular lymphocytes, *Blood*, 82, 1, 1993.

246. Oshimi, K., Yamada, O., Kaneko, T., et al., Laboratory findings and clinical courses of 33 patients with granular lymphocyte-proliferative disorders, *Leukemia*, 7, 782, 1993.

247. Hoffman, R., Kopel, S., Hsu, S., Dainiak, N., and Zanjani, E., T cell chronic lymphocytic leukemia: presence in bone marrow and peripheral blood of cells that suppress erythropoiesis *in vitro*, *Blood*, 52, 255, 1978.

248. Nagasawa, T., Abe, T., and Nakagawa, T., Pure red cell aplasia and hypogammaglobulinemia associated with Tr-cell chronic lymphocytic leukemia, *Blood*, 57, 1025, 1981.

249. Linch, D., Cawley, J., Worman, C., et al., Abnormalities of T-cell subsets in patients with neutropenia and an excess of lymphocytes in the bone marrow, *Br. J. Haematol.*, 48, 137, 1981.

250. Barton, J., Prasthofer, E., Egan, M., Heck, J.L.W., Koopman, W., and Grossi, C., Rheumatoid arthritis associated with expanded populations of granular lymphocytes, *Ann. Int. Med.*, 104, 314, 1986.

251. Freimark, B., Lanier, L., Phillips, J., Quertermous, T., and Fox, R., Comparison of T-cell receptor gene rearrangements in patients with large granular T cell leukemia and Felty's syndrome, *J. Immunol.*, 138, 1724, 1987.

252. Loughran, J.T.P., Starkebaum, G., Kidd, P., and Neiman, P., Clonal proliferation of large granular lymphocytes in rheumatoid arthritis, *Arthritis Rheum.*, 31, 31, 1988.

253. Saway, P., Prasthofer, E., and Barton, J., Prevalence of granular lymphocyte proliferation in patients with rheumatoid arthritis and neutropenia, *Am. J. Med.*, 86, 303, 1989.

254. Ahern, M., Roberts-Thomson, P., Bradley, J., Story, C., and Seshadri, P., Phenotypic and genotypic analysis of mononuclear cells from patients with Felty's syndrome, *Ann Rheumatic Dis.*, 49, 103, 1990.

255. Gonzalez-Chambers, R., Przepiorka, D., Winkelstein, A., et al., Lymphocyte subsets associated with T-cell receptor beta-chain gene rearrangement in patients with rheumatoid arthritis and neutropenia, *Arthritis Rheum.*, 35, 516, 1992.

256. Centers for Disease Control and Prevention U.S.P.H.S. Working Group, Guidelines for counseling persons infected with human T-lymphotropic virus type I (HTLV-1) and type II (HTLV-II), *Ann. Intern. Med.*, 118, 448, 1993.

257. Waldmann, T., Greene, W., Sarin, P., et al., Functional and phenotypic comparison of human T-cell leukemia/lymphoma virus positive adult T-cell leukemia with human T-cell leukemia/lymphoma virus negative Sezary leukemia and their distinction using anti-Tac, *J. Clin. Invest.*, 73, 1711, 1984.

258. Morimoto, C., Matsuyama, T., Oshige, C., et al., Functional and phenotypic studies of Japanese adult T-cell leukemia cells, *J. Clin. Invest.*, 75, 836, 1985.

259. Haynes, B., Metzgar, R., Minna, J., and Bunn, P., Phenotypic characterization of cutaneous T-cell lymphoma. *N. Engl. J. Med.*, 304, 1319, 1981.

260. Kung, P., Berger, C., Goldstein, G., LoGerfo, P., and Edelson, R., Cutaneous T-cell lymphoma: characterization by monoclonal antibodies, *Blood*, 57, 261, 1981.

261. Schroff, R., Foon, K., Billing, R., and Fahey, J., Immunologic classification of lymphocytic leukemias based on monoclonal antibody-define cell surface antigens, *Blood*, 59, 207, 1982.

262. Braylan, R. and Benson, N., Flow cytometric analysis of lymphomas, *Arch. Path. Lab. Med.*, 113, 627, 1989.

263. Batata, A. and Shen, B., Diagnostic value of clonality of surface immunoglobulin light and heavy chains in malignant lymphoproliferative disorders, *Am. J. Hematol.*, 43, 265, 1993.

264. De Martini, R., Turner, R., Boone, D., Lukes, R., and Parker, J., Lymphocyte immunophenotyping of B- cell lymphomas: a flow cytometric analysis of neoplastic and nonneoplastic cells in 271 cases, *Clin. Immunol. Immunopath.*, 49, 365, 1988.

265. Slymen, D., Miller, T., Lippman, S., et al., Immunobiologic factors predictive of clinical outcome of diffuse large-cell lymphoma, *J. Clin. Oncol.*, 8, 986, 1990.

266. Schmid, C., Pan, L., Diss, T., and Isaacson, P., Expression of B-cell antigens by Hodgkin's and Reed- Sternberg cells, *Am. J. Pathol.*, 139, 701, 1991.

267. Kadin, M., Muramoto, L., and Said, J., Expression of T-cell antigens on Reed-Sternberg cells in a subset of patients with nodular sclerosing and mixed cellularity Hodgkin's disease, *Am. J. Pathol.*, 130, 345, 1988.

268. Casey, T., Olson, S., Cousar, J., and Collins, R., Immunophenotypes of Reed-Sternberg cells: a study of 19 cases of Hodgkin's disease in plastic-embedded sections, *Blood*, 74, 2624, 1989.

269. Hsu, S., Yang, K., and Jaffe, E., Phenotypic expression of Hodgkin's and Reed-Sternberg cells in Hodgkin's disease, *Am. J. Path.*, 118, 209, 1985.

270. Poppema, S., The nature of the lymphocytes surrounding Reed-Sternberg cells in nodular lymphocyte predominance and in other types of Hodgkin's disease, *Am. J. Pathol.*, 135, 351, 1989.

271. Diehl, V., von Kalle, C., Fonatsch, C., Tesch, H., Juecker, M., and Schaadt, M., The cell of origin in Hodgkin's disease, *Semin. Oncol.*, 17, 660, 1990.

272. Stein, H., Mason, D., Gerdes, J., et al., The expression of the Hodgkin's disease associated antigen Ki-1 in reactive and neoplastic lymphoid tissue: evidence that Reed-Sternberg cells and histiocytic malignancies are derived from activated lymphoid cells, *Blood*, 66, 848, 1985.

273. Delabie, J., Ceuppens, J., Vandenberghe, P., de Boer, M., Coorevits, L., and De Wolf-Peeters, C., The B7/BB1 antigen is expressed by Reed Sternberg Cells of Hodgkin's disease and contributes to the stimulating capacity of Hodgkin's disease derived cell lines, *Blood*, 82, 2845, 1993.

274. Kamel, O., Gelb, A., Shibuya, R., and Warnke, R., Leu 7 (CD57) reactivity distinguishes nodular lymphocyte predominance Hodgkin's disease from nodular sclerosing Hodgkin's disease, T-cell-rich B-cell lymphoma and follicular lymphoma, *Am. J. Pathol.*, 142, 541, 1993.

275. Ellis, P., Hart, D., Colls, B., Nimmo, J., MacDonald, J., Angus H., Hodgkin's cells express a novel pattern of adhesion molecules, *Clin. Exp. Immunol.*, 90, 117, 1992.

Chapter **12**

RELEVANCE OF ANTIBODY SCREENING AND CROSSMATCHING IN SOLID ORGAN TRANSPLANTATION

Andrea A. Zachary and John M. Hart

CONTENTS

0-8493-0134-3/97/$0.00+$.50
© 1997 by CRC Press LLC

I. INTRODUCTION

Early reports correlating a positive crossmatch between recipient serum and donor lymphocytes with hyperacute rejection of transplanted kidneys,[1-3] led to establishing tests of recipient sera as the standard of practice in transplantation. In the U.S., tests for donor-reactive antibody are required by federal regulations.[4] The large body of data accumulated over the past 25 years not only provides insight into the relevance of various antibody characteristics and the utility of various assays, but also elucidates the many unanswered questions and potential avenues of investigation. The first part of this chapter will review some data on antibodies and graft outcome. The second and third sections will discuss the establishment of test protocols and the interpretation of test results.

II. BACKGROUND

The numerous published studies on alloreactive antibodies in transplantation permit few definitive and unqualified statements to be made about the relevance of these antibodies to transplant outcome or the way(s) in which these antibodies should be tested. Areas of controversy include: (1) the level of sensitivity needed for crossmatch tests for renal transplantation; (2) the relevance of B-cell crossmatches; (3) the importance of crossmatch tests for nonrenal transplantation; (4) the relevance of the immunoglobulin class and subclass of donor-reactive antibodies; (5) the significance of historical antibodies — i.e., antibodies present previously, but not at the time of transplantation; (6) the techniques and type of analyses to be performed for serum screening; and (7) the appropriate frequency and timing of serum screening. For any of these controversies, one may find published data to support each of the varying points of view. Further, rarely, if ever, can one find even a single report of a perfect correlation between the presence of donor-reactive antibody and clinical outcome. This apparent ambiguity is due, in large part, to the extensive variability in the studies conducted. Variability may be in the age of the specimen used for the pretransplant crossmatch, whether or not the specificity of donor-reactive antibody was determined and confirmed, whether immunoglobulin class of donor-reactive antibody was identified, the type(s) of cells tested, the techniques used, and the clinical endpoints evaluated. The interpretation of these studies is further complicated by variability in transplantation including the type of organ transplanted, whether the transplant was a primary or a regraft, the degree of HLA mismatch, and the immunosuppression protocol.

Despite the number of variables, when the data from reported studies are considered collectively, a few themes emerge. These are that: (1) HLA-specific antibodies (i.e., specific for donor HLA antigens) that are present in the recipient at the time of transplant or that develop and persist after transplantation are serious risk factors that diminish graft function and graft survival significantly; (2) antibodies specific for HLA class II antigens (HLA-DR and -DQ) are as detrimental as those specific for class I antigens (HLA-A, -B, -C); (3) the degree of risk resulting from HLA-specific antibodies varies among immunoglobulin classes with IgG antibodies representing the most serious risk; (4) HLA-specific antibody appears to be detrimental in transplants of all organ types; and (5) the risk represented by HLA-specific antibodies is ameliorated by the production of anti-idiotypic antibodies specific for the HLA antibodies.

A. Donor Reactive Antibody

Since the early reports of hyperacute rejection of kidneys transplanted in the face of a positive lymphocytotoxicity crossmatch,[1-3] there have been numerous attempts to assess the extent of risk presented by donor-reactive antibody. Some have examined the risk of any lymphocytotoxic antibody present in the recipient, as assessed by reactivity of patients' sera with lymphocytes from a panel of individuals.[5-7] These studies have looked at correlations between graft survival and panel reactive antibody (PRA), expressed as the percentage of the panel with which a serum gives a positive reaction. Mjörnstedt et al.[8] found a 37% decrease in the 1 year survival of renal grafts among patients with PRA>50 compared to those with PRA<10. A similar difference in 5-year survival was found, by others,[9] in heart transplant recipients who had PRA>25 vs. those with PRA ≤10. An increase in the incidence or severity of rejection has also been reported for heart transplant recipients with lymphocytotoxic antibody.[10,11] However, there have been numerous reports of a failure to find differences in graft survival or rejection among patients differentiated by the presence of antibody or PRA value, particularly in heart[12-14] and liver[15,16] transplantation. The presence of lymphocytotoxic antibodies does not guarantee donor-specific reactivity; therefore, it is not surprising that the crossmatch test is a better predictor of graft outcome than is antibody screening.

The report by Patel and Terasaki showed that 80% of kidneys transplanted when the pretransplant crossmatch (XM) was positive would suffer hyperacute rejection. Although these early tests were performed with a technique of rather low sensitivity, they provided a means to prevent most, but not all hyperacute rejections. Subsequently, more sensitive techniques were employed in attempts not only to prevent all hyperacute rejections but also to improve graft survival rates at 1 or more years. Techniques* that have been used include: variations of the lymphocytotoxicity test that incorporate wash steps, change incubation time(s) and/or temperature(s), and/or add an antiglobulin reagent; flow cytometry; and a variety of other methods such as antibody-dependent cellular cytotoxicity and Western blotting. Two of the most sensitive techniques are the antiglobulin-augmented lymphocytotoxicity (AHG)[17] and flow cytometry.[18-20] Studies employing more sensitive techniques have shown, predominantly but not uniformly, that a positive crossmatch predicts poorer graft survival and increased frequency and severity of rejection episodes. Multiple studies in renal transplantation have shown correlations between positive AHG or flow cytometric crossmatches and decreased graft survival at 1 or more years.[21-24] The differences have ranged from as little as 14% (66 vs. 53%)[22] to as much as 46% (77 vs. 31%),[23] with bigger differences occurring in regrafts vs. primary grafts. In some studies,[25-27] the effect of a

---

* *Authors' note.* While the literature is replete with a variety of terms, such as "standard" and "NIH" for the various XM techniques, we have avoided using these terms for a number of reasons. First, even a cursory review of the methods described in published reports will reveal that there is no "standard" technique. Further, the last NIH publication of histocompatibility techniques occurred nearly 20 years ago and has been replaced with more up-to-date manuals by both the American Society for Histocompatibility and Immunogenetics[166] and the South-Eastern Organ Procurement Organization.[167] We have chosen to use more descriptive terms found in the ASHI Laboratory Manual. The interested reader is advised to obtain precise descriptions of the techniques from the methods sections of the publications cited here.

more sensitive crossmatch technique was seen only in regrafts. The benefits of more sensitive crossmatch techniques have also been demonstrated using other clinical criteria. In an early study, Cook et al.[28] showed that flow cytometry vs. the basic XM was a better predictor of early (1 month) graft failure for any renal transplant (33 vs. 8%) but, in particular, the regraft (56 vs. 21%). These findings have been substantiated by others who found three-fold increases in 1-month graft failure[29,30] and fivefold differences in 2-month graft failure[31] in patients with positive vs. negative flow cytometric crossmatch. In other studies, a crossmatch positive only by a more sensitive technique correlated with an increased number of rejection episodes[26,32] or a shorter time to a rejection episode.[33]

Until recently, crossmatches were not routinely performed for transplants of organs other than the kidney because of more severe time constraints. These time constraints are no longer relevant, since improvements in technology now permit reliable testing to be performed on blood samples obtained prior to organ recovery. Data from retrospective and, more recently, prospective studies have shown that positive crossmatches correlate with diminished graft survival and function for all transplanted organs that have been studied, and that more sensitive crossmatch techniques can identify patients at risk better than can techniques of low sensitivity. A correlation between reduced graft survival at 1 or more years and a positive crossmatch has been demonstrated for both heart[11,12,14,34] and liver[16,35-37] transplants. Further, there are data that indicate, for both heart and liver transplants, that a positive crossmatch may predict early rejection,[38-41] increased severity or frequency of rejection episodes,[42,43] and even hyperacute rejection.[44,45] In contrast, some studies have shown no significant benefit from a more sensitive crossmatch in renal transplantation[46,47] or from any crossmatch in heart[9,48] or liver.[15,49-51] transplantation. This apparent conflict in findings may be due, in part, to the failure to take into account the specificity or isotype of the antibody giving a positive reaction or whether the antibody is present at the time of transplant.

The predictive value of crossmatches using B lymphocytes has been equally controversial. Early studies showed that either there was no difference in outcome between patients with a positive vs. a negative B-cell crossmatch[52-54] or that a positive B-cell crossmatch predicted improved graft survival.[55-57] However, with improved test protocols and techniques, there has been an increasing number of reports demonstrating diminished outcome for patients with a positive B-cell crossmatch. Noreen et al.[58] showed a reduction in 1- and 2-year graft survival of 14 to 15% in 728 primary renal transplant patients with a positive B cell crossmatch. Similarly, Russ[59] found that 1-year graft survival in 192 renal transplant patients was 79% for those with a negative B-cell crossmatch, but only 42% for those with a positive B-cell crossmatch.

In an early study, Lazda et al.[60] found that the diminished 1-year graft survival in patients with a positive vs. a negative B-cell crossmatch (40 vs. 56%) was overcome by the use of cyclosporine therapy. However, more recently they[61] have found that positive B-cell crossmatches, performed by flow cytometry, predict a significant reduction in 1-year graft survival (63 vs. ≥90%) when a positive reaction is defined as fluorescence shift of greater than 50 channels compared to when it is less than 50 channels. Bunke et al.[62] found that a positive B-cell crossmatch in heart transplant recipients was associated with early graft loss, death, increased numbers of rejection episodes, and the need for higher levels of immunosuppression.

Among the reports showing a benefit from crossmatch testing, there are no perfect correlations between test results and transplant outcome. That is, not all patients with a positive crossmatch have diminished graft survival or function nor do all patients with diminished graft function or survival have a positive crossmatch. Thus, two types of error can occur in the interpretation of the crossmatch test: (1) failing to identify the high risk transplant; and (2) preventing a transplant that is not high risk. Further, as noted above, there are reports that suggest that crossmatches of increased sensitivity do not provide a benefit in renal transplantation and reports that show no correlation between crossmatch results and graft survival in nonrenal transplants. These data suggest that some, but not all, antibodies are relevant to transplant outcome and that additional criteria must be considered to permit a meaningful interpretation of the crossmatch outcome. They also suggest that posttransplant events, such as development of new antibody or the down-regulation of antibody, also need to be examined.

B. HLA-Specific Antibodies

1. Pretransplant Antibody

Several studies have determined the specificity of donor-reactive antibody. These studies have shown that the level of risk correlates, significantly, with the presence of HLA-specific antibody. In a thorough analysis of the antibodies of 15 renal transplant recipients who had negative T-cell and positive B-cell crossmatches at the time of transplant, Taylor et al.[63] found that none of the patients with HLA-specific antibody had grafts surviving to 1 year. In similar studies, Karuppan et al.[64,65] used flow cytometry with blocking by monoclonal antibodies to determine, retrospectively, the presence of HLA-specific antibodies present in sera from patients who had crossmatches performed by lymphocytotoxicity (CYT) testing at the time of transplant. There were 11 patients with positive B-cell CYT crossmatches, 14 patients with negative B-cell CYT crossmatches and early acute rejection, 12 patients with no immunologic complications, and 5 patients with early graft loss attributed to nonimmunologic causes. All 11 patients with positive B-cell CYT crossmatches had HLA-specific antibody, and of these patients, 9 lost their grafts within 2 months and 2 patients had grafts surviving at 1 year. Among the 14 patients with negative B-cell CYT crossmatches and early acute rejection, 12 patients lost their grafts within days and 2 had grafts functioning at 1 year. HLA-specific antibody was detected by flow cytometry in 11 of these 12 patients, but not in patients with good graft function or with nonimmunologic graft loss. Thus, all 21 patients with early graft loss had HLA-specific antibodies, and only 1 of 22 patients with HLA-specific antibody had a functioning graft at 1 year. In an effort to diminish the number of positive crossmatches due to non-HLA antibodies, Wang et al.[66] performed flow cytometric crossmatches using donor platelets as target cells for 74 renal transplant recipients. They found that of 19 recipients with a positive platelet crossmatch, 5 of 11 (45%) primary transplants and 5 of 8 (63%) regrafts failed within 1 month but that only 8 of 55 (15%) of those with a negative platelet crossmatch had grafts that failed in the first month. HLA-Cw antigens usually are considered less immunogenic than the HLA-A and B antigens, most likely because of their reduced expression on tissues. However, even the rare antibody specific for HLA-Cw antigens can be problematic, as demonstrated by the hyperacute rejection of a renal graft due to antibody specific for the donor's HLA-Cw5 antigen.[67]

The lower incidence of sensitization to HLA antigens among patients with nonrenal end stage organ disease has limited the information on the significance of HLA-specific presensitization in transplants of other organs. However, the data available indicate that HLA-specific antibodies may be detrimental to any type of transplanted organ or tissue. Following the hyperacute rejection of a transplanted heart by a patient with a positive crossmatch, Weil et al.[44] found that absorption of the recipient's serum with pooled platelets abrogated reactivity in the crossmatch, providing putative identification of the antibody as specific for donor HLA class I antigens. Fenoglio et al.[39] examined the survival of 25 heart transplant recipients who had HLA-specific antibody. Graft survival in 23 recipients who had antibody specific for HLA antigens not found in the donor was comparable to recipients who had no antibody. In contrast, the 2 patients who had antibody specific for donor HLA antigens experienced acute rejection of the graft. Preliminary data indicate that antibody specific for donor HLA antigens is also deleterious to other types of transplanted organs. Donaldson et al.,[68] observed that, in liver transplantation, antibody specific for HLA class I antigens occurred only in patients with vanishing bile duct syndrome. Karuppan et al.[69] found a significant decrease in 1-year survival of liver transplants among patients with a positive (40%) vs. a negative crossmatch (83%). The difference in graft survival was even more dramatic when they determined the specificity of antibodies that resulted in a positive crossmatch. In those with antibodies **not** specific for HLA, 1-year graft survival was 75%, while among patients with HLA-specific antibody, 1-year graft survival was only 16%. Peltenberg et al.[70] reported an accelerated acute rejection of a combined pancreas–spleen graft that was performed in a patient with a positive pretransplant crossmatch. HLA specificity of the antibody was putatively determined by platelet absorption. Taken collectively, these data demonstrate that the correlation between the results of crossmatch tests and graft outcome increases dramatically when one determines antibody specificity and that antibody specific for donor HLA antigens is a significant contraindication to transplantation.

2. HLA Class II-Specific Antibody

It is widely accepted that antibody specific for HLA class I antigens usually constitutes a significant risk factor in transplantation. However, the relevance of class II-specific antibody remained unclear for a long time. This was due, in part, to the increased sensitivity of B cells to nonspecific antibody and to the type of antibody response that occurs, most often, in sensitized patients. Karuppan et al.[69] have postulated that poor correlations between B-cell crossmatch outcome and graft survival, particularly in liver transplantation, can be explained by the occurrence of positive crossmatches due to non-HLA-specific antibody, such as those that occur during viral infection. HLA-specific antibodies in patients awaiting transplantation are most often directed against class I antigens or class I and class II antigens, but rarely against class II antigens only. This is not surprising since the allogeneic tissue to which a patient may be exposed via transfusion, transplantation, or pregnancy rarely differs from the patient only in class II antigens. In a review of more than 600 patients on a renal transplant waiting list, Zachary[71] found that 90% of those with class II-specific antibody also had antibody specific for HLA class I antigens. Because patients rarely have antibody specific only for class II and transplants are rarely mismatched only for class II antigens, cases of graft failure mediated by class II-specific antibody have not been as obvious as for class I-specific antibody. There is now a large body of data indicating that both class I-specific and class II-specific antibodies are significant risks to transplant outcome. In renal transplantation, there have been at least 7 reported cases of hyperacute rejection[72-75] and 15 cases of accelerated rejection[59,65,75-78] due to class II-specific antibodies. Karuppan et al.[69] also observed a severe rejection of a liver transplant, mediated by class II-specific antibody, that led to death of the patient 15 days posttransplant.

Further, it appears from some of these reports that antibodies specific for HLA-DQ are as capable of mediating rapid, humoral rejection as are anti-HLA-DR antibodies. As with class I-specific antibody, the effects of class II-specific antibody are not always immediate but may, instead, be reflected in significantly reduced 1-year graft survival, increased numbers of rejection episodes, diminished graft function, and the need for higher levels of immunosuppressive agents. When Taylor et al.[63] evaluated patients with crossmatches that were positive with B cells and negative with T cells, they found that 1-year graft survival among patients with non-HLA-specific antibody was 82% (56/68) but only 50% (4/8) among patient with class II-specific antibody. Similar results were observed in a smaller group of patients by Ten Hoor et al.,[79] who found that 2 of 3 patients with non-HLA-specific antibody but only 4 of 13 patients with class II-specific antibody had renal grafts functioning at 1 year. In a study of 165 recipients of primary, cadaveric renal grafts, Sirchia et al.[80] found that 3-year graft survival in patients with DR-specific antibody was only 38% compared to 80% in patients without DR-specific antibody. Lederer et al.[81] observed the occurrence of class II-specific antibody in more than half (44 of 86) of renal transplant patients with early graft dysfunction. Thus it appears that antibody specific for donor class II antigens is a significant risk factor that has been underestimated because many patients with such antibody also have class I-specific antibody.

However, there remain cases in which good graft function is obtained in the face of a positive crossmatch due to donor HLA-specific antibody. Such cases suggest that additional properties of the antibodies may be relevant to graft outcome. These properties include: the immunoglobulin class of the antibody; the timing of occurrence (historic vs. at the time of transplant vs. post-transplant) of the antibody; and other factors that may diminish or eliminate the impact of the antibody.

C. Factors Affecting the Risk Represented by HLA-Specific Antibody

1. Immunoglobulin Isotype

When the immunoglobulin class of antibody causing a positive crossmatch is examined, without respect to antibody specificity, the data suggest that there is a greater risk associated with IgG than with IgM antibody. Early studies [54,55] of positive B-cell crossmatches differentiated by warm (37°C) vs. cold (5°C) incubations showed poorer 1-year renal graft survival when positive crossmatches occurred at warm temperatures than when they occurred only at 5°C. Differential reactivity of IgG and IgM at these temperatures suggested that the immunoglobulin class of the antibody may have been important. In studies using reducing agents that inactivate IgM antibodies preferentially, 1-year renal graft survival was shown to be significantly lower for positive crossmatches that could not be abrogated by treating sera with reducing agents than for crossmatches inactivated by such treatment.[23,24,63,82] Similar results have been demonstrated in both heart[10,34,48] and liver[83] transplantation. Autoantibodies are most often IgM antibodies, and these antibodies have been demonstrated in numerous studies not to have a deleterious effect on transplant outcome.[84-89] It is likely that many studies demonstrating the lack of relevance of IgM antibodies reflected the presence of autoantibodies. The importance of immunoglobulin class of antidonor HLA-specific antibodies remains to be resolved. Unfortunately, there are limited data available on this issue, and although there is consensus that IgG anti-HLA antibodies are a significant risk factor, the data on IgM HLA-specific antibodies are less conclusive.

Taylor et al.[63] demonstrated that 1-year graft survival of renal transplants was better in patients with HLA-specific antibody of the IgM class (65%) than in patients with IgG HLA-specific antibody (31%), but was lower than in patients without antibody (82%), suggesting IgM HLA-specific antibodies represented a risk factor of intermediate strength. Karuppan et al.[65] observed a 14% graft loss in patients with non-HLA-specific antibody vs. those with HLA-specific antibody whose graft loss was 33% if the antibody class was IgM and 73% if the antibody was IgG. Similarly, Ten Hoor et al.[79] found that among patients with HLA-specific antibody, 1-year graft survival was better if the antibody was IgM (81%) than if it was IgG (42%), but that the graft survival among those with IgM antibody was poorer in regraft patients (67%) than in primary graft patients (88%). Others[90] have observed that increased rejection correlated with any HLA-specific antibody but was more frequent among those whose antibody was IgG than among those whose antibody was IgM. In studies of HLA-specific antibodies occurring after heart transplantation, Smith et al.[13] saw a significant correlation between increased rejection episodes and HLA specificity of antibody, regardless of the immunoglobulin isotype. Also, Karuppan et al.[69] found that 1-year graft survival in liver transplantation correlated with HLA specificity, regardless of immunoglobulin class. Clearly, more information is needed to determine the risk represented by HLA-specific antibodies of the IgM class. Although other classes of antibodies have not been studied extensively, Koka and co-workers[91,92] have made an interesting observation on the potential relevance of IgA antibodies. They saw improved survival of renal grafts in patients with HLA-specific antibodies of the IgA class compared to those without these antibodies.

2. Timing of Antibody Response

Of great interest has been the importance of antibodies that were present previously, but not at the time of transplant, and of antibodies that develop or persist following transplantation. For more than 15 years, the belief in the laws of immunologic memory dictated that a positive crossmatch with any serum, regardless of the number of years it antedated the transplant, was a contraindication to renal transplantation. That bastion of immunologic dogma was destroyed when Cardella et al.[93] reported successful transplantation in the face of a historic positive crossmatch. This report represented a dramatic increase in the potential for transplantation for patients who were once, but are no longer, highly sensitized. Further, long-term follow-up confirmed their initial findings.[94] The American Society for Histocompatibility and Immunogenetics[95] conducted a survey of such transplants to evaluate various factors that might affect graft outcome. The survey included 260 kidney transplants, 130 each of primary and regrafts, and found no correlation between graft failure and either peak PRA (either historic or current serum specimens) or the amount of time between the last serum giving a positive crossmatch and the date of transplant. More recently, Guerin et al.[96] found no difference in graft survival between a group of 36 renal transplant patients with a historic positive and current negative crossmatch and patients with no positive crossmatch. Cristol et al.[97] saw no differences in 2-year renal graft survival among patients with PRA>50%, whether or not they had a historic positive crossmatch. These studies did not determine the specificity of the antibody producing a positive crossmatch. Barger et al.[98] refined the approach by examining 111 regrafts of kidney transplants and found that there was no difference in graft survival among 103 patients who had either no positive crossmatch and/or no repeat mismatched antigen. However, 7 of 8 patients who had both a historic positive crossmatch and a repeated mismatched antigen lost their graft within 45 days. This suggested that historic antibody specific for an HLA antigen present in the current donor might be a contraindication to transplantation. This concept is supported by three additional studies. Chapman et al.[99] found that, among 42 renal transplant patients with historic positive but current negative crossmatches, 26 of the positive crossmatches were due to autoantibodies, 7 were due to HLA-specific antibody of the IgM class, and 7 to IgG anti-HLA antibodies with graft survival of 65%, 57%, and 0%, respectively. Taylor et al.[63] found that 1-year renal graft survival among patients with a historic positive crossmatch was 82% when the antibody was not specific for HLA and 51% when the antibody was HLA specific. Finally, in a small study of 10 patients, Ten Hoor et al.[79] found 1-year graft survival of patients with historic positive crossmatches due to HLA-specific and nonspecific antibodies to be 29% and 100%, respectively. The current perspective of the Toronto group[100] is that historic antibodies are not a risk factor for primary renal transplants but are considered a risk factor for regraft patients, particularly those who lost a previous graft within 90 days following transplantation.

There are many variable factors that may explain these apparently conflicting results, including the nature of the sensitizing events that provoked the earlier antibody response, the immunoglobulin class and specificity of the historic antibody, the nature and frequency of intervening sensitizing events, the sensitivity of the crossmatch technique used, and the immunosuppression protocol. In turn, these factors may be related to how the patient's immune system has regulated the antibody response, i.e., whether the antibody production has simply become senescent or has been actively down-regulated or suppressed. Unfortunately, this is an area in which minimal investigation has been carried out and has been focused, to a large extent, on the posttransplant period.

3. Posttransplant Antibody

Transfusion, transplantation, and pregnancy are the best known routes of humoral sensitization to HLA antigens. The nature and course of the humoral response to these events varies with the type of event, the circumstances, and the individual. Transplantation and renal transplantation, in particular, seems to provoke the most vigorous humoral response and antibody can be found in serum samples obtained within 72 hours of donor nephrectomy of most patients who experience graft failure due to rejection. The development of HLA-specific antibody following transplantation has not been widely studied due, in large part, to the cost of such testing for which reimbursement is not readily available in the U.S. Halloran et al.[101,102] have noted an unusual pattern of rejection occurring in cyclosporine treated patients who have class I-specific antibody. This rejection is characterized by acute tubular necrosis without edema or tenderness of the kidney, endothelial injury in the microvasculature, mild to moderate complement deposition, moderate infiltration of monocytes, and infiltration of neutrophils. They have proposed that this rejection is mediated by class I-specific antibody and that the inability to detect such antibody in biopsy sections is due to inadequacy of the technique. They tested serum specimens, obtained weekly for 3 months, from 64 renal transplant patients for the presence of class I-specific antibody. All of the patients were negative for antibody prior to transplantation. Following transplantation, 13 patients developed antibody. All 13 patients experienced rejection episodes, 80% of which were severe, and five (38%) lost their grafts. In contrast, of the 51 patients who did not develop antibody during the course of the study, only 41% experienced rejection, the rejections were severe in only 32% of the cases, and only two (4%) of these patients lost their grafts. The differences between the two groups of patients were all highly significant. Similar findings have been reported by Barr et al.[103] They found that renal transplant recipients who developed HLA-specific antibody following transplantation had lower 5-year graft survival than did patients without antibody (53 vs. 70%) and a higher incidence of chronic rejection compared to patients without antibody (27 vs. 13%). Al-Hussein[104] found that the development of antibody in the 2 week period following transplantation was predictive of severe rejection episodes. Somewhat different results were obtained by Lobo et al.,[105] who followed 129 renal transplant patients for the development of donor-reactive, IgG lymphocytotoxic antibodies. They found that of 19 patients who developed lymphocytotoxic antibody following transplantation, 15 (79%) lost their grafts to acute rejection but none lost grafts to chronic rejection, while graft loss due to acute and chronic rejection among 110 patients without antibody was 5% and 10%, respectively. However, antibody specificity was not determined in this study. Scornik et al.[106] followed 50 consecutive, cadaveric renal transplant recipients by flow cytometry. Donor-reactive antibody appeared in 40% of those experiencing rejection and in only 9% of those without rejection. Interestingly, two thirds of the patients with antibody and rejection had IgG antibody with or without IgM antibody, but one third of these patients had IgM antibody only.

The development of HLA-specific antibodies appears to be relevant in transplants of other organs as well. Investigators at Columbia University have conducted a multiyear follow-up of heart transplant patients for the development of antibody, tested initially by lymphocytotoxicity methods and more recently by flow cytometry. In earlier work,[39] they found a significant difference in 4-year graft survival of heart transplant patients with antibody that developed or persisted after transplantation vs. those without antibody (59 vs. 90%). In three 5-year studies of a larger group of patients, this difference in graft survival persisted but was not as dramatic.[39,103] However, they also found that atherosclerosis occurred in 15% of patients with antibody but in none of the patients without antibody, and that there was a correlation between the presence of antibody and episodes of acute cellular rejection. Smith et al.[13] determined graft outcome with respect to specificity and immunoglobulin isotype of lymphocytotoxic antibody present after heart transplantation. Sixty-seven of 82 patients had antibody and of these, the isotype was IgM only in 39 patients and IgG with or without IgM in the other 28. Of the 67, 33 had antibody to HLA antigens not present in the donor. They found that there was no correlation between rejection and the presence of antibody, regardless of the immunoglobulin class of the antibody. Further they found that there was no difference in patient survival for those who had positive vs. negative posttransplant donor crossmatches. The sera of 24 of the patients with positive crossmatches were screened for HLA specificity, and of these, 18 were found to be HLA-specific: 1 for class I only, 5 for class II, and 12 for both. Patients with positive crossmatches and HLA-specific antibody had a significantly higher occurrence of rejection episodes regardless of the isotype or class specificity of the antibody. Rose et al.[107] evaluated the impact of the breadth (as measured by PRA) and duration of anti-HLA antibody production in 240 heart transplants. They found that there was little difference in 3-year graft survival between patients whose antibodies persisted at least 1 year but remained at PRA<10 (100%) compared to those with PRA>10, but whose antibodies persisted 6 months or less (91%). In contrast, when the PRA was greater than 10% and the antibodies persisted beyond 6 months, 3-year graft survival dropped to 70%. Further, atherosclerosis was present in 14% of those with antibody, but in only 4% of those without antibody. Not surprisingly, others[108] have found that the development of antibody after heart transplantation is relevant to outcome only if the antibody is specific for donor HLA antigens. In liver transplantation, Manez et al.[109] have observed that the relevance of a positive crossmatch might be determined by the persistence of antidonor HLA antibody after transplantation. They saw that graft survival of 14 of 22 patients whose antibody disappeared after transplantation was comparable to those with a negative crossmatch, while graft and patient survival were poor in the seven patients whose antibody persisted. Karuppan et al.[69] saw that 1-year graft survival in patients who developed antibody following liver transplantation was 60% if the antibody was HLA-specific and 83% if the antibody was not HLA specific. Two of the patients who developed HLA-specific antibody after transplantation lost their grafts within 10 days. Recently, Schulman et al.[110] reported that 3-year survival was significantly lower among lung transplant patients who developed HLA-specific antibody after transplantation than among those who did not. Further, they found a significant correlation between the development of obliterative bronchiolitis and the production of HLA-specific antibody.

4. Anti-Idiotypic Antibody

It appears that a major factor determining graft survival among patients who developed antidonor HLA antibody after transplantation is the persistence of the antibody.[111] There is increasing evidence that the factor determining graft survival may be the development of anti-idiotypic antibodies specific for the patient's anti-HLA antibodies. Hardy et al.[112] followed antibody production in 330 cadaveric renal and 170 heart transplant patients for at least 1 year. They found three patterns of HLA antibody production: (1) consistent presence of anti-HLA antibody; (2) cyclic variation of anti-HLA antibody without the occurrence of anti-idiotypic antibody; and (3) cyclic appearance of anti-HLA antibody with development of anti-idiotypic antibody. Two-year graft survival was dramatically different for the three types of antibody patterns in both renal and heart transplant recipients. Two-year graft survival for groups 1, 2, and 3 were 47%, 36%, and 100%, respectively, in renal transplant recipients, and 56%, 71%, and 100%, respectively, in heart transplant recipients. They also noted that no anti-idiotypic antibody was found in patients undergoing chronic rejection. Five-year follow-up of patients by this group[113] revealed that patients who develop anti-idiotypic antibody had five-year graft survival as good as patients who never develop antibody for both heart (80 vs. 86%) and kidney transplantation (100%). In contrast, patients who develop anti-HLA antibody but do not develop anti-idiotypic antibody have significantly reduced 5-year graft survival (57% in heart and 58% in kidney patients). Similarly, Ramounau-Pigout et al.[114] found that four patients with anti-idiotypic antibody had successful renal grafts, but that the transplants failed in three of five patients with anti-HLA antibody but no anti-idiotypic antibody. The value of anti-idiotypic antibody was demonstrated, dramatically, by the case study of a patient who had hyperacutely rejected a first kidney transplant.[115] This patient went on to produce anti-idiotypic antibody and was successfully transplanted with a second graft that, amazingly, shared mismatched antigens with the first donor. In another case report,[116] it was shown that successful heart transplantation occurred in a woman who had antibody specific for HLA-A2, as the result of three pregnancies. The donor had the A2 antigen and, in addition, had three other class I antigens (B17, B44, and Cw6) that were also present in the patient's husband. The A2-specific antibody disappeared on the 17th week posttransplant, at which time anti-idiotypic antibody was identified through blocking studies. Biopsies exhibited no evidence of humoral rejection and the patient had good graft function at the last reported follow-up (29 months). These findings are supported by an animal study in which production of anti-idiotypic antibodies by Lewis rats was achieved by immunizing the rats with IgG and IgM fractions of serum from other Lewis rats that had been hyperimmunized with skin grafts from ACI rats.[117] Survival of transplanted ACI hearts was significantly better in the rats immunized with the immunoglobulin preparations (11.2 ± 0.7 days) compared to control rats (6.4 ± 0.5 days). Production of anti-idiotypic antibodies following liver transplantation in humans has also been reported.[118]

D. Antibodies Specific for Antigens Other Than HLA

The occurrence of accelerated and other antibody-mediated graft rejection and the identification of non-MHC tissue-specific antigens in animal models has provoked interest in other antigen systems that might be targets of humoral rejection in transplantation (reviewed by Steinmuller[119]). Antigens present on vascular endothelial cells (VEC) have been proposed to account for graft loss in patients without HLA-specific antibody and in patients receiving transplants from HLA identical donors.[120,121] Cerilli et al.[122] observed that six of seven renal transplant patients with irreversible rejection occurring within 72 hours and four of five patients with early, reversible rejection had VEC antibodies reactive with donor cells, while these antibodies could be found in only 5 of 43 patients who had a benign course. Examined another way, of 15 patients with VEC antibody, 5 (33%) had graft loss while 9 (67%) did not. Yard et al.[123] tested sera from 64 renal transplant patients against cultured umbilical vein endothelial cells derived from 10 subjects, using the antibody-dependent cell-mediated cytotoxicity assay. They found that 5 of 10 patients who had antibody reactive with these cells had vascular rejection and lost their grafts within 50 days. In contrast, vascular rejection was seen in only 4 of the 54 patients without antibody. The apparent expression of the VEC antigens on monocytes provoked an interest in performing monocyte crossmatches, and cases have been reported in which antibody reactive with monocytes but not with T or B lymphocytes was found in patients experiencing early, humoral graft rejection.[124] Both monocytes and endothelial cells present technical problems in the crossmatch because of their fragility and broad antigen repertoire. Endothelial cells pose additional difficulties in access and isolation. To overcome these problems, one group has used skin as a target tissue for the crossmatch test because of a strong possibility of antigens shared with endothelial cells (reviewed in Moraes et al.[125]). In early studies, they obtained a perfect correlation between crossmatch outcome and graft failure in 25 patients who were all negative by the antiglobulin lymphocytotoxicity (CYT) crossmatch.

Another approach has been to look for antibodies reactive with tissue from the transplanted organ. Joyce et al.[126] found that eluates from rejected kidneys contained antibodies to HLA antigens, monocytes, endothelial cells, and kidney cells. After removal of HLA-specific antibodies, they were able to identify antibodies reactive with a 90- to 100 kDa kidney protein. However, it was not possible to determine if this antibody was involved in the graft rejection. Evans et al.[127] also looked for antibodies binding to kidney using pre-anastomosis biopsies. They found such antibodies in 13 of 70 patients, but did not see a correlation between the presence or staining pattern of the antibodies and graft outcome. However, when they followed antibody after transplantation, they found a high rate of graft failure (71%) in patients with persistent antibody compared to the rate of graft failure in patients with transient antibody (17%). Although the presence of kidney-reactive antibody did not correlate with the presence of lymphocytotoxic antibodies in the serum, they found that antibodies eluted from seven of eight rejected kidneys were HLA specific. Dunn et al.[128] examined antibodies before and after heart transplantation in 22 patients, using a myocardial protein extract in a Western blotting technique. They found a correlation between severe or frequent rejection episodes and the presence, before transplantation, of antibodies reactive with the protein extract. All patients had a negative lymphocyte crossmatch before transplantation.

III. PROTOCOLS

The best patient care is achieved when the patient's humoral response is assessed, the immunologic risk to the patient is estimated, and that risk estimate is applied to determining treatment. Achieving these goals requires the selection of appropriate tests, correct interpretation of test results, and evaluation of a variety of factors including the information provided by the test results, the patient's immunologic history, the suitability and likelihood of success of available treatment options, and the level of risk acceptable. In the development of laboratory protocols, one should consider the risk factors to be assessed, the technology and expertise available, the applicability of the test results to clinical management of the patient, and the cost and logistics of various test methods.

A. Assessment of Risk Factors

The studies cited above provide a means to assess the degree of risk associated with various parameters of lymphocyte-reactive antibody. Antibody specific for class I (HLA-A, -B, -C) and/or class II (HLA-DR, -DQ) antigens, present at the time of transplantation in sufficient strength to be detected by techniques of lower sensitivity, i.e., lymphocytotoxicity techniques that do **not** include an antiglobulin reagent, represent the most serious risk factor and are a contraindication to renal transplantation. While there are fewer data for transplants of other organs, the studies of heart and liver transplants strongly suggest that HLA-specific antibodies are a significant risk factor in transplants of those organs also. Perhaps because of the nature of the organs, the time course of rejection of hearts and livers is different from that of kidneys. Although patients awaiting heart or liver transplantation may demonstrate lymphocytotoxic antibody, the antibody is often nonspecific, induced by medication (e.g., antiarrythmics such as procainamide[129] are known to induce autoantibody production) or viral infections. The occurrence of HLA-specific antibodies, prior to transplantation, has been less frequent among patients with end-stage heart or liver disease than among patients awaiting kidney transplantation, probably because the latter group has a greater proportion of previously transplanted patients and has, at least historically, had a higher frequency of blood transfusions. Even less is known about the risk associated with HLA-specific antibody in transplants of other organs. However, it is reasonable to project that as more patients are evaluated and antibody specificity is carefully defined, HLA-specific antibody will be established as a major risk factor in transplants of all vascularized organs.

Low levels of HLA-specific antibody, i.e., those detected by B-cell, antiglobulin, or flow cytometric techniques, and antibodies of different immunoglobulin classes present at the time of transplant appear to represent different degrees of risk, depending on the transplant history of the patient. Antibodies detected only by these more sensitive methods correlate with early graft loss in regrafts and with an increase in the number and severity of rejections in primary grafts. This may be due to a difference between primary and regraft patients in clonal expansion of HLA-specific cells, as proposed by Scornik,[130] or a shift in the relative amounts of IgG vs. IgM antibodies. There is consensus that IgG antibodies are a risk, but the importance of IgM antibodies is not clearly defined. Perhaps it is not the presence but the course of IgM antibodies, i.e., whether class switch to IgG occurs after transplantation, that is important. Then, IgM antibodies would not be a risk factor but a marker representing a potential for risk.

It is difficult to assess the risk of antibodies that were present historically but are not present at the time of transplant. There is no consensus about the relative importance of either the amount of time between last antibody occurrence and transplant or HLA specificity of the historic antibody. An enticing concept to account for differences among patients is the occurrence of anti-idiotypic antibody, which varies among patients. In a study of antigen-specific transfusions in patients with historic antibody, Zachary et al.[131] found that recall of antibody not only varied among patients but also among antibodies of different specificity in individual patients. However, as noted above, the Toronto group considers early loss (within 90 days) of a previous graft to be the only risk factor associated with a historic positive cross-match.[100]

There are convincing data that the development and persistence, following transplantation, of antibody specific for donor HLA antigens contributes to chronic rejection, the development of atherosclerosis in heart transplants, and early graft loss. It is unfortunate that posttransplant testing is not reimbursable under Medicare coverage, because early intervention in patients at risk could enhance graft survival which, in turn, would result in significant cost savings, improve patient survival and quality of life, and reduce the imbalance between the number of donor organs available and the number needed.

It is quite possible, even likely, that antibodies to other antigen systems such as VEC antigens and organ specific antigens are quite important in transplantation. Like the HLA class II-specific antibodies, their importance is probably overshadowed by HLA class I-specific antibody. Although tests of these antibodies may be most important in the well-matched transplant, they have not been incorporated as routine tests in most clinical laboratories because of the technical obstacles they present, the cost of such testing, and the time constraints on testing of cadaver donors.

Risk factors associated with humoral sensitization to HLA antigens may be increased or diminished by other factors, including sensitizing events (transfusion and pregnancy), type and amount of immunosuppression, the genotype of the patient, and HLA match of the transplant. The risk represented by HLA-specific antibody may vary from patient to patient and situation to situation. For example, certain immunosuppression protocols may overcome some or all of the risk associated with very low levels of antibody. However, these protocols may not be suitable for all patients or in all situations. There are probably other, as yet unidentified, factors that impact on the risk represented by HLA antibodies. Therefore, no single test protocol will benefit all patients equally and it is usually necessary to have multiple protocols to accommodate different categories of patients. Further, as the conditions relevant to a particular patient change, the laboratory scientist should customize testing whenever it is appropriate and possible.

Protocols for testing sera should eliminate unacceptable risks to the patient and permit a meaningful interpretation of the crossmatch test (i.e., permit identification of those situations where transplant is contraindicated and those where it is not). Protocol selection may be constrained by the cost of, time involved in, and the technical and scientific expertise required to perform and interpret the results of some tests. Table 1 is a summary of the risk factors discussed here.

B. Selection of Test Methods

The various test methods, including the multiple variations of the lymphocytotoxicity test, flow cytometry, and enzyme-linked immunosorbent assay (ELISA), differ in their sensitivity. The degree of acceptable risk is one factor to consider in selecting a method of appropriate sensitivity. For example, if the only risk considered unacceptable is that of hyperacute rejection, a technique of lower sensitivity is adequate. A second factor to consider is the degree to which an individual patient or type of patient is at risk for graft rejection. For example, regraft

TABLE 1

Risk Associated with Various Properties of HLA-Specific Antibody

Factor	Property	Comments	Effect
Titer at time of transplant	High	High risk	Hyperacute or accelerated rejection
	Low	Primary grafts	Increased number and severity of rejection episodes[a]
		Regrafts	Early graft loss
Immunoglobulin class	IgG	High risk	Early rejection[a]
	IgM	May be a greater risk in regrafts	Not clearly established
Timing of occurrence: Historic[b]	Transplant history	Primary grafts — not resolved, but majority of data favor low or no risk	
		Regrafts — high risk for repeat mismatches and in patients with early loss of a previous graft	Early humoral rejection, increased number and severity of rejection episodes
	Immunoglobulin class	Unclear, but IgG may be a higher risk factor than IgM	
	Time to last positive	No known correlation	
Posttransplant	All	High risk if anti-idiotype is not produced	Early graft loss, chronic rejection[a]

[a] Atherosclerosis in heart transplants; vanishing bile duct syndrome in liver transplants; obliterative bronchiolitis in lung transplants.

[b] Not evaluated in non-renal transplants.

patients are at higher risk for graft rejection than are those receiving a primary graft. Because patients differ in the degree to which they are at risk, it is appropriate to use different techniques to offset that risk, particularly in the crossmatch test. A third factor to consider, in antibody screening, is the extent of sensitization of an individual or, more precisely, the antibody content of their serum. For example, using the sensitive antiglobulin technique to screen sera from highly sensitized patients may result in a panreactivity that necessitates testing against an extremely large and impractical number of phenotypes in order to determine antibody specificity. It has been argued that the technique used for the crossmatch test should also be used for screening sera. On the face of it, that argument is logical. It has been demonstrated that both the antiglobulin and flow cytometric techniques, used in many laboratories for the crossmatch test, reveal the presence of antibodies not detected by other methods,[17,132] either because the antibodies are in a titer too low for detection or because they are of an immunoglobulin class that activates complement inefficiently. However, both of these techniques are time-consuming. Further, for the nonsensitized patient and the highly sensitized patient, the extra time invested in these techniques may yield little additional information.

It is possible to achieve a compromise that minimizes both risk and effort. Rodey et al.[133] and Fuller[132] have shown that patients who are highly sensitized, in particular those sensitized by transplantation, generally have a limited number of antibodies and that these antibodies are specific for public determinants shared by the so-called cross-reactive groups (CREGS). They have demonstrated that these antibodies are seen in their entirety in the antiglobulin technique but often react sporadically with all or some members of the CREG when tested with techniques of lower sensitivity. Then, for sensitized patients, particularly those who have had a previous transplant, one may make certain assumptions regarding the antibody specificities detected using less sensitive techniques. By correlating the specificities of the antibodies identified with the best-fitting crossreactive groups,[132,133] one may simulate the results that would be obtained with the antiglobulin test. Alternatively, the antiglobulin test could be performed on selected serum specimens, to determine if the antibody specificities seen with techniques of lower sensitivity are, in fact, specific for public determinants. Another approach to identifying CREG antibodies is to absorb serum with platelets bearing either one of the antigens for which antibodies have been detected or an antigen that is a member of the CREG but for which antibodies have not been seen. However, if such absorption abrogates reactivity with all the antigens in the CREG, it is not possible to determine if the serum contained a single antibody specific for a public epitope or multiple antibodies which must all be present to achieve lysis in the cytotoxicity assay. The ability to remove antibody of one (or more) specificity by absorption with antigens of another specificity is the CYNAP[135] (cytotoxicity negative absorption positive) phenomenon and reflects an inherent flaw in the cytotoxicity assay. That is, that there must be sufficient antibody of the right immunoglobulin class and subclass to achieve lysis in the absence of an antiglobulin reagent. Techniques that determine antibody binding, such as flow cytometry and ELISA, overcome these shortcomings.

C. Antibody-Binding Assays

Shroyer et al.[136] have described a flow cytometric screening protocol that utilizes cells pooled from six individuals with distinct HLA phenotypes. They have shown that antibody reactive with cells from only one of the six subjects can be detected. Although the use of this technique would be facilitated by using cytometers equipped with carriers that hold multiple samples, it would be cumbersome and, potentially, costly for testing large numbers of serum specimens on a regular basis. Further, it does not permit, readily, precise definition of antibody specificity. Several investigators[137-141] have developed methods for isolating soluble HLA class I antigens and testing them in an ELISA assay. There are multiple potential advantages to this method: (1) elimination of the need for viable lymphocytes; (2) a sensitivity comparable to that of the antiglobulin assay or greater; (3) detection of immunoglobulin classes that do not activate complement readily; (4) elimination of test variability contributed by the complement component; (5) the possibility of partial automation; (6) elimination of scoring variability, with use of an ELISA plate reader; and, importantly, (7) elimination of reactivity due to antibody (ies) specific for antigens other than HLA.

At present, three commercial kits for testing for HLA-specific antibodies using soluble HLA antigens in an ELISA assay are available. Two kits are designed for screening sera and one kit is for performing crossmatch tests. One of the antibody screening kits, PRA-STAT™*, utilizes soluble HLA class I antigens captured from the eluates of 46 transformed cell lines. The other antibody screening kit, Quik-Screen™**, uses pooled, soluble class I antigens extracted from platelets obtained from 600 individuals, representing three racial groups (African-American, Caucasian, and Hispanic/Latino). The tests have different objectives, with that of PRA-STAT being determination of antibody specificity and that of QuikScreen being detection of antibody. Different groups have reported varied findings in the evaluation of PRA-STAT vs. cytotoxicity testing. Buelow et al.[142] reported results obtained in a multicenter study in which 102 serum specimens from patients awaiting renal transplantation were tested by PRA-STAT (PS) in six labs and by basic or one- or two-wash lymphocytotoxicity in five of the same labs. Interlaboratory reproducibility for PRA values obtained by PS were very high ($r = 0.89$–0.96), and there was a high correlation, between PS and CYT, for PRA values obtained for 61 sera that were positive by CYT. Comparison of specificities detected by the two assays revealed that: (1) the 2 assays defined the same specificity(ies) in 9 sera

---

* Trademark of SangStat Medical Corporation, Menlo Park, CA.
** Trademark of GTI, Brookfield, WI.

(19.2%); (2) for 11 sera (23.4%), some but not all specificities were the same in the two assays; (3) there were 11 sera (23.4%) in which specificities were found by PS but not CYT; (4) there were 12 sera (25.5.%) in which specificities were defined by CYT but not PS; and (5) different specificities were defined in the 2 assays for 4 sera (8.5%). Bryan et al.[143] compared PS to results obtained with the antiglobulin modification of the cytoxicity test (AHG). They found a lower correlation (r = 0.42) between the two assays in the PRA values obtained. In tests of 230 sera from prospective transplant patients, they found that PS defined more antibody specificities (383) than did AHG (266), and that only 28 of the specificities were concordant in the 2 assays. They also found that PS identified a minority of antibody specificities assigned by cytotoxicity testing to 29 reagent-typing sera, although not all of these antibodies were established to be IgG, the only isotype detected by PRA-STAT. Zachary et al.[144] tested sera from different groups of patients, multiparous females, and healthy, non-sensitized individuals using PS and 2 different cytotoxicty techniques, the basic and the antiglobulin test. They found a high correlation (r = 0.78) between PS and CYT for the detection of IgG antibodies. Analysis of antibody specificity of 66 sera reactive in both assays revealed that identical specificities were identified by both assays in 18% of the sera, 27% of the sera had more specificities identified by PS than by CYT, 8% had more specificities identified by CYT, and 47% had different specificities identified in the 2 assays with overlap in about half of these. They observed that sera from three nonsensitized males, which were consistently negative when tested against lymphocytes by antiglobulin lymphocytotototoxicity and flow cytometry, were consistently positive in the PS test. They also found that the presence of IgM, HLA-specific antibody could affect test results in PS. It is not surprising that tests of lymphocytes and those of soluble antigens yield different results. Further, it should be noted that these disparities are not unlike those that exist in the results of different cytotoxicity assays and even between laboratories using the same cytotoxicity assay. Several factors should be taken into account when evaluating this assay for routine, clinical use. PRA-STAT has FDA approval. The investigator using the kit is unable, at present, to validate the contents of the trays. That is, are all antigens of the reported phenotype present? Are the assigned phenotypes correct? The manufacturer performs quality control assays to assure a minimal protein content in the extracts of the culture supernatants. However, it is possible for mutations to occur that would abrogate expression of one or more of the HLA genes. Further, there is no way, at present, for the user to validate the phenotypes.

There are fewer reports on the QuikScreen kit. Preliminary data from Lucas et al.[145] indicated that the sensitivity of the assay was comparable to that of the antiglobulin method, at a minimum, and that there was a good correlation in the detection of HLA-specific antibody between the results obtained by QuikScreen and those obtained by cytotoxicity testing. Bryan et al.[143] have evaluated antibody screening using soluble antigens extracted from pooled platelets in their own test system. They found a good correlation (r = 0.77) between ELISA and AHG in the detection of antibody and between the OD ratios and PRA values obtained by the two tests, respectively. Further studies by Lucas et al.[146] have found this system to provide a rapid method of detecting the presence of HLA class I-specific antibody at an appreciably reduced cost. The low cost and short turn-around time of the test make it particularly advantageous in two situations: (1) for testing nonsensitized patients or groups of patients who have a low incidence of sensitization, where screening against a panel of lymphocytes represents a high cost/benefit ratio; and (2) when it is important to know, rapidly, whether or not a patient has HLA-specific antibody, such as for patients being added to a transplant waiting list or patient suspected of experiencing humoral rejection. The QuikScreen kit is also FDA approved. Some of the same caveats and recommendations given for PRA-STAT also apply to this test.

Both PRA-STAT and QuikScreen have a notable limitation and a significant advantage. Namely, neither assay detects class II-specific antibodies, but both assays are immune to interference by cytotoxic drugs (such as OKT3 and antilymphocyte globulin). These authors have used both assays successfully to evaluate the presence of HLA-specific antibody in patients being treated with such agents. Current federal regulations require that serum screening tests use lymphocytes as targets. However, since these regulations no longer mandate monthly screening, assays using soluble antigens may be used as adjuncts to lymphocyte assays. Finally, the data from the evaluations of these assays are preliminary. Because of the tremendous potential to expedite testing, increase sensitivity above many cytotoxicity assays, and eliminate reactions with non-HLA-specific antibody, the histocompatibility community should continue to explore these assays and generate data, and the manufacturers should use these data to bring the products to their full potential.

In addition to the potential advantages of using soluble antigens for antibody screening, application of this technology to donor cross-matches has the potential to overcome problems that arise, frequently, in tests of cadaver donors. Many laboratories perform histocompatibility tests of cadaver donors prior to organ recovery in order to minimize cold ischemia time. However, there is often a limited amount of blood available for testing. Even when lymph nodes and/or spleen are used, the expression of HLA antigens may be reduced because of various

TABLE 2

Advantages and Disadvantages of Various Test Methods

Test Method	Advantages	Disadvantages
Lymphocytotoxicity: low sensitivity (basic, one wash, extended incubation)	Rapid Does not require additional reagents or equipment	Detects only those antibodies efficient at activating complement High risk of missing low titer antibodies
Lymphocytotoxicity: antiglobulin modification	Very sensitive Detects antibodies that do not activate complement readily Can differentiate immunoglobulin class with specific conjugates	Extends test time Requires preparation and use of additional reagent May result in nonspecific killing of cells with borderline viability
Flow cytometry	Very sensitive Permits simultaneous assessment of multiple factors (lymphocyte subset, immunoglobulin class, etc.)	Requires expensive equipment Increased reagent expense Additional technical expertise necessary Not well-suited to high volume testing
ELISA using soluble HLA antigens	High sensitivity Partial automation Eliminates need for viable cells Eliminates use of complement Rapid Results unaffected by presence of therapeutic cytotoxic antibodies	Currently available commercial kits do not detect class II-specific antibodies Federal regulations require use of lymphocyte targets Experience base is limited, at present Further clarification of quality control requirements is needed

medications given the donor, and cell viability can be reduced by improper handling and maintenance of tissues during transport.[147] CROSS-STAT™,* is an FDA approved, commercially available crossmatch kit. Buelow et al.[148] have reported that a parallel study conducted in four laboratories revealed a high (99%) concordance among the laboratories and a level of sensitivity comparable to flow cytometry. The kit is applicable to class I testing only. The advantages and disadvantages of the antibody detection methods used routinely in clinical laboratories are provided in Table 2.

---

* Trademark of SangStat Medical Corporation, Menlo Park, CA.

D. Blocking/Removal of Non-HLA-Specific Antibodies

There are several methods available to differentiate HLA-specific antibodies from those of other specificities and to determine immunoglobulin isotype. Among renal and cardiac patients awaiting transplantation, autoantibodies are among the most prevalent non-HLA antibodies and can be detected, readily, by performing a crossmatch with autologous cells. When such antibodies are present, it is necessary to remove the autoantibody to be able to determine if allogeneic antibodies are also present. The most specific approach is to absorb the serum with autologous mononuclear cells. Because many autoantibodies are IgM, some laboratories simply treat the sera to inactivate IgM. The obvious danger of such a policy is that IgM HLA-specific antibodies would also be destroyed. Whether or not one considers IgM HLA-specific antibodies to be a risk factor, knowledge of their presence might be important for selecting test and treatment protocols. Other non-HLA-specific antibodies may arise during the course of viral infection. It is more difficult to remove these antibodies because their specificity is rarely known. Sumitran-Karuppan and Möller[149] have treated sera with soluble HLA class I and class II molecules to verify the HLA specificity of antibodies reactive in crossmatch tests. Therapeutic antibodies, such as OKT3 and ALG, are reactive in lymphocytotoxicity assays and must be removed or blocked in order to detect HLA-specific antibodies. However, antibodies of nonhuman origin do not interfere with antibody binding assays such as flow cytometric tests or ELISA.

E. Isotype Determination

Inactivation of IgM antibodies with reducing agents such as dithiothreitol (DTT)[150] and dithioerythretol (DTE) or by incubating sera at 63°C[151] and parallel testing of treated and untreated aliquots of serum have been used to differentiate IgG and IgM antibodies. DTT and DTE have certain disadvantages: (1) they will also reduce IgG antibodies to some extent;[99] (2) both agents are carcinogenic; and (3) the amount of serum treated must be sufficient to minimize the effect of dilution. Neither reducing agents nor heating will abrogate, completely, the reactivity of high-titered IgM antibodies.[151] More precise identification of immunoglobulin class can be achieved by using conjugates specific for the different classes in adherence assays such as flow cytometry or ELISA. Other methods to identify and purify different immunoglobulin classes, such as Western blotting and column chromatography, are very useful in research applications, but, generally, not for routine clinical testing.

F. Antibody Screening: Timing of Tests

1. Pretransplant Testing

A. Renal Transplantation

Prior to the availability of recombinant erythropoietin, it had been standard practice to screen samples obtained monthly from patients. Reduced sensitization rates resulting from less frequent blood transfusions, pressure to contain costs, and increasing workloads resulting from the ongoing growth of waiting lists have prompted an interest in less frequent screening. The Histocompatibility Committee of the United Network for Organ Sharing conducted a survey to determine the extent of fluctuation in sensitization as measured by panel reactive antibody. They* found two groups of patients, those with PRA≤10% and those with PRA≥80%, in which PRA fluctuations were infrequent, and who might be candidates for reduced frequency screening. However, there is some risk involved in adopting such a practice. First, the use of erythropoietin has not eliminated transfusions completely, and reliable information about transfusion events often is not available to the laboratory. The unrecognized occurrence of a sensitizing transfusion could lead to a positive crossmatch, and the clinical relevance of this crossmatch would be difficult to interpret without antibody screening data. Second, the potential for sensitization by infectious agents has not been evaluated thoroughly. The protein products of several microorganisms, including certain enteric bacteria, Epstein Barr virus, and cytomegalovirus, have been shown to have sequence homology and, in some cases, serologic crossreactivity, with certain HLA molecules. It has not been established that infection with these microbes can lead to HLA sensitization, but there are reports suggesting the possibility of sensitization other than through transfusion, transplantation, or pregnancy. Lepage[152] reported detecting an HLA-specific antibody in a nontransfused, nontransplanted male. One of us[153] also observed IgM, HLA-specific antibodies occurring in two males who had no known source of sensitization. There have also been reports[154-156] of increases in PRA in patients who were being treated with erythropoietin and not receiving transfusions. Rather than forfeit potentially valuable information by screening at less frequent intervals, it may be a better practice to perform the routine screening procedure at less frequent intervals and to test sera from the intervening months using less elaborate and costly procedures, such as testing pooled lymphocytes or soluble antigens. Either approach is appropriate only for patient groups known to have infrequent fluctuations in their antibody.

---

* Report of the Histocompatibility Committee to the UNOS Board of Directors, September 30, 1993.

B. Transplants of Other Organs

The incidence of sensitized patients among those awaiting transplants of other organs is lower than among renal transplant candidates and, in many centers, these patients are not screened regularly for antibody. In practice, many laboratories receive only a single serum specimen on each patient, usually obtained at the time the patient is placed on the waiting list. This serum may be months old at the time the patient is translanted, which may explain, in part, the lack of correlation, reported by some, between graft outcome and antibody levels or crossmatch test results. The data demonstrating the serious risk posed by HLA-specific antibody indicate that patients awaiting transplantation of an organ other than the kidney should be tested for antibody either: (1) following any known sensitizing event; or (2) at regular intervals (no less than quarterly) in the absence of reliable information about sensitizing events. As with other patients at low risk for sensitization, these tests could be performed using less elaborate and costly procedures aimed at screening for the presence of antibody. More elaborate testing could be limited to those specimens shown to have antibody.

2. Posttransplant Testing

There are overwhelming data indicating that the development and persistence of donor HLA-specific antibody following transplantation significantly increases the risk of early graft loss and may contribute to the chronic rejection process. It is unfortunate that the lack of reimbursement for posttransplant testing has prohibited its routine use, particularly since the potential for improving graft survival, if realized, would more than offset the cost of testing. At the time of this writing, a study is being conducted by the American Society for Histocompatibility and Immunogenetics to assess the efficacy of various methods of posttransplant testing and to determine their relevance to graft outcome. Hopefully, the results of this study will establish, conclusively and unequivocally, the value of posttransplant testing.

G. Tests for Anti-Idiotypic Antibodies

Tests for anti-idiotypic antibodies specific for HLA antibodies are neither routine tests in most laboratories nor reimbursable. Nonetheless, the data from a few centers indicate that these tests warrant further evaluation, not only because they may correlate with superior graft outcome, but also because identification of the factors that determine their production represents the possibility for manipulating the immune response.

H. Crossmatch Tests: Selection of Serum Specimens

1. Renal Transplantation

Prior to the reports by Cardella et al.[93,94] of safe transplantation in the face of a crossmatch positive with historical serum but negative with current serum, it had been standard practice to include a selection of historical sera representative of the patient's sensitization along with a current serum in the crossmatch test and to consider a positive crossmatch with any specimen a contraindication to transplantation. At present, there are conflicting data regarding the factors that determine when an historic positive crossmatch is safe and when it is not. Factors that may be relevant to the risk associated with an historic positive crossmatch include: (1) the transplant history of the regraft patient — i.e., whether or not the patient experienced an early immunologic loss of a previous graft; (2) the antibody history of the patient, in particular the antibody specificity, degree of fluctuation in antibody, and response to transfusion; (3) the sensitivity of the crossmatch technique; (4) the degree of HLA mismatch; (5) the time between the most recent positive crossmatch and transplant; (6) the isotype of the antibody giving a positive crossmatch; and (7) the immunosuppression protocol. Regardless of what historic positive crossmatches are considered acceptable, the historic sera should be tested, since the information may be useful in fine-tuning the crossmatch policy and in determining patient treatment protocols.

These same factors are relevant to determining what is meant by a current serum. Additionally, the acceptable age of a current serum is affected by the occurrence of a recent sensitizing event since it may take 2 weeks for a humoral response to such an event to be detectable.

2. Transplantation of Other Organs

In addition to being required by federal regulations, the data demonstrating the risk of graft failure posed by donor HLA-specific antibody dictate that a crossmatch should be performed prior to transplantation for all sensitized patients. As noted above, the only serum sample available to the laboratory may be months old and a crossmatch using this sample is likely to be meaningless. If the transplant center provides serum samples following sensitizing events or at regular intervals, the sample present in the laboratory is adequate. Alternatively, when histocompatibility testing is performed prior to organ recovery, there is, often, sufficient time to obtain a serum specimen from the patient who is the primary candidate for transplantation. In any event, given the risk of graft failure due to sensitization to HLA and the shortage of donor organs, every attempt should be made to utilize a serum specimen that represents the patient's sensitization to donor HLA antigens at the time of transplant.

TABLE 3

Ancillary Techniques

Technique	Application	Comments
Absorption with autologous mononuclear cells or platelets	Removal of autoantibodies	Permits detection and characterization of alloantibodies May be difficult to obtain sufficient cells for absorption
Incubation of serum at 63°C for 10 min	IgM inactivation	May produce inaccurate results in ELISA assays
Treatment with reducing agents (DTT or DTE)	IgM inactivation	Some dilution of test serum occurs Agents are carcinogenic May affect IgG antibodies
Blocking with soluble HLA molecules	Abrogate reactivity of HLA-specific antibodies	Requires preparation of soluble molecules May require titration of serum
Absorption with pooled platelets	Removal of class I-specific antibodies	Most commonly used technique for evaluating class II-specific antibodies
Tests for anti-idiotypic antibody	Determine basis for reduction of PRA	May be useful in determining risk associated with historic positive crossmatch and in predicting posttransplant course

3. Posttransplant Specimens

As with antibody screening, reimbursement for posttransplant crossmatches is usually unavailable. However, from a medical standpoint, a crossmatch test with a posttransplant specimen is indicated whenever humoral rejection is suspected. Further, reported studies indicate that crossmatch testing or antibody screening at regular intervals following transplantation may detect humoral rejection before it is manifested in clinical symptoms.

Table 3 provides a listing of some specialized techniques and Table 4 identifies required and recommended specimens for testing.

IV. INTERPRETATION OF TEST RESULTS

A. Antibody Screening

Four types of data may be generated from antibody screening tests: (1) presence or absence of antibody; (2) immunoglobulin isotype; (3) the percent panel reactive antibody, i.e., the frequency of positive reactions;

TABLE 4

Serum Sample Selection

Period	Test	Transplant	Samples	Comments
Pre-Tx[a]	Antibody screen	Renal	Initial work-up Nonsensitized patients: monthly or following a sensitizing event Sensitized patients: monthly	Required by federal regulations Periodic testing required by federal regulations Authors recommend monthly testing Required by federal regulations
		Nonrenal	At initial work-up and following sensitizing event	Requirement is implicit in crossmatch regulations
	Crossmatch	Renal	1. Current specimen 2. Historic specimens considered a risk factor	Current specimen required by federal regulations Tests of historic specimens may provide useful information even if not considered a contraindication to transplant
		Nonrenal	Current specimen	Testing before transplantation is required by fed reg except in emergency circumstances
Post-Tx	Donor crossmatch or other test to detect antibody	Any	1, 2, 3, and 4 weeks, 2 months, quarterly thereafter or when rejection is suspected	Highly recommended for high risk renal transplants; may be useful for all transplants
	Antibody screen for specificity	Any	Whenever knowledge of antibody specificity is needed	Particularly important when donor cells are not available

[a] Transplant.

and (4) HLA specificity. The presence or absence of antibody is determined by all types of assays, but in assays that use pooled targets (lymphocytes or soluble antigens) this is the only information obtained. In the latter case, positive reactivity indicates that further testing against a panel of appropriate HLA phenotypes should be performed. The relevance of immunoglobulin isotype to graft outcome has been discussed at length above, and will not be covered further here. It is the opinion of the authors and of others that the PRA statistic is of limited value. First, even a casual review of the literature will indicate that the particular PRA values that are considered to define low, moderate, and high levels of sensitization are inconsistent and somewhat arbitrary. Second, if the panel of phenotypes used to test sera is not consistent, fluctuations in PRA may be more a reflection of panel variability than of changes in extent of sensitization. Third, changes in antibody specificity may occur without appreciable or noticeable changes in PRA. Fourth, PRA values obtained with panels comprised of phenotypes selected to represent all or most HLA antigens do not provide an accurate assessment of the frequency with which positive crossmatches will occur. Even panels of individuals selected at random, unless they include a large number of individuals, are rarely representative of the donor population because of the high degree of HLA heterogeneity in all populations.[157] Finally, as noted above, PRA is a poor predictor of risk to graft outcome.

HLA specificity of antibodies may be the single most important type of information derived from serum screening tests. This information can be applied to: (1) determining the likelihood of a positive crossmatch;[158-161] (2) identifying safe and unsafe antigens;[162] (3) interpreting crossmatch results; and (4) preventing unnecessary shipment of organs and unnecessary crossmatch testing. Antibody specificity is crucial to evaluating the relevance of a positive crossmatch, particularly when the crossmatch procedure does not restrict positive reactions to HLA-specific antibodies.

Determination of antibody specificity, most frequently, is based on a statistically significant correlation between pattern of serum reactivity and the pattern of a particular HLA antigen in the panel.[134,163] Precise definition of antibody specificity may be affected by: (1) the presence of multiple antibodies; (2) the antigen composition and size of the panel of target phenotypes; (3) the way in which HLA antigens are defined; and (4) the targets used in the assay. When multiple antibodies are present, those antibodies specific for antigens present in higher numbers in the panel may mask the recognition of antibodies to less frequent antigens. This problem will be diminished, to some extent, by using panels that are large and have distinguishable patterns for all antigens. Testing sera at multiple dilutions may also enhance the ability to determine antibody specificities. When multiple antibodies are present, it is not uncommon for the different antibodies to have different titers. Then, by subtracting the specificities recognized at higher dilutions, it may be possible to define the specificity in the remaining positive reactions. Finally, absorption of the serum with cells from a single individual can assist in defining antibody specificities. It should be noted that tests of absorbed serum can be interpreted meaningfully only when tests of the serum use techniques that overcome the CYNAP phenomenon, such as the antiglobulin test, ELISA, and flow cytometry. Recognition of antibody specificity requires that the panel have antigen patterns that are clearly distinguishable. Linkage disequilibrium, the nonrandom association of alleles of linked loci, in the HLA system makes it difficult to achieve this goal. For example, individuals who have the B8 antigen frequently also have the A1 antigen. If this is true for all B8⁺ individuals in the panel, an antibody specific for B8 would always be masked by antibody to A1. Achieving distinguishable patterns even for the majority of HLA antigens requires using a panel comprised of multiple individuals (usually at least 50). Identification of antibody specificity can be facilitated by defining the panel according to known antigenic epitopes,[132,164,165] rather than by HLA antigen assignments. An antibody specific for a determinant common to all members of a crossreactive group may not achieve a correlation with each member of the group adequate to assign the multiple specificities, but may be readily recognized by a correlation with the common epitope.

The interpretation of test results may be affected by the targets used in the assay. If the targets are soluble HLA class I antigens, the test would fail to reveal the presence of antibody specific for class II. On the other hand, class II-specific antibodies might be mistaken for antibodies specific for class I antigens when the target cells include both T and B lymphocytes. In tests against B lymphocytes, class I-specific antibodies would give positive reactions unless these antibodies have been removed by platelet absorption. Finally, the interpretation of the results of serum screening tests should not be based solely on computer-assigned antibody specificities. Since most antibody screen protocols incorporate some compromises to accommodate time constraints, the need for cost containment, and personnel availability, a final interpretation of the results should utilize expert knowledge of the HLA system, familiarity with the patient's antibody history and previous sensitizing events, and an appreciation of the limitations of the test protocol.

B. Crossmatch Tests

Meaningful interpretation of crossmatch tests requires knowledge of the patient's antibody history, including HLA specificity and immunoglobulin isotype, an understanding of the risk factors represented by the crossmatch results, familiarity with technique used, information regarding recent events that may have affected sensitization and antibody specificity, knowledge of the level of acceptable risk, and an appreciation of the risk factors of the individual patient. Since no single technique has been shown to have a perfect correlation with transplant outcome, risk factors vary among patients, and treatment protocols vary among transplant programs, it would be presumptuous to attempt to dictate rules for interpreting the results of crossmatch tests. The laboratory scientist must assess the level of risk according to the information available to provide an interpretation to the clinical practitioner. The ability to interpret crossmatch results in a way that provides the clinician with useful information is what defines the expert in the field of histocompatibility.

REFERENCES

1. Williams, G.M., Hume, D.M., Hudson, R.P., Morris, P.J., Kano, K., and Milgrom, F., Hyperacute renal-homograft rejection in man, *N. Engl. J. Med.*, 279, 611, 1968.
2. Patel, R. and Terasaki, P.I., Significance of the positive cross match test in kidney transplantation, *N. Engl. J. Med.*, 280, 735, 1969.
3. Kissmeyer-Nielsen, F., Olsen, F., Peterson, V., and Fjeldborg, O., Hyperacute rejection of kidney allografts associated with preexisting humoral antibodies against donor cells, *Lancet*, 2, 662, 1966.
4. Federal Register, DHHS, HCFA, PHS (42CFR Part 493), February 28, 1992.
5. Iwaki, Y. and Terasaki, P.I., Sensitization effect, in *Clinical Transplants*, Terasaki, P.I., Ed., UCLA Tissue Typing Laboratory, Los Angeles, 1986, 257.
6. Opelz, G.,for the Collaborative Transplant Study, Effect of HLA matching, blood transfusion, and presensitzation in cyclosporine treated kidney transplant recipients, *Transplant. Proc.*, 17, 2179, 1985.
7. Iwaki, Y. and Terasaki, P.I., Effect of sensitization on kidney allografts, in *Clinical Kidney Transplants 1985*, Terasaki, P.I., Ed., UCLA Tissue Typing Laboratory, Los Angeles, 1985, 139.
8. Mjörnstedt, L., Konar, J., Nyberg, G., Olausson, M., Sandberg, L., and Karlberg, I., Renal transplantation in patients with lymphocytotoxic antibodies — a 5-year experience from a single centre, *Transplant. Proc.*, 24, 333, 1992.
9. Lavee, J., Kormos, R.L., Duquesnoy, R.J., Zerbe, T.R., Armitage, J.M., Vanek, M., Hardesty, R.L. and Griffith, B.P., Influence of panel-reactive antibody and lymphocytotoxic crossmatch on survival after heart transplantation, *J. Heart Lung Transplant.*, 10, 921, 1991.
10. McKenzie, F.N., Tadros, N., Stiller, C., Keown, P., Sinclair, N. and Kostuk, W., Influence of donor-recipient lymphocyte crossmatch and ABO status on rejection risk in cardiac transplantation, *Transplant. Proc.*, 19, 3439, 1987.
11. Zerbe, T.R., Arena, V.C., Kormos, R.L., Griffith, B.P., Hardesty, R.L., and Duquesnoy, R.J., Histocompatibility and other risk factors for histological rejection of human cardiac allografts during the first three months following transplantation, *Transplantation*, 52, 485, 1991.

12. McCloskey, D., Festenstein, H., Banner, N., Hawes, R., Holmes, J., Khaghani, A., Smith, J., and Yacoub, M., The effect of HLA lymphocytotoxic antibody status and crossmatch result on cardiac transplant survival, *Transplant. Proc.*, 21, 804, 1989.

13. Smith, J.D., Danskine, A.J., Rose, M.L., and Yacoub, M.H., Specificity of lymphocytotoxic antibodies formed after cardiac transplantation and correlation with rejection episodes, *Transplantation*, 53, 1358, 1992.

14. Smith, J.D., Danskine, A.J., Laylor, R.M., Rose, M.L., and Yacoub, M.H., The effect of panel reactive antibodies and the donor specific crossmatch on graft survival after heart and heart-lung transplantation, *Transplant Immunol.*, 1, 60, 1993.

15. Gordon, R.D., Fung, J.J., Markus, B., Fox, I., Iwatsuki, S., Esquivel, C.O., Tzakis, A., Todo, S., and Starzl, T.E., The antibody crossmatch in liver transplantation, *Surgery*, 100, 705, 1986.

16. Donaldson, P.T., Thomson, L.J., Heads, A., Underhill, J.A., Vaughan, R.W., Rolando, N., and Williams, R., IgG donor-specific crossmatches are not associated with graft rejection or poor graft survival after liver transplantation, *Transplantation*, 60, 1016, 1995.

17. Zachary, A.A., Klingman, L., Thorne, N., Smerglia, A.R., and Teresi, G.A., Variations of the lymphocytotoxicity test: an evaluation of sensitivity and specificity, *Transplantation*, 60, 498, 1995.

18. Garovoy, M.R., Rheinschmidt, M.A., and Bigos, M., Flow cytometry analysis: a high technology crossmatch technique facilitating transplantation, *Transplant. Proc.*, 15, 1939, 1983.

19. Bray, R.A., Flow cytometry in the transplant laboratory, *Ann. N.Y. Acad. Sci.*, 677, 138, 1996.

20. Bray, R.A., Lebeck, L.K., and Gebel, H.M., The flow cytometric crossmatch, *Transplantation*, 48, 834, 1989.

21. Gaston, R.S., Shroyer, T.W., Hudson, S.L., Deierhoi, M.H., Laskow, D.A., Barber, W.H., Julian, B.A., Curtis, J.J., Barger, B.O., and Diethelm, A.G., Renal retransplantation: the role of race, quadruple immunosuppression, and the flow cytometry cross-match, *Transplantation*, 57, 47, 1994.

22. Talbot, D., White, M., Shenton, B.K., Bell, A., Forsythe, J.L.R., Proud, G. and Taylor, R.M.R., Flow cytometric crossmatching in renal transplantation — the long term outcome, *Transplant. Immunol.*, 3, 352, 1995.

23. Kerman, R.H., Kimball, P.M., van Buren, C.T., Lewis, R.M., DeVera, V., Baghdahsarian, V., Heydari, A., and Kahan, B.D., AHG and DTE/AHG procedure identification of crossmatch-appropriate donor-recipient pairings that result in improved graft survival, *Transplantation*, 51, 316, 1991.

24. Martin, S., Liggett, H., Robson, A., Connolly, J., and Johnson, R.W., The association between a positive T and B cell flow cytometry crossmatch and renal transplant failure, *Transplant. Immunol.*, 1, 270, 1993.

25. Kerman, R.H., van Buren, C.T., Lewis, R.M., de Vera, V., Baghdahsarian, V., Gerolami, K., and Kahan, B.D., Improved graft survival for flow cytometry and antihuman globulin crossmatch-negative retransplant recipients, *Transplantation*, 49, 52, 1990.

26. Johnson, A., Hallman, J., Alijani, M.R., Melhorn, N., Lim, L.Y., Jenson, A.B., and Helfrich, G.B., A prospective study of the clinical relevance of the current serum antiglobulin-augmented T cell crossmatch in renal transplant recipients, *Transplant. Proc.*, 19, 792, 1987.

27. Sridhar, N.R., Munda, R., Balakrishnan, K., and First, M.R., Evaluation of flow cytometric crossmatching in renal allograft recipients, *Nephron*, 62, 262, 1992.

28. Cook, D.J., Terasaki, P.I., Iwaki, Y., Terashita, G.Y., and Lau, M., An approach to reducing early kidney transplant failure by flow cytometry crossmatching, *Clin. Transplant.*, 1, 253, 1987.

29. Ogura, K., Terasaki, P.I., Johnson, C., Mendez, R., Rosenthal, J.T., Ettenger, R., Martin, D.C., Dainko, E., Cohen, L., Mackett, T., Berne, T., Barba, L., and Lieberman, E., The significance of a positive flow cytometry crossmatch test in primary kidney transplantation, *Transplantation*, 56, 294, 1993.

30. Ogura, K., Koyama, H., Takemoto, S., Chia, J., Johnson, C. and Terasaki, P.I., Flow cytometry crossmatching for kidney transplantation, *Transplant. Proc.*, 25, 245, 1993.

31. Mahoney, R.J., Ault, K.A., Given, S.R., Adams, R.J., Breggia, A.C., Paris, P.A., Palomaki, G.E., Hitchcox, S.A., White, B.W., Himmelfarb, J., and Leeber, D.A., The flow cytometric crossmatch and early renal transplant loss, *Transplantation*, 49, 527, 1990.

32. Lazda, V.A., Pollak, R., Mozes, M.F., and Jonasson, O., The relationship between flow cytometer crossmatch results and subsequent rejection episodes in cadaver renal allograft recipients, *Transplantation*, 45, 562, 1988.

33. Stratta, R.J., Mason, B., Lorentzen, D.F., Sollinger, H.W., D'Alessandreo, A.M., Pirsch, J.D., Kalayoglu, M. and Belzer, F.O., Cadaveric renal transplantation with quadruple immunosuppression in patients with a positive antiglobulin crossmatch, *Transplantation*, 47, 282, 1989.

34. Ratkovec, R.M., Hammond, E.H., O'Connell, J.B., Bristow, M.R., DeWitt, C.W., Richenbacher, W.E., Millar, R.C., and Renlund, D.G., Outcome of cardiac transplant recipients with a positive donor-specific crossmatch — preliminary results with plasmapheresis, *Transplantation*, 54, 651, 1992.

35. Nikaein, A., Backman, L., Jennings, L., Levy, M.F., Goldstein, R., Gonwa, T., Stone, M.J., and Klintmalm, G., HLA compatibility and liver transplant outcome, *Transplantation*, 7, 786, 1994.

36. Demetris, A.J., Nakamura, K., Yagihashi, A., Iwaki, Y., Takaya, S., Hartman, G.G., Murase, N., Bronsther, O., Manez, R., Fung, J.J., and Starzl, T.E., A clinicopathological study of human liver allograft recipients harboring preformed IgG lymphocytotoxic antibodies, *Hepatology*, 16, 671, 1992.

37. Talbot, D., Bell, A., Shenton, B.K., Al Hussein, K., Manas, D., Gibbs, P., and Thick, M., The flow cytometric crossmatch in liver transplantation, *Transplantation*, 59, 737, 1995.

38. Ogura, K., Terasaki, P.I., Koyama, H., Chia, J., Imagawa, D.K., and Busuttil, R.W., High one-month liver graft failure rates in flow cytometry crossmatch-positive recipients, *Clin.Transplant.*, 8, 111, 1994.

39. Fenoglio, J., Ho, E., Reed, E., Rose, E., Smith, C., Reemstma, K., Marboe, C., and Suciu-Foca, N., Anti-HLA antibodies and heart allograft survival, *Transplant. Proc.*, 21, 807, 1989.

40. Takaya, S., Iwaki, Y., and Starzl, T.E., Liver transplantation in positive cytotoxic crossmatch cases using FK506, high-dose steroids, and prostaglandin E1, *Transplantation*, 54, 927, 1992.

41. Takaya, S., Duquesnoy, R., Iwaki, Y., Demetris, J., Yagihashi, A., Bronsther, O., Iwatsuki, S., and Starzl, T.E., Positive crossmatch in primary human liver allografts under cyclosporine or FK506 therapy, *Transplant. Proc.*, 23, 396, 1991.

42. Shenton, B.K., Glenville, B.E., Mitcheson, A.E., Coates, E., Talbot, D., Givan, A.L., Kirk, A., and Dark, J.H., Use of flow cytometric crossmatching in cardiac transplantation, *Transplant. Proc.*, 23, 1153, 1991.

43. Nakamura, K., Yagihashi, A., Iwaki, Y., Hartman, G.G., Murase, N., Bronsther, O., Manez, R., Fung, J.J., Iwatsuki, S., Starzl, T.E., and Demetris, A.J., The lymphocytotoxic crossmatch in liver transplantation: a clinicopathologic analysis, *Transplant. Proc.*, 23, 3021, 1991.

44. Weil, R.I., Clarke, D.R., Iwaki, Y., Porter, K.A., Koep, L.J., Paton, B.C., Terasaki, P.I., and Starzl, T.E., Hyperacute rejection of a transplanted human heart, *Transplantation*, 32, 71, 1981.

45. Batts, K.P., Moore, S.B., Perkins, J.D., Wiesner, R.H., Grambsch, P.M., and Krom, R.A.F., Influence of positive lymphocyte crossmatch and HLA mismatching on vanishing bile duct syndrome in human liver allografts, *Transplantation*, 45, 376, 1988.

46. Dafoe, D.C., Bromberg, J.S., Grossman, R.A., Tomaszewski, J.E., Zmijewski, C.M., Perloff, L.J., Naji, A., Asplund, M.W., Alfrey, E.J., Sack, M., Zellers, L., Kearns, J., and Barker, C.F., Renal transplantation despite a positive anti-globulin crossmatch with and without prophylactic OKT3, *Transplantation*, 51, 762, 1991.

47. Thistlethwaite, J.R.J., Heffron, T.G., Stevens, L., Buckingham, M., Stuart, J.K., and Stuart, F.P., The use of the T-cell flow cytometry crossmatch to evaluate the significance of positive B-cell serologic crossmatches in cadaveric donor renal transplantation, *Transplant. Proc.*, 22, 1897, 1990.

48. Kerman, R.H., Kimball, P., Scheinen, S., Radovancevic, B., van Buren, C.T., Kahan, B.D., and Frazier, O.H., The relationship among donor-recipient HLA mismatches, rejection, and death from coronary artery disease in cardiac transplant recipients, *Transplantation*, 57, 884, 1994.

49. Gordon, R.D., Fung, J.J., Iwatsuki, S., Duquesnoy, R.J., and Starzl, T.E., Immunological factors influencing liver graft survival, *Gastroenterol. Clin. North Am.*, 17, 53, 1988.

50. Iwatsuki, S., Ratsin, B.S., and Shaw, B.W.J., Liver transplantation against T cell-positive warm crossmatches, *Transplant. Proc.*, 16, 1427, 1984.

51. Lay, G., Schallon, D., Klein, A., Hopkins, K.A., Zachary, A.A., and Leffell, M.S.,The effect of HLA match and antibody on liver transplant outcome, *Human Immunol.*, 44 (S1), 110, 1995.

52. Ettenger, R.B., Uittenbogaart, C.H., Pennisi, A.J., Malekzadeh, M.H., and Fine, R.N., Long-term cadaver allograft survival in the recipient with a positive B lymphocyte crossmatch, *Transplantation*, 27, 315, 1979.

53. Jeannet, M., Benzonana, G., and Arni, I., Donor-specific B and T lymphocyte antibodies and kidney graft survival, *Transplantation*, 31, 160, 1981.

54. Schäfer, A.J., Hasert, K., and Opelz, G., for the Collaborative Transplant Study, Collaborative Transplant Study crossmatch and antibody project, *Transplant. Proc.*, 17, 2469, 1985.

55. Ayoub, G., Park, M.S., Terasaki, P.I., Iwaki, Y., and Opelz, G., B cell antibodies and crossmatching, *Transplantation*, 29, 227, 1980.

56. Lobo, P.I., Westervelt, J.F.B., and Rudolf, L., Kidney transplantation across positive B and T cell crossmatches, *Transplantation*, 26, 84, 1978.

57. D'Apice, A.J.F. and Tait, B.D., Improved survival and function of renal transplants with positive B cell crossmatches, *Transplantation*, 27, 324, 1979.

58. Noreen, H., van der Hagen, E., Bach, F.H., Fryd, D., Ascher, N., Simmons, R.L., and Najarian, J.S., Renal allograft survival in patients with positive donor-specific B lymphocyte crossmatches, *Transplant. Proc*, 19, 780, 1987.

59. Russ, G.R., Nicholls, C., Sheldon, A., and Hay, J., Positive B lymphocyte crossmatch and glomerular rejection in renal transplant recipients, *Transplant. Proc.*, 19, 785, 1987.

60. Lazda, V.A., Pollak, R., Mozes, M.F., and Jonasson, O., Positive B cell crossmatches in highly sensitized patients — influence of antibody specificity on renal transplant outcome, *Transplant. Proc*, 19, 782, 1987.

61. Lazda, V.A., Identification of patients at risk for inferior renal allograft outcome by a strongly positive B cell flow cytometry crossmatch, *Transplantation*, 57, 964, 1994.

62. Bunke, M., Ganzel, B., Klein, J.B., and Oldfather, J., The effect if a positive B cell crossmatch on early rejection in cardiac transplant recipients, *Transplantation*, 56, 758, 1993.

63. Taylor, C.J., Chapman, J.R., Ting, A., and Morris, P.J., Characterization of lympho-cytotoxic antibodies causing a positive crossmatch in renal transplantation, *Transplantation*, 48, 953, 1989.

64. Karuppan, S., Ohlman, S., and Möller, E., The occurrence of cytotoxic and non-complement-fixing antibodies in the crossmatch serum of patient with early acute rejection episodes, *Transplantation*, 54, 839, 1992.

65. Karuppan, S.S., Lindholm, A., and Möller, E., Fewer acute rejection episodes and improved outcome in kidney-transplanted patients with selection criteria based on crossmatching, *Transplantation*, 53, 666, 1992.

66. Wang, G.X., Terashita, G.Y., and Terasaki, P.I., Platelet crossmatching to kidney transplants by flow cytometry, *Transplantation*, 48, 959, 1989.

67. Chapman, J.R., Taylor, C.J., Ting, A., and Morris, P.J., Hyperacute rejection of a renal allograft in the presence of anti-HLA-Cw5 antibody, *Transplantation*, 42, 91, 1986.

68. Donaldson, P.T., Alexander, G.J.M., O'Grady, J.G., Neuberger, J., Portmann, B., Thick, M., Davis, M., and Calne, R.Y., Evidence for an immune response to HLA class I antigens in the vanishing bile duct syndrome after liver transplantation, *Lancet*, 1, 945, 1987.

69. Karuppan, S., Ericzon, B.G., and Möller, E., Relevance of a positive crossmatch in liver transplantation, *Transplant.Int.*, 4, 18, 1991.

70. Peltenberg, H.G., Tiebosch, A., and van den Berg-Loonen, P.M., A positive T cell crossmatch and accelerated acute rejection of a pancreas-spleen allograft, *Transplantation*, 53, 226, 1991.

71. Zachary, A.A., The technique and application of B cell crossmatches in renal trans-plantation, presented at the SEOPF Annu. Meeting, May 10, 1989, Savannah, GA.

72. Ahern, A.T., Artruc, S.B., DellaPelle, P., Cosimi, A.B., Russell, P.S., Colvin, R.B., and Fuller, T.C., Hyperacute rejection of HLA-AB-identical renal allorgrafts asso-ciated with B lymphocyte and endothelial reactive antibodies, *Transplantation*, 33, 103, 1982.

73. Berg, B. and Möller, E., Immediate rejection of a HLA-A,B compatible HLA-DR incompatible kidney with a positive donor-recipient B cell crossmatch, *Scand. J. Urol. Nephrol.*, 54, 36, 1980.

74. Braun, W.E., Dejelo, C., and Williams, T., B cell crossmatch in renal transplantation, *Lancet*, 2, 241, 1977.

75. Scornik, J.C., LeFor, W.M., Cicciarelli, J.C., Brunson, M.E., Bogaard, T., Howard, R.J., Ackermann, J.R.W., Mendez, R., Shires, D.L.J., and Pfaff, W.W., Hyperacute and acute kidney graft rejection due to antibodies against B cells, *Transplantation*, 54, 61, 1992.

76. Albrechtsen, D., Flatmark, A., and Jervell, J., Significance of HLA-D/DR matching in renal transplantation, *Lancet*, 1, 1126, 1978.

77. Mohanakumar, T., Rhodes, C., Mendez-Picon, G., Goldman, M., Moncore, C., and Lee, H., Renal allograft rejection associated with presensitization to HLA-DR antigens, *Transplantation*, 31, 93, 1981.

78. van Rood, J.J., Persijn, G.G., and van Leeuwen, A., A new strategy to improve kidney graft survival: the induction of CML nonresponsiveness, *Transplant. Proc.*, 11, 736, 1979.

79. Ten Hoor, G.M., Coopmans, M., and Allebes, W.A., Specificity and Ig class of preformed alloantibodies causing a positive crossmatch in renal transplantation, *Transplantation*, 56, 298, 1993.

80. Sirchia, G., Mercuriali, F., Scalamogna, M., Rosso di San Secondo, V., Pizzi, C., Poli, F., Fortis, C., and Greppi, N., Preexistent anti-HLA-DR antibodies and kidney graft survival, *Transplant. Proc.*, 11, 950, 1979.

81. Lederer, S.R., Schneeberger, H., Albert, E., Johnson, J.P., Gruber, R., Land, W., Burkhardt, K., Hillebrand, G., and Feucht, H.E., Early renal graft dysfunction, *Transplantation*, 61, 313, 1996.

82. Talbot, D., Cavanagh, G., Coates, E., Givan, A.L., Shenton, B.K., Lennard, T.W.J., Proud, G., and Taylor, R.M.R., Improved graft outcome and reduced complications due to flow cytometric crossmatching and DR matching in renal transplantation, *Transplantation*, 53, 925, 1992.

83. Katz, S.M., Kimball, P.M., Ozaki, C., Monsour, H., Clark, J., Cavazos, D., Kahan, B.D., Wood, R.P., and Kerman, R.H., Positive pretransplant crossmatches predict early graft loss in liver allograft recipients, *Transplantation*, 57, 616, 1994.

84. Barger, B., Shroyer, T.W., Hudson, S.L., Deierhoi, M.H., Barber, W.H., Curtis, J.J., Julian, B.A., Luke, R.G., and Diethelm, A.G., Successful renal allografts in recipients with crossmatch-positive, dithioerythritol-treated negative sera, *Transplantation*, 47, 240, 1989.

85. Cross, D.E., Greiner, R., and Whittier, F.C., Importance of the autocontrol crossmatch in human renal transplantation, *Transplantation*, 21, 307, 1976.

86. Reekers, P., Lucassen-Hermans, R., Koene, R.A.P. and Kunst, V.A.J.M., Autolymphocytotoxic antibodies and kidney transplantation, *Lancet*, 1, 1063, 1977.

87. Ting, A. and Morris, P.J., Renal transplantation and B-cell cross-matches with autoantibodies and alloantibodies, *Lancet*, 2, 1095, 1977.

88. Ting, A. and Morris, P.J., Successful transplantation with a positive T and B cell crossmatch due to autoreactive antibodies, *Tissue Antigens*, 21, 219, 1983.

89. Ettenger, R.B., Jordan, S.C., and Fine, R.N., Cadaver renal transplant outcome in recipients with autolymphocytotoxic antibodies, *Transplantation*, 35, 429, 1983.

90. Piazza, A., Torlone, N., Valeri, M., Paggi, E., Monaco, P.I., Provenzani, L., Tisone, G., Adorno, D., and Casciani, C.V., Antidonor-HLA antibodies and soluble HLA antigens after kidney transplantation, *Transplant. Proc.*, 25, 3279, 1993.

91. Koka, P., Anti-HLA antibodies: detection and effect on renal transplant function, *Transplant. Proc.*, 25, 243, 1993.

92. Koka, P., Chia, D., Terasaki, P.I., Chan, H., Chia, J., and Ozawa, M., The role of IgA anti-HLA class I antibodies in kidney transplant survival, *Transplantation*, 56, 207, 1993.

93. Cardella, C.J., Falk, J.A., Nicholson, M.J., Harding, M., and Cook, G.T., Successful renal transplantation in patients with T-cell reactivity to donor, *Lancet*, 2, 1240, 1982.

94. Cardella, C.J., Falk, J.A., Halloran, P., Robinette, M., Arbus, G., and Bear, R., Renal transplantation in patients with a positive crossmatch on non-current sera: long-term follow-up, *Transplant. Proc.*, 17, 626, 1985.

95. Goeken, N., for the ASHI Clinical Affairs Committee, Outcome of renal transplantation following a positive crossmatch with historical sera: the second analysis of the ASHI survey, *Transplant. Proc.*, 17, 2443, 1985.

96. Guerin, C., Pomier, G., Fleuru, H., Laverne, S., Le Petit, J.C., and Berthoux, F.C., Differential crossmatch in renal transplantation: allopositive historical crossmatch (B and/or T) but current T-cell negative crossmatch, *Transplant. Proc.*, 22, 2286, 1990.

97. Cristol, J.P., Mourad, G., Argiles, A., Seignalet, J., Iborra, F., Ramounau-Pigot, A., Chong, G., and Mion, C., Negative crossmatch on current sera and good HLA matching are the main requirements for renal transplantation in highly sensitized patients, *Transplant. Proc.*, 24, 2470, 1992.

98. Barger, B.O., Shroyer, T.W., Hudson, S.L., Deierhoi, M.H., Barber, W.H., Curtis, J.J., Julian, B.A., Luke, R.G., and Diethelm, A.G., Early graft loss in cyclosporine A-treated cadaveric renal allograft recipients receiving retransplants against previous mismatched HLA-A, -B, -DR donor antigens, *Transplant. Proc.*, 20, 170, 1988.

99. Chapman, J.R., Taylor, C.J., Ting, A., and Morris, P.J., Immunoglobulin class and specificity of antibodies causing positive T cell crossmatches: relationship to renal transplant outcome, *Transplantation*, 42, 608, 1986.

100. Wade, J.F. and Cardella, C., personal communication, 1996.

101. Halloran, P.F., Wadgymar, A., Ritchie, S., Falk, J., Solez, K., and Srinivasa, N.S., The significance of the anti-class I antibody response. I. Clincal and pathologic features of anti-class I-mediated rejection, *Transplantation*, 49, 85, 1990.

102. Halloran, P.F., Schlaut, J., Solez, K., and Srinivasa, N.S., The significance of the anti-class I response. II. Clinical and pathologic features of renal transplants with anti-class I-like antibody, *Transplantation*, 53, 50, 1992.

103. Barr, M.L., Cohen, D.J., Benvenisty, A.I., Hardy, M., Reemtsma, K., Rose, E.A., Marboe, C.C., D'Agati, V., Suciu-Foca, N., and Reed, E., Effect of anti-HLA antibodies on the long-term survival of heart and kidney allografts, *Transplant. Proc.*, 25, 262, 1993.

104. Al-Hussein, K.A., Shenton, B.K., Bell, A., Talbot, D., White, M.D., Clark, K.R., Rigg, K.M., Forsythe, J., Proud, G., and Taylor, R.M.R., Value of flow cytometric monitoring of posttransplant antibody status in renal transplantation, *Transplant. Proc.*, 25, 259, 1993.

105. Lobo, P.I., Spencer, C.E., Stevenson, W.C., and Pruett, T.L., Evidence demonstrating poor kidney graft survival when acute rejections are associated with IgG donor-specific lymphocytotoxin, *Transplantation*, 59, 357, 1995.

106. Scornik, J.C., Salomon, D.R., Lim, P.B., Howard, R.J., and Pfaff, W.W., Posttransplant antidonor antibodies and graft rejection. Evaluation by two-color flow cytometry, *Transplantation*, 47, 287, 1989.

107. Rose, E.A., Pepino, P., Barr, M.L., Smith, C.G., Ratner, A.J., Ho, E., and Berger, C., Relation of HLA antibodies and graft atherosclerosis in human cardiac allograft recipients, *J. Heart Lung Transplant.*, 11, S120, 1992.

108. George, J.F., Kirklin, J.K., Shroyer, T.W., Naftel, D.C., Bourge, R.C., McGiffin, D.C., White-Williams, C., and Noreuil, T., Utility of posttransplantation panel-reactive antibody measurements for the prediction of rejection frequency and survival of heart transplant recipients, *J. Heart Lung Transplant.*, 14, 856, 1995.

109. Manez, R., Kobayashi, M., Takaya, S., Bronsther, O., Kramer, D., Bonet, H., Iwaki, Y., Fung, J.J., Demetris, A.J., and Starzl, T.E., Humoral rejection associated with antidonor lymphocytotoxic antibodies following liver transplantation, *Transplant. Proc.*, 25, 888, 1993.

110. Schulman, L.L., Ho, E.K., Reed, E.F., McGregor, C., Smith, C.R., Rose, E.A., and Suciu-Foca, N.M., Immunologic monitoring in lung allograft recipients, *Transplantation*, 61, 252, 1996.

111. Suciu-Foca, N., Reed, E., D'Agati, V.D., Ho, E., Cohen, D.J., Benvenisty, A.I., McCabe, R., Brensilver, J.M., King, D.W., and Hardy, M.A., Soluble HLA antigens, anti-HLA antibodies, and antiidiotypic antibodies in the circulation of renal transplant recipients, *Transplantation*, 51, 593, 1991.

112. Hardy, M.A., Suciu-Foca, N., Reed, E., Benvenisty, A.I., Smith, C., Rose, E., and Reemstma, K., Immunomodulation of kidney and heart transplants by anti-idiotypic antibodies, *Ann. Surg.*, 214, 522, 1991.

113. Reed, E., Ho, E., Cohen, D.J., Ramey, W., Marboe, C., D'Agati, V., Rose, E.A., Hardy, M., and Suciu-Foca, N., Anti-idiotypic antibodies specific for HLA in heart and kidney allograft recipients, *Immunol. Res.*, 12, 1, 1993.

114. Ramounau-Pigot, A., Mourad, G., Cristol, J.P., Argiles, A., and Seignalet, J., Role of anti-idiotypic antibodies in sensitized patients awaiting renal transplantation, *Transplant. Proc.*, 24, 2496, 1992.

115. Rodey, G. and Phelan, D., Association of anti-idiotypic antibody with successful second transplant of a kidney sharing antigens with previously hyperacutely rejected first kidney, *Transplantation*, 49, 54, 1989.

116. Braun, W.E., Klingman, L., Stewart, R.W., Ratliff, N., Tubbs, R., Zachary, A.A., Teresi, G.A., Rincon, G., and Protiva, D., Two major serologic events in a successful cardiac transplant recipient — circumvention of hyperacute rejection despite a positive donor T lymphocyte crossmatch and late appearance of probable antiidiotypic antibody, *Transplantation*, 46, 153, 1988.

117. Wasfie, T., Reed, E., Suciu-Foca, N., and Hardy, M.A., Production of antiidiotypic antibodies in the rat: *in vitro* characterization of specificity and correlation with *in vivo* specific suppression of cardiac allograft immune reaction across major histocompatibility complex, *Surgery*, 108, 431, 1990.

118. Chauhan, B., Phelan, D.L., Marsh, J.W., and Mohanakumar, T., Characterization of antiidiotypic antibodies to donor HLA that develop after liver transplantation, *Transplantation*, 56, 443, 1993.

119. Steinmuller, D., Tissue-specific and tissue-restricted histocompatibility antigens, *Immunol. Today*, 5, 234, 1984.

120. Paul, L.C., van Es, L.A., van Rood, J.J., van Leeuwen, A., de la Riviere, A.B., and de Graeff, J., Antibodies directed against antigens on the endothelium of peritubular capillaries in patients with rejecting renal allografts, *Transplantation*, 27, 175, 1979.

121. Paul, L.C., Baldwin, W., and van Es, L., Vascular endothelial alloantigens in renal transplantation, *Transplantation*, 40, 117, 1985.

122. Cerilli, J., Clarke, J., Doolin, T., Cerilli, G., and Brasile, L., The significance of a donor-specific vessel crossmatch in renal transplantation, *Transplantation*, 46, 359, 1988.

123. Yard, B., Spruyt-Gerritse, M., Claas, F., Thorogood, J., Bruijn, J.A., Paape, M.E., Stein, S.Y., van Es, L.A., van Bockel, J.H., Kooymans-Coutinho, M., Daha, M.R., and van der Woude, F.J., The clinical significance of allospecific antibodies against endothelial cells detected with an antibody-dependent cellular cytotoxicity assay for vascular rejection and graft loss after renal transplantation, *Transplantation*, 55, 1287, 1993.

124. Leichter, H.E., Ettenger, R.B., Robertson, L., and Fine, R.N., Significance of the monocyte crossmatch in living-related transplantation, *Child. Nephrol. Urol.*, 10, 186, 1990.

125. Moraes, J.R.,Luo, Y.,Moraes, M.E., and Stastny, P., Clinical relevance of antibodies to non-HLA antigens in organ transplantation, in *Clinics in Laboratory Medicine*, W.B. Saunders, Philadelphia, 1991, 621.

126. Joyce, S., Flye, M.W., and Mohanakumar, T., Characterization of kidney cell-specific, non-major histocompatibility complex alloantigen using antibodies eluted from rejected human renal allografts, *Transplantation*, 46, 362, 1988.

127. Evans, P.R., Trickett, L.P., Gosney, A.R., Hodges, E., Shires, S., Wilson, P.J., MacIver, A.G., Gardner, B., Slapak, M., and Smith, J.L., Detection of kidney reactive antibodies at crossmatch in renal transplant recipients, *Transplantation*, 46, 844, 1988.

128. Dunn, M.J., Rose, M.L., Latif, N., Bradd, S., Lovegrove, C., Seymour, C., Pomerance, A., and Yacoub, M.H., Demonstration by Western blotting of antiheart antibodies before and after cardiac transplantation, *Transplantation*, 51, 806, 1991.

129. Bluestein, H.G., Zvaifler, N.J., Weisman, M.H., and Shapiro, R.F., Lymphocyte alteration by procainamide: relation to drug-induced lupus erythematosus syndrome, *Lancet*, 2, 816, 1979.

130. Scornik, J.C., Brunson, M.E., Howard, R.J., and Pfaff, W.W., Alloimmunization, memory, and the interpretation of crossmatch results for renal transplantation, *Transplantation*, 54, 389, 1992.

131. Zachary, A.A., Braun, W.E., and Murphy, N.M., unpublished data, 1981.

132. Fuller, T.C., Monitoring HLA alloimunization. Analysis of HLA alloantibodies in the serum of prospective transplant recipients, in *Clinics in Laboratory Medicine*, W.B. Saunders, Philadelphia, 1991, 551.

133. Rodey, G.E., Neylan, J.F., Whelchel, J.D., Revels, K.W., and Bray, R.A., Epitope specificity of class I alloantibodies. I. Frequency analysis of antibodies to private vs. public specificities in potential transplant recipients, *Human Immunol.*, 39, 272, 1994.

134. Duquesnoy, R.J., White, L.T., Fierst, J.W., Vanek, M., Banner, B.F., Iwaki, Y., and Starzl, T.E., Multiscreen serum analysis of highly sensitized renal dialysis patients for antibodies toward public and private class I HLA determinants, *Transplantation*, 50, 427, 1990.

135. Yunis, E.J.,Ward, F.E., and Amos, D.B., Observations of the CNAP phenomenon, in *Histocompatibility Testing 1970*, Terasaki, P.I., Ed., Williams & Wilkins, Baltimore, 1971, 352.

136. Shroyer, T.W., Deierhoi, M.H., Mink, C.A., Cagle, L.R., Hudson, S.L., Rhea, S.D., and Diethelm, A.G., A rapid flow cytometry assay for HLA antibody detection using a pooled cell panel covering 14 serological crossreacting groups, *Transplantation*, 59, 626, 1995.

137. Kao, K.J., Scornik, J.C., and Small, S.J., Enzyme-linked immunoassay for anti-HLA antibodies — an alternative to panel studies by lymphocytotoxicity, *Transplantation*, 55, 192, 1993.

138. Doxiadis, I., Westhoff, U., and Grosse-Wilde, H., Quantification of soluble HLA class I gene products by enzyme linked immunosorbent assay, *Blut*, 59, 449, 1989.

139. Shimizu, B., Sra, K., Ferrone, S., and Pouletty, P., sHLA-STAT class I, an ELISA for quantification of HLA antigens in serum, *Human Immunol.*, 32, 289, 1991.

140. Pouletty, C., Mercier, I., Glanville, L., Tomavo, N., Igoudin, L., Pouletty, P., and Buelow, R., Typing of a panel of soluble HLA class I antigens by ELISA, *Human Immunol.*, 40, 218, 1994.

141. Gelder, F.B., McDonald, J.C., Landreneau, M.D., McMillan, R.W. and Aultman, D.F., Identification, characterization, and quantitation of soluble HLA antigens in the circulation and peritoneal dialysate of renal patients, *Ann. Surg.*, 213, 591, 1991.

142. Buelow, R., Mercier, I., Glanville, L., Regan, J., Ellingson, L., Janda, G., Claas, F., Colombe, B., Gelder, F., Grosse-Wilde, H., Orosz, C., Westhoff, U., Voegeler, U., Monteiro, F., and Pouletty, P., Detection of panel reactive anti-HLA class I antibodies by enzyme-linked immunosorbent assay or lymphocytotoxicity: results of a blinded, controlled multicenter study, *Human Immunol.*, 44, 1, 1995.

143. Bryan, C.F., Baier, K.A., Fora-Ginter, F., Shield III, C.F., Warady, B.A., Aeder, M.I., Borkon, M., Estep, T.H., Forster, J., Landreneau, M.D., Luger, A.M., Nelson, P.W., Ross, G., and Pierce, G.E., Detection of HLA IgG antibodies by two enzyme-linked immunoassays, solubilized HLA class I and PRA-STAT, *Transplantation*, 60, 1588, 1995.

144. Zachary, A.A., Griffin, J., Lucas, D.P., Hart, J.M., and Leffell, M.S., Evaluation of HLA antibodies with the PRA-STAT test: an ELISA test using soluble HLA class I molecules, *Transplantation*, 60, 1600, 1995.

145. Lucas, D.P., Carruth, W., Leffell, M.S., and Zachary, A.A., Evaluation of the Quik-Screen HLA antibody screening system, *Human Immunol.*, 44 (S1), 132, 1995.

146. Lucas, D.P., Paparounis, M., Myers, L., Hart, J.M., and Zachary, A.A., Detection of HLA Class I-Specific Antibodies by the QuikScreen™ ELISA Test, submitted to *Clin. Lab. Immunol.*, 1996.

147. Jacobbi, L.M., Guidelines for specimen collection, storage, and transportation, in *ASHI Laboratory Manual*, 3rd ed., Phelan D.L., Mickelson E.M., Noreen H.S., Shroyer T.W., Cluff D.M., and Nikaein A., Eds., ASHI, Lenexa, KS, 1993, I.A.1.1.

148. Buelow, R., Chiang, T., Monteiro, F., Cornejo, M.C., Ellingson, L., Claas, F., Gaber, O., Gelder, F., Kotb, M., Orosz, C., and Pouletty, P., Soluble HLA antigens and ELISA — a new technology for crossmatch testing, *Transplantation*, 60, 1594, 1995.

149. Sumitran-Karuppan, S. and Möller, E., Specific inhibition of HLA class I and II antibodies by soluble antigens — a method for the identification of antibody specificity in sera from alloimmunized individuals, *Transplantation*, 58, 713, 1994.

150. Olson, P.R., Weiben, J., and O'Leary, J.J., A simple technique for the inactivation of IgM antibodies using dithiothreitol, *Vox Sanguinis*, 30, 149, 1976.

151. Thorne, N., Klingman, L.L., Teresi, G.A., and Cook, D.J., Effects of heat inactivation and DTT treatment of serum on immunoglobulin binding, *Human Immunol.*, 37 (S1), 123, 1993.

152. Lepage, V., Degos, L., and Dausset, J., A "natural" anti-HLA-A2 antibody reacting with homozygous cells, *Tissue Antigens*, 8, 139, 1976.

153. Zachary, A.A., unpublished data, 1990.

154. Braun, W.E., Paganini, E.P., and Zachary, A.A., Potential impact of recombinant erythropoietin (Epo) on patient sensitization, in *Visuals of the Clinical Histocompatibility Workshop*, Terasaki, P., Ed., One Lambda, Inc., Los Angeles, 1989, 16.

155. Paganini, E.P., Braun, W.E., Latham, D., and Abdulhadi, M.H., Renal transplantation: results in hemodialysis patients previously treated with recombinant human erythropoietin, *ASAIO Transactions*, 35, 535, 1989.

156. Phelan, D.L., Hibbett, S., Wetter, L., Hanto, D.W., and Mohanakumar, T. Recombinant erythropoietin: does it really effect sensitization?, *Transplant. Proc.*, 23, 409, 1991.

157. Leffell, M.S., Steinberg, A.G., Bias, W.B., Machan, C.H., and Zachary, A.A., The distribution of HLA antigens and phenotypes among donors and patients in the UNOS registry, *Transplantation*, 58, 1119, 1994.

158. Zachary, A.A. and Braun, W.E., Calculation of a predictive value for transplantation. *Transplantation*, 39, 316, 1985.

159. Zachary, A.A. and Steinberg, A.G., Statistical analysis of HLA population data, in *Manual of Clinical Laboratory Immunology*, 5th ed., Rose, N.L., Ed., American Society for Microbiology, Washington, D.C., 1996, in press.

160. Claas, F.H.J., de Waal, L.P., Beelen, J., Reekers, P., Berg-Loonen, P.V.D., de Gast, E.,D'Amaro, J., Persijn, G.G., Zantvoort, F., and van Rood, J.J., Transplantation of highly sensitized patients on the basis of acceptable HLA-A and B mismatches, in *Clinical Transplants 1989*, Terasaki, P. Ed., UCLA Tissue Typing Laboratory, Los Angeles, 1989, 185.

161. Oldfather, J.W., Anderson, C.B., Phelan, D.L., Cross, D.E., Luger, A.M., and Rodey, G.E., Prediction of crossmatch outcome in highly sensitized dialysis patients based on the identification of serum HLA antibodies, *Transplantation*, 42, 267, 1986.

162. Thompson, J.S., Bryne, J.E., Hempel, H.O., Oldfather, J.W., Green, W.F., Crow, D.O., Sanfilippo, F., MacQueen, J.M., McCalmon, R.N., and Helman, S.W., Computer algorithm that predicts both acceptable and unacceptable private and public HLA class I antigens in highly sensitized patients, *Transplant. Proc.*, 25, 251, 1993.

163. Zachary, A.A., Murphy, N.B., Smerglia, A.R., and Braun, W.E., Screening sera for HLA antibodies, in *Manual of Clinical Laboratory Immunology*, 3rd ed., Rose N.R., Friedman H., and Fahey J.L., Eds., American Society for Microbiology, Washington, D.C. 1986, 824.

164. Laundy, G.J. and Bradley, B.A., The predictive value of epitope analysis in highly sensitized patients awaiting renal transplantation, *Transplantation*, 59, 1207, 1995.

165. Duquesnoy, R.J., White, L.T., Iwaki, Y., and Vanek, M., Multiscreen analysis of high PRA sera for antibodies towards public and private class I antigens: implication for computer-predicted acceptable donors for kidney transplant candidates, *Transplant. Proc.*, 23, 387, 1991.

166. Phelan, D.L., Micleelson, E.M., Noreen, H.S., Shroger, T.W., Cluff, D.M., and Nikaein, A., Eds., *ASHI Laboratory Manual*, 3rd ed., ASHI, Lenexa, KS, 1993.

167. Tardiff, G.N. and MacQueen, J.M., Eds., *Tissue Typing Reference Manual*, South-Eastern Organ Procurement Foundation, Richmond, VA, 1993.

Chapter **13**

DNA-BASED TYPING OF HLA FOR TRANSPLANTATION

Carolyn Katovich Hurley

CONTENTS

Each individual expresses six different HLA molecules, HLA-A, -B, -C (class I molecules), -DR, -DQ, and -DP (class II molecules). These molecules are encoded by the most polymorphic genetic loci yet known in man.[1] The large number of HLA alleles found in the human population is thought to be maintained because the HLA molecules are used by the cells of the immune system to discriminate between self and nonself.

I. HLA GENES

The genes (or loci) encoding one chain of the HLA class I molecules (the heavy chain) and both chains (alpha and beta) of the HLA class II molecules are clustered in one region of human chromosome 6, termed the major histocompatibility complex (MHC) (Figure 1). The products of the A, B, and C loci associate with the product of the β-2 microglobulin locus to form the class I molecules (Figure 2A). The products of alpha (A) and beta (B) loci of DR, DQ, and DP associate with one another to form the class II molecules (Figure 3A). For example, the product of the DQB1 locus, the DQ beta chain, associates with the product of the DQA1 locus, the DQ α chain, to form a DQ molecule.

At the DNA level, the HLA loci have multiple alternate forms (alleles). Tables 1 through 3 list the alleles of the class I heavy chain loci. β-2 Microglobulin is not polymorphic. Alleles of the A and B loci of the class II molecules are listed in Tables 4 through 6. Each individual carries two copies, that is, two alleles, of each locus. The total number of alleles present in the entire human population at each locus differs.[2] For example, there have been over 100 alleles described at the DRB1 locus, but only two alleles described for the DRA locus (Table 4). Thus, each individual carries a limited set of HLA alleles (e.g., 2 HLA-A locus alleles, 2 HLA-B locus alleles, 2 HLA-C locus alleles, etc.), while the entire population carries a very diverse and extensive collection of HLA alleles. This is in contrast to immunoglobulin and T-cell receptor diversity

HUMAN MHC
HLA

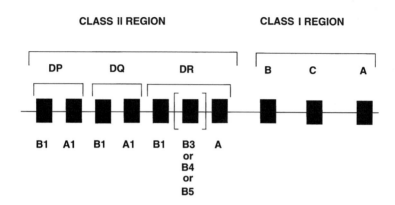

Figure 1

A diagram of the human major histocompatibility gene complex (MHC) on chromosome 6, showing the loci encoding the HLA class I and class II molecules. The class I loci, A, B, and C, encode the heavy chains of the three class I molecules, HLA-A, HLA-B, and HLA-C. Within the class II region, the A and Al loci encode the class II α chains, while the B1, B3, B4, and B5 loci encode the class II beta chains. The DRB3, DRB4, and DRB5 loci are in brackets to indicate that not all HLA gene complexes contain these loci. This will be described in Figure 7. The HLA gene complex on chromosome 6 is termed a "haplotype." Each individual carries two copies of chromosome 6 and, hence, two HLA haplotypes.

in which a single individual can generate an enormous and diverse array of antigen receptors by recombining gene segments and by somatic mutation. Because many HLA alleles exist in the population, most outbred individuals carry two different alleles at a locus and are heterozygous. Individuals who carry two identical alleles at a locus are homozygous for that locus.

Each HLA allele is designated by the name of the locus (Figure 2B, 3B) followed by an asterisk and a number indicating the allele. For example, A*0201 is an allele of the HLA-A locus, while DQA1*0601 is an allele of the HLA-DQ α chain locus. The first two numbers in the numerical designation of each allele are often based on the serologic type of the resultant protein (allelic product) (discussed below) and/or the structural similarity to other alleles. For example, the HLA-A molecule encoded by the A*0201 allele bears the A2 serological specificity. As a second example, the DRB1*0103 allele bears structural similarity to alleles encoding molecules bearing the DR1 serological specificity (e.g., DRB1*0101); however, the DR molecule encoded by DRB1*0103 is not typed as DR1 serologically. The last two numbers in the allele designation refer to the order in which the gene sequence

CLASS I REGION

A.

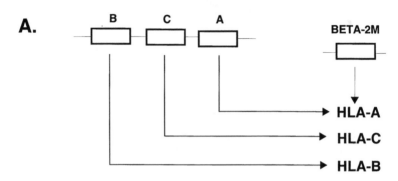

B.

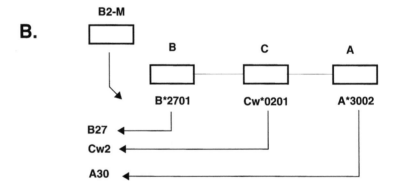

Figure 2

(A) A diagram of the region of the MHC which encodes one of the two polypeptide chains of the HLA-A, -B, and -C molecules. β-2 Microglobulin, which forms the remainder of each HLA molecule, is encoded on another chromosome. (B) An example of the alleles that might be carried at each class I locus on one haplotype of an individual. The alleles, A*3002, B*2701, Cw*0201 encode heavy chains which associate with β-2 microglobulin. The three class I molecules expressed, A30(19), B27, and Cw2, are identified using alloantisera described in a later section.

was determined. For example, A*0201 was the first HLA-A2 allele to be sequenced and A*0202 was the second. New alleles are described in yearly reports of the World Health Organization (WHO) HLA nomenclature committee.[2,4]

CLASS II REGION

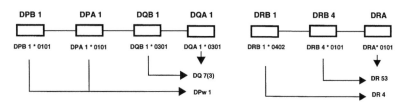

Figure 3

(A) A diagram of the region of the MHC which encodes the HLA class II molecules. The alpha chains encoded by the DRA, DQA1, and DPA1 loci associate with beta chains encoded by the DRB1, DQB1, and DPB1 loci, respectively. Individuals may differ in the number of DR beta chain loci within each haplotype. If a second DR beta chain locus is present (i.e., , either DRB3, DRB4, or DRB5), the beta chain encoded by that locus will associate with the product of the DRA locus to form a second, expressed DR molecule. The MHC also contains nonfunctional loci (pseudogenes) which do not encode HLA molecules and loci which encode HLA molecules, expressed in specific tissues at specific times. These loci (e.g., HLA-G, -DRB2, -DQB2, -DPA2, -DPB2) are not considered in matching for transplantation. (B) An example of the alleles that might be carried at each class II locus on a haplotype of an individual. The allele, DRB1*0402, encodes a beta chain which associates with the α chain encoded by the DRA locus to form a DR molecule which is identified using alloantisera as DR4 (serologic types are described below). The allele, DRB4*0101, encodes a beta chain which associates with the α chain encoded by the DRA locus to form a DR molecule identified using alloantisera as DR53. Thus, this individual expresses both DR4 and DR53 molecules. The allele, DQB1*0301, encodes a beta chain which associates with the α chain encoded by the DQA1*0301 allele to form a DQ molecule identified using alloantisera as DQ7(3). The allele, DPB1*0101, encodes a beta chain which associates with the α chain encoded by the DPA1*0101 allele to form a DPw1 molecule. Alloantisera defining DP molecules are rare. The frequency of association between different alleles such as DQA1*0301 and DQB1*0301 in the human population is discussed in Tables 10 through 14.

TABLE 1

HLA-A Alleles and Their Serologic Designation[a,b]

HLA Alleles	Serologic Specificity
A*0101	A1
A*0102	A1
A*0201	A2
A*0202	A2
A*0203	A203
A*0204	A2
A*0205	A2
A*0206	A2
A*0207	A2
A*0208	A2
A*0209	A2
A*0210	A210
A*0211	A2
A*0212	A2
A*0213	A2
A*0301	A3
A*0302	A3
A*1101	A11
A*1102	A11
A*2301	A23(9)[c]
A*2401	A24(9)
A*2402	A24(9)
A*2403	A2403
A*2501	A25(10)
A*2601	A26(10)
A*2602	A26(10)
A*2603	A26(10)
A*2604	A26(10)
A*2901	A29(19)
A*2902	A29(19)
A*3001	A30(19)
A*3002	A30(19)
A*3003	A30(19)
A*31011[d]	A31(19)
A*31012	A31(19)
A*3201	A32(19)
A*3301	A33(19)
A*3302	A33(19)
A*3401	A34(10)
A*3402	A34(10)
A*3601	A36
A*4301	A43
A*6601	A66(10)
A*6602	A66(10)
A*68011	A68(28)
A*68012	A68(28)
A*6802	A68(28)
A*6901	A69(28)
A*7401	A74(19)
A*8001	Not defined[e]

TABLE 1 (continued)

HLA-A Alleles and Their Serologic Designation[a,b]

---

a   It is likely that the number of HLA-A alleles will in-
    crease as more individuals are studied. Alleles are
    defined by DNA sequencing. An annual summary of
    allele sequences is published in *Human Immunology,
    Tissue Antigens,* and *Immunogenetics.*
b   Each row in the table lists an HLA-A allele and the
    associated serologic specificity. For example, individ-
    uals carrying the A*0101 allele are serologically typed
    as A1.
c   The number in () defines the broad serologic specific-
    ity. This is described in Table 8.
d   The fifth digit indicates a nucleotide change that cre-
    ates a new allele but does not change the protein se-
    quence of the molecule. These differences are not
    considered important for transplantation matching.
e   The HLA-A molecule encoded by this allele has not
    yet received a WHO nomenclature assignment.

From Bodmer, J. G. et al., *Tissue Antigens,* 44, 1, 1994.
Published with permission of Munksgaard International
Publishers Ltd., Copenhagen, Denmark.

TABLE 2

HLA-B Alleles and Their Serologic Designation[a,b]

HLA Alleles	Serologic Specificity
B*0701	B7
B*0702	B7
B*0703	B703
B*0704	B7
B*0801	B8
B*1301	B13
B*1302	B13
B*1401	B14
B*1402	B65(14)[c]
B*1501	B62(15)
B*1502	B75(15)
B*1503	B72(70)
B*1504	B62(15)
B*1505	B62(15)
B*1506	B62(15)
B*1507	B62(15)
B*1508	B62(15)
B*1509	B70
B*1510	B71(70)
B*1511	B15
B*1512	B76(15)
B*1513	B77(15)
B*1514	B76(15)
B*1515	B62(15)

TABLE 2 (continued)

HLA-B Alleles and Their Serologic Designation[a,b]

HLA Alleles	Serologic Specificity
B*1516	B63(15)
B*1517	B63(15)
B*1518	Not defined[d]
B*1519	B76(15)
B*1520	B62(15)
B*1801	B18
B*1802	B18
B*2701	B27
B*2702	B27
B*2703	B27
B*2704	B27
B*27051[e]	B27
B*27052	B27
B*2706	B27
B*2707	B27
B*2708	Not defined
B*3501	B35
B*3502	B35
B*3503	B35
B*3504	B35
B*3505	B35
B*3506	B35
B*3507	B35
B*3508	B35
B*3701	B37
B*3801	B38(16)
B*3802	B38(16)
B*39011	B3901
B*39013	B3901
B*39021	B3902
B*39022	B3902
B*3903	B39(16)
B*3904	B39(16)
B*40011	B60(40)
B*40012	B60(40)
B*4002	B40
B*4003	B40
B*4004	B40
B*4005	B4005
B*4006	B61(40)
B*4101	B41
B*4201	B42
B*4401	B44(12)
B*4402	B44(12)
B*4403	B44(12)
B*4404	B44(12)
B*4501	B45(12)
B*4601	B46
B*4701	B47

TABLE 2 (continued)

HLA-B Alleles and Their Serologic Designation[a,b]

HLA Alleles	Serologic Specificity
B*4801	B48
B*4802	B48
B*4901	B49(21)
B*5001	B50(21)
B*5101	B51(5)
B*5102	B5102
B*5103	B5103
B*5104	B51(5)
B*5105	B51(5)
B*52011	B52(5)
B*52012	B52(5)
B*5301	B53
B*5401	B54(22)
B*5501	B55(22)
B*5502	B55(22)
B*5601	B56(22)
B*5602	B56(22)
B*5701	B57(17)
B*5702	B57(17)
B*5801	B58(17)
B*5901	B59
B*6701	B67
B*7301	B73
B*7801	B7801
B*7901[f]	Renamed as B*1518

[a] It is likely that the number of HLA-B alleles will increase as more individuals are studied. Alleles are defined by DNA sequencing. An annual summary of allele sequences is published in *Human Immunology, Tissue Antigens,* and *Immunogenetics.*

[b] Each row in the table lists the HLA-B allele and its associated serologic specificity or antigen. For example, individuals who carry a B*0701 allele are serologically typed as B7.

[c] The number in () defines the broad serologic specificity. This is described in Table 8.

[d] The HLA-B molecule encoded by this allele is not identified by a serologic reagent.

[e] The fifth digit indicates a nucleotide change that creates a new allele but does not change the protein sequence. These differences are not considered important for transplantation matching.

[f] This designation is no longer valid. The allele has been renamed as B*1518.

From Bodmer, J. G. et al., *Tissue Antigens,* 44, 1, 1994. Published with permission of Munksgaard International Publishers Ltd., Copenhagen, Denmark.

TABLE 3

HLA-C Alleles and Their Serologic Designation[a,b]

HLA Alleles	Serologic Specificity
Cw*0101	Cw1
Cw*0102	Cw1
Cw*0201	Cw2
Cw*02021[c]	Cw2
Cw*02022	Cw2
Cw*0301	Cw3
Cw*0302	Cw3
Cw*0303	Cw3
Cw*0304	Cw3
Cw*0401	Cw4
Cw*0402	Cw4
Cw*0501	Cw5
Cw*0601	Cw6
Cw*0602	Cw6
Cw*0701	Cw7
Cw*0702	Cw7
Cw*0703	Cw7
Cw*0801	Cw8
Cw*0802	Cw8
Cw*0803	Cw8
Cw*1201	Not defined[d]
Cw*12021	Not defined
Cw*12022	Not defined
Cw*1203	Not defined
Cw*1301	Not defined
Cw*1401	Not defined
Cw*1402	Not defined
Cw*1501	Not defined
Cw*1502	Not defined
Cw*1503	Not defined
Cw*1504	Not defined
Cw*1601	Not defined
Cw*1602	Not defined
Cw*1701	Not defined

[a] It is likely that the number of HLA-C alleles will increase as more individuals are studied. Alleles are defined by DNA sequencing. An annual summary of allele sequences is published in *Human Immunology, Tissue Antigens*, and *Immunogenetics*.

[b] Each row in the table lists the HLA-C allele and its associated serologic specificity. For example, individuals who carry a Cw*0101 allele are serologically typed as Cw1.

[c] The fifth digit indicates a nucleotide change that creates a new allele but does not change the protein sequence of the antigen. These differences are not considered important for transplantation matching.

[d] The HLA-C molecule encoded by this allele is not defined by a serologic reagent.

From Bodmer, J. G. et al., *Tissue Antigens*, 44, 1, 1994. Published with permission of Munksgaard International Publishers Ltd., Copenhagen, Denmark.

TABLE 4

HLA-DR Alleles and Their Serologic Designation[a,b]

HLA Alleles	Serologic Specificity
DRA*0101[c]	Not defined[d]
DRA*0102	Not defined
DRB1*0101[e]	DR1
DRB1*0102	DR1
DRB1*0103	DR103
DRB1*0104	DR1
DRB1*1501	DR15(2)[f]
DRB1*15021[g]	DR15(2)
DRB1*15022	DR15(2)
DRB1*1503	DR15(2)
DRB1*1504	DR15(2)
DRB1*1601	DR16(2)
DRB1*1602	DR16(2)
DRB1*1603	Not defined
DRB1*1604	DR16(2)
DRB1*1605	Not defined
DRB1*1606	DR2
DRB1*03011	DR17(3)
DRB1*03012	DR17(3)
DRB1*0302	DR18(3)
DRB1*0303	DR18(3)
DRB1*0304	DR3
DRB1*0401	DR4
DRB1*0402	DR4
DRB1*0403	DR4
DRB1*0404	DR4
DRB1*0405	DR4
DRB1*0406	DR4
DRB1*0407	DR4
DRB1*0408	DR4
DRB1*0409	DR4
DRB1*0410	DR4
DRB1*0411	DR4
DRB1*0412	DR4
DRB1*0413	DR4
DRB1*0414	DR4
DRB1*0415	DR4
DRB1*0416	DR4
DRB1*0417	DR4
DRB1*0418	DR4
DRB1*0419	DR4
DRB1*11011	DR11(5)
DRB1*11012	DR11(5)
DRB1*1102	DR11(5)
DRB1*1103	DR11(5)
DRB1*11041	DR11(5)
DRB1*11042	DR11(5)
DRB1*1105	DR11(5)
DRB1*1106	DR11(5)

TABLE 4 (continued)

HLA-DR Alleles and Their Serologic Designation[a,b]

HLA Alleles	Serologic Specificity
DRB1*1107	Not defined
DRB1*11081	DR11(5)
DRB1*11082	DR11(5)
DRB1*1109	DR11(5)
DRB1*1110	Not defined
DRB1*1111	Not defined
DRB1*1112	Not defined
DRB1*1113	Not defined
DRB1*1201	DR12(5)
DRB1*1202	DR12(5)
DRB1*1203	DR12(5)
DRB1*1301	DR13(6)
DRB1*1302	DR13(6)
DRB1*1303	DR13(6)
DRB1*1304	DR13(6)
DRB1*1305	DR13(6)
DRB1*1306	DR13(6)
DRB1*1307	Not defined
DRB1*1308	DR13(6)
DRB1*1309	Not defined
DRB1*1310	DR13(6)
DRB1*1311	DR13(6)
DRB1*1312	Not defined
DRB1*1313	Not defined
DRB1*1401	DR14(6)
DRB1*1402	DR14(6)
DRB1*1403	DR1403
DRB1*1404	DR1404
DRB1*1405	DR14(6)
DRB1*1406	DR14(6)
DRB1*1407	DR14(6)
DRB1*1408	DR14(6)
DRB1*1409	DR14(6)
DRB1*1410	Not defined
DRB1*1411	Not defined
DRB1*1412	Not defined
DRB1*1413	Not defined
DRB1*1414	Not defined
DRB1*1415	Not defined
DRB1*1416	Not defined
DRB1*1417	Not defined
DRB1*0701	DR7
DRB1*0801	DR8
DRB1*08021	DR8
DRB1*08022	DR8
DRB1*08031	DR8
DRB1*08032	DR8
DRB1*08041	DR8
DRB1*08042	DR8

TABLE 4 (continued)

HLA-DR Alleles and Their Serologic Designation[a,b]

HLA Alleles	Serologic Specificity
DRB1*0805	DR8
DRB1*0806	DR8
DRB1*0807	DR8
DRB1*0808	DR8
DRB1*0809	DR8
DRB1*0810	DR8
DRB1*0811	DR8
DRB1*09011	DR9
DRB1*09012	DR9
DRB1*1001	DR10
DRB3*0101[h]	DR52
DRB3*0201	DR52
DRB3*0202	DR52
DRB3*0301	DR52
DRB4*01011[i]	DR53
DRB4*01012N[j]	Not expressed
DRB4*0102	DR53
DRB4*0103	DR53
DRB5*0101[k]	DR51
DRB5*0102	DR51
DRB5*0201	DR51
DRB5*0202	DR51
DRB5*0203	DR51

[a] It is likely that the number of HLA-DR alleles will increase as more individuals are studied. Alleles are defined by DNA sequencing. An annual summary of allele sequences is published in *Human Immunology, Tissue Antigens*, and *Immunogenetics*.

[b] Each row in the table lists the DR allele and its associated serologic specificity. For example, individuals who carry a DRB1*0101 allele are serologically typed as DR1.

[c] Alleles of the DRA locus. The differences between these DR alpha chain alleles are not considered important for transplantation matching. The associations of specific DRA alleles with specific DRB1 alleles are described by Kimura et al.[3]

[d] "Not defined" indicates an allele which is not defined by serologic reagents.

[e] Alleles of the DRB1 locus. Every haplotype described to date contains a DRB1 locus.

[f] The number in ( ) defines the broad serologic specificity. This is described in Table 8.

[g] The fifth digit indicates a nucleotide change that creates a new allele but does not change the protein sequence of the molecule. These differences are not considered important for transplantation matching.

[h] Alleles of the DRB3 locus, the second expressed DR molecule in haplotypes encoding DR17(3), DR18(3), DR11(5), DR12(5), DR13(6), and DR14(6). See Figure 7 for further discussion.

[i] Alleles of the DRB4 locus, the second expressed DR molecule in haplotypes encoding DR4, DR7, and DR9. See Figure 7 for further discussion.

[j] N indicates a null allele which does not encode a DR53 molecule.

[k] Alleles of the DRB5 locus, the second expressed DR molecule in haplotypes encoding DR15(2) and DR16(2). This second molecule is sometimes termed DR51. See Figure 7 for further discussion.

From Bodmer, J. G. et al., *Tissue Antigens*, 44, 1, 1994. Published with permission of Munksgaard International Publishers Ltd., Copenhagen, Denmark.

TABLE 5

HLA-DQ Alleles and Their Serologic Designation[a,b]

HLA Alleles	Serologic Specificity
DQA1*0101[c]	Not defined[d]
DQA1*0102	Not defined
DQA1*0103	Not defined
DQA1*0104	Not defined
DQA1*0201	Not defined
DQA1*03011[e]	Not defined
DQA1*03012	Not defined
DQA1*0302	Not defined
DQA1*0401	Not defined
DQA1*0501	Not defined
DQA1*05011	Not defined
DQA1*05012	Not defined
DQA1*05013	Not defined
DQA1*0502	Not defined
DQA1*0601	Not defined
DQB1*0501[f]	DQ5(1)[g]
DQB1*0502	DQ5(1)
DQB1*05031	DQ5(1)
DQB1*05032	DQ5(1)
DQB1*0504	Not defined[h]
DQB1*06011	DQ6(1)
DQB1*06012	DQ6(1)
DQB1*0602	DQ6(1)
DQB1*0603	DQ6(1)
DQB1*0604	DQ6(1)
DQB1*06051	DQ6(1)
DQB1*06052	DQ6(1)
DQB1*0606	Not defined
DQB1*0607	Not defined
DQB1*0608	Not defined
DQB1*0609	Not defined
DQB1*0201	DQ2
DQB1*0202	DQ2
DQB1*0301	DQ7(3)
DQB1*0302	DQ8(3)
DQB1*03031	DQ9(3)
DQB1*03032	DQ9(3)
DQB1*0304	DQ7(3)
DQB1*0305	Not defined
DQB1*0401	DQ4
DQB1*0402	DQ4

[a] It is likely that the number of HLA-DQ alleles will increase as more individuals are studied. Alleles are defined by DNA sequencing. An annual summary of allele
sequences is published in *Human Immunology, Tissue Antigens,* and *Immunogenetics.*

[b] Each row in the table lists a DQ allele and its associated
serologic specificity. For example, individuals who carry
a DQB1*0501 allele are serologically typed as DQ5(1).

TABLE 5

HLA-DQ Alleles and Their Serologic Designation[a,b]

c	Allele of the DQA1 locus which encodes the DQ alpha chain.
d	While it is likely that serologic reagents define a DQ alpha/DQ beta chain combination, it is thought that the DQ beta chain is the major contributor to the serologic type.
e	The fifth digit indicates a nucleotide change that creates a new allele but does not change the protein sequence of the molecule. These differences are not considered important for transplantation matching.
f	Allele of the DQB1 locus which encodes the DQ beta chain.
g	The number in () defines the broad serologic specificity. This is described in Table 8.
h	"Not defined" indicates a DQB1 allele which is not defined by serologic reagents.

From Bodmer J. G. et al., *Tissue Antigens,* 44, 1, 1994. Published with permission of Munksgaard International Publishers Ltd., Copenhagen, Denmark.

TABLE 6

HLA-DP Alleles and Their Cellular Designation[a,b]

HLA Alleles	Cellular Specificity[c]
DPA1*0101[d]	Not defined[e]
DPA1*0102	Not defined
DPA1*0103	Not defined
DPA1*0201	Not defined
DPA1*02021[f]	Not defined
DPA1*02022	Not defined
DPA1*0301	Not defined
DPA1*0401	Not defined
DPB1*01011[g]	DPw1
DPB1*01012	DPw1
DPB1*0201	DPw2
DPB1*02011	DPw2
DPB1*02012	DPw2
DPB1*0202	DPw2
DPB1*0301	DPw3
DPB1*0401	DPw4
DPB1*0402	DPw4
DPB1*0501	DPw5
DPB1*0601	DPw6
DPB1*0801	Not defined
DPB1*0901	Not defined
DPB1*1001	Not defined
DPB1*11011	Not defined
DPB1*11012	Not defined

TABLE 6 (continued)

HLA-DP Alleles and Their Cellular Designation[a,b]

HLA Alleles	Cellular Specificity[c]
DPB1*1301	Not defined
DPB1*1401	Not defined
DPB1*1501	Not defined
DPB1*1601	Not defined
DPB1*1701	Not defined
DPB1*1801	Not defined
DPB1*1901	Not defined
DPB1*20011	Not defined
DPB1*20012	Not defined
DPB1*2101	Not defined
DPB1*2201	Not defined
DPB1*2301	Not defined
DPB1*2401	Not defined
DPB1*2501	Not defined
DPB1*26011	Not defined
DPB1*26012	Not defined
DPB1*2701	Not defined
DPB1*2801	Not defined
DPB1*2901	Not defined
DPB1*3001	Not defined
DPB1*3101	Not defined
DPB1*3201	Not defined
DPB1*3301	Not defined
DPB1*3401	Not defined
DPB1*3501	Not defined
DPB1*3601	Not defined
DPB1*3701	Not defined
DPB1*3801	Not defined
DPB1*3901	Not defined
DPB1*4001	Not defined
DPB1*4101	Not defined
DPB1*4401	Not defined
DPB1*4501	Not defined
DPB1*4601	Not defined
DPB1*4701	Not defined
DPB1*4801	Not defined
DPB1*4901	Not defined
DPB1*5001	Not defined
DPB1*5101	Not defined
DPB1*5201	Not defined
DPB1*5301	Not defined
DPB1*5401	Not defined
DPB1*5501	Not defined

[a] It is likely that the number of HLA-DP alleles will increase as more individuals are studied. Alleles are defined by DNA sequencing. An annual summary of allele sequences is published in *Human Immunology, Tissue Antigens,* and *Immunogenetics.*

TABLE 6 (continued)

HLA-DP Alleles and Their Cellular Designation[a,b]

HLA Alleles	Cellular Specificity[c]

[b] Each row in the table lists a DP allele and its associated cellular specificity. For example, individuals who carry a DPB1*0101 allele are typed as DPw1 using cellular reagents.

[c] Alloantisera that define DP types are rare, and these molecules have been defined using cellular typing reagents (primed lymphocyte lines). Only a few of these reagents have been generated, so that many alleles are not defined by cellular types.

[d] Allele of the DPA1 gene which specifies the DP alpha chain. Alleles of DPA1 are currently not considered in matching for transplant.

[e] This allele is not defined by a cellular reagent.

[f] The fifth digit indicates a nucleotide change that creates a new allele but does not change the protein sequence of the molecule. These differences are not considered important for transplantation matching.

[g] Allele of the DPB1 gene which specifies the DP antigen.

From Bodmer, J. G. et al., *Tissue Antigens*, 44, 1, 1994. Published with permission of Munksgaard International Publishers Ltd., Copenhagen, Denmark.

The differences among HLA proteins are localized to the amino-terminal region of these molecules. Thus, class I polymorphism is predominantly found in the first 180 amino acids of the heavy chain, while class II polymorphism is found in the first 90 to 95 amino acids of alpha and/or beta chains. At the DNA level, where each HLA locus is divided into multiple exons (each encoding a region of the molecule), this diversity is focused in exons 2 and 3 for the class I loci and exon 2 for the class II loci (Figure 4). DNA-based testing methods target these regions of polymorphism in order to identify the HLA alleles in a process called "HLA typing."

II. SEROLOGIC TYPING

The polymorphism present in HLA alleles is reflected in the HLA proteins expressed on cell surfaces. The HLA molecules are detected serologically using human alloantisera or monoclonal antibodies in a microcytoxicity assay. These alloantisera define serologic specificities localized on five of the HLA molecules, HLA-A, -B, -C, -DR, and -DQ (Table 7).[4] Alloantisera defining HLA-DP molecules are rare. Each serologic specificity (or HLA type) is designated by a letter indicating the HLA molecule and a number. For example, A1 is a serologic specificity

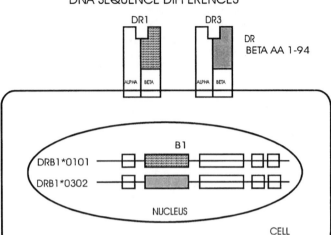

Figure 4

The diagram indicates the polymorphic region of the HLA-DR molecules (DR beta chain amino acids 1 to 94) (shaded gray and black) that is detected by serologic and cellular typing reagents. The corresponding exons in the DRB1 gene which encodes the polymorphic regions are shaded gray and black. DNA-based typing utilizing DNA as a starting material detects sequence differences in this region of the DNA.

localized on an HLA-A molecule, while B5 is a serologic specificity localized on an HLA-B molecule. There are many possible HLA types in the human population. For example, there are 27 possible HLA-A types listed in Table 7. It is also common to utilize the term "antigen" or "specificity" to refer to an HLA type (e.g., HLA-A1 antigen, HLA-B5 specificity).

The number of different HLA molecules detected by each alloantiserum depends on the specificity of the alloantiserum used in the assay. Some alloantisera define clusters of HLA molecules that share structural similarity and that are indistinguishable using that particular alloantiserum (Figure 5, Table 8). For example, the A9 specificity is located on molecules bearing either A23 or A24 specificities. Thus, the specificity A23 is often called a "split" of the broad specificity A9 and can be also written as A23(9). An individual typing as A23 using A23-specific alloantisera would also type as A9 using A9-specific alloantisera.

Different HLA alleles can encode molecules which are serologically indistinguishable (Tables 1 through 5). For example, the sixteen DRB1*11 alleles (DRB1*11011, DRB1*1102, DRB1*1103, etc.) encode molecules which type serologically as DR11. Figure 6 compares the number of HLA-DR types identified by serology to the number of types defined using molecular biology typing methods. The inability of currently

TABLE 7

Complete Listing of Recognized HLA
Specificities Defined by Serology[a]

A	B	C	DR	DQ
A1	B5	Cw1[b]	DR1	DQ1
A2	B7	Cw2	DR103	DQ2
A203	B703	Cw3	DR2	DQ3
A210	B8	Cw4	DR3	DQ4
A3	B12	Cw5	DR4	DQ5(1)
A9	B13	Cw6	DR5	DQ6(1)
A10	B14	Cw7	DR6	DQ7(3)
A11	B15	Cw8	DR7	DQ8(3)
A19	B16	Cw9(w3)	DR8	DQ9(3)
A23(9)[c]	B17	Cw10(w3)	DR9	
A24(9)	B18		DR10	
A2403	B21		DR11(5)	
A25(10)	B22		DR12(5)	
A26(10)	B27		DR13(6)	
A28	B35		DR14(6)	
A29(19)	B37		DR1403	
A30(19)	B38(16)		DR1404	
A31(19)	B39(16)		DR15(2)	
A32(19)	B3901		DR16(2)	
A33(19)	B3902		DR17(3)	
A34(10)	B40		DR18(3)	
A36	B4005			
A43	B41		DR51[d]	
A66(10)	B42			
A68(28)	B44(12)		DR52[d]	
A69(28)	B45(12)			
A74(19)	B46		DR53[d]	
	B47			
	B48			
	B49(21)			
	B50(21)			
	B51(5)			
	B5102			
	B5103			
	B52(5)			
	B53			
	B54(22)			
	B55(22)			
	B56(22)			
	B57(17)			
	B58(17)			
	B59			
	B60(40)			
	B61(40)			
	B62(15)			
	B63(15)			
	B64(14)			
	B65(14)			

TABLE 7 (continued)

Complete Listing of Recognized HLA
Specificities Defined by Serology[a]

A	B	C	DR	DQ
	B67			
	B70			
	B71(70)			
	B72(70)			
	B73			
	B75(15)			
	B76(15)			
	B77(15)			
	B7801			
	Bw4[e]			
	Bw6[e]			

[a] Each column of the table is independent and unrelated to the other columns.

[b] "w" is added to avoid confusion with the complement genes.

[c] () indicates the broad serologic specificity as described in Table 8. The serologic type may be listed without the broad specificity. For example, both A23(9) and A23 are correct designations.

[d] DR51, DR52, and DR53 are serologic specificities associated with a number of DR serologic types as described in Figure 7.

[e] Bw4 and Bw6 are serologic specificities found on multiple B and A molecules.

From Bodmer, J. G. et al., *Human Immunol.*, 34, 4, 1992. Published with permission of Munksgaard International Publishers Ltd., Copenhagen, Denmark.

available serologic reagents to discriminate all of the products of the HLA alleles is one of the major reasons for the shift in HLA typing methodologies toward DNA-based typing methods.[5,6] The problem is particularly acute when typing some population groups. For example, African-Americans frequently express class I and class II allelic products which are difficult to identify with the currently available serologic reagents.[7] Other problems associated with serologic typing are the difficulty in obtaining human alloantisera for typing and the difficulty in obtaining sufficient numbers of the appropriate cells for typing from some patients, such as patients with leukemia.

III. CELLULAR TYPING

Cellular assays such as the mixed lymphocyte culture (MLC) can be used to determine the HLA class II types of an individual and/or to measure the HLA class II disparity between two individuals (HLA

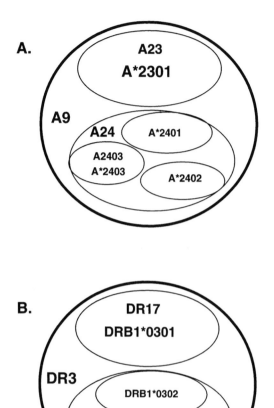

Figure 5

The Venn diagrams illustrate the serologic relationship between a broad specificity and a serologic split and the relationship between serologic types and the alleles encoding these HLA molecules. The alloantisera used in HLA serologic typing are not standardized. Each typing laboratory may use commercially available sera from several sources or may rely on their own alloantisera acquisition program to obtain reagents. Thus, the reagents used by each typing laboratory may vary, and laboratories will differ in their ability to define all WHO-designated serologic specificities listed in Table 7. (A) Depending on the ability of the typing reagents utilized to define serologic splits, two individuals may appear to have different HLA types (A23 vs. A24) or the same HLA type (A9). Serologic reagents can not detect the difference in the antigens encoded by A*2401 and A*2402 alleles; however, a serologic reagent has been identified which can specifically detect the the product of the A*2403 allele. This serologic type is defined as A2403 (Table 8). (B) Depending on the ability of the typing reagents utilized to define serologic splits, the two individuals may appear to have different HLA types (DR17 vs. DR18) or the same HLA type (DR3). Serologic reagents can not detect the difference in the DR18 antigens encoded by DRB1*0302 and DRB1*0303 alleles. The importance of matching at each level of resolution (alleles vs. serologic splits vs. broad specificities) for transplantation is discussed in a later section.

TABLE 8

Serologic Splits and Associated Antigens[a,b]

Original Broad Specificities	Splits	Associated Antigens[c]
A2		A203, A210
A9	A23, A24	A2403
A10	A25, A26, A34, A66	
A19	A29, A30, A31, A32, A33, A74	
A28	A68, A69	
B5	B51, B52	
B7		B703
B12	B44, B45	
B14	B64, B65	
B15	B62, B63, B75, B76, B77	
B16	B38, B39	B3901, B3902
B17	B57, B58	
B21	B49, B50	B4005
B22	B54, B55, B56	
B40	B60, B61	
B70	B71, B72	
Cw3	Cw9, Cw10	
DR1		DR103
DR2	DR15, DR16	
DR3	DR17, DR18	
DR5	DR11, DR12	
DR6	DR13, DR14	DR1403, DR1404
DQ1	DQ5, DQ6	
DQ3	DQ7, DQ8, DQ9	

[a] Each row of the table lists a broad specificity and its associated splits and antigens. For example, A203 and A210 antigens are subdivisions of A2.

[b] The clinical relevance of defining splits and associated antigens for HLA matching for transplantation is discussed later in the chapter.

[c] The associated antigens can be considered splits of the broad serologic specificity. These serologic specificities detect the product of a specific HLA allele that falls within a serologic cluster. For example, the A203 serologic specificity is located on a molecule encoded by an allele in the A2 family, A*0203.

From Bodmer, J. G. et al., *Human Immunol.*, 34, 4, 1992. Published with permission of Munksgaard International Publishers Ltd., Copenhagen, Denmark.

matching). A cellular assay is more sensitive in detecting HLA differences than serologic typing, since even minor amino acid differences not recognized by alloantisera can cause stimulation of T lymphocytes. For example, an individual typed as DR4 using serologic reagents may express one of several cellularly defined Dw types (Table 9). One drawback to cellular assays for HLA typing is the difficulty in generating and maintaining cellular typing reagents (i.e., cryopreserved functional viable lymphocytes). One drawback to the MLC for HLA matching of donor and recipient is the inconsistency in experimental results in determining HLA matching or predicting graft vs. host disease.[8,9] It is for these reasons that cellular assays are being replaced by DNA-based typing methods.[8-11]

RESOLUTION ACHIEVED IN HLA TESTING

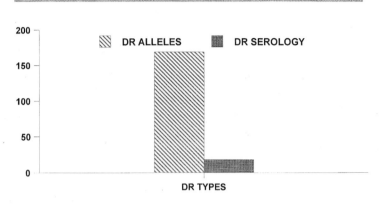

Figure 6

A comparison of the number of serologic types detected (shaded bar) and the number of DNA-based types (alleles) detected (striped bar) for HLA-DR. Alleles are identified by DNA sequencing and represent the true extent of HLA diversity present in the human population.

IV. ADDITIONAL COMPLEXITY OF THE HLA SYSTEM

Both the number and the kinds of genes in the MHC can differ in different individuals. One major difference is the number of DR beta chain loci that encode a protein product within the MHC (or within an HLA haplotype).[4] As shown in Figure 7, some haplotypes express the product of only one DRB locus (DRB1). These haplotypes are found in individuals who carry DRB1 loci which encode DR1, DR8, or DR10 alleles. Other haplotypes contain two loci which encode DR beta chains. These haplotypes contain a DRB1 locus and a second DRB locus. Depending on the haplotype, one of three potential second loci may be present, DRB3, DRB4, or DRB5. These haplotypes encode two different DR molecules and, since the association of a specific DRB1 allele with an allele at a specific second DRB locus is usually fixed, the combination of DR molecules encoded by a haplotype is predictable (Table 10). Therefore, individuals who express a DR4 molecule will also express a DR53 molecule and carry a DR4 beta chain allele (e.g., DRB1*0403) and a DR53 beta chain allele (e.g., DRB4*0101). Figure 7 and Table 10 describe specific DRB1/DRB3, DRB1/DRB4, and DRB1/DRB5 associations. Specific DRB1/DQB1 and DQA1/DQB1 associations are also common (Tables 11, 12).

There are exceptions to these associations. For example, some DR7 haplotypes carry a DRB4 allele, but it is not expressed as a DR53

TABLE 9

HLA-DR Serologic Specificities and Their Associated Cellular Specificities[a]

HLA-DR	Cellular Specificity
DR1	Dw1, Dw20
DR2	Dw2, Dw12, Dw21, Dw22
DR3	Dw3
DR4	Dw4, Dw10, Dw13, Dw14, Dw15
DR11(5)	Dw5
DR13(6)	Dw6, Dw18(w6), Dw19(w6)
DR14(6)	Dw9, Dw16
DR7	Dw7, Dw11(w7), Dw17(w7)
DR8	Dw8
DR9	Dw23
DR52	Dw24, Dw25, Dw26[b]

[a] Each row in the table shows the association between a serologically defined DR type and a cellularly defined type. For example, DR1 individuals can be typed using cellular reagents as either Dw1 or Dw20. It is also likely that some individuals typed as DR1 would express other cellular types; however, the reagents needed to define those types have not been generated or have not received a W.H.O. designation. Cellular typing is being replaced by nucleic acid-based typing methods.

[b] Dw24, Dw25, and Dw26 are sometimes termed DR52a, DR52b, and DR52c, respectively.

From Bodmer, J. G. et al., *Human Immunol.*, 34, 4, 1992. Published with permission of Munksgaard International Publishers Ltd., Copenhagen, Denmark.

molecule on the cell surface. In a second example, a haplotype has been identified which encodes a DRB1*1501 allele but does not appear to contain a DRB5 locus. In a final example, in Caucasians, DRB1*0901 is usually found in association with DQB1*0303, while in African-Americans, DRB1*0901 is usually found with DQB1*0201.

The tendency for certain alleles at two loci to occur significantly more frequently in the same haplotype than would be expected on the basis of chance alone is called "linkage disequilibrium." The best known example of linkage disequilibrium for an entire MHC haplotype is the A1, Cw7, B8, DR3, DR52, DQ2 haplotype in Caucasoids, which occurs approximately four times more frequently than would be expected by chance. It is thought that these "extended haplotypes" account for at least 30% of normal Caucasian haplotypes.[1] These haplotypes carry very similar, probably identical, alleles, even when they are found in apparently unrelated individuals(Tables 13, 14).[12] Thus, it is easier to find an unrelated individual who is an HLA match for a patient carrying common extended haplotypes.

Frequencies of HLA alleles and haplotypes differ significantly among ethnic populations (Table 15).[14] Therefore, it is more likely that individuals will find an HLA match for a transplant within their own ethnic group. For example, an African-American carrying a DRB1*0302 allele is much more likely to find a donor within the African-American population, where the percent of DR3 individuals carrying the DRB1*0302 allele is 29.9%, than in the Caucasian or Oriental populations where the frequency of that allele is much lower (0.9% and 0.0%)(Table 15).[13] In addition, some populations such as African-Americans show extensive HLA diversity in comparison to other populations such as Japanese.[14-15] Some of this diversity results from admixture of populations groups.

V. HLA MATCHING FOR TRANSPLANTATION

From an HLA-matching standpoint, the best bone marrow donor is either self (if the malignancy is not one of the hematopoietic system) or a monozygotic twin. Since this is usually not possible, an HLA identical sibling donor is the next choice (Figure 8). The use of a sibling donor also increases the probability that non-HLA loci which might affect transplantation success and which are not yet well defined (i.e., minor histocompatibility loci), are more likely to be matched.[16] However, since most (~60%) patients do not have an HLA-matched sibling and because of the success with transplants of HLA-matched unrelated bone marrow donors, national registries of unrelated bone marrow donors have been developed around the world.[17-18] Such a registry is the National Marrow Donor Program in the U.S. which contains over 1.6 million HLA-typed donors.[19]

For solid organ transplants, similar criteria are used for finding a match. For living related kidney donors, the choice is based on decreasing order of histocompatibility: (1) monozygotic twin; (2) HLA-identical siblings; (3) HLA-haploidentical siblings; (4) HLA-haploidentical child or parent; and (5) first-order relatives, grandparents, aunts, uncles, or cousins, preferably haploidentical. As definition of HLA antigens has become better refined, it appears that cadaveric renal allografts that are serologically identical for HLA-A, B, and DR (i.e., 6-antigen match) survive as well as grafts from genotypically HLA identical siblings.[20] Thus, the United Network for Organ Sharing (UNOS) requires mandatory sharing of phenotypically identical cadaveric kidneys.

The level of HLA typing resolution required probably differs for bone marrow and solid organ transplants. It is likely that higher resolution of HLA types is required to match donor and recipient for bone

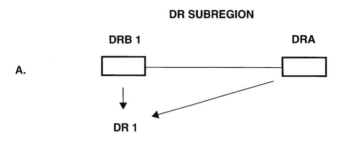

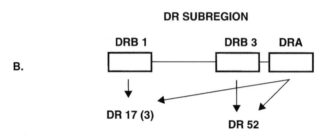

Figure 7
Haplotypes differ in the number of DR beta chain loci present. (A) Haplotypes which
contain a gene encoding a DR1 antigen contain only one functional DR beta chain locus,
DRB1. These haplotypes encode only a single DR molecule. This is also true for haplotypes encoding DR8 and DR10 antigens. (B) Haplotypes which contain a gene encoding
a DR17(3) antigen contain two functional DR beta chain loci, DRB1 and DRB3. These
haplotypes encode two different DR molecules, DR17(3) and DR52. This is also true for
haplotypes encoding DR18(3), DR11(5), DR12(5), DR13(6), and DR14(6) antigens. All of
these haplotypes express DR52 in conjunction with another DR molecule (e.g., DR13(6)
and DR52). (C) Haplotypes which contain a gene encoding a DR7 antigen contain two
functional DR beta chain loci, DRB1 and DRB4. These haplotypes encode two different
DR molecules, DR7 and DR53. This is also true for haplotypes encoding DR4 and DR9
antigens. All of these haplotypes express DR53 in conjunction with another DR molecule
(e.g., DR9 and DR53). (D) Haplotypes which contain a gene encoding a DR15(2) antigen
contain two functional DR beta chain loci, DRB1 and DRB5. These haplotypes encode
two different DR molecules, DR15(2) and DR51. This is also true for haplotypes which
encode a DR16(2) antigen.

marrow transplantation than is required for solid organ transplantation. Preliminary data suggest that matching donor and recipient for
HLA-DRB1 alleles is important to decrease the risk of graft vs. host
disease,[21] although the importance of matching alleles at other loci is
not yet clear.[22-23]

DR SUBREGION

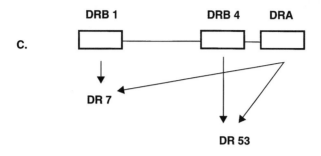

DR SUBREGION

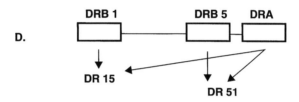

Figure 7 (continued)

TABLE 10

Examples of Associations of DRB1 with DRB3/4/5 Alleles[a,b,c]

DRB1*	DRB3/DRB4/DRB5[d]
0101	None
0101	B5*0101
0102	None
0103	None
0301	B3*0101
0301	B3*0202
0302	B3*0101
0303	B3*0101
0401	B4*0101
0402	B4*0101
0403	B4*0101
0404	B4*0101
0405	B4*0101
0406	B4*0101
0407	B4*0101
0408	B4*0101
0409	B4*0101
0410	B4*0101
0411	B4*0101
0412	B4*0101
0701	B4*0101[e]
0801	None
0802	None

TABLE 10 (continued)

Examples of Associations of DRB1 with DRB3/4/5 Alleles[a,b,c]

DRB1*	DRB3/DRB4/DRB5[d]
0803	None
0803	None
0804	None
0804	None
0805	None
0901	B4*0101
1001	None
1101	B3*0202
1102	B3*0202
1103	B3*0202
1104	B3*0202
1201	B3*0101
1201	B3*0202
1202	B3*0301
1301	B3*0101
1301	B3*0202
1302	B3*0301
1303	B3*0101
1303	B3*0202
1304	B3*0202
1305	B3*0202
1401	B3*0202
1402	B3*0101
1403	B3*0101
1403	B3*0202
1404	B3*0101
1404	B3*0202
1405	B3*0101
1405	B3*0202
1406	B3*0202
1407	B3*0202
1408	B3*0101
1408	B3*0202
1409	B3*0101
1410	B3*0101
1501	B5*0101
1501	None
1502	B5*0102
1503	B5*0101
1601	B5*0201
1602	B5*0202

[a] This is only a partial listing of the associations between DRB1 alleles and DRB3/4/5 alleles.

[b] Each row of the table shows the observed association between a specific DRB1 allele and a second DR allele as described in Figure 7.

[c] The associations can vary in different ethnic populations.

[d] The entry of "none" in the column indicates that an associated second DR allele is not present.

[e] DRB1*0701 can be found in association with either a DRB4*0101 allele or a DRB4*0101 allele that is not expressed.

Table provided by F. M. Robbins, Georgetown University, Washington, D.C.

TABLE 11

Examples of Associations between DRB1 and DQB1 Alleles[a,b,c]

DRB1*	DQB1*
0101	0501
0102	0501
0103	0301
0103	0501
0301	0201
0302	0402
0303	0402
0401	0301
0401	0302
0402	0302
0403	0302
0404	0302
0404	0402
0405	0401
0405	0503
0406	0301
0407	0301
0407	0302
0408	0301
0408	0302
0409	0401
0410	0401
0410	0402
0411	0302
0412	0401
0412	0402
0701	0201
0701	0303
0801	0402
0802	0402
0803	0301
0803	0601
0804	0301
0804	0402
0805	0402
0806	0301
0806	0602
0901	0201
0901	0303
1001	0501
1101	0502
1101	0301
1102	0301
1103	0301
1104	0301
1104	0603
1105	0602
1201	0301
1202	0301

TABLE 11 (continued)

Examples of Associations between DRB1 and DQB1 Alleles[a,b,c]

DRB1*	DQB1*
1301	0603
1302	0604
1302	0605
1303	0301
1304	0201
1304	0301
1305	0301
1305	0603
1401	0503
1402	0301
1402	0302
1403	0301
1404	0503
1405	0503
1406	0301
1407	0502
1407	0503
1408	0503
1409	0402
1410	0402
1501	0602
1502	0601
1503	0602
1601	0502
1602	0301

[a] This is only a partial listing of the associations observed between DRB1 and DQB1 alleles.
[b] Each row of the table shows the observed associations between a specific DRB1 allele and a DQB1 allele.
[c] The associations can vary in different ethnic populations.

Table provided by F.M. Robbins, Georgetown University, Washington, D.C.

VI. AMPLIFIED DNA SERVES AS A TEMPLATE FOR DNA-BASED TYPING

With the advent of rapid and reliable methods for the isolation and identification of HLA genes and the determination of the nucleotide sequences of HLA alleles, it has become possible to use DNA-based methods for HLA typing (Table 16). All DNA-based typing methods focus on identifying segments of the sequence of the nucleotide pairs comprising each allele and utilize denaturation and reannealing of the A-T and G-C nucleotide base pairs to achieve sensitivity and specificity. DNA-based typing of class II alleles, HLA-DR, -DQ, and -DP, is now a commonly used technique in HLA-typing laboratories, while DNA-based

TABLE 12

Examples of DQ Alpha and Beta Allele
Combinations Encoded by a Haplotype[a,b]

DQ Serologic Specificities	DQA1*	DQB1*
DQ5(1)	0101	0501
DQ5(1)	0101	0502
DQ5(1)	0101	0503
DQ5(1)	0102	0501
DQ5(1)	0102	0502
DQ5(1)	0102	0504
DQ5(1)	0104	0501
DQ5(1)	0104	0503
DQ6(1)	0101	0603
DQ6(1)	0102	0602
DQ6(1)	0102	0604
DQ6(1)	0102	0605
DQ6(1)	0103	0601
DQ6(1)	0103	0603
DQ2	0201	0201
DQ2	0501	0201
DQ2	0301	0201
DQ7(3)	0301	0301
DQ7(3)	0301	0302
DQ7(3)	0401	0301
DQ7(3)	0501	0301
DQ7(3)	0601	0301
DQ8(3)	0301	0302
DQ8(3)	0302	0302
DQ9(3)	0201	0303
DQ9(3)	0301	0303
DQ4	0301	0401
DQ4	0401	0402

[a] Each row in this table lists observed DQA1 and
DQB1 allele combinations encoded by a haplotype and their associated serologic type. For example, DQA1*0101 and DQB1*0501 alleles are
often found on the same haplotype. Individuals
that carry these alleles will express a DQ5(1) serologic type.

[b] This listing is not complete. Other DQA1/DQB1
associations have been described.

typing of class I alleles, HLA-A, -B, and -C, is just beginning to be
utilized. Although DNA-based HLA typing has been in practice only
a few years, its reproducibility in large-scale typing using blind controls
has been extraordinary[24] and is one reason for the transition from
serology to DNA-based HLA typing.

While either DNA or RNA can be used for typing, DNA is more
stable and is the template of choice for the amplification reaction. Any
cell with a nucleus can be used as a source of DNA for typing. Cell

TABLE 13

HLA-B, -DR, -DQ Haplotypes with High Positive
Disequilibrium[a]

DRB1*[b]	DQA1*[b]	DQB1*[b]	HLA-B[c]
1501	0102	0602	7
0301	0501	0201	8
0701	0201	0201	13
0701	0201	0303	17
0401	0301	0301	12
0401	0301	0302	15
0404	0301	0302	27
1302	0102	0604	35
0404	0301	0302	40
0101	0101	0501	35
0801	04/06[e]	04[e]	35
0401	0301	0301	15
0701	0201	0201	12

Note: From a study of the CEPH families.
[a] Each row of the table lists alleles which are found encoded by
     a single haplotype. For example, one common haplotype carries
     DRB1*1501, DQA1*0102, DQB1*0602, and HLA-B7 alleles.
[b] Allele identified by nucleic-acid based typing.
[c] Antigen identified by serologic typing.
[d] The specific allele has not been identified.
From Begovich, A. B. et al., *J. Immunol.*, 148, 249, 1992, copyright
1992, by the *Journal of Immunology*. With permission.

TABLE 14

HLA-DR, -DQ, -DP Haplotypes with High Positive
Disequilibrium[a]

DRB1*	DQA1*	DQB1*	DPB1*
0701	0201	0201	1701
1302	0102	0604	0301
0404	0301	0302	0601
0701	0201	0201	1101
0401	0301	0301	0401
1501	0102	0602	0401
1501	0102	0602	0501
0101	0101	0501	0402

Note: From a study of the CEPH families.
[a] Each row of the table lists alleles which are found encoded by
     a single haplotype. For example, one common haplotype carries
     DRB1*0701, DQA1*0201, DQB1*0201, and DPB1*1701 alleles.
From Begovich, A. B., *J. Immunol.*, 148, 249, 1992, copyright 1992
by *Journal of Immunology*. With permission.

TABLE 15

DRB1 Allele Distributions in Three Population Groups[a,b]

Serologic Group	DRB1 Allele	Black %[c]	Caucasian %	Oriental %
DR3	0301	70.1	99.1	100.0
	0302	29.9	0.9	0.0
DR11	1101	56.1	54.8	96.4
	1102	34.8	3.2	0.0
	1103	0.0	2.2	0.0
	1104	9.1	39.8	3.6
DR13	1301	26.8	46.8	8.7
	1302	52.8	36.0	77.7
	1303	17.9	13.4	13.6
	1304	2.5	0.0	0.0
	1305	5.7	3.8	0.0
DR8	0801	6.5	78.3	0.0
	0802	12.9	1.7	26.7
	0803	0.0	16.7	73.3
	0804	80.6	3.3	0.0

[a] Only some of the DRB1 alleles are included in this table.

[b] The distribution of alleles differs in different human populations. Even within a population group, the distribution may vary. Thus, the distribution of DRB1 alleles in Orientals may differ among populations from Korea, China, and Japan.

[c] The percent of each DRB1 allele within a serologic group is indicated for each population group. As new alleles are discovered, the percent distribution will alter. For example, when this study was carried out, DRB1*0303 had not yet been described. It is likely that some of the individuals classified as DRB1*0302 actually carry the DRB1*0303 allele.

From Fernandez-Vina, M. A., et al., in *HLA 1991*, Vol. 1, Tsuji, K., Aizawa, M., and Sasazuki, T., Eds., Oxford University Press, New York, 1992, 471. With permission.

lines such B lymphoblastoid cell lines can be cultured in the laboratory and provide an inexhaustible supply of DNA. These lines are often used to provide reference DNA for quality control of the typing procedures.

DNA is usually prepared from a small quantity (0.5 to 2 ml) of whole blood. Many different protocols can be used to isolate DNA from cells. One protocol uses Triton X-100 (a detergent) to lyse the cell membrane, releasing the nuclei.[25] If the starting material is whole blood, these nuclei must be washed extensively to remove any hemoglobin released by the red blood cells. The heme portion of hemoglobin interferes with the gene amplification reaction used to determine HLA types. The nuclei are lysed using another detergent, Tween-20. The DNA is freed from the proteins bound to it by treatment with proteinase K, an enzyme which destroys proteins. The proteinase K is later destroyed by incubation of the DNA at high temperatures (90°C). It is important to deactivate the proteinase K because it can degrade the enzyme used in the HLA typing reaction. Commercial kits are also available for the preparation of DNA.

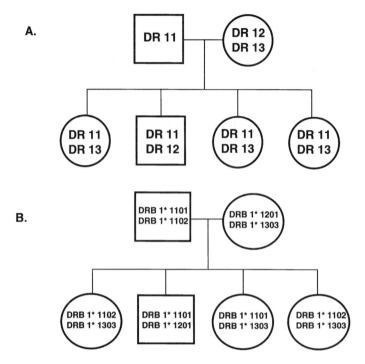

Figure 8

Inheritance of HLA alleles in a family as monitored by: (A) Serologic typing. (B) DNA-based typing. The resolution obtained by DNA-based typing allows the identification of siblings carrying identical DR alleles. The presence of two DRB1*11 alleles and a DRB1*13 allele, an allele easily misidentified, requires high resolution analysis to identify alleles within the family. This level of resolution would not be required if the parents had expressed DRB1 alleles in each of four easily distinguished serologic groups (e.g., DR1, DR11, DR12, and DR7) and typing at the serologic level (low resolution) alone would be sufficient to identify HLA-matched siblings.

TABLE 16

Methods of DNA-Based HLA Typing

Sequence specific oligonucleotide probe hybridization (SSOPH)
PCR — restriction fragment length polymorphism (RFLP)
Sequence-specific priming (SSP)/allele refractory mutation system (ARMS)
DNA sequencing
Sequence specific conformational polymorphism
Heteroduplex typing

The sensitivity and specificity of the HLA typing procedure is enhanced greatly by the amplification of DNA encoding HLA genes using a technique termed the "polymerase chain reaction" or PCR.[26] In this patented process, a pair of synthetic single-stranded oligonucleotides

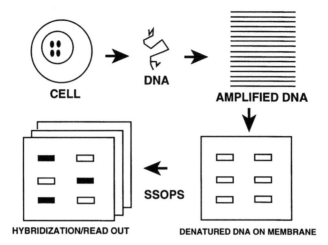

Figure 9
A diagram of the sequence-specific oligonucleotide typing process including preparation of DNA, amplification of the HLA gene being identified, attachment of amplified DNA to a solid support, and hybridization with a panel of sequence specific oligonucleotide probes.

(primers) containing sequences complementary to those found flanking a specific HLA gene are utilized in combination with a thermostable DNA polymerase to generate millions of copies of that gene for use in the HLA typing reaction. Many typing techniques utilize primer sequences that are complementary to all alleles at an HLA locus; other typing procedures utilize primer sets that are complementary to only a subset of alleles at a locus. The amplification reaction is performed by varying the temperature of the reaction mix causing: (1) denaturation of the DNA; (2) annealing of the primers to the denatured DNA; and (3) DNA synthesis by attachment of nucleotides onto the annealed primers. This three-step cycle is repeated approximately 30 times, each time doubling the number of DNA strands. Annealing of the primers to complementary sequences in sample DNA during the PCR reaction uses hybridization conditions that guarantee that the primers will hybridize to perfectly matched sequences and not to sequences of other loci or other alleles that are not matched. By adjusting the temperature of the annealing component of the PCR reaction, the typing laboratory can control the specificity of the amplification.

VII. SEQUENCE-SPECIFIC OLIGONUCLEOTIDE HYBRIDIZATION

It has been possible to use hybridization of synthetic sequence-specific single-stranded oligonucleotide probes (SSOP) to amplified denatured DNA to identify alleles (e.g., References 27 to 29). The use of several different oligonucleotides to define a specific HLA allele may be required when no unique sequence can be identified. This is especially true for the typing of DPB1 alleles, which often share variable region sequences.[30] A set of oligonucleotides capable of identifying each potential allele or a subset of potential alleles is hybridized to denatured PCR-amplified DNA attached to a solid support (Figure 9). Hybridization conditions are adjusted so that each oligonucleotide will anneal only to HLA alleles carrying a sequence complementary to the oligonucleotide probe. The oligonucleotides are labeled with radioisotope or, more commonly, with a nonisotopic tag for detection (see Reference 31). After visualization, the pattern of hybridization can be read to determine the alleles present. The SSOP method is often used in situations where many samples are typed in large batches.[24] Modifications in the procedure to convert it to a microtiter well format allow a single DNA sample to be tested with multiple probes to facilitate the typing of a small number of samples (e.g., References 32 and 33). Commercial kits using the SSOP method are available.

In a related procedure, termed the "reverse dot blot," the oligonucleotide probes are bound to a solid support (e.g., Reference 34). DNA from the samples to be tested is amplified using primers labeled with biotin. The amplified DNA is then hybridized to the immobilized probes which contain sequences complementary to sequences found in the alleles potentially present in the DNA. After visualization (using an avidin-linked detection system), the pattern of hybridization is used to determine the alleles present. The reverse dot blot procedure procedure is useful for typing any number of samples, and commercial kits utilizing this method are available.

VIII. PCR-RESTRICTION FRAGMENT LENGTH POLYMORPHISM (RFLP)

If two alleles differ for a sequence which alters a restriction enzyme site, the amplified DNA fragment can be tested for cleavage with the restriction enzyme. The resultant DNA fragments are then analyzed by gel electrophoresis. While this approach is limited by the presence of restriction enzyme sites, the PCR-RFLP method has been used to identify HLA types and can used as a supplementary technique.[35]

IX. SEQUENCE-SPECIFIC PRIMING

Another method of identification of HLA alleles uses sequence-specific primers (SSP) in the PCR reaction (sometimes termed ARMS,

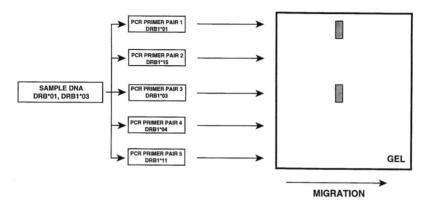

Figure 10
Diagram of the use of sequence specific primers. Since the DNA sample tested carries DRB1*01 and DRB1*03 alleles, the DNA will only amplify with the primer sets specific for DRB1*01 and DRB1*03, and not the other primer sets. Amplification is detected by gel electrophoresis.

allele refractory mutation system) (e.g., References 36 to 39). The primers anneal to a subset of HLA alleles with sequences complementary to the primer sequences (Figure 10). In the subsequent PCR reaction, only these selected alleles are amplified under carefully controlled conditions. DNA amplified by the primers is identified following gel electrophoresis, and the pattern amplification is used to determine HLA types. The SSP procedure is useful in typing a small number of samples, and commercial kits are available.

X. DNA SEQUENCING

Another method of identification of HLA alleles involves the direct determination of the DNA sequences of the HLA alleles carried by an individual. Sequencing is labor intensive and highly complex but will be used more frequently in the future to determine the level of HLA match between bone marrow transplant patients and their prospective donors (see References 40 and 41). While all other DNA-based techniques can miss sequence polymorphisms that are not tested for with primers and/or probes, sequencing will identify all of the differences present in the region analyzed. In this process, PCR is utilized to amplify the gene of interest, and the amplified DNA is sequenced directly without cloning the DNA into a vector. Since most individuals are heterozygous at HLA loci, sequence-specific primers may be chosen to amplify a single allele at the locus to be tested. Alternatively, a mixture of alleles may be amplified and sequenced and analysis of polymorphic nucleotide positions used to identify the alleles present.[42]

Automated DNA sequencers facilitate the acquisition and analysis of the sequence data.

XI. SEQUENCE-SPECIFIC CONFORMATIONAL POLYMORPHISM OR HETERODUPLEX TYPING FOR MATCHING DONOR AND RECIPIENT

Amplified DNA can be denatured and the single strands electrophoresed in an acrylamide gel. The mobilities of single-stranded DNA fragments in the gel differ depending on their sequences, an observation termed sequence-specific conformational polymorphism (SSCP) (see Reference 43). Comparison of the single-stranded DNA patterns between patient and potential donor can be analyzed to estimate the allele match. Alternatively, denatured single-stranded DNA can be allowed to reanneal prior to electrophoresis. In this protocol, termed "heteroduplex analysis," amplified single-stranded DNA from a heterozygote (A–A' and a–a', where A and A' are complementary strands of one allele) will reanneal to form homoduplexes (A–A' and a–a') and heteroduplexes (A–a' and a–A'). The mobilities of the reannealed fragments vary depending on their sequences, and comparison of the patterns between patient and potential donor can be analyzed to estimate the allele match.[44-45] The electrophoresis patterns obtained by both SSCP and heteroduplex analysis can be complex, so the methods are most effectively used to determine if a patient and potential donor exhibit the same pattern of fragments and are potentially matched for the alleles at that locus. Identification of the specific HLA alleles present is more difficult.

XII. QUALITY CONTROL AND QUALITY ASSURANCE

The specificity of DNA-based typing is controlled, in large measure, by the conditions of annealing of synthetic primers and probes to denatured DNA. Under stringent conditions of temperature and salt, primers and probes will anneal to perfectly matched complementary sequences, but not to imperfectly matched sequences. Alterations in the reaction conditions may lead to nonspecific priming during DNA synthesis reactions involved in PCR amplification and DNA sequencing as well as nonspecific hybridization of probes. Specificity can be monitored by the use of reference DNA carrying well-defined HLA alleles. A second major concern in DNA-based typing is contamination of samples with previously amplified DNA. Thus, it is critical for laboratories to prevent contamination by segregation of pre- and

TABLE 17

Levels of Resolution of DNA Typing Results

Low Resolution or Serologic Level	Intermediate Resolution	High Resolution or Allele Level Resolution
DRB1*04	DRB1*0402 or DRB1*0414	DRB1*0402
DRB1*11	DRB1*1101 or DRB1*1104	DRB1*1104

post-amplification processes and to continually monitor the level of contamination. A final concern is the quality of the DNA template. Poor templates may result in amplification failure during the polymerase chain reaction. Typing methods such as sequence-specific priming utilize the presence or absence of amplification to identify HLA types. Thus, it is important to add controls to SSP protocols to monitor template quality and to interpret amplification negative results. Standards and protocols for DNA-based HLA testing are published by the American Society for Histocompatibility and Immunogenetics.[46]

XIII. LEVEL OF RESOLUTION OF DNA-BASED TYPING

The level of resolution obtained by DNA-typing methods is controlled by the choice and number of primers and/or probes used in the assay. This may depend on the purpose of the typing (e.g., large-scale bone marrow registry typing vs. typing of an actual bone marrow donor/recipient combination), the time available for carrying out the typing, the cost of the typing, and the expertise of the laboratory. For example, typing of a cadaveric kidney donor requires results to be obtained in 3 to 6 h. Most DNA-based typing methods can produce a typing result in this time frame; however, the level of resolution obtained in that time will be limited.

Low resolution (or generic or serologic) level DNA-based typing produces a result which is similar in appearance and detail to a serologic type (Table 17). For example, a DNA-defined type, DRB1*04 or DRB1*04XX, is the equivalent of the serologic type DR4. The "XX" indicates that the allele was not further defined. At this level of resolution, it is not possible to determine which of the over 20 DRB1*04 alleles is carried by the individual being tested. Although serologic typing is as informative as low resolution typing, the results are more reliable with DNA-based typing. Intermediate resolution level DNA-based typing may narrow down the choices by listing several different possibilities for the type of an individual, for example, DRB1*0402 or DRB1*0414. Finally, high resolution level (or allele level) DNA-based typing identifies the specific allele carried by an individual (e.g., DRB1*0402).

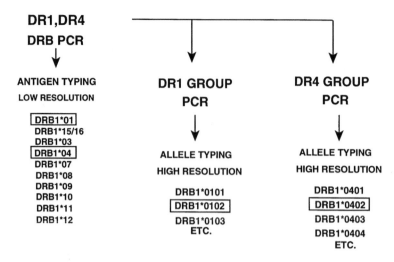

Figure 11

Diagram of a two-step amplification protocol for identification of HLA alleles. Amplification of DNA with primers which amplify all DRB1 alleles followed by hybridization of the amplified DNA to a panel of sequence specific oligonucleotide probes will identify a low resolution HLA type, DRB1*01 and DRB1*04. The DNA is then amplified with primers specific for either DRB1*01 alleles or DRB1*04 alleles. Hybridization with a panel of oligonucleotide probes which distinguish among alleles of DRB1*01 is used to identify the allele as DRB1*0102. Likewise, hybridization with a panel of oligonucleotide probes which distinguish among alleles of DRB1*04 is used to identify the allele as DRB1*0402.

The similarity among HLA loci and alleles adds complexity to the identification of HLA molecules and genes. It is thought that these loci arose by duplication of a single primordial gene and diversified through mutation and exchange of genetic segments among alleles and loci.[47] The "patchwork" nature of many of the HLA alleles means that DNA-based typing approaches often must utilize a multistep approach to identify HLA alleles (Figure 11). In this approach, a PCR primer set is chosen which amplifies all alleles at a locus. Using a panel of oligonucleotide probes, a low or intermediate resolution result is obtained. Based on these results, primers are selected which amplify only a subset of alleles to obtain amplification of only one of the two alleles present in an individual (e.g., Reference 27, 48, and 49). A second set of oligonucleotide probes is then used to identify the allele present.

XIV. CORRELATION OF DNA-BASED AND SEROLOGIC TYPING DATA

Although errors can occur in both serologic and DNA-based typings, discrepancies in HLA typing results can also arise due to differences in

TABLE 18

Sources of Potential Discrepancies in Nucleic Acid vs. Serologic Assignments[a]

Nucleic Acid Typing Assignment	Serologic Assignment	Explanation
DRB1*0103 or DRB1*01	No DR1 serologic type identified	The serologic reagent defining the DRB1*0103-encoded molecule, DR103, was not readily available on serologic typing trays until recently
DRB4*0101	No DR53 serologic type identified	Some DRB4*0101 alleles are not expressed as proteins at the cell surface
DRB1*1304	DR11	Some DR11 and DR13 molecules share sequence homology; the serologic definition depends on the alloantisera utilized[b]
DRB1*1102	DR13	Some DR11 and DR13 molecules share sequence homology; the serologic definition depends on the alloantisera utilized[b]
No DRB3 allele identified	DR52	DR8 molecules carry DR52 serologic determinants but the regions of the DRB3 gene detected by nucleic-acid based typing reagents is missing in these haplotypes

[a] Each row lists the nucleic acid typing assignment, the serologic assignment for the same sample, and the explanation of the discrepancy between the two typing methods.
[b] The alloantisera used in HLA typing are not standardized. Thus, the reagents used by each typing laboratory will vary and laboratories will differ in their ability to define serologic specificities.

typing methodologies. It is, therefore, critical to include an expert in histocompatibility testing in the interpretation of HLA typing results and in the selection of an organ donor. Table 18 lists some of the differences in HLA-DR typing results that may be encountered.

XV. THE IMPLICATIONS FOR HLA MATCHING

DNA-based typing methods for HLA typing reveal the extensive HLA diversity present within human populations. With this level of resolution, it is likely that it will be difficult to identify an HLA-matched donor for some individuals. Current research is focused on the importance and level of matching required for each locus.[23] It is likely that matching alleles at every HLA locus will not be critical. In addition, efforts must turn toward defining approaches toward intelligent HLA mismatching in transplantation. In the case of bone marrow transplantation, this means matching to decrease graft rejection and graft vs. host disease, while retaining graft vs. host disease effects with effective engraftment and reconstitution of immune responses. In solid organ transplantation, this means engraftment and long-term function of the transplanted organ with minimal immunosuppressive therapy.

REFERENCES

1. Johnson, A.H., Hurley, C.K., Hartzman, R., Yunis, E., and Alper, C., The major histocompatibility complex of man, in *Clinical Diagnosis and Management*, 18th ed., Henry, J.B., Ed., W. B. Saunders, Philadelphia, 1991, 761.
2. Bodmer, J. G., Marsh, S. G. E., Albert, E. D., Bodmer, W. F., Dupont, B., Erlich, H. A., Mach, B., Mayr, W. R., Parham, P., Sasazuki, T., Schreuder, G. M. T., Strominger, J. L., Svejgaard, A., and Terasaki, P. I., Nomenclature for factors of the HLA system, 1994, *Tissue Antigens*, 44, 1, 1994.
3. Kimura, A., Dong, R.-P., Harada, H., and Sasazuki, T., DNA typing of HLA Class II genes in B-lymphoblastoid cell lines homozygous for HLA, *Tissue Antigens*, 40, 5, 1992.
4. Bodmer, J. G., Marsh, S. G. E., Albert, E. D., Bodmer, W. F., Dupont, B., Erlich, H. A., Mach, B., Mayr, W. R., Parham, P., Sasazuki, T., Schreuder, G. M. T., Strominger, J. L., Svejgaard, A., and Terasaki, P. I., Nomenclature for factors of the HLA system, 1991, *Human Immunol.*, 34, 4, 1992.
5. Tiercy, J. M., Morel, C., Freidel, A.C., Zwahlen, R., Gebuhrer, L., Betuel, H., Jeannet, M., and Mach, B., Selection of unrelated donors for bone marrow transplantation is improved by HLA class II genotyping with oligonucleotide hybridization, *Proc. Natl. Acad. Sci. U.S.A.*, 88, 7121, 1991.
6. Tiercy, J. M., Goumaz, C., Mach, B., and Jeannet, M., Application of HLA-DR oligotyping to 110 kidney transplant patients with doubtful serological typing, *Transplantation*, 51, 1110, 1991.
7. Opelz, G., Wujciak, T., Schwarz, V., Back, D., Mytilineos, J., and Scherer, S., Collaborative transplant Study analysis of graft survival in blacks, *Transplant. Proc.*, 25, 2443, 1993.
8. Mickelson, E. M., Bartsch, G. E., Hansen, J. A., and Dupont, B., The MLC assay as a test for HLA-D region compatibility between patients and unrelated donors: results of a National Marrow Donor Program involving multiple centers, *Tissue Antigens*, 42, 465, 1993.
9. Mickelson, E. M., Guthrie, L. A., Etzioni, R., Anasetti, C., Martin, P. J., and Hansen, J. A., Role of the mixed lymphocyte culture (MLC) reaction in marrow donor selection: matching for transplants from related haploidentical donors, *Tissue Antigens*, 44, 83, 1994.
10. Baxter-Lowe, L. A., Eckels, D. D., Ash, R., Casper, J., Hunter, J. B., and Gorski, J., The predictive value of HLA-DR oligotyping for MLC responses, *Transplantation*, 53, 1352, 1992.
11. Termijtelen, A., Erlich, H. A., Braun, L. A., Verduyn, W., Drabbels, J. J. M., Schroeijers, W. E. M., van Rood, J. J., de Koster, H. S., and Giphart, M. J., Oligonucleotide typing is a perfect tool to identify antigens stimulatory in the mixed lymphocyte culture, *Human Immunol.*, 31, 241, 1991.
12. Begovich, A. B., McClure, G. R., Suraj, V. C., Helmuth, R. C., Fildes, N., Bugawan, T., Erlich, H. A., and Klitz, W., Polymorphism, recombination, and linkage disequilibrium within the HLA class II region, *J. Immunol.*, 148, 249, 1992.

13. Fernandez-Vina, M. A., Tiercy, J. M., Tonai, R., Katovich-Hurley, C., Tsai, J., and Stastny, P., W3.10 DNA typing of DRB1 and DRB3 DR52-related specificities, in *HLA 1991*, Vol. 1, Tsuji, K., Aizawa, M., and Sasazuki, T., Eds, Oxford University Press, New York, 1992, 471.

14. Imanishi, T., Akaza, T., Kimura, A., Tokunaga, K., and Gojobori, T., Allele and haplotype frequencies for HLA and complement loci in various ethnic groups, in *HLA 1991*, Vol. I, Tsuji, K., Aizawa, M., and Sasazuki, T., Eds., Oxford University Press, New York, 1992, 1065.

15. Olerup, O., Troye-Blomberg, M., Schreuder, G. M. T., and Riley, E.M., HLA-DR and -DQ gene polymorphism in West Africans is twice as extensive as in North European Caucasians: evolutionary implications, *Proc. Natl. Acad. Sci. U.S.A.*, 88, 8480, 1991.

16. Marijt, E. A. F., Veenhof, W. F. J., Goulmy, E., Kluck, P. M. C., Brand, A., Willemze, R., Van Rood, J. J., and Falkenburg, J. H. F., Multiple minor histocompatibility antigens disparities between a recipient and four HLA-identical potential sibling donors for bone marrow transplantation, *Human Immunol.*, 37, 221, 1993.

17. Beatty, P. G., Dahlberg, S., Mickelson, E. M., Nisperos, B., Opelz, G., Martin, P. J., and Hansen, J. A., Probability of finding HLA-matched unrelated marrow donors, *Transplantation*, 45, 714, 1988.

18. Kernan, N. A., Bartsch, G., Ash, R. C., Beatty, P. G., Champlin, R., Filipovich, A., Gajewski, J., Hansen, J. A., Henslee-Downey, J., McCullough, J. et al., Analysis of 462 transplantations from unrelated donors facilitated by the National Marrow Donor Program, *N. Engl. J. Med.*, 328, 593, 1993.

19. Perkins, H. A. and Hansen, J. A., The U.S. National Marrow Donor Program, *Am. J. Pediatr. Hematol. Oncol.*, 16, 30, 1994.

20. Terasaki, P. I., Cecka, J. M., Cho, Y., Cicciarelli, J., Cohn, M., Gjertson, D., Lim, E. et al., Overview, in *Clinical Transplants 1990*, Terasaki, P., Ed., UCLA Tissue Typing Laboratory, Los Angeles, 1991, 585.

21. Hansen J. A., Anasetti C., Petersdorf, E., and Martin P. J., Marrow transplants from unrelated donors, *Transplant. Proc.*, 26, 1710, 1994.

22. Petersdorf, E. W., Smith, A. J., Mickelson, E. M., Longton, G. M., Anasetti, C., Choo, S. Y., Martin, P. J., and Hansen, J. A., Influence of HLA-DQB1 disparity on the development of acute graft-versus-host disease following unrelated donor marrow transplantation, *Transplant. Proc.*, 25, 1230, 1993.

23. Beatty, P.G., Anasetti, C., Hansen, J.A. et al., Marrow transplantation from unrelated donors for treatment of hematologic malignancies: effect of mismatching for one HLA locus, *Blood*, 81, 249, 1993.

24. Ng J., Hurley C. K, Baxter-Lowe L. A., Chopek M., Coppo, P.A., Hegland, J., KuKuruga, D., Monos, D., Rosner, G., Schmeckpeper, B., Yang, S. Y., Dupont, B., and Hartzman R. J., Large-scale oligonucleotide typing for HLA-DRB1/3/4 and HLA-DQB1 is highly accurate, specific, and reliable, *Tissue Antigens*, 42, 473, 1993.

25. Kawasaki, E.S. Sample preparation from blood, cells and other fluids, in *PCR Protocols: A Guide to Methods and Application*, Innis M.A., Gelfand, D.H., Sninsky, J.J., and White, T.J., Eds., Academic Press, New York, 1990, 146.

26. Saiki, R. K., Gelfand, D. H., Stoffel, S., Scharf, S. J., Higuchi, R., Horn, G. T., Mullis, K.B., and Erlich, H. A., Primer-directed enzymatic amplification of DNA with a thermostable DNA polymerase, *Science*, 239, 487, 1988.

27. Gao, X., Fernandez-Vina, M., Shumway, W., and Stastny, P., DNA typing for class II HLA antigens with allele-specific or group-specific amplification. I. Typing for subsets of HLA-DR4, *Human Immunol.*, 27, 40, 1990.

28. Molkentin, J., Gorski, J., and Baxter-Lowe, L. A., Detection of 14 HLA-DQB1 alleles by oligotyping, *Human Immunol.*, 31, 114, 1991.

29. Allen, M., Liu, L., and Gyllensten, U., A comprehensive polymerase chain reaction-oligonucleotide typing system for the HLA class I A locus, *Human Immunol.,* 40, 25, 1994.

30. Bugawan, T. L., Begovich, A. B., and Erlich, H. A., Rapid HLA-DPB typing using enzymatically amplified DNA and nonradioactive sequence-specific oligonucleotide probes, *Immunogenetics,* 32, 231, 1990.

31. Shaffer, A. L., Falk-Wade, J. A., Tortorelli, V., Cigan, A., Carter, C., Hassan, K., and Hurley, C. K., HLA-DRw52-associated DRB1 alleles: identification using polymerase chain reaction-amplified DNA, sequence-specific oligonucleotide probes, and a chemiluminescent detection system, *Tissue Antigens,* 39, 84, 1992.

32. Lazaro, A., Fernandez-Vina, M., Liu, Z., and Stastny, P., Enzyme-linked DNA oligotyping: a practical method for clinical HLA-DNA typing, *Human Immunol.,* 36, 243, 1993.

33. Kostyu, D. D., Pfohl, J., Ward, F. E., Lee, J. Murray, A., and Amos, D. B., Rapid HLA-DR oligotyping by an enzyme-linked immunosorbent assay performed in microtiter trays, *Human Immunol.,* 38, 1488, 1993.

34. Bugawan, T. L., Apple, R., and Erlich, H. A., A method for typing polymorphism at the HLA-A locus using PCR amplification and immobilized oligonucleotide probes, *Tissue Antigens,* 44, 137, 1994.

35. Salazar, M., Yunis, J. J., Delgado, M.B., Bing, D., and Yunis, E. J., HLA-DQB1 allele typing by a new PCR-RFLP method: correlation with a PCR-SSO method, *Tissue Antigens,* 40, 116, 1992.

36. Olerup, O. and Zetterquist, H., HLA-DR typing by PCR amplification with sequence specific primers (PCR-SSP) in 2 hours: an alternative to serological DR typing in clinical practice including donor-recipient matching in cadaveric transplantations, *Tissue Antigens,* 39, 225, 1992.

37. Zetterquist, H. and Olerup, O., Identification of the *HLA-DRB1*04, -DRB1*07,* and *-DRB1*09* alleles by PCR amplification with sequence-specific primers (PCR-SSP) in 2 hours, *Human Immunol.,* 34, 64, 1992.

38. Bunce, M. and Welsh, K. I., Rapid DNA typing for HLA-C using sequence specific primers (PCR-SSP): identification of serological and non-serologically defined HLA-C alleles including several new alleles, *Tissue Antigens,* 43, 7, 1994.

39. Sadler, A. M., Petronzelli, F., Krausa, P., Marsh, S. G. E., Guttridge, M. G., Browning, M. J., and Bodmer, J., Low resolution DNA typing for HLA-B using sequence-specific primers in allele- or group-specific ARMS/PCR, *Tissue Antigens,* 44, 148, 1994.

40. Spurkland, A., Knutsen, I., Markussen, G., Vartdal, F., Egeland, T., and Thorsby, E., HLA matching of unrelated bone marrow transplant pairs: direct sequencing of *in vitro* amplified HLA-DRB1 and -DQB1 genes using magnetic beads as solid support, *Tissue Antigens,* 41, 155, 1993.

41. Petersdorf, E.W., Stanley, J .F., Martin, P. J., and Hansen, J. A., Molecular diversity of the HLA-C locus in unrelated marrow transplantation, *Tissue Antigens,* 44, 93, 1994.

42. Versluis, L.F., Rozemuller, E., Tonks, S., Marsh, S. G. E., Bouwens, A. G. M., Bodmer, J. G., and Tilanus, M. G. J., High-resolution HLA-DPB typing based upon computerized analysis of data obtained by fluorescent sequencing of the amplified polymorphic exon 2, *Human Immunol.,* 38, 277, 1993.

43. Hoshino, S., Kimura, A., Fukuda, Y., Dohi, K., and Sasazuki, T., Polymerase chain reaction-single-strand conformation polymorphism analysis of polymorphism in DPA1 and DPB1 genes, A simple, economical, and rapid method for histocompatibility testing, *Human Immunol.,* 33, 98, 1992.

44. Summers, C., Morling, F., Taylor, M., Yin, J. L., and Stevens, R., Donor-recipient HLA class I bone marrow transplant matching by multilocus heteroduplex analysis, *Transplantation,* 58, 628, 1994.

45. Sorrentino, R., Potolicchio, I., Ferrara, G.B., and Tosi, R., A new approach to HLA-DPB1 typing combining DNA heteroduplex analysis with allele-specific amplification and enzyme restriction, *Immunogenetics*, 36, 248, 1992.

46. Hurley, C.K. and Yang, S.Y., Quality assurance and quality control for amplification-based typing, in *American Society for Histocompatibility and Immunogenetics Procedure Manual*, 1994.

47. Parham, P., Lomen, C. E., Lawlor, D. A., Ways, J. P., Holmes, N., Coppin, H. L., Salter, R. D., Wan, A. M., and Ennis, P. D., Nature of polymorphism in HLA-A, -B, and -C molecules, *Proc. Natl. Acad. Sci. U.S.A.*, 85, 4005, 1988.

48. Gao, X., Moraes, J. R., Miller, S., and Stastny, P., DNA typing for class II HLA antigens with allele-specific or group-specific amplification. V. Typing for subsets of HLA-DR1 and DR'Br, *Human Immunol.*, 30, 147, 1991.

49. Fernandez-Vina, M., Shumway, W., and Stastny, P., DNA typing for class II HLA antigens with allele-specific or group-specific amplification. II. Typing for alleles of the DRw52-associated group, *Human Immunol.*, 28, 51, 1990.

Chapter 14

METHODS FOR THE ANALYSIS OF THE HUMAN T-CELL RECEPTOR (TCR) REPERTOIRE IN HEALTH AND DISEASE

Pradip N. Akolkar, Beena Gulwani-Akolkar, and Jack Silver

CONTENTS

0-8493-0134-3/97/$0.00+$.50
© 1997 by CRC Press LLC

I. T LYMPHOCYTES IN THE IMMUNE SYSTEM

The development of immune responses in vertebrates requires the specific recognition of foreign substances by cells of the immune system. This specific recognition is mediated by lymphocytes divided into two main groups, B and T cells. B lymphocytes recognize soluble antigens such as proteins or molecules on the surface of pathogens using a cell surface receptor that essentially consists of a membrane form of an antibody molecule.[1-6] The recognition of antigen by B cells is highly dependent upon conformation; B-cell receptors that recognize a protein in its native conformation will, in general, fail to recognize the same protein when it is denatured.[2] In contrast, immunization of an animal with a protein in its native conformation will elicit T cells that can recognize the protein reintroduced to the animal in either native or denatured form. This is because T cells recognize foreign antigen only after processing of the protein, by antigen-presenting cells (APC), i.e., macrophages or B cells, into smaller peptides.[7,8] These peptides are then presented on the cell surface of the APC in combination with MHC (major histocompatibility complex) molecules to the T-cell receptor (TCR).[9] Peptides derived from proteins synthesized inside the APC (e.g., virally derived proteins) are normally presented to T cells by class I MHC products and consist of eight or nine amino acids.[10-14] In contrast, peptides derived from proteins that have become internalized by APC, by phagocytosis, for example, are presented to T cells by class II MHC molecules and can range in size from 15 to 20 amino acids.[13,15] Thus, because of the way that T cells "see" antigen, the TCR on the surface of the T cell must recognize not only the specific peptide but also the class I or class II MHC molecule (Figure 1). In most T cells (>90%) this receptor consists of a heterodimer composed of two polypeptide chains designated α and β. A minor population of T cells express an alternate receptor composed of the γ and δ polypeptides.

T lymphocytes are a heterogeneous population of cells phenotypically distinguishable on the basis of function and expression of cell surface markers such as CD4 and CD8. CD8+ cells, which comprise about 30 to 35% of peripheral blood T cells, represent the cytotoxic/suppressor population of T cells. In contrast, CD4+ cells, which represent about 60% of the total peripheral blood T-cell population, represent the

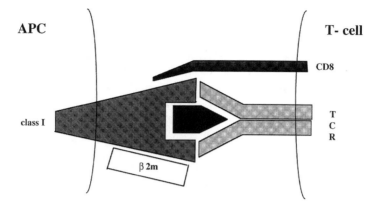

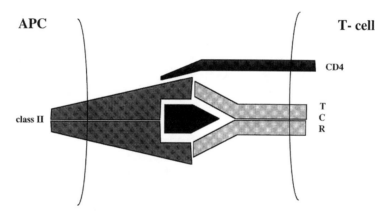

Figure 1
Interaction of MHC molecules on APC with T cells. Top: MHC class I molecules with bound peptide antigen interact with the T-cell receptor (TCR) and the coreceptor CD8. Bottom: MHC class II molecules with bound peptide antigen interact with the T-cell receptor (TCR) and the coreceptor CD4.

"helper" T-cell population; they "help" B cells to produce antibody and are necessary for the differentiation of immature CD8+ T cells to "killer" cells. For both groups of cells the CD4+ and CD8+ cell surface markers act as coreceptors in antigen recognition and interact specifically with class II and class I molecules, respectively, expressed by APC (Figure 1). CD4+ cells can be further subdivided into Th1 and Th2 cells, based on their ability to produce various lymphokines.[16,17] However, no cell surface markers distinguishing Th1 and Th2 cells have been described so far.

In addition to these subdivisions, both CD4+ and CD8+ T cells can be divided into a CD45RA+ and a CD45RO+ population. Thirty to 45% of CD4+ cells and 15 to 25% of CD8+ cells express CD45RO in the normal

T-cell population.[18,19] The surface markers CD45RA and CD45RO represent structurally distinct isoforms of a transmembrane tyrosine phosphatase that plays an important role in thymocyte maturation and T-cell activation and function.[20-23] The expression of CD45RA and CD45RO has been thought to be associated with "virgin" and "memory" cells, respectively.[24] However, recent studies suggest that expression of CD45RA more closely correlates with the state of responsiveness of the T cell. Thus, with time, activated/memory T cells return to a state of quiescence or hyporesponsiveness and express high levels of CD45RA. Therefore, not all CD45RA+ T cells are virgins.[25,26] Within the CD4+ population, CD45RO+ cells mediate proliferative responses to recall antigens and can support B-cell differentiation, whereas the CD8+ CD45RO+ subpopulation contains precursors that mediate memory-dependent cytotoxicity.[22]

In addition to single-positive (SP) T cells (CD4+ or CD8+), a small proportion of T cells in the peripheral blood do not express either the CD4 or CD8 marker and, hence, are called double negative (DN) T cells.[27] Most DN cells express the γδ receptor, but a small population of T cells that are DN instead express the αβ receptor. γδ T cells, which comprise 1 to 3% of the peripheral blood T-cell population, show a preponderance of reactivity to bacterial antigens and are thought to represent the first line of defense against bacteria. αβ DN T cells represent about 1% of peripheral blood T cells. Although their function is still unknown, they are present in the peripheral blood of all individuals and have been reported to increase in some pathological conditions such as systemic lupus erythematosis SLE or graft vs. host disease.[27-29]

II. THE T-CELL ANTIGEN RECEPTOR

The antigen receptor of circulating mature T cells is a heterodimer made up of two glycoproteins of highly variable structure that is clonally distributed and noncovalently associated with the CD3 complex.[1-6] Two types of T-cell receptors exist, one composed of α and β chains and another comprising γ and δ chains. Like immunoglobulin genes, the TCR genes are split in germline DNA into a number of gene segments comprising V, D, J, and C segments that recombine in developing T cells to form a functional TCR gene.[30]

A. The αβ T-Cell Receptor

The αβ heterodimer is the most common antigen receptor on human T cells and is present on over 95% of peripheral blood T cells.[6,30]

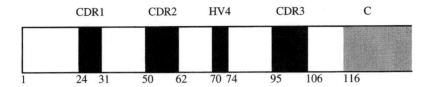

Figure 2
Schematic diagram of TCR Vβ polypeptide showing the hypervariable (HV) regions. The HV1, 2 and 3 regions correspond to the canonical complementarity-determining regions (CDR)1, 2, and 3, respectively. The HV4 region is thought to be involved in the interaction of Vβ chains with superantigen.

The development and maturation of T cells bearing the αβ heterodimer take place predominantly in the thymus.[3,4] Mature T cells bearing the αβ heterodimer recognize antigen when presented in association with either MHC class I or class II antigens. Like immunoglobulins (Ig), the α and β chains consist of variable (amino acids 1 to 116 for both α and β chains, Kabat et al. numbering system[31]) and constant (amino acids 117 to 259 for α chain and 117 to 295 for β chain) regions. Furthermore, like immunoglobulin variable (V) regions, the TCR V segments also show regions of hypervariability. Using a modified Wu-Kabat variability plot, Jores et al.[32] have shown that there are four regions of hypervariability in TCR β chains corresponding to aa 24 to 31, 50 to 62, 70 to 74 and 96 to 105 (Figure 2). However, unlike Ig V regions, precise identification of the complementarity determining regions (CDR), those regions of TCR V segments that interact directly with the antigen/MHC complex, has been difficult.[31-34] By using Ig V regions as a model, Jores et al.[32] and Chothia et al.[34] could identify framework regions of the T-cell receptor and define three complementarity determining regions (CDR1, aa 24 to 31; CDR2, aa 47 to 60; CDR3, aa 96 to 105) which comprise the putative peptide/MHC binding site. The first two, which are relatively less variable, are thought to be involved primarily in the interaction of the T-cell receptor with MHC proteins, whereas the third, CDR3, is thought to interact primarily with peptide (Figure 2). The fourth hypervariable region of the Vβ chain (aa 70 to 74) is thought to be involved in interactions with superantigens.[32,35]

The entire α and β (γ and δ) polypeptides are encoded by discontinuous gene segments that rearrange specifically in T cells during development. The portion of the Vβ chain that contains CDR1 and CDR2 (aa 1 to 102) is germline encoded and is represented in germline DNA by at least 63 different Vβ gene segments, at least 11 of which are nonfunctional because of premature termination codons.[36-39] These 63 Vβ segments can be grouped into 25 families, consisting of one or more members that are at least 75% identical in DNA sequence (Table 1). In

TABLE 1

Actual and Functional Size of Human Vβ Gene Families

Vβ Family	No. of Genes	No. of Functional Genes
1	1	1
2	2	1
3	1	1
4	2	1
5	6	6
6	9	7
7	3	3
8	5	3
9	2	1
10	2	1
11	2	1
12	3	3
13	9	9
14	1	1
15	1	1
16	1	1
17	1	1
18	1	1
19	2	1
20	1	1
21	3	3
22	1	1
23	1	1
24	1	1
25	1	1

contrast, the CDR3 (aa 96 to 105), which shows the greatest variability in terms of length and sequence, is represented by the V–D–J junctional region formed by the recombination of V, D, and J segments and can be further diversified by several additional mechanisms (see below). There are two groups of Dβ/Jβ segments, each of which is associated with a separate Cβ segment. Recombination of a Vβ segment with one of the two groups of Dβ/Jβ segments commits the RNA transcript to utilization of that particular Cβ segment. The two Cβ segments are highly homologous, differing in only four amino acids, and are thought to serve similar functions. Thus, a complete β chain is derived by recombination of one of 52 functional Vβ segments with one of the two Dβ segments and one of the 13 Jβ segments (Figure 3A), all of which are located on chromosome 7 at 7q35.[5,6,30,40] In a similar way, a functional α chain is derived by recombination between one of approximately 50 Vα segments, grouped into 29 families,[41] and one of over 70 Jα gene segments (Figure 3B). The entire TCR α gene complex is located on chromosome 14 at 14q11 and includes a single Cα segment.[5,6,30]

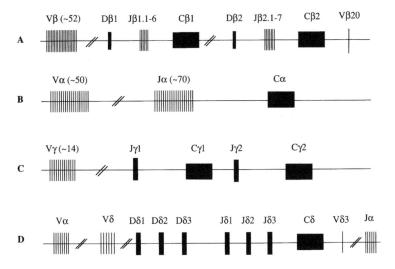

Figure 3

Genomic organization of the TCR genes. (A) β chain, (B) α chain, (C) γ chain, and (D) δ chain. V, variable segments; D, diversity segments; J, joining segments, and C, constant region segments. Note that the Vβ20 gene segment is located downstream of the Cβ2 segment.

B. The γδ T-Cell Receptor

A small percentage of T cells express a receptor composed of a γδ heterodimer instead of the αβ receptor. These cells usually lack both the CD4 and CD8 markers, although a small percentage of γδ⁺ T cells do express CD8 on their cell surface. In mice, distinct γδ T-cell subsets have been shown to develop in fetal thymus, adult thymus, and, independently of the thymus, in intestinal epithelia.[42-46] γδ Cells display cytotoxic activity and secrete lymphokines suggesting that they have most, if not all, of the effector functions of αβ T cells. γδ T cells may or may not require self MHC for recognition of antigen.[43,44] The γ chain gene complex is located on the short arm of chromosome 7. There are about 14 Vγ segments, 8 of which are functional, located upstream of two Jγ segments, each of which is associated with its own constant region segment (Figure 3C, 30). The human δ chain gene complex lies between the Vα- and Jα-segment complexes (Figure 3D). There are three Vδ segments, three Dδ segments, and three Jδ segments linked to a single constant region. Up to three Dδ segments may be used in a single transcript.[5]

TABLE 2

Generation of TCR Diversity

	Alpha	Beta
V gene segments	50	52
D gene segments	–	2
J gene segments	70	13
Ds in three reading frames	–	+
N region addition	+	++
Junctional diversity	+++	+++
Combinatorial joining	V × J	V × D × J
	50 × 70	52 × 2 × 13
Total	3,500	1,352
Combinatorial association	4.73×10^6	

III. THE T-CELL RECEPTOR REPERTOIRE

As described above, functional TCRs are derived from the recombination of various V, D, and J gene segments. In man, there are approximately 50 V and over 70 J gene segments for the α chain.[5,30,41,47] Similarly, for the β chain there are about 52 V, 2 D, and 13 J gene segments, divided into two groups of 6 and 7 Jβ segments, designated Jβ1.1 to 1.6 and Jβ2.1 to 2.7, respectively.[5,30,39,47] Any one of the Vα segments can, in theory, combine with any Jα-gene segment to form a functional Vα segment. Similarly, any one of the Vβ segments can combine with either of the Dβ segments (Dβ1.1 or Dβ2.1) and any one of the Jβ segments to form a functional Vβ segment. Occasionally both Dβ segments are used by the Vβ chain. Thus, recombination events can generate a vast array of Vα and Vβ chains (Table 2). This diversity can be further increased by combinatorial pairing of the functional α and β chains resulting, in theory, in about 5×10^6 combinations of αβ heterodimers (Table 2). Further diversification can occur by several additional mechanisms, such as junctional diversity that allows the V–D and D–J joining to occur in any one of three possible frames (Figure 4). Furthermore, the insertion of 0–6 nucleotides at the ends during V–J/V–D–J recombiation adds an additional degree of diversity (Figure 5). Thus, as many as 10^9 to 10^{11} different TCRs can, in theory, be formed by a combination of these mechanisms.

The TCR repertoire of an individual can be defined as the entire array of different TCRs normally present in any one organ or tissue (e.g., peripheral blood, spleen, gut) or which is used in response to an antigen. Although the theoretical TCR repertoire of an individual can be vast, in practice it is likely to be much smaller because of positive and negative selection mechanisms (see below). Furthermore, the

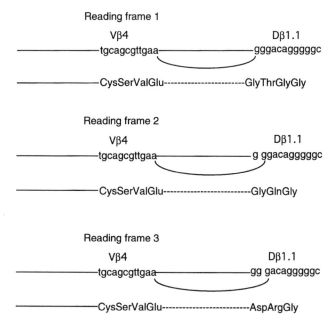

Figure 4
TCR diversity generated by recombination of the Vβ and Dβ gene segments in three different reading frames.

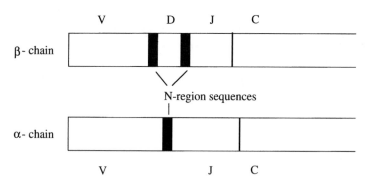

Figure 5
Generation of diversity by the insertion of N-region sequences during the recombination of V–(D)–J segments.

requirements for specific antigen recognition can drastically limit the TCR repertoire used in response to a specific antigen. Nevertheless, even a repertoire limited by these factors can still be substantially large, with estimates that range from 10^4 for an antigen-specific response to

10^9 for an unselected repertoire. Because of this enormity, "short cut" methods have been devised to gain a "window" on TCR usage that might be representative of the entire T-cell population of an individual, and which would allow one to distinguish between the utilization of very similar or disparate repertoires by different individuals or by different antigens. These methods range from the tedious, but highly specific methods of T-cell cloning, followed by DNA sequence analysis, to the more crude but rapid analyses of Vβ-, Vα-, or Jβ-segment utilization by qPCR (quantitative polymerase chain reaction, see below) or hybridization with oligonucleotide probes. However, before the methods that have been employed to assess the TCR repertoire are reviewed, it is instructive to first discuss some of the factors that can influence the functional TCR repertoire.

IV. FACTORS THAT INFLUENCE THE TCR REPERTOIRE

At least three factors, two of which are genetic, can potentially influence the human TCR repertoire.

A. Germline Polymorphism

Allelic variants differing by one or a few amino acids have now been described for Vβ1, Vβ2, Vβ5.3, Vβ6.1, 6.5, 6.7, Vβ13.4, Vβ15, Vβ20, and Vβ21.[4,38,39,48-54] Some of these changes localize to CDR1 or CDR2[49,50] and, thus, could potentially alter the ability to recognize specific peptide/MHC complexes. Others result in either premature termination codons (Vβ20[48,51]) or amino acid substitutions that preclude formation of a functional T-cell receptor (Vβ6.1[39]). In one recently described example, a mutation in the recombination signal region of Vβ3 genes results in very different levels of Vβ3.[53] In another case (Vβ6.7), allelic variation in the fourth hypervariable region (HVR4), which is thought to be involved in the interaction between superantigens and the TCR, results in two alleles that differ in their ability to respond to the superantigen SEE.[35,52] These and other allelic variants could, obviously, have a major impact on the available TCR repertoire, and could potentially have important health implications, especially if they were involved in mediating normal immune responses to a pathogen or abnormal autoimmune responses to a self-antigen. An additional polymorphism that has been described for the TCR β locus involves a 30-kb insertion/deletion.[55,56] This segment is now known to include several additional Vβ segments (Vβ7.3, 9.2, 13.2; see Reference 57).

B. Thymic Selection

During the development of T cells in the thymus, the TCR repertoire undergoes a selection process. This occurs during the maturation of double positive (DP), i.e., $CD4^+CD8^+$, thymocytes to single positive (SP), i.e., $CD4^+$ or $CD8^+$, T cells. During this transition from DP to SP, in a process known as positive selection which is not entirely understood, cells whose TCR have the potential to recognize foreign peptides presented by self-MHC class I molecules are allowed to mature into $CD8^+$ SP cells. Similarly, cells whose TCR have the potential to recognize peptides presented by self-MHC class II molecules are selected as $CD4^+$ SP cells. Those T cells selected by this process are, in general, incapable of recognizing the same peptides presented by nonself MHC molecules. In this way, the vast number of T cells that can potentially recognize foreign peptides presented by any allelic form of MHC molecule are culled so that only a small portion of all of the possible TCR is ever used. In addition to "positive" selection, a process known as "negative" selection occurs in which T cells whose TCR have the potential to recognize self-antigens presented by self-MHC are eliminated. Although, in general, this process eliminates only a small portion of the potential TCR repertoire, clonal deletion by endogenous "superantigens," which in most cases have been identified as retroviral proteins, can lead to elimination of major portions of the potential repertoire.[58,59] However, such endogenous "superantigens" have so far only been described in mice.

C. Antigen Exposure

Exposure of naive T cells to antigen leads to activation and clonal expansion. Thus, an individual's TCR repertoire at any point in time may be a function of recent exposure to various antigens and pathogens. In addition, some disease processes appear to alter the "normal" TCR repertoire (Table 3), so that it is important to have a good medical history of the individual when interpreting the results of TCR repertoire analysis. Furthermore, some T cells are long-lived and thus, alteration of the TCR repertoire by any of these factors can also lead to a permanent change in the TCR repertoire. As a result, the TCR repertoires of older individuals tend to deviate more from the normal "naive" repertoire. Several studies suggest that these changes are especially pronounced in the $CD8^+$ population.[132,133] Attempts have been made to avoid the effects of prior antigen exposure when analyzing the TCR repertoire by prior selection for CD45RO⁻ ("naive") cells. However, even this does not provide for an accurate measure of the repertoire,

TABLE 3

TCR Repertoire in Disease

Method Used	Cells Analyzed	Results	Author (Ref.)
Rheumatoid Arthritis			
Oligonucleotide PCR	Synovial fluid (SF) T cells	Expansion of Vβ14	Paliard et al. (60)
Oligonucleotide PCR	IL-2R⁺ T cells of synovial tissue	Over expression of Vβ13, 14, 17	Howell et al. (61)
Oligonucleotide PCR	Synovial T cells, PBL	Polyclonal Vα	Olive et al. (62)
Oligonucleotide PCR	SF T cells	Dominant Vβ7	Sottini et al. (63)
Inverse PCR	SF T cells	Vβ2, polyclonal Vα	Uematsu et al. (64)
Anchored PCR	SF T cells	Biased Vα usage	Pluschke et al. (65)
Oligonuclotide PCR	SF T cells	Heterogeneity in Vβ restricted Vα usage	Bucht et al. (66)
Oligonucleotide PCR	SF T cells, PBL	Increased Vα10, 15, 18, and Vβ4, 5, 13 in SF	Lunardi et al. (67)
Oligonucleotide PCR	SF T cells, PBL	Heterogeneity in Vβ	Williams et al. (68)
Oligonucleotide PCR	SF T cells, PBL	Increased Vβ6	Weyand et al. (69)
Oligonucleotide PCR	SF T cells	Vγ2 clonal expansion	Doherty et al. (70)
Oligonucleotide PCR	Synovial membrane, T-cells	Increased Vδ2	Olive et al. (71)
Oligonucleotide PCR	Synovial membrane, T cells	No bias in Vγ, increased Vδ1	Olive et al. (72)
Oligonucleotide PCR	Synovial membrane, T cells	Vγ-clonal expansion	Olive et al. (73)
Oligonucleotide PCR	SF T cells	No bias in Vβ	Dedeoglu et al. (74)
Anchored PCR	SF T cells	Biased Vβ usage	Pluschke et al. (75)
Oligonucleotide PCR	BCG reactive T-cell clones from SF	Increased Vβ8	Wilson et al. (76)
Oligonucleotide PCR	SF T cells, PBL	No change	Davey et al. (77)
Oligonucleotide PCR	SF T cells, PBL	Increased Vβ 6, 14, 15 in SF	Jenkins et al. (78)
Anchored PCR	PB T cells	No specific expansion	Kohsaka et al. (79)
Mab	SF T cells, PBL	No change	Posnett et al. (80)
Mab	PB T cells	Increased Vα12.1	Der Simonian et al. (81)
Mab	Synovial tissue	Biased use of Vβ	Gudmundsson et al. (82)
Mab	T-cell clones from SF	No Change	Korthauer et al. (83)

Method	Tissue/Cells	Finding	Reference
Mab	Synovial membrane	Increased Vδ1	Shen et al. (84)
Mab	SF T cells, PBL	Increased Vα2 in SF	Broker et al. (85)
Multiple Sclerosis			
Oligonucleotide PCR	T cells from brain	Increased Vβ12.1	Oksenberg et al. (86)
Oligonucleotide PCR	MS plaque tissue	Polyclonal	Wucherpfennig et al. (87)
Oligonucleotide PCR	MS plaque tissue	Clonal expansion of Vδ1, Vδ2 and Vγ2	Wucherpfennig et al. (88)
Oligonucleotide PCR	PBL, CSF	Increased Vβ12	Birnbaum et al. (89)
Oligonucleotide PCR	PBL	Skewed Vβ repertoire	Utz et al. (90)
Oligonucleotide PCR	MS plaque tissue	Increased Vβ5.2	Oksenberg et al. (91)
Oligonucleotide PCR	CSF	Clonal expansion of γδ cells	Shimonkevitz et al. (92)
Oligonucleotide PCR	T cells from brain	Increased Vδ2 and Vγ2	Hvas et al. (93)
Oligonucleotide PCR	CSF, PBL	Increased Vβ1, 2, 5, 18	Chou et al. (94)
Oligonucleotide PCR	PBL	No specific change	Roth et al. (95)
Sarcoidosis			
Oligonucleotide PCR	PBL, lung T cells	No specific change	Bellocq et al. (96)
Mab	T cells from bronchoalveolar lavage fluid	Increased Vα2.3 in HLA DR3 individuals	Grunewald et al. (97)
Autoimmune Thyroid Disease			
Oligonucleotide PCR	Intrathyroid T cells	Restricted Vα usage	Davies et al. (98)
Grave's Disease			
Oligonucleotide PCR	PBL	No change	McIntosh et al. (99)
Myasthenia Gravis			
Mab	PBL	Increased Vβ12	Grunewald et al. (100)

TABLE 3 (continued)

TCR Repertoire in Disease

Method Used	Cells Analyzed	Results	Author (Ref.)
Sjögren's Syndrome			
Oligonucleotide PCR	T cells in lips	Predominant expression of Vβ13	Sumida et al. (101)
Oligonucleotide PCR	T-cells in lips	Predominant expression of Vβ13	Yonaha et al. (102)
Kawasaki Disease			
Oligonucleotide PCR	PBL	Elevated levels of Vβ2 and Vβ8.1	Abe et al. (103)
Mab	PBL	Polyclonal expansion of Vβ2 and Vβ8 T-cells	Abe et al. (104)
Crohn's Disease			
Oligonucleotide PCR	PBL	No change	Gulwani-Akolkar et al. (105)
Mab	PBL	Increased Vβ8	Posnett et al. (106)
Mab	PBL, lamina propria lymphocytes	No change	Shalon et al. (107)

TABLE 3 (continued)

TCR Repertoire in Disease

Method Used	SA/Ag	Cells Analyzed	Results	Author (Ref.)
Superantigens				
Oligonucleotide PCR	SEB	PBL	Increased Vβ 3,12, 14,15,17,20	Choi et al. (108)
	SEC2		Increased Vβ 12,13.1 13.2,14,15,17,20	
	SEE		Increased Vβ Vβ 5.1,6,8,18	
	EXT		Increased Vβ 2	
	TSST		Increased Vβ 2	
Oligonucleotide PCR	Toxic shock syndrome	PBL	Increased Vβ 2	Choi et al. (109)
Oligonucleotide PCR	Staph M Protein	PBL	Increased V β2,4	Tomqi et al. (110)
Mab	SEA	PBL	No change	Kappler et al. (111)
	SEB	Increased Vβ 12		
	SEC1	Increased Vβ 12		
	SEC2	Increased Vβ 12		
	SEC3	Increased Vβ 5,12		
	SED	Increased Vβ 5,12		
	SEE	Increased Vβ 8		
	EAFT	No change		
	TSST	No change		
Mab	MAM	PBL	Increased Vβ17	Friedman et al. (112)
Mab	Rabies	PBL	Increased Vβ 8.0	Lafon et al. (113)

TABLE 3 (continued)

TCR Repertoire in Disease

Method Used	SA/Ag	Cells Analyzed	Results	Author (Ref.)
Viral Infections				
Oligonucleotide PCR	HIV	PBL	Reduced expression of Vβ14, 15, 16, 17, 18, 19, 20	Imberti et al. (114)
Oligonucleotide PCR	HIV	PBL Lymphnodes	Altered TCR repertoire	Soudeyns et al. (115)
Mab	HIV	PBL	Increased Vβ5.3	Dalgleish et al. (116)
Mab	HIV	PBL	Reduced Vβ5.1, 12 and Vα2	Bansal et al. (117)
Mab	HIV	PBL	Reduced Vβ5.1, 12 and Vα2	Bansal et al. (118)
Mab	EBV	PBL	Increased Vδ1	Orsini et al. (119)
Mab	HIV	PBL	Increased Vβ13, 21	Rebai et al. (120)
Bacterial Infections				
Oligonucleotide PCR	*M. leprae*	T-cells lesions	Increased Vβ6, 12, 14 and 19	Wang et al. (121)
Oligonucleotide PCR	*M. leprae*	T-cells lesions	Skewed Vβ usage	Uyemura et al. (122)
Oligonucleotide PCR	*M. leprae*	T-cells lesions	Expansion of Vδ1	Uyemura et al. (123)
Oligonucleotide PCR	*M. tuberculosis*	PBL	Expansion of Vβ8	Ohmen et al. (124)
Leukemias and Lymphomas				
Oligonucleotide PCR	Hodgkin's disease	TIL	No bias	Xerri et al. (125)
Oligonucleotide PCR	Leukemia	PBL	No bias	Kasten-Sportes et al. (126)
Mab	Cutaneous T-cell lymphoma	Biopsy	Reactive T cells Vβ5	Hunt et al. (127)
Mab	T-cell lymphomas	Biopsy	29% showed restricted V-gene usage	Poppema et al. (128)
Mab	Cutaneous T-cell lymphoma	Biopsy	10/16 expressed Vβ8	Jack et al. (129)
Mab	T-cell lymphomas	Malignant cells	Increased Vβ5,12 and Vα2	Smith et al. (130)
Mab	T-cell lymphomas	Malignant cells	Increased Vα2	Ohshima et al. (131)

since several studies suggest that activated ("memory") T cells can lose the CD45RO marker over time,[19,24-26] and, thus, will contaminate the "naive" pool of T cells. It should also be noted that the TCR repertoire can vary among the different organs of the body. For example, T cells in peripheral blood and in the intestine appear to have different TCR repertoires. This may be due to differences in the antigens to which these cells have been exposed or, as has been suggested for IEL (intraepithelial lymphocytes) in the intestine, to the lack of thymic selection.[134]

V. ANALYSIS OF THE TCR REPERTOIRE WITH V-SEGMENT-SPECIFIC Mab

The employment of Mab technology has led to the development of reagents capable of detecting and specifically distinguishing between TCR expressing different V segments.[112,135-143] By combining these reagents with fluorescence–activated cell sorting (FACS) or flow cytometry, it is now possible to analyze, quantitate, and isolate subpopulations of T cells bearing different TCR. Numerous Mab against specific Vα and Vβ segments are now commercially available, although Vβ-specific reagents predominate. A listing of the reagents available and their specificity is provided in Table 4. Some of the Mab recognize selected members of a Vα or Vβ family, while others appear to recognize all of the members within a particular V-segment family. For some, the precise specificity is still being determined. Furthermore, the influence of Vα or Jβ segments on the recognition of specific Vβ segments by Vβ-specific Mab is still unknown in most cases, leaving open the possibility that receptors with particular combinations of VαVβ or VβJβ segments may go unrecognized even by Mab that are specific for that particular Vβ segment.

Blood is the most common source of lymphoid cells used for analysis. In general, lymphocytes are separated from other cells prior to staining, and this is achieved by density gradient separation on Ficoll-Hypaque. Preparation of lymphocytes from lymphoid tissue other than blood requires additional processing. In general, lymphoid tissues are relatively easy to dissociate by teasing or forcing the tissue through a mesh. The resulting cell suspension is processed in a manner similar to blood for purification of lymphocytes.

T cells are stained with V-segment-specific Mab, either by the direct method in which the Mab is directly conjugated to a fluorochrome or, by the indirect method in which the fluorochrome is attached to a second step reagent, i.e., goat antimouse Ig, which in turn binds to the Mab. Each of these techniques has its own advantages and disadvantages for flow cytometry. Direct staining is technically simpler and, in general, results in less nonspecific staining. However, it lacks the signal

TABLE 4

List of Commercially Available V-Segment Specific Mab Reagents

Name	Antibody Clone	Specificity	Source
TCR Vβ2	E22E72	All members of Vβ2 family	Immunotech
TCR Vβ3	LE89	Vβ3.1 and Vβ3.2	Immunotech
TCR Vβ5.2	36213	Vβ5.2	Immunotech
TCR Vβ5.3	3D11	Vβ5.3	Immunotech
TCR Vβ8	56C5	Vβ8.1 and Vβ8.2	Immunotech
TCR Vβ13.5	JU74	Vβ13.5	Immunotech
TCR Vβ17	BA62	Vβ17.1 and 17.2	Immunotech
TCR Vβ19	E17.5F3	Vβ19.1	Immunotech
TCR Vβ21	1G125	Vβ21.6	Immunotech
TCR Vβ22	Immu546	Vβ22.1	Immunotech
TCR VγI	23D12	VγI-2, VγI-3, VγI-4	Immunotech
TCR Vγ9	Immu360	Vγ9	Immunotech
TCR Vδ1	Immu515	Vδ1	Immunotech
TCR Vδ2	Immu389	Vδ2	Immunotech
βV3	8F10	Vβ3.1	T Cell Diagnostics
βV5(a)	1C1	Vβ5.3 and 5.2	T Cell Diagnostics
βV5(b)	W112	Vβ5.3	T Cell Diagnostics
βV5(c)	LC4	Vβ5.1	T Cell Diagnostics
βV6(a)	OT145	Vβ6.7	T Cell Diagnostics
βV7	3C5	Vβ7.1	T Cell Diagnostics
βV8(a)	16G8	Vβ8	T Cell Diagnostics
βV8(b)	MX6	Vβ8	T Cell Diagnostics
βV12(a)	S511	Vβ12.1	T Cell Diagnostics
βV13	BAM13	Vβ13.1 and 13.3	T Cell Diagnostics
βV16	Tamaya1.2	Vβ16	T Cell Diagnostics
βV17	C1	Vβ17	T Cell Diagnostics
βV18	BA62	Vβ18	T Cell Diagnostics
βV20	ELL1.4	Vβ20	T Cell Diagnostics
βV21	IG.125	Vβ21.3	T Cell Diagnostics
αV2(a)	F1	Vα2.3	T Cell Diagnostics
αV12(a)	6D6	Vα12.1	T Cell Diagnostics
δV1(a)	TS8	Vδ1	T Cell Diagnostics
δV2(a)	15D	Vδ2	T Cell Diagnostics
γV1.4	4A11	Vγ1.4	T Cell Diagnostics
γV2(a)	7A5	Vγ2.0	T Cell Diagnostics

amplification that can be achieved with the indirect method where multiple second-step reagent molecules bind to a single TCR-specific molecule. Other factors to be considered at the time of staining the cells include the use of saturating amounts of reagents, the possible effects of temperature, the metabolic activity of the cells, and the time required to achieve equilibrium. Generally, it is preferable to stain lymphocytes in the cold and/or in the presence of inhibitors of metabolism, such as sodium azide. It is generally agreed that equilibrium of binding occurs rapidly (15 to 30 min) under the conditions used for staining cells. It is also advisable to use F(ab)$_2$ fragments to reduce nonspecific binding when indirect staining is used.

It has become increasingly common to employ staining protocols utilizing several different chromophores to allow the detection of two or more cell surface markers simultaneously. For immunofluorescence, the choice of fluorochrome for double or triple staining is critical. Until recently, the only practical choices were to use fluorescein isothiocynate and an analogue of rhodamine known as Texas red. This combination required the use of two lasers for maximum excitation of·both dyes and for complete separation of the emissions. With the introduction of phycoerythrin, it is now possible to use a single laser source for the two different dyes. Successful analysis requires that the positive cells be clearly resolvable from negative cells. Control samples are generally used to define the negative population. For indirect immunofluorescence, the control may be an irrelevant Mab or buffer followed by the second-stage reagent. With direct staining, the control usually consists of a directly conjugated irrelevant Mab of the same isotype.

Although double and triple staining of cells by the direct method is usually the method of choice, most of the V-segment-specific Mab, unfortunately, are not available in directly labeled form. Although this situation may change in the near future, it places severe limitations on the ability to define the repertoire in subpopulations of T cells. One method for circumventing this problem is to use magnetic beads in combination with a Mab to one of the cell surface markers of interest, e.g., CD4+ or CD8+, to first isolate the desired subpopulation before staining with the V-segment-specific Mab. The Mab used to first isolate the desired cell population may be either directly coupled to the magnetic beads or, in a method analogous to indirect immunoprecipitation or indirect staining, can be used in combination with magnetic beads to which goat-antimouse Ig has been coupled. We have successfully used these methods to compare the TCR repertoires of CD4+ and CD8+ cells.[105,144,145] Another way of getting around this problem is to take advantage of the fact that most of the Vβ-specific Mab are of the γ1 or γ2 subclass. By combining a directly labeled reagent (e.g., anti-CD4) which is of one subclass, e.g., γ1, with V-segment-specific Mab of another subclass, e.g., γ2, and rat-antimouse IgG2 directly labeled with a different fluorochrome, it is possible to perform two-color staining of T cells.[146]

VI. ANALYSIS OF THE TCR REPERTOIRE BY THE QUANTITATIVE POLYMERASE CHAIN REACTION

The quantitative polymerase chain reaction (qPCR) is a method for rapidly amplifying a portion of DNA where, usually, only sequences in the flanking regions are completely known.[147-152] In this way, DNA of mutant proteins, allelic variants, and individual members of multigene

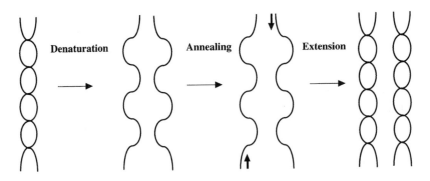

Figure 6
The polymerase chain reaction. The basic PCR cycle consists of three steps: denaturation of DNA at high temperature, annealing of the oligonucleotide primers, and enzymatic extension of the primers. During PCR, the concentration of the targeted DNA increases geometrically.

families can be rapidly isolated and characterized. The template DNA can be derived from clinical, laboratory, forensic, or archeological samples and requires minimal purification. Amplification of DNA by PCR is based on the repetition of three reactions (Figure 6). In the first, DNA is denatured by heating to a high temperature (95°C) to dissociate the two strands of DNA. In the second step, the temperature is lowered to allow the annealing of specific oligonucleotide primers, ranging in size from 14 to 25 bases, to their complementary sequences on the opposite strands of the template DNA. Thus, two primers, a "forward" and a "reverse" primer are required for any PCR. The third step involves extension of the primers with DNA polymerase. Because the primers are present in the reaction at large molar concentrations, the formation of primer-DNA complexes is favored over the reassociation of the two template DNA strands. The end product is then denatured again for another cycle. Typically, 25 to 35 cycles are sufficient to amplify the product of interest by a factor of 10^9.

By combining PCR with V-segment-specific forward primers and constant (C) region reverse primers and performing the reaction on cDNA derived from T-cell RNA, it is possible to amplify the expressed TCR repertoire of any one individual or subpopulation of T cells. In addition, by appropriately modifying conditions, PCR can be used to semiquantitate the amount of RNA corresponding to a particular sequence or V-segment family. This method, known as qPCR, has been used successfully to analyze the human TCR repertoire in many different situations; qPCR has been used to assess V-segment usage in different antigen responses and in defining the Vβ segments that are recognized by, and respond to, superantigens (Table 3). However, its greatest contribution has been in defining the changes in TCR repertoire that accompany a variety of disease processes (Table 3). Thus, for example, qPCR has been used to characterize T cells derived from the peripheral blood and pathological lesions of patients with autoimmune diseases or with bacterial or viral infections (see Table 3). In addition, PCR has been used to define TCR in tumor-infiltrating lymphocytes.[153-155] Described below is the protocol used by us for the analysis of the Vα and Vβ repertoire in CD4+ and CD8+ cells.[27,144,145]

T-cell subsets are purified using Mab-coupled immunomagnetic beads and total RNA is extracted from the bound cells with RNAzol-B.[156] The RNA is reverse transcribed into cDNA using either oligo dT, random hexamers or a C-region-specific oligonucleotide reverse primer. In our hands, downstream C-region primers have worked best for preparing the first strand cDNA template (Cβ-3 in Table 5). The cDNA is then amplified with a V-segment-specific primer and a second, nested (upstream of the first C-region primer, Cβ-2R in Table 5), constant-region primer (Figure 7). The sequences of the V-segment-specific primers and those used for preparing cDNA are given in Tables 5 and 6. However, other V-segment-specific primers have been used by other investigators.[157-159] As a control and for purposes of quantitation, when Vβ segments are analyzed by qPCR, a constant-region segment of the α chain is usually coamplified simultaneously using two Cα-chain-specific primers (Table 5). Of course, this also requires that a Cα-region reverse primer be used in the preparation of α chain cDNA at the same time that β chain cDNA is reverse-transcribed. Similarly, when Vα segments are analyzed by qPCR, a C-region segment of the β chain is coamplified. Using the primers shown in Table 5, the sizes of the amplified Vβ–specific segments range from 170 to 220 bp, whereas the control C-region segment of the Cα chain is 315 bp long. Similarly, using the primers shown in Table 6, the sizes of the amplified Vα-specific segments range in size from 320 to 410, whereas the control C-region segment of the Cβ chain is 510 bp long.

For quantitation, the amplifications are performed using reverse primers labeled with ^{32}P at the 5′ end. The amplified products are separated on 8.0% polyacrylamide gels (6.0% for Vα segments), dried under vacuum, and exposed to X-ray film. Examples of the amplification of Vβ and Vα segments by PCR are shown below (Figures 8 and 9). By using the autoradiograms for alignment, the amplified Cα (or Cβ) and Vβ (or Vα) bands are excised from the gel and the amount of radioactivity incorporated determined by liquid scintillation counting. Alternatively, commercial phosphorimagers may be used to quantitate the amount of radioactivity in each band; however, we have found that quantitation using the manual method is equally accurate. To correct for the efficiency of amplification in each well, the cpm in each V-segment band is normalized to the C-segment band. The relative amount of each V segment is then expressed as a percent of the total

TABLE 5

PCR Primers for Vβ Analysis

Vβ1	5'-GCACAACAGTTCCCTGACTTGCAC-3'
Vβ2	5'-TCATCAACCATGCAAGCCTGACCT-3'
Vβ3	5'-GTCTCTAGAGAGAAGAAGGAGCGC-3'
Vβ4	5'-ACATATGAGAGTGGATTTGTCATT-3'
Vβ5.1	5'-ATACTTCAGTGAGACACAGAGAAAC-3'
Vβ5.2	5'-TTCCCTAACTATAGCTCTGAGCTG-3'
Vβ6	5'-AGGCCTGAGGGATCCGTCTC-3'
Vβ7	5'-CCTGAATGCCCCAACAGCTCTC-3'
Vβ8	5'-ATTTACTTTAACAACAACGTTCCG-3'
Vβ9	5'-CCTAAATCTCCAGACAAAGCTCAC-3'
Vβ10	5'-CTCCAAAAACTCATCCTGTACCTT-3'
Vβ11	5'-TCAACACAGTCTCCAGAATAAGGACG-3'
Vβ12	5'-AAAGGAGAAGTCTCAGAT-3'
Vβ13.1	5'-CAAGGAGAAGTCCCCAAT-3'
Vβ13.2	5'-GGTGAGGGTACAACTGCC-3'
Vβ14	5'-GTCTCTCGAAAAGAGAAGAGGAAT-3'
Vβ15	5'-AGTGTCTCTCGACAGGCACAGGCT-3'
Vβ16	5'-AAAGAGTCTAAACAGGATGAGTCC-3'
Vβ17	5'-CAGATAGTAAATGACTTTCAG-3'
Vβ18	5'-GATGAGTCAGGAATGCCAAAGGAA-3'
Vβ19	5'-CAATGCCCCAAGAACGCACCCTGC-3'
Vβ20	5'-AGCTCTGAGGTGCCCCAGAATCTC-3'
Cβ–3	5'-TTCTGATGGCTCAAACAC-3'
Cβ–2R	5' -ACAGCGACCTCGGGTGGGAA -3'
5'Cα	5'-GAACCCTGACCCTGCCGTGTACC-3'
3'Cα	5'-TCATGTTTCAAAGCTTTTCTCGAC-3'

cpm incorporated in all the V segments after normalizing to the C-segment counts.

A number of precautions must be taken to ensure that the results obtained by this procedure are sufficiently quantitative. First, it is mandatory that one establishes and uses conditions in which PCR amplification proceeds exponentially at a constant efficiency so that the PCR signal is proportional to the amount of input RNA for each V segment. Otherwise, at high cycle number and/or high concentrations of RNA it is possible to reach conditions where the PCR signal begins to plateau and is no longer proportional to the amount of RNA present.[160] Thus, it is extremely important, when quantitating the relative usage of different Vβ (or Vα) segments by this procedure, that the appropriate dilutions of cDNA and the number of PCR cycles be calibrated so that the PCR signal correlates in a fairly linear fashion with the amount of input RNA. This can be done by performing the PCR at variable numbers of cycles, using increasing amounts of cDNA and examining whether the signal increases proportionately. We have found that 30 PCR cycles used together with approximately 100 ng of T-cell RNA provides signals that correlate well with the amount of input RNA (see

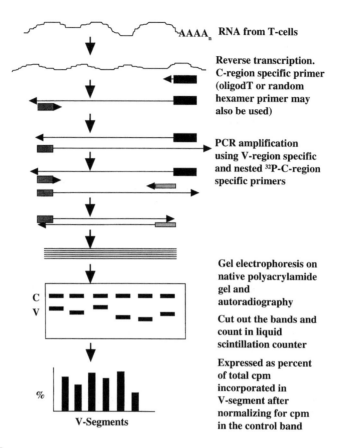

Figure 7
Schematic diagram of RT (reverse transcriptase)-PCR used for quantitating TCR V-segment usage.

Figure 10). However, it is important to remember that the relative RNA values obtained after qPCR for each V segment do not necessarily reflect the actual values of V-segment-specific RNA present before amplification. This is because the various V-segment-specific primers do not amplify with the same efficiency. However, if necessary, the absolute amount of any specific V segment can be determined by competitive PCR.[161,162] Alternatively, the number of T cells expressing that particular V segment can be determined with V- segment-specific Mab, although this procedure also has its limitations (see above). In most cases, this is not important, since the investigator is usually interested only in determining whether the repertoires of two individuals or subpopulations of T cells are different or whether some pathological or environmental factor has led to an alteration of the repertoire. It does mean, however, that, when the repertoires of any two samples that the

TABLE 6

PCR Primers for Vα Analysis

Vα1	5'-CTGAGGTGCAACTACTCA-3'
Vα2	5'-GTGTTCCCAGAGGGAGCCATTGCC-3'
Vα3	5'-GGTGAACAGTCAACAGGGAGA-3'
Vα4	5'-ACAAGCATTACTGTACTCCTA-3'
Vα5	5'-GGCCCTGAACATTCAGGA-3'
Vα6	5'-GTCACTTTCTAGCCTGCTGA-3'
Vα7	5'-GGAGAGATGTGGAGATAAA-3'
Vα8	5'-GGAGAGATGTGGAGCAGCATC-3'
Vα9	5'-ATCTCAGTGCTTGTGATAATA-3'
Vα10	5'-ACCCAGCTGGTGGAGCAGAGCCCT-3'
Vα11	5'-AGAAAGCAAGGACCAAGTGTT-3'
Vα12	5'-CAGAAGGTAACTCAAGCGCAGACT-3'
Vα13	5'-GCTTATGAGAACACTGCGT-3'
Vα14	5'-GCAGCTTCCCTTCCAGCAAT-3'
Vα15	5'-AGAACCTGACTGCCCAGGAA-3'
Vα16	5'-CATCTCCATGGACTCATATGA-3'
Vα17	5'-GACTATACTAACACAGCATGT-3'
Vα19	5'-AAATGAAGTGGAGCAGAGTCCTCAGAAGCT-3'
Vα20	5'-AGCTAAGACCACCCAGCCCATC-3'
Vα21	5'-ACAGCAAGTTAAGCAAAATTCACCA-3'
Vα23	5'-AAACAGGAGGTGACACAGATTCCTGCAGCT-3'
Vα24	5'-TCAATGCAATTATACAGTGAG-3'
Vα25	5'-TTCAAGCATATTTAACACCTG-3'
Vα26	5'-GCACGTCATCAAAGACGTTATATGGCTTAT-3'
Vα27	5'-CCACTTCAGACAGACTGTATT-3'
Vα28	5'-AAGTGACTAACTTTCGAAGCC-3'
Vα29	5'-CCTCCAAGGCTTTATATTCTG-3'
Cα1R	5'-GGTACACGGCAGGGTCAGGGTT-3'
Cα2R	5'-ACAGACTTGTCACTGGAT-3'
Cβ1	5'-TTCCCACCCGAGGTCGCTGT-3'
Cβ4	5'-ATCCTTTCTCTTGACCATGGC-3'

Vβ Segment

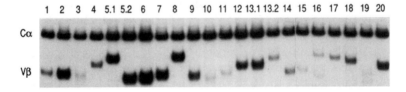

Figure 8

A representative autoradiogram of PCR-amplified Vβ segments. The Cα segment was coamplified in each reaction. The values for Vβ segments were normalized to the Cα value in each lane.

Vα segment

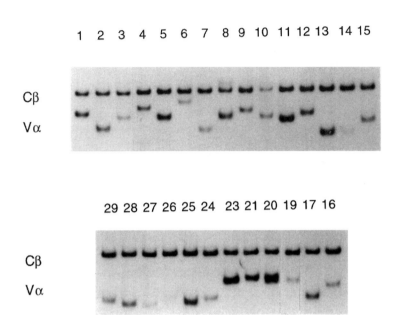

Figure 9

A representative autoradiogram of PCR amplified Vα segments. The Cβ segment was coamplified in each reaction. The values for Vα segments were normalized to the Cβ value in each lane. (From Gulwani-Akolkar, B. et al., *J. Immunol.*, 154, 3843, 1995. Copyright 1995. The American Association of Immunologists. With permission.)

investigator wishes to compare are determined, the oligonucleotide primers should be the same and should preferably come from the same oligonucleotide synthesis. Furthermore, as pointed out above, the PCR signals in both samples should be roughly proportional to the amount of input RNA. In addition, in order to relate the relative qPCR signals for each V segment to each other, it is necessary that the signals be normalized with respect to some internal standard RNA (e.g., Cα or Cβ; see above). This is extremely important because minute differences in a number of variables affecting amplification efficiency (e.g., position in automated cycling device) can dramatically alter product yield.[163]

Finally, to have a fair degree of confidence in any observed differences in repertoires, it is mandatory that the analysis by qPCR be reproducible. Although qPCR is notorious for being irreproducible, we have made several modifications to the procedure used by most other investigators to increase its reliability. These modifications include the utilization of acrylamide rather than agarose gels to analyze the qPCR

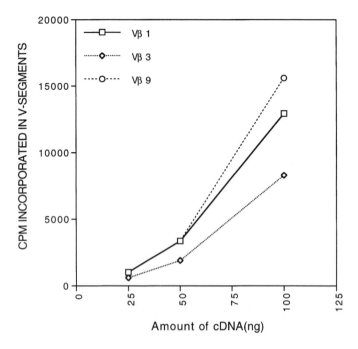

Figure 10
Proportionality of qPCR signal to amount of input RNA. Total RNA from T cells was reverse-transcribed to cDNA, and aliquots were amplified using Vβ-segment-specific primers.

products. This step was instituted because we have found that there are numerous artifactual bands as well as bands due to cross-priming of inappropriate Vβ segments that are difficult, if not impossible, to resolve on agarose gels; by using acrylamide gels, the correct Vβ segments can be readily separated from those that have been inappropriately amplified. Furthermore, to provide an additional degree of specificity a second, nested Cβ(Cα)-region primer, which is different from the Cβ(Cα) primer used to make cDNA, is used to amplify the Vβ(Vα)-specific products. These modifications result in a qPCR that is highly reproducible. Indeed, duplicate analyses of the same RNA show less than 15% variation on average (Figure 11).

It should also be kept in mind that although qPCR can provide rapid and relatively reliable data on V segment usage, it does not provide any information regarding the sequences of the TCR that are being amplified. This can be accomplished, however, simply by cloning and sequencing the PCR-amplified material. A more serious drawback to qPCR analysis of the TCR repertoire is that only known V-segment families with known upstream V-segment-specific sequences can be amplified. Thus, for Vα, where some of the segments have yet to be

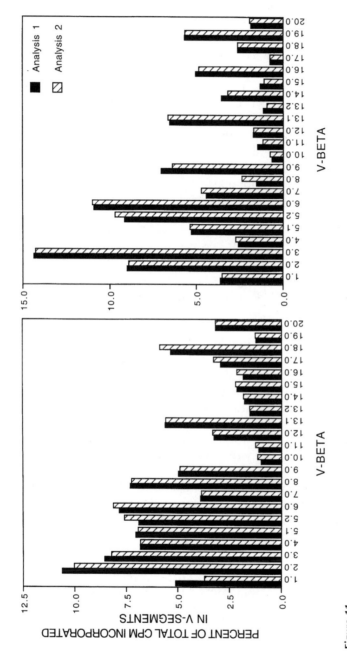

Figure 11
Reproducibility of modified qPCR analysis. Repeat analysis of the same RNA sample using Vβ-specific primers.

identified, qPCR may, by itself, not be sufficient to analyze the entire TCR repertoire.

Although each method for analysis of the TCR repertoire (V-specific qPCR or Mab) has its own advocates and adherents, it is fair to say that both methods, in combination, provide the greatest and most comprehensive amounts of information. This is because each method, depending upon the circumstances and V segment of interest, may have its own advantages and disadvantages (Table 7). For example, as noted above, the number of family members with which a Vβ-specific Mab reacts is often uncertain, as is the influence of Vα or Jβ segments on Vβ-specific reactivity. Furthermore, some Vβ-specific Mab react with one, but not the other, allele of selected Vβ segments.[137] In contrast, in qPCR one can usually, although not always, design oligonucleotide primers that are specific for one member of a multimember family, e.g., Vβ5.1 and 5.2, and mutations in V segments generating multiple allelic forms will not, in general, affect the PCR. On the other hand, some Vβ-specific Mab have been used very successfully to distinguish individual members of multimember V-segment families (e.g., Vβ13.1 and 13.2; see Table 4), and Mab that can distinguish allelic forms of V segments that differ functionally, e.g., in response to a superantigen, can be very useful (e.g., Mab OT145 that distinguishes Vβ6.7a and Vβ6.7b; see Reference 35 and Table 4). In any event, the major differences in these two methods, in terms of advantages or disadvantages, is that with Mab one can easily and rapidly get an accurate representation of the number of T cells expressing a particular V segment, whereas qPCR, by the very nature of being able to amplify small amounts of material, makes it possible to determine the repertoire in situations where there may not be sufficient material to thoroughly analyze the repertoire. Furthermore, analysis with V-segment-specific Mab of the various V segments that comprise the repertoire requires the existence of such Mab, which is not always the case, whereas with qPCR, all that is required for repertoire analysis is knowledge of the DNA sequences of the V segments that make up the repertoire. Thus, although in some situations it may be preferable to use either qPCR or Mab for analysis of the TCR repertoire, in many cases it may be advantageous to use a combination of both methods.

VII. DETERMINATION OF OLIGOCLONALITY

Determination of oligoclonality in any T-cell response has, in the past, been a very laborious procedure and required extensive sequence analysis of multiple TCR cDNA clones. Recently, a novel method has been devised which allows the rapid assessment of oligoclonality.[132] This procedure involves amplification of TCR by V-segment-specific

TABLE 7

Comparison of V-Segment-Specific Mab and qPCR for Analysis of the TCR Repertoire

V-Segment-Specific Mab

Advantages
1. Rapid and technically simple
2. Accurately reflects number of T cells expressing specific V segment
3. Can, in some instances, easily distinguish between individual members of multimember V-segment families (e.g., Vβ13.1 and Vβ13.2)
4. Can, in some instances, distinguish between TCR alleles which are functionally different (e.g., Vβ6.7a and Vβ6.7b)

Disadvantages
1. Requires more material than qPCR
2. Lack of reagents for most Vα and many Vβ segments
3. May not distinguish between individual members of multimember V-segment families
4. Reactivity may vary, depending upon presence or absence of particular forms of other TCR elements (e.g., Vα or Jβ)

qPCR

Advantages
1. Requires much less material than Mab
2. Many more Vα and Vβ segments can be analyzed
3. Can distinguish between individual members of multimember V-segment families
4. Is not, in general, dependent upon presence of particular alleles

Disadvantages
1. Technically difficult and laborious
2. Does not necessarily reflect actual number of T cells expressing particular V segments
3. Cannot, in most cases, distinguish between alleles which are functionally different

TABLE 8

"Nested" PCR Primers for Detecting Oligoclonality by CDR3 Sizing

Vβ1	5'-C TCA GCT TTG TAT TTC TGT G-3'
Vβ2	5'-CAA CCA TGC AAG CCT GAC CT-3'
Vβ3	5'-AGA GAG AAG AAG GAG CGC TT-3'
Vβ4	5'-ACA TAT GAG AGT GGA TTT GTC ATT-3'
Vβ5	5'-C TCG GCC CT(G or C) TAT CTC TGT G-3'
Vβ6	5'-C TC(G or C or A) GCC (G or A)TG TAT CTC TGT G-3'
Vβ7	5'-C TC(G or A) GCC CTG TAT CTC TGC G-3'
Vβ8	5'-C TCA GCT GTG TAC TTC TGT G-3'
Vβ9	5'-CCT AAA TCT CCA GAC AAA GCT CAC-3'
Vβ10	5'-C ACA GCA CTG TAT TTC TGT G-3'
Vβ11	5'-T ACC TCT CAG TAC CTC TGT G-3'
Vβ12/13	5'-G ACA TCT GTG TAC TTC TGT G-3'
Vβ14	5'-CTC GAA AAG AGA AGA GGA ATT-3'
Vβ15	5'-G ACA GCT CTT TAC TTC TGT G-3'
Vβ16	5'-TTC TGG AGT TTA TTT CTG TG-3'
Vβ17	5'-GAC AGC TTT CTA TCT CTG TG-3'
Vβ18	5'-T TCG GCA G(G or C)T TAT TTC TGT G-3'
Vβ19	5'-C ACG GCA CTG TAT CTC TGT G-3'
Vβ20	5'-C TCT GGC TTC TAT CTC TGT G-3'

PCR, followed by electrophoresis on a DNA-sequencing gel resulting in the resolution of products differing by a single codon. Briefly, total RNA is reverse-transcribed into cDNA and amplified by PCR using the V-segment-specific forward primers and a C-region reverse primer, as described above for qPCR. An aliquot of the amplified material is then used for a second round of amplification using the same C-region-specific reverse primer and new forward primers (Table 8) which are nested 3' to the first V-segment-specific primers. For the second amplification the C-region reverse primer is labeled with ^{32}P. The amplified products are then electrophoresed on a conventional DNA sequencing gel and visualized by autoradiography. This two-step amplification procedure results in TCR fragments that are about 150 bp in size and consist predominantly of the V–D–J junctional region and a fixed number of upstream V-region and downstream C-region nucleotides (Figure 12). More importantly, each V segment amplified in this way migrates as a series of bands differing by multiples of 3 bp (equivalent to one amino acid), with each band representing a mixture of V segments of differing sequence but having the identical CDR3 size (Figure 13). Usually one observes anywhere from 4 to 10 bands representing V segments of differing CDR3 size. This diversity in CDR3 size reflects differential use of D and J region segments and differing degrees of N region addition for each V segment specifically amplified (see above, section on generation of TCR diversity). In a polyclonal response, the bands display a Poisson distribution in terms of intensity in which the major bands represent CDR3 sizes of 6 to 12 amino acids

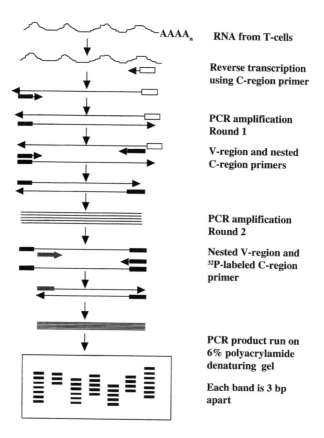

Figure 12
Schematic flow chart for analysis of oligoclonality as determined by CDR3 length analysis of TCR V segments.

(Figure 12). However, when a V segment-specific response is oligoclonal, one or a few bands of disproportionate intensity are seen, and these oligoclonal bands are usually found to consist of a single DNA sequence.[132] The intensity of the bands or degree of oligoclonality can then be quantitated using commercially available phosphorimagers.

VIII. DETERMINATION OF CDR3 OLIGOCLONALITY WITH RESPECT TO JB USAGE

As described in the earlier sections the Jβ segment plays an important role in determining TCR antigen specificity since a portion of it (the 5′ end) constitutes part of the CDR3 region. By combining methods for amplifying specific Jβ segments with those for Vβ segments it is possible to greatly enhance the resolution and sensitivity for detection

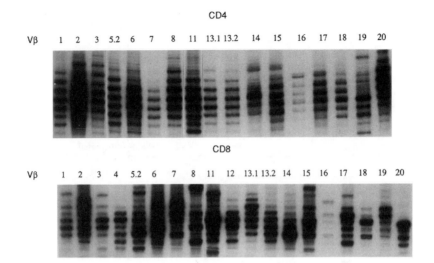

Figure 13

A representative autoradiogram of CDR3 length analysis used to determine oligoclonality in TCR V segments. Note the high level of oligoclonality in CD8⁺ cells compared to CD4⁺ cells. (From Akolkar, P.N. et al., *Clin. Immunol. Immunopath.*, 75, 155, 1995. With permission.)

TABLE 9

PCR Primers for Jβ-Specific CDR3 Length Analysis

Jβ	
1.1	5′-AACTGTGAGTCTGGTGCCTT-3′
1.2	5′-ACGGTTAACCTGGTCCCCGA-3′
1.3	5′-CTCTACAACAGTGAGCCAAC-3′
1.4	5′-GACAGAGAGCTGGGTTCCAC-3′
1.5	5′-TGGAGAGTCGAGTCCCATCA-3′
1.6	5′-TGAGCCTGGTCCCATTCCCA-3′
2.1	5′-CCTCTAGCACGGTGAGCCGT-3′
2.2	5′-TACGGTCAGCCTAGAGCCTT-3′
2.3	5′-CTGTCAGCCGGGTGCCTGGG-3′
2.4	5′-CTGAGAGCCGGGTCCCGGCG-3′
2.5	5′-CCTCGAGCACCAGGAGCCGC-3′
2.6	5′-CCTGCTGCCGGCCCCGAAAG-3′
2.7	5′-TGACCGTGAGCCTGGTGCCC-3′

of oligoclonality. Thus, by using Jβ-specific primers that amplify only a single Jβ segment, Vβ segments can be resolved not only on the basis of CDR3 size but also on the basis of Jβ usage. Briefly, total RNA is reverse transcribed into cDNA and first amplified by PCR using a Vβ-specific forward primer and a C-region reverse primer as described above for conventional qPCR. An aliquot of the amplified material then

| 1.1 | 1.2 | 1.3 | 1.4 | 1.5 | 1.6 | 2.1 | 2.2 | 2.3 | 2.4 | 2.5 | 2.6 | 2.7 |

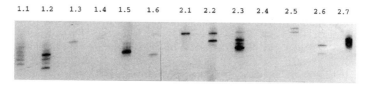

Figure 14

CDR3 length analysis of a Vβ segment amplified using different Jβ-segment-specific primers.

serves as a template for a second round of PCR which uses the same Vβ-specific primer as used in the first round but which is now labeled with ^{32}P, and a Jβ-specific primer instead of the Cβ primer. The Jβ-specific primers (Table 9) for each of the 13 Jβ segments (Jβ 1.1–1.6 and Jβ2.1–2.7) are 16-mers designed to minimize cross-priming with other Jβ segments. The conditions for the second round of PCR are, denaturation at 95°C for 30 s, annealing at 60°C for 30 s, and extension at 72°C for 45 s. After 20–25 cycles the amplified products are electrophoresed on a conventional sequencing gel and visualized by autoradiography.

This two-step amplification results in TCR fragments that are about 120 bp in size with each Vβ-Jβ segment migrating as a series of bands differing by multiples of 3 bp (Figure 14). We have successfully used this method to demonstrate oligoclonality in T cells when it was not readily apparent by the conventional method for CDR3 length analysis.[164] It should also be noted that this method not only increases the ability to detect oligoclonality, but also, at the same time, defines the Jβ segment being used when oligoclonality is observed.

REFERENCES

1. Paul, W.E., *Fundamental Immunology*, Raven Press, New York, 1993.
2. Abbas, A.K., Lichtman, A.H., and Pober, J.S., *Cellular and Molecular Immunology*, W.B. Saunders, Philadelphia, 1991.
3. Marrack, P. and Kappler, J., The T cell Receptor. *Science*, 238, 1073, 1987.
4. Kronenberg, M., Siu, G., Hood, L., and Shastri, N., The molecular genetics of the T-cell antigen receptor and T-cell antigen recognition, *Annu. Rev. Immunol.*, 4, 529, 1986.
5. Davis, M.M. and Bjorkman, P.J., T-cell antigen receptor genes and T-cell recognition, *Nature*, 334, 395, 1988.
6. Unanue, E.R. and Allen, P.M., The basis for the immunoregulatory role of macrophages and other accessory cells, *Science*, 236, 551, 1987.
7. Allen, P.M., Antigen processing at the molecular level, *Immunol. Today*, 8, 270, 1987.
8. Unanue, E.R. and Allen, P.M., Biochemistry and biology of antigen presentation by macrophages. *Cell Immunol.*, 99, 3, 1986.

9. Babbitt, B.P., Allen, P.M., Matsueda, G., Haber, E., and Unanue, E.R., Binding of immunogenic peptides to Ia histocompatibility molecules, *Nature*, 317, 359, 1985.

10. Madden, D.R., Gorga, J.C., Strominger, J.L., and Wiley, D.C., The structure of HLA-B27 reveals nonamer self-peptides bound in an extended conformation, *Nature*, 353, 321, 1992.

11. Jardetzky, T.S., Lane, W.S., Robinson, M.A., Madden, D.R., and Wiley, D.C., Identification of self peptides bound to purified HLA-B27, *Nature*, 353, 326, 1991.

12. Bjorkman, P.J., Saper, M.A., Samraoui, B., Bennett, W.S., Strominger, J.L., and Wiley, D.C., The foreign antigen binding site and T cell recognition regions of class I histocompatibility antigens, *Nature*, 329, 512, 1987.

13. Bjorkman, P.J., Saper, M.A., Samraoui, B., Bennett, W.S., Strominger, J.L., and Wiley, D.C., Structure of the human class I histocompatibility antigen, HLA-A2, *Nature*, 329, 506, 1987 .

14. Benjamin, R.J., Madrigal, J.A., and Parham, P., Peptide binding to empty HLA-B27 molecules of viable human cells. *Nature*, 351, 74, 1991.

15. Rudensky, A.Y., Preston-Hurlburt, P., Hong, S.C., Barlow, A. and Janeway, C.A., Jr., Sequence analysis of peptides bound to MHC class II molecules, *Nature*, 353, 622, 1991.

16. Seder, R.A. and Paul, W.E., Acquisition of lymphokine-producing phenotype by CD4+ T cells, *Annu. Rev. Immunol.*,12, 635, 1994.

17. Romagnani, S., Lymphokine production by human T cells in disease states, *Annu. Rev. Immunol.*,12, 227, 1994.

18. Terry, L.A., Brown, M.H., and Beverley, P.C.L., The monoclonal antibody, UCHL1, recognizes a 180,000 MW component of the human leukocyte-common antigen, CD45, *Immunology*, 64, 331, 1988.

19. Jones, R.A., Richard, S.J., Roberts, B.E., Child, J.A., and Scott, C.S., Phenotypic switch from CD45RA+ to CD45RA− by normal blood T cells is associated with increased HLA-ABC expression for CD4+ and CD8+ populations but not for the NK-associated CD4-CD8dim+ or CD4- CD8- fractions, *Immunology*, 70, 55, 1990 .

20. Trowbridge, I.S. and Thomas, M.L., CD45: an emerging role as a protein tyrosine phosphatase required for lymphocyte activation and development, *Annu. Rev. Immunol.*, 12, 85, 1994.

21. Mason, D. and Powrie, F., Memory CD4+ T cells in man form two distinct subpopulations, defined by their expression of isoforms of the leukocyte common antigen, CD45, *Immunology*, 70, 427, 1990.

22. Donovan, J.A. and Koretzky, G.A., CD45 and the immune response, *J. Am. Soc. Nephrol.*, 4, 976, 1993.

23. Bryne, J.A., Butler, J.L., and Cooper, M.D., Differential activation requirements for virgin and memory T cells, *J. Immunol.*,141, 3249, 1988.

24. Akbar, A.N., Terry, L., Timms, A., Beverly, P.C.L., and Jannosy, G., Loss of CD45R and gain of UCHL1 reactivity is a feature of primed T cells, *J. Immunol.*,140, 1435, 1988.

25. Rothstein, D., Yamada, A., Schlossman, S.F., and Morimoto, C., Cyclic regulation of CD45 isoform expression in a long term human CD4+CD45RA+ T cell line, *J. Immunol.*, 146, 1175, 1991.

26. Ligthstone, L. and Marvel, J., CD45RA+ T cells: not simple virgins, *Clin. Sci.*, 85, 515, 1993.

27. Niehues, T., Gulwani-Akolkar, B., Akolkar, P.N., Tax, W., and Silver, J. Unique phenotype and distinct TCR Vβ Repertoire in human peripheral blood αβTCR+, CD4-, and CD8- double negative T cells, *J. Immunol.*, 173, 1072, 1994.

28. Wirt, D.P., Brooks, E.G., Vaidya, S., Klimpel, G.R., Waldmann, T.A., and Goldblum, R.M., Novel T-lymphocyte population in combined immunodeficiency with features of graft-versus-host disease, *N. Engl. J. Med.*, 321, 370, 1989.

29. Shivakumar, S.G., Tsokos, C., and Datta, S.K., T-cell receptor αβ expressing double-negative (CD4⁻CD8⁻) and CD8⁻ T helper cells n humans augment the production of pathogenic anti-DNA autoantibodies associated with lupus nephritis, *J. Immunol.*, 143, 103, 1989.

30. Mak, T.W., Caccia, N., Reis, M., Ohashi, P., Sangster, R., Kimura, N., and Toyonaga, B., Genes encoding the α, β, and γ chains of the human T cell antigen receptor, *J. Infect. Dis.*, 155, 418, 1987.

31. Kabat, E.A., Wu, T.T., Perry, H.M., Gottesman, K.S., and Foeller, C. Sequences of proteins of immunological interest, U.S. Dept. of Healthand Human Services, Public Health Service National Institutes of Health, 1991, 5th ed.

32. Jores, R., Alzari, M., and Meo, T. Resolution of hypervariable regions in TCR β chains by a modified Wu-Kubat index of amino acid diversity, *Proc. Natl. Acad. Sci. U.S.A.*, 87, 9138, 1990 .

33. Bougueleret, L., and Claverie, J.M. Variability analysis of the human and mouse T-cell receptor β chains, *Immunogenetics*, 26, 304, 1987.

34. Chothia, C., Boswell, D.R., and Lesk, A.M., The outline structure of the T-cell αβ receptor, *EMBO J.*, 7, 3745, 1988.

35. Prasher, Y., Li, Y., Kubinec, J.S., Jones, N., and Posnett, D.N., A monoclonal antibody (OT145) specific for the T cell antigen receptor V beta 6.7a allele detects an epitope related to a proposed superantigen-binding site, *J. Immunol.*, 147, 3441, 1992.

36. Robinson, M.A., The human T-cell receptor β-chain gene complex contains at least 57 variable gene segments, *J. Immunol.*, 146, 4392, 1991.

37. Robinson, M.A., Mitchell, M.P., Wei, S., Day, C.D., Zhao, T.M., and Concannon, P., Organization of human T-cell receptor β-chain genes: cluster of Vβ genes are present on chromosomes 7 and 9, *Proc. Natl. Acad. Sci. U.S.A.*, 90, 2433, 1993 .

38. Robinson, M.A. and Concannon, P. Organization of the human TCRB gene complex, in *T Cell Receptor*, Bell, J., Owen, M. J., and Simpson, E., Oxford Press, Oxford, 1995, 269.

39. Barron, K.S. and Robinson, M.R., The human T-cell receptor variable gene segment, TCRBV6S1, has two null alleles, *Human Immunol.*, 40, 17, 1994.

40. Davis, M.M., Molecular genetics of the T cell-receptor beta chain, *Annu. Rev. Immunol.*, 3, 537, 1985.

41. Roman-Roman, S., Ferradini, L., Azocar, J., Genevee, C., Hercend, T., and Trievel, F., Studies on the human T-cell receptor αβ variable region genes. I. Identification of 7 additional $V_α$ and 14 $J_α$ gene segments, *Eur. J. Immunol.*, 21, 927, 1994.

42. Groh, V., Porcelli, S., Fabbi, M., Lanier, L.I., Picker, I.J,. Anderson, T., Warnke, R.A., Bhan, A.K., Strominger, J.L., and Brenner, M. Human lymphocytes bearing T-cell receptor gamma delta are phenotypically diverse and evenly distributed throughout the lymphoid system, *J. Exp. Med.*, 169, 1277, 1989.

43. Brenner, M.B., McLean, J., Scheft, H., Warnke, R.A., Jones, N., and Strominger, J.L., Characterization and expression of human αβ T cell receptor by using a framework monoclonal antibody, *J. Immunol.*, 138, 1502, 1986.

44. Hass, W., Peereira, P., and Tonegawa, S., Gamma/Delta Cells, *Annu. Rev. Immunol.*, 11, 637, 1993.

45. Raulet, D.H., The structure, function, and molecular genetics of the γ/δ T-cell receptor, *Annu. Rev. Immunol.*, 7,175, 1989.

46. Brenner, B.M., Strominger, J.L., and Krangel, M.S. The γδ T-cell receptor, *Adv. Immunol.*, 43, 133, 1988.

47. Moss, P., Rosenberg, M., and Bell, J., The human T-cell receptor in health and disease, *Annu. Rev. Immunol.*, 10, 71, 1992.

48. Malhotra, U., Spielman, R., and Concannon, P., Variability in T-cell receptor Vβ gene usage in human peripheral blood lymphocytes. Studies of identical twins, siblings, and insulin-dependent diabetes mellitus patients, *J. Immunol.*, 149, 1802, 1992.

49. Gomolka, M., Epplen, C., Buitkamp, J., and Epplen, J.T., Novel members and germline polymorphisms in the human T-cell receptor Vβ6 family, *Immunogenetics*, 37, 257, 1993.

50. Hansen, T., Ronningen, K.S., Polski, R., Kimura, A., and Thorsby, E., Coding region polymorphisms of human T-cell receptor Vβ 6.9 and Vβ 21.4, *Scan J. Immunol.*, 36, 285, 1992.

51. Charmley, P., Wang, K., Hood, L., and Nickerson D.A., Identification and physical mapping of a polymorphic human T-cell receptor Vβ gene with a frequent null allele, *J. Exp. Med.*, 177,135-143, 1993.

52. Li, U., Szabo, P., Robinson, M.A., Dong, B., Posnett, D.N., Allelic variations in the human T-cell receptor V beta 6.7 gene products, *J. Exp Med.*, 171, 221, 1990.

53. Posnett, D.N., Vissinga, C.S., Pambuccian, C., Wei, S, Robinson, M.A., Kostyu, D., and Concannon, P., Level of human TCRBY351 (V beta 3) expression correlates with allelic polymorphism in the spacer region of the recombination signal sequence, *J. Exp. Med.*, 179, 1707, 1994.

54. Li, Y., Wong, A., Szabo, P., and Posnett, D.N., Human Tcrb-V6.10 is a pseudogene with Alu reptitive sequences in the promoter region, *Immunogenetics*, 37, 347, 1993.

55. Robinson, M.A., Allelic sequence variations in the hypervariable region of a T-cell receptor β chain: correlation with restriction fragment length polymorphism in human families and populations, *Proc. Natl. Acad. Sci. U.S.A.*, 86, 9422, 1989

56. Robinson, M.A. and Kindt, T.J., Segregation of polymorphic T-cell receptor genes in human families, *Proc. Natl. Acad. Sci. U.S.A.*, 82, 3804, 1985.

57. Zhao, T.M., Whitaker, S.E., and Robinson, M.A., A genetically determined insertion/deletion related polymorphism in human T-cell receptor β chain (TCRB) inludes functional variable gene segments, *J. Exp. Med.*, 180, 1405, 1994.

58. Herman, A., Kappler, J.W., Marrack, P., and Pullen, A.M., Superantigens: mechanism of T cell stimulation and role in immune responses, *Annu. Rev. Immunol.*, 9, 745,1991.

59. Janeway Jr, C.A., Yagi, J., Conrad, P.J., Katz, M.E., Jones, B., Vroegop, S., and Buxser, S., T-cell responses to Mls and to bacterial proteins that mimic its behavior, *Immunol. Rev.*, 107, 61, 1989.

60. Paliard, X., West, S.G., Lafferty, J.A., Clements, J.R., Kappler, J.W., Marrack, P., and Kotzin, B.L., Evidence for the effects of a superantigen in rheumatoid arthritis, *Science*, 253, 325, 1991.

61. Howell, M.D., Diveley, J.P., Lundeen, K.A., Esty, A., Winters, S.T., Carlo, D.J., and Brostoff, W.W., Limited T-cell β-chain heterogeneity among interleukin 2 receptor-positive synovial T cells suggests a role for superantigen in rheumatoid arthritis, *Proc. Natl. Acad. Sci. U.S.A.*, 88, 10921, 1991.

62. Olive, C., Gatenby, P.A., and Serjeantson, S.W., Analysis of T-cell receptor V alpha with rheumatoid arthritis, *Immunol. Cell Biol.*, 69, 349, 1991.

63. Sottini, A., Imberti, L., Gorla, R., Cattaneo, R., and Primi, D., Restricted expression of T-cell receptor V beta but not V alpha genes in rheumatoid arthritis, *Eur. J. Immunol.*, 21(2), 461, 1991.

64. Uematsu, Y., Wege, H., Strauss, A., Ott, M., Bannwarth, W., Lanchbury, J., Panayi, G., and Steinmetz, M., The T-cell receptor repertoire in the synovial fluid of a patient with rheumatoid arthritis is polyclonal, *Proc. Natl. Acad. Sci. U.S.A.*, 88, 8534, 1991.

65. Pluschke, G., Ginter, A., Taube, H., Melchers, I., Peters H.H., and Krawinkel, U., Analysis of T-cell receptor V beta regions expressed by rheumatoid synovial T lymphocytes, *Immunobiology*, 188, 330, 1993.

66. Bucht, A., Oksenberg, J.R., Lindblad, S., Gronberg, A., Steinman, L., and Klareskog, L., Characterization of T-cell receptor alpha beta repertoire in synovial tissue from different temporal phases of rheumatoid arthritis, *Scand. J. Immunol.*, 35(2), 159, 1992.

67. Lunardi, C., Marguerie, C., and So, A.K., An altered repertoire of T-cell receptor V gene expression by rheumatoid synovial fluid T lymphocytes, *Clin. Exp. Immunol.*, 90, 440, 1992.

68. Williams, W.V., Fang, Q., Demarco, D., Von Feldt, J., Zurier R.B., and Weiner, D.B., Restricted heterogeneity of T-cell receptor transcripts in rheumatoid synovium, *J. Clin. Invest.*, 90, 326, 1992.

69. Weyand, C.M., Oppitz, U., Hicok, K., and Goronzy, J.J., Selection of T-cell receptor V beta elements by HLA-DR determinants predisposing to rheumatoid arthritis, *Arthritis Rheum.*, 35, 990, 1992.

70. Doherty, P.J., Silverman, E.D., Laxer, R.M., Yang, S.X., and Pan, S., T cell receptor V beta usage in synovial fluid of children with arthritis, *J. Rheumatol.*, 19, 468, 1992.

71. Olive, C., Gatenby, P.A., and Serjeantson, S.W., Evidence for oligoclonality of T-cell receptor delta chain transcripts expressed in rheumatoid arthritis patients, *Eur. J. Immunol.*, 22, 2587, 1992.

72. Olive, C., Gatenby, P.A., and Serjeantson, S.W., Variable gene usage of T-cell receptor gamma- and delta-chain transcripts expressed in synovia and peripheral blood of patients with rheumatoid arthritis, *Clin. Exp. Immunol.*, 87, 172, 1992.

73. Olive, C., Gatenby, P.A., and Serjeanston, S.W., Molecular characterization of the V gamma 9 T-cell receptor repertoire expressed in patients with rheumatoid arthritis, *Eur. J. Immunol.*, 22, 2901, 1992.

74. Dedeoglu, F., Kaymaz, H., Seaver, N., Schluter, S.F., Yocum, D.E., and Marchalonis, J.J., Lack of preferential V beta usage in synovial T cells of rheumatoid arthritis patients, *Immunol. Res.*, 12, 12, 1993.

75. Pluschke, G., Ginter, A., Taube, H., Melchers, I., Peter, H.H., and Krawinkel, U., Analysis of T-cell receptor V beta regions expressed by rheumatoid synovial T lymphocytes, *Immunobiology*, 188, 330, 1993.

76. Wilson, K. B., Quayle, A.J., Suleyman, S., Kjeldsen-Kraugh, J., Forre, O., Natvig, J.B., and Capra, J.D., Heterogeneity of the TCR repertoire in synovial fluid T lymphocytes responding to BCG in a patient with early rheumatoid arthritis, *Scand. J. Immunol.*, 38, 102, 1993.

77. Davey, M.P. and Munkirs, D.D., Patterns of T-cell receptor variable beta gene expression by synovial fluid and peripheral blood T-cells in rheumatoid arthritis, *Clin. Immunol. Immunopathol.*, 68, 79, 1993.

78. Jenkins, R.N., Nikaein, A., Zimmermann, A., Meek, K., and Lipsky, P.E., T-cell receptor V beta gene bias in rheumatoid arthritis, *J. Clin. Invest.*, 92, 2688, 1993.

79. Kohsaka, H., Taniguchi, A., Chen, P.P., Ollier, W.E., and Carson, D.A., The expressed T-cell receptor V gene repertoire of rheumatoid arthritis monozygotic twins: rapid analysis by anchored polymeras chain reaction and enzyme-linked immunosorbent assay, *Eur. J. Immunol.*, 23, 1895, 1993.

80. Posnett, D.N., Gottlieb, A., Bussel, J.B., Friedman, S.M., Chiorazzi, N., Li, Y, Szabo, P., Farid, N.R. and Robinson, M.A., T cell antigen receptors in autoimmunity, *J. Immunol.*, 140, 1963, 1988

81. Der Simonian, H., Band, H., and Brenner, M.D., Increased frequency of T-cell receptor V alpha 12.1 expression on DC8$^+$ T cells: evidence that V alpha participates in shaping the peripheral T cell repertoire, *J. Exp. Med.*, 174, 639, 1991.

82. Gudmundsson, S., Ronnelid, J., Karlsson-Parra, A., Lysholm, J., Gudbjornsson, B., Widenfalk, B., Janson, C.H., and Klareskog, L., T-cell receptor V-gene usage in synovial fluid and synovial tissue from RA patients, *Scand. J. Immunol.*, 36, 681, 1992.

83. Korthauer, U., Hennerkes, B., Menninger, H., Mages, H.W., Zacher, J., Potocnik, A.J., Emmrich, F., and Kroczek, R.A., Oligoclonal T cells in rheumatoid arthritis; identification strategy and molecular characterization of a clonal T-cell receptor, *Scand. J. Immunol.*, 36, 855, 1992.

84. Shen, Y., Li, S., Quayle, A.J., Mellbye, O.J., Natvig, J.B., and Forre, O., TCR gamma/delta+ cell subsets in the synovial membranes of patients with rheumatoid arthritis and juvenile rheumatoid arthritis, *Scand. J. Immunol.*, 36, 533, 1992.

85. Broker, B.M., Korthauer, U., Heppt, P., Weseloh, G., de la Camp, R., Kroczek, R.A., and Emmrich, F., Biased T cell receptor V gene usage in rheumatoid arthritis. Oligoclonal expansion of T cells expressing V alpha 2 genes in synovial fluid but not in peripheral blood, *Arthritis Rheum.*, 36, 1234, 1993.

86. Oksenberg, J.R., Stuart, S., Begovich, A.B., Bell, R.B., Erlich, H.A., Steinman, L., and Bernard, C.C., Limited heterogeneity of re-arranged T-cell receptor V alpha transcripts in brains of multiple sclerosis patients, *Nature*, 345, 344, 1990.

87. Wucherpgfennig, K.W., Newcombe, J., Li, H., Keddy, C., Cuzner, M.L., and Hafler, D.A., T-cell receptor V alpha-V beta repertoire and cytokine gene expression in active multiple sclerosis lesions, *J. Exp. Med.*, 175, 993, 1992.

88. Wusherpfennig, K.W., Newcombe, J., Hong, L., Keddy, C., Cuzner, M.L., and Hafler, D.A., γδ T-cell receptor repertoire in acute multiple sclerosis lesions, *Proc. Natl. Acad. Sci. U.S.A.*, 89, 4588, 1992.

89. Birnbaum, G. and van Ness, B., Quantitation of T-cell receptor V beta chain expression on lymphocytes from blood, brain, and spinal fluid in patients with multiple sclerosis and other neurological diseases, *Ann. Neurol.*, 32, 24,1992.

90. Utz, U., Biddison, W.E., McFarland, H.F., McFarland, D.E., Flerlage, M., and Martin, R., Skewed T-cell receptor repertoire in genetically identical twins correlates with multiple sclerosis, *Nature*, 364, 243, 1993.

91. Oksenberg, J.R., Panzara, M.A., Begovich, A.B., Mitchell, D., Erlich, H.A., Murray, R.S., Shimonkevitz, M.S., Rothbard, J., Bernard, C.C.A., and Steinman, L., Selection for T-cell receptor Vβ–Dβ–Jβ gene rearrangements with specificity for a myelin basis protein peptide in brain lesions of multiple sclerosis, *Nature*, 362, 68, 1993.

92. Shimonkevitz, R., Colburn, D., Burnham, J.S., Murray, R.S., and Kotzin, B.L., Clonal expansions of activated gamma/delta T cells in recent-onset multiple sclerosis, *Proc. Natl. Acad. Sci. U.S.A.*, 90, 923, 1993.

93. Hvas, J., Oksenberg, J.R., Fernando, R., Steinman, L., and Bernard, C.C., Gamma delta T-cell receptor repertoire in brain lesions of patients with multiple sclerosis, *J. Neuroimmunol.*, 46, 225, 1993.

94. Chou, Y.K., Buenafe, A.C., Dedrick, R., Morrison, W.J., Bourdette, D.N., Whitham, R., Atherton, J., Lane, J., Spoor, E., Hashim, G.A. et al., T-cell receptor V beta gene usage in the recognition of myelin basic protein by cerebrospinal fluid- and blood-derived T cells from patients with multiple sclerosis, *J. Neurosci. Res.*, 37, 169, 1994.

95. Roth, M.P., Riond, J., Champagane, E., Essaket, S., Cambon- Thomsen, A., Clayton, J., Clanet, M. and Coppin, H., TCRB-V gene usage in monozygotic twins discordant for multiple sclerosis, *Immunogenetics*, 39, 281,1994.

96. Grunewald, J., Janson, C.H., Eklund, A., Ohrn, M., Olerup, O., Persson, U., and Wigzell, H., Restricted V alpha 2.3 gene usage by CD4+ T lymphocytes in bronchoalveolar lavage fluid from sarcoidosis patients correlates with HJLA-DR3, *Eur. J. Immunol.*, 22, 129, 1992.

97. Bellocq, A., Lecossier, D., Pierre-Audigler, C., Tazi, A., Valerye, D., and Hance, A.J., T-cell receptor repertoire of T lymphocytes recovered from the lung and blood of patients with sarcoidosis, *Am. J. Respir. Crit. Care Med.*, 149, 646, 1994.

98. Davis, T.F., Martin, A., Concepcion, E.S., Graves, P., Cohen, L., and Ben-Nun, A., Evidence of limited variability of antigen receptors on intrathyroidal T cells in autoimmune thyroid disease, *N. Engl. J. Med.*, 238, 1991.

99. McIntosh, R.S., Tandon, N., Pickerill, A.P., Davies, R., Barnett, D., and Weetman, A.P., The gamma delta T cell repertoire in Grave's disease and multinodular goitre, *Clin. Exp. Immunol.*,94, 474, 1993.

100. Grunewald, J., Ahlberg, R., Lefvert, A.K., Der Simonlan, H., Wigzell, H., and Janson, C.H., Abnormal T-cell expansion and V-gene usage in myasthenia gravis patients, *Scand . J. Immunol.*, 34, 161, 1991.
101. Sumida, T., Yonaha, F., Maeda, T., Tanabe, E., Koike, T., Tomioka, H., and Yoshida, S., T-cell receptor repertoire of infiltrating T cells in lips of Sjogren's syndrome patients, *J. Clin. Invest.*, 89, 681, 1992.
102. Yonaha, F., Sumida, T., Maeda, T., Tomioka, H., Koike, T., and Yoshida, S., Restricted junctional usage of T-cell receptor V beta 2 and V beta 13 genes, which are overrepresented on infiltrating T cells in the lips of patients with Sjogren's syndrome, *Arthritis Rheum.*, 35, 1362, 1992.
103. Abe, J., Kotzin, B.L., Meissner, Melish, M.E., Takahashi, M., Fulton, D., Romagne, F., Maliessen, B. and Leung, D.Y.M., Characterization of T cell repertoire changes in acute Kawasaki disease, *J. Exp. Med.*, 177, 791, 1993.
104. Abe, J., Kotzin, L., Jujo, K., Melish, M.E., Glode, M.P., Kohsaka, T., and Leung, D.Y.M., Selective expansion of T cells expressing T-cell receptor variable regions Vβ2 and Vβ8 in Kawasaki disease, *Proc. Natl. Acad. Sci. U.S.A.*, 89, 4066, 1992.
105. Gulwani-Akolkar, B., Shalon, L., Akolkar, P.N., Fisher, S.E., and Silver, J., Analysis of the peripheral blood T-cell receptor (TCR) repertoire in monozygotic twins discordant for crohn's disease, *Autoimmunity*, 17, 242, 1994.
106. Posnett, D.N., Schmelkin, I., Burton, D.A., August, A., McGrath, H., and Mayer, L.F., T cell antigen receptor V gene usage. Increases in Vβ8+ T cells in Crohn's disease, *J. Clin. Invest.*, 85, 1770, 1990.
107. Shalon, L., Gulwani-Akolkar, B., Fisher, S.E., Akolkar, P., Panja, A., Mayer, L., and Silver, J., An altered T-cell receptor repertoire in Crohn's disease, *Autoimmunity*, 17, 301, 1994.
108. Choi, Y., Kotzin, B., Herron, L., Callahan, J., Marrack, P., and Kappler, J., Interaction of *Staphylococcus aureus* toxin "superantigens" with human T cells, *Proc. Natl. Acad. Sci. U.S.A.*, 86, 8941, 1989.
109. Choi, Y., Lafferty, J.A., Clements, J.R., Todd, J.K., Gelfand, E.W., Kappler, P.M. and Kotzin, B.L., Selective expression of T cells expressing Vβ2 in toxic shock syndrome, *J. Exp. Med.*, 172, 981, 1990.
110. Tomai, M.A., Aelion, J.A., Dockter, M.E., Majumdar, G., Spinella, D.G., and Kotb, M., T-cell receptor V gene usage by human T cells stimulated with the superantigen streptococcol M protein, *J. Exp. Med.*, 174, 285, 1991.
111. Kappler, J., Kotzin, B., Herron, L., Gelfand, E.W., Bigler, R.D., Boylston, S.C., Posnett, D.N., Choi, Y., and Marrack, P., Vβ-Specific stimulation of human T cells by staphylococcal toxins, *Science*, 244, 811, 1989.
112. Friedman, S.M., Crow, M.K., Tumang, J.R., Tumang, M., Xu, Y., Hodtsev, A.S., Cole, B.C., and Posnett, D.N., Characterization of human T cells reactive with the *Mycoplasma arthritidis*-derived superantigen (MAM): the T-cell receptor gene product expressed by a large fraction of MAM-reactive human T cells, *J. Exp. Med.*, 174, 891, 1991.
113. Lafon, M., Lafage, M., Martinex-Arends, A., Ramirez, R., Vuiller, F., Charron, D., Lotteau, V., and Scott-Algara, D., Evidence for a viral superantigen in humans, *Nature*, 358, 507, 1992.
114. Imberti, L., Sottini, A., Bettinardi, A., Puoti, M., and Primi, D., Selective depletion in HIV infection of T cells that bear specific T-cell receptorβ sequences, *Science*, 254, 860, 1991.
115. Soudeyns, H. Rebai, N., Pantaleo, G.,Ciurli, C., Boghossian T. Sekaly, R.P., and Fauci, A.S., The T-cell receptor Vβ repertoire in HIV infection and disease, *Semin. Immunol.*, 5, 175, 1993.
116. Dalgleish, A.G., Wilson, S., Gompels, M., Ludlam, C., Gazzard, B., Coates, A.M., and Habeshaw, J., T-cell receptor variable gene products and early HIV-1 infection, *Lancet*, 339, 823, 1992.

117. Bansal, A.S., Green, L.M., Pumphrey, R.S.H., and Mandal, B., T cells, V genes, and HIV, *Lancet*, 339, 1604, 1992.

118. Bansal, A.S., Green, L.M., Khoo, S.H., Pumphrey, R.S., Haeney, M.R., and Mandal, B.X., HIV induces deletion of T-cell receptor variable gene product-specfic T cells, *Clin. Exp. Immunol.*, 94, 17, 1993.

119. Orsini, D.L.M., Res, P.C.M., Van Laar, J.M., Muller, L.M., Soprano, A.E.L., Kooy, Y.M.C., Tak, P.O., and Koning, F., A subset of Vδ1+ T cells proliferates in response to Epstein-Barr virus-transformed B Cells *in vitro*. *Scand. J. Immunol.*, 38, 335, 1993.

120. Rebai, N., Pantaleo, G., Demarest, J.F., Ciurli, C., Soudeyns, H., Adelsberger, J.W., Vaccarezza, M., Walker, R.E., Sekaly, R.P., and Fauci, A.S., Analysis of the T-cell receptor beta-chain variable-region (V beta) repertoire in monozygotic twins discordant for human immunodeficiency virus: evidence for perturbations of specific V beta segments in CD4+ T cells of the virus-positive twins, *Proc. Natl. Acad. Sci. U.S.A.*, 91, 1529, 1994.

121. Wang, X.-H., Ohmen, J.D., Uyemura, K., Rea, T.H., Kronenbert, M., and Modlin, R.L., Selection of T lymphocytes bearing limited T-cell receptor β chains in the response to a human pathogen, *Proc. Natl. Acad. Sci., U.S.A.*, 90, 188, 1993.

122. Uyemura, K., Ohmen, J.D., Grisso, C.L., Sieling, P.A., Wyzykowski, R., Reisinger, D.M., Rea, T.H., and Modlin, R.L., Limited T-cell receptor beta-chain diversity of a T-helper cell type 1-like response to *Mycobacterium leprae*, *Infect. Immun.*, 60, 4542, 1992.

123. Uyemura, K., Ha, C.T., Ohmen, J.D., Rea, T.H., and Modln, R.L., Selective expansion of V delta 1 + T cells from leprosy skin lesions, *J. Invest. Dermatol.*, 99, 848, 1992.

124. Ohmen, J.D., Barnes, P.F., Grisso, C.L., Bloom, B.R., and Modlin, R.L., Evidence for a superantigen in human tuberculosis, *Immunity*, 1, 25, 1994.

125. Xerri, L., Mathoulin, M.P., Birg, F., Bouabdallah, R., Stoppa, A.M., and Hassoun, J., Heterogeneity of rearranged T-cell receptor V-alpha and V-beta transcripts in tumor-infiltrating lymphocytes from Hodgkin's disease and non-Hodgkin's lymphoma, *Am. J. Clin. Pathol.*, 101, 76, 1994.

126. Kasten-Sportes, C., Zaknoen, S., Steis, R.G., Chan, W.C., Winton, E.F., and Waldmann, T.A., T-cell receptor gene rearrangement in T-cell large granular leukocyte leukemia: preferential V alpha but diverse J alpha usage in one of five patients, *Blood*, 83, 767, 1994.

127. Hunt, S.J., Charley, M.R., and Jegasothy, B.V., Cutaneous T-cell lymphoma: utility of antibodies to the variable regions of the human T-cell antigen receptor, *J. Am. Acad. Dermatol.*, 26, 552, 1992.

128. Poppema, S. and Hepperle, B., Restricted V gene usage in T-cell lymphomas as detected by anti-T-cell receptor variable region reagents, *Am. J. Pathol.*, 138, 1479, 1991.

129. Jack, A.S., Boylston, A.W., Carrel, S., and Grigor, I., Cutaneous T- cell lymphoma cells employ a restricted range of T-cell antigen receptor variable region genes, *Am. J. Pathol.*, 136, 17, 1990.

130. Smith, J.L., Lane A.C., Hodges, E., Reynolds, W.M., Howell, W.M., Jones, D.B., and Janson, C.H., T-cell receptor variable (V) gene usage by lymphoid populations in T-cell lymphoma, *J. Pathol.*, 166,109,1992.

131. Ohshima, K., Kikuchi, M., Yoneda S., Kobari, S., Sumiyosi, Y., Takeshita M., and Kimura, M., Restriction of T-cell receptor variable region in lymph nodes of adult T-cell leukemia/lymphoma, *Hematol. Oncol.*, 11,147,1993.

132. Hingorani, R., Choi, I.-H., Akolkar, P., Gulwani-Akolkar, B., Pergolizzi, R., Silver, J., and Gregersen, P.K., Clonal predominance of T-cell receptors within the CD8+ CD45R0+ subset in norman human subjects, *J. Immunol.*, 151, 5762, 1993.

133. Posnett D.N., Sinha, R., Kabak, S., and Russo C., Clonal populations of T cells in normal elderly humans: the T cell equivalent to "benign monclonal gammapathy," *J. Exp. Med.*, 179, 609, 1994.
134. Poussier, P. and Julius, M., Thymus independent T cell development and selection in the intestinal epithelium, *Annu. Rev. Immunol.*, 12, 521, 1994.
135. Bigler, R.D., Posnett, D.N., and Chiorazzi, N., Stimulation of a subset of normal resting T lymphocytes by a monoclonal antibody to a crossreactive determinant of the human T cell antigen receptor, *J. Exp. Med.*, 161, 1450, 1985.
136. Wang, C.Y., Bushkin, Y., Pica, R., Lane, C., McGrath, H., and Posnett, D.N., Stimulation and expansion of a human T cell subpopulation by a monoclonal antibody to T-cell receptor molecule, *Hybridoma*, 5, 179, 1986.
137. Posnett, D.N., Wang, C.Y., and Friedman, S., Inherited polymorphism of the human T cell antigen receptor detected by a monoclonal antibody. *Proc. Natl. Acad. Sci. U.S.A.*, 83, 7888, 1986.
138. Acuto, O., Campen, T.J., Royer, H.D., Hussey, R.E., Poole, C.B., and Reinherz, E.L., Molecular analysis of T-cell receptor (Ti) variable region (V) gene expression. Evidence that a single Ti β V gene family can be used in formation of V domains of phenotypically and functionally diverse T-cell populations, *J. Exp. Med.*, 161, 1326, 1985.
139. Maecker, H.T. and Levy, R., Prevalence of antigen receptor variants in human T cell lines and tumors. *J. Immunol.*, 142, 1395, 1989.
140. Tian, W.T., Skibbens, R., Kubinec, J., Henry, L., Ko, J.-L., Yeh, G., and Ip, S., Monoclonal antibodies specific to human T cell antigen receptor Vβ gene products, *FASEB J.*, 3, A486,1989 .
141. Janson, C.H., Tehrani, M.J., Mellstedt, H., and Wigzell, H., Anti-idiotypic monoclonal antibody to a T cell chronic lymphatic leukemia. Characterization of the antibody, *in vitro* effector functions and results of therapy, *Cancer Immunol. and Immunother.*, 28, 225, 1989.
142. DerSimonian, H., Band, H., and Brenner, M.B., Increased frequency of T-cell receptor Vα12.1 expression on CD8+ T cells: evidence that Vα participates in shaping the peripheral T cell repertoire, *J. Exp. Med.*, 174, 639, 1991.
143. Devaux, B., Bjorkman, P.J., Stevenson, C., Greif, W., Elliott, J.F., Sagerstrom, C., Clayberger, C., Krensky, A.M., and Davis, M.M., Generations of monoclonal antibodies against soluble human T-cell receptor polypeptides, *Eur. J. Immunol.*, 21, 2111, 1991.
144. Gulwani-Aklolkar, B., Posnett, D.N., Janson, C.H., Grunewald, J., Wigzell, H., Akolkar, P., Gregersen, P.K., and Silver, J., T-cell receptor V-segment frequencies in peripheral blood T cells correlate with human leukocyte antigen type, *J. Exp Med.*, 174, 1139, 1991.
145. Akolkar, P.N., Gulwani-Akolkar, B., Pergolizzi, R., Bigler, R.D., and Silver, J., Influence of HLA genes on T-cell receptor V-segment frequencies and expression levels in peripheral blood lymphocytes, *J. Immunol.*, 150, 2761, 1993.
146. Soudeyns, H., Routy, J.-P. and Sekaly, R. Comparative analysis of the T-cell receptor Vβ repertoire in various lymphoid tissues from HIV-infected patients:evidence for an HIV associated superantigen, *Leukemia*, 8(s1), 95, 1994.
147. Saiki, R.K., Scharf, S., Faloona, F., Mullis K.B., Horn, G.T., Erlich, H.A., and Arnheim, N., Enzymatic amplification of β-globin genomic sequences and restriction site analysis for diagnosis of sickle cell anemia, *Science*, 230, 1350, 1985.
148. Erlich H.A., Gelfand, D., and Sninsky J.J., Recent advances in the polymerase chain reaction, *Science*, 252, 1643, 1991.
149. Mullis, K.B. and Faloona, F.A., Specific synthesis of NDNA *in vitro* via a polymerase-catalyzed chain reaction. *Methods Enzymol.*, 155, 335, 1987.

150. Mulder, J., McKinney, N., Christopherson, C., Sninsky, J., Greenfield, L., and Kwok, S., Rapid and simple PCR assay for quantitation of human immunodefiency virus type 1 RNA in plasma: application to acute retroviral infection, *J. Clin. Microbiol.*, 32, 292, 1994.

151. Saiki R.K., Bugawan, T.L., Horn, G.T. Mullis, K.B., and Erlich H.A., Analysis of enzymatically amplified beta-globin and HLA-DQ alpha DNA with allele-specific oligonucleotide probes, *Nature*, 324, 163, 1986.

152. Bugawan, T.L, Begovich A.B., and Erlich H.A., Rapid HLA-DPB typing using enzymatically amplified DNA and nonradioactive sequence-specific oligonucleotide probes, *Immunogenetics*, 32, 231, 1990.

153. Peoples, G.E., Davey M.P., Goedegebuure, P.S., Schoof, D.D., and Eberlein, T.J., T-cell receptor Vβ2 and Vβ6 mediate tumor-specific cytotoxicity by tumor-infiltrating lymphocytes in ovarian cancer, *J. Immunol.*, 141, 5472, 1993.

154. Puisieux, I., Even, H., Pannetier, C., Jotereau, F., Favrot, M., and Kourilsky, P., Oligoclonality of tumor-infiltrating lymphocytes from human melanomas, *J. Immunol.*, 153, 2807, 1994.

155. Farace, F., Orlanducci, F., Dietrich P.-Y., Gaudin, C., Angevin, E., Courtier, M.-H., Bayle, C., Hercend, T., and Triebel, F., T cell repertoire in patients with B chronic lymphocytic leukemia, *J. Immunol.*, 153, 4281, 1994.

156. Chomczynski, P. and Sacchi, N., Single-step method of RNA isolation by acid guanidinium thiocyanate-phenol-chloroform extraction, *Anal. Biochem.*, 162, 156, 1987.

157. Genevee, C., Diu, A., Nierat, J, Caignard, A., Dietrich, P.-V., Ferradini, L., Roman-Roman, S., Triebel, F., and Hercend, T., An experimentally validated panel of subfamily-specific oligonucleotide primers ($V_\alpha 1$-w29/$V_\beta 1$-24) for the study of human T-cell receptor variable V gene segment usage by polymerase chain reaction, *Eur. J. Immunol.*, 22, 1261, 1992.

158. Lopez, D. and deCastro Lopez, J.A., T-cell receptor Vβ gene usage in a human alloreactive response, *J. Exp. Med.*, 171, 1189, 1990.

159. Hall, B.L. and Finn, O.J., PCR-based analysis of the T-cell receptor Vβ multigene family: experimental parameters affecting its validity, *Biotechniques*, 13, 248, 1992.

160. Graziosi, C. Pantaleo, G., Gantt, K.R., Fortin, J.-P, Demarst, J.F., Cohen, O.J., Sekaly, R.P., and Fauci, A.S., Lack of evidence for dichotomy of $T_h 1$ and $T_h 2$ predominance in HIV-infected individuals, *Science*, 265, 248, 1994.

161. Wang, A.M., Doyle, M.V., and Mark, D.F., Quantitation of mRNA by the polymerase chain reaction, *Proc. Natl. Acad. Sci. U.S.A.*, 86, 9717, 1989.

162. de Kant, E., Rochlitz C.F., and Herrman, R., Gene expression analysis by a competitive and differential PCR with antisense competitors, *Biotechniques*, 17, 934, 1994.

163. Linz, U., Thermocycler temperature variation invalidates PCR results, *Biotechniques*, 9, 286, 1990.

164. Gulwani-Akolkar, B., Akolkar, P.N., Minassian, A., McKinley, M., Fisher, S. and Silver, J., CD4+ cell oligoclonality in Crohn's disease: Evidence for an antigen-specific response, *Human Immunol.*, 48, 114, 1996.

INDEX

A

ABC (ATP-binding cassette family), 29
Accessory cells, 3, 4, 6. *See also* Killer cells;
    Natural killer cells
AccuProbe, 156, 158, 159
Acinetobacter, 205
Acquired hemolytic anemia, 50, 114, 119
Acquired immunodeficiency syndrome.
    See AIDS
Acquisition, 385
Actin, 112
Actin dysfunction, 327, 329
Activated memory cells, 427
Activated natural killer cells (A-NK),
    374
Acute cellular rejection, 489
Acute graft rejection, 489
Acute leukemia, 428–439
Acute lymphoblastic leukemia (ALL),
    429, 430–434
Acute myeloid leukemia (AML), 431,
    434–436
Acute poststreptococcal
    glomerulonephritis (APSGN),
    287, 288, 289, 290
Adaptive immune system, 345
ADCC. *See* Antibody-dependent, cell-
    mediated cytotoxicity
Adenovirus, 189
Adhesion
    of leukocytes. *See* Adhesion molecules;
        Leukocyte adhesion deficiency
    of neutrophils and monocytes, 320,
        323
    of pathogens, 37
Adhesion molecules, 5, 6–7, 10
    deficiencies in, 49
    of immunoglobulin superfamily, 7–9,
        10, 12
    integrins and, 12
    role in lymphocyte emigration and
        antigen recognition, 32–33
    of selectins, integrin and address in
        families, 9, 11–12
Adhesion receptors, 323
Admixture, 545
Adrenalitis, 115, 119
Adressin family of adhesion molecules, 9,
    11, 33
Adult T-cell leukemia/lymphoma (ATL),
    459
Agammaglobulinemia, X-linked, 49, 78,
    101
Age factors, autoantibody increase, 113
Agglutination, 120. *See also* Latex
    agglutination
AHG (antiglobulin-augmented
    lymphocytotoxicity), 480, 499, 500
AIDS, 48
    increase in tuberculosis and, 184
    interferons in clinical applications, 248,
        249
    limitations of serological techniques
        with, 129–130
    Mycobacterium genovense in liver of
        infected individuals, 201
Alanine aminotransferase enzymes
    (ALT), 194
Alcohol intoxication, neutrophil
    dysfunction and, 337
Alkaline phosphatase, 164, 165
ALL (acute lymphoblastic leukemia), 429,
    430–434
Allele refractory mutation system
    (ARMS), 556–557
Allelic variants, 576
Allergic encephalomyelitis, 118
Allergic reactions, 37
Allophycocyanin (APC), 395